# The Thumb

Sang Hyun Woo
Editor

# The Thumb

## A Guide to Surgical Management

Springer

*Editor*
Sang Hyun Woo
W Institute for Hand and Reconstructive Microsurgery
Department of Plastic and Reconstructive Surgery
W Hospital
Daegu
South Korea

ISBN 978-981-10-4399-4 ISBN 978-981-10-4400-7 (eBook)
https://doi.org/10.1007/978-981-10-4400-7

Library of Congress Control Number: 2018963300



This Springer imprint is published by the registered company Springer Nature Singapore Pte Ltd.
The registered company address is: 152 Beach Road, #21-01/04 Gateway East, Singapore 189721, Singapore

# Preface

With so many advances in our understanding of and success in thumb surgery, the need to provide a comprehensive up-to-date text has been long overdue. Thanks to the hard work of all contributors, we have been able to provide detailed explanations, photographs, and surgical results to this comprehensive book on *The Thumb* with the intent of improving physician practice and enhancing surgical outcomes. The inclusion of visual descriptions of each and every available techniques relating to thumb surgeries aims to equip students, residents, fellows, and experienced physicians alike with the knowledge and confidence they need to make expedient decisions in the process of achieving the most favorable results possible for their patients. From the basic anatomy; deformities and other anomalies in the thumb; problems in the bone, joint, tendon, and nerves; tumors; and, of course, replantation and reconstruction, this is a very special book with many special interests.

The surgeons who have collaborated on this book are at the cutting edge of their field and are world class in their practice, research, and surgical acumen. It is to them that we owe a great debt of gratitude. Even, our staffs of hand surgeons at W Hospital include Young Woo Kim, Hee Chan Ahn, Ho Jun Cheon, Dong Ho Kang, Hyun Jae Nam, Myung Jae Yoo, Young Seok Lee, and Tae Kyung Lee. Their hard work in carrying out elective and all night or weekend emergency operations in over 10,000 cases a year truly make them the dream team.

Many thanks go to Professors Jae Sung Seo and Sung Jung Kim for their mental support and also to my respected mentors, Professor Jung Hyun Seul, See Ho Choi, and Joo-Chul Ihn. Much appreciation goes to all contributors including the teachers of hand surgery, Professor Tsu Min Tsai and Luis R. Scheker in Louisville, Professor Ulrich Lanz in Munich, Professor Fu-Chan Wei in Linkou, Professor Suk Joon Oh and Professor Kwan Chul Tark in Korea.

My gratitude goes out to my publisher and helpers, Vinoth Kuppan and Dinesh Vinayagam, in being patient with this exhaustive process and to Andrew Miller in his proofreading and revisions to help you, the reader, understand all that is in front of you.

Finally, I am indebted to all my family who had to endure the many nights I spent toiling away in the creation of this book and also in my absence as I carried out surgeries on too many nights and weekends to even consider counting.

I have dedicated my working life to helping those with developmental anomalies and those involved in trauma regain as close to 100% physical functionality as possible, the thumb playing perhaps the most important role of all in the futures of my patients. It is with this that I trust you will follow suit and use the contents of this text to the best of your abilities.

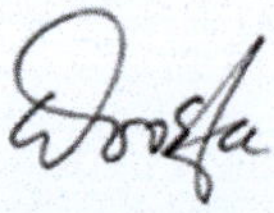

Daegu, South Korea
July 30, 2018

Sang Hyun Woo, MD, PhD

# Contents

# Part I

# Introduction

# History of "Making a Thumb"

1

Suk Joon Oh

The thumb plays an important role in hand function. Daily tasks involving pinch, grip, grasp, and precision handling are more easily accomplished with an opposable thumb. The causes of thumb deficiency are traumatic loss and congenital anomalies.

Attempts to restore thumb function were recorded as early as 1874, when Huguier [1] reported on the phalangization of the thumb metacarpal, which was carried out by deepening the first web space [2]. In 1900, Nicoladoni [3] described a reconstruction procedure following traumatic amputation of the thumb in which a staged, pedicled transfer of the great toe was performed [2]. Development of microsurgical techniques allowed successful transfer of a toe to a thumb in monkeys in 1965 [4] and in a human in 1966 [5].

The loss of a thumb results in a notable functional impairment. Multiple reconstructive procedures have been described to address these deficits. Compared with no reconstruction, any procedure is of benefit. However, each of the described methods offers subtle benefits and downsides and may be more applicable in certain situations. A reconstructed thumb ideally will (1) have adequate length; (2) have a sensate, nontender tip; (3) have stability; and (4) be positioned to meet the other digits, with an adequate first web space [6]. *Littler* [7] analyzed these attributes and believed that although all of them are important, strategic positioning of the thumb is the key factor to achieving optimal function. Emphasizing this, he stated, "It is not the full length of the thumb, nor its great strength and movement, but rather its strategic position relative to the fingers and the integrity of the specialized terminal pulp tissue which determines prehensile status."

## Traumatic Thumb Defect

Lister [8] divided thumb defects into four groups: (1) acceptable length with poor soft tissue coverage; (2) subtotal amputation with questionable remaining length; (3) total amputation with preservation of the basal joint; and (4) total amputation with loss of the basal joint.

1. Amputation at or distal to the interphalangeal (IP) joint rarely results in a functional deficit. These cases require a sensate and supple tip, which can be provided by glabrous and nonglabrous skin flaps. Glabrous flaps include Moberg, V-Y advancement [9], Littler's neurovascular island [10], free toe pulp transfer [11], and partial hallux transfer [12]. Nonglabrous skin flaps include the first dorsal metacarpal artery (Foucher) [13], cross-finger [14, 15],

S. J. Oh (✉)
Hallym University College of Medicine, Chuncheon, South Korea

Department of Plastic and Burn Reconstructive Surgery, Bestian Seoul Hospital, Seoul, South Korea


S. H. Woo (ed.), *The Thumb*, https://doi.org/10.1007/978-981-10-4400-7_1

dorso-ulnar or dorso-radial, and distant or free flaps such as the distally based posterior island interosseous flap [16], reverse radial forearm flap [17], free groin flaps [18], and free neurovascular medial plantar flaps [19].

2. Proximal amputation of the proximal phalanx inevitably results in reduced hand span, difficulty grasping large objects, and fine pinch limitations. Distal proximal phalanx amputations often suffice with web-deepening procedures.

   Procedures that provide relative lengthening without true lengthening have been termed "phalangization" and use local, regional, distant pedicled, or free flaps to deepen the web space. Flap options include Z-plasty (single [20], four-flap [21]), dorsal rotation [22], and regional or free flaps including posterior interosseous artery flap, reverse radial forearm flap, groin flap [23], first web space free flap of the foot [24], and free medial plantar flap [19] (Fig. 1.1a–c). In an on-top plasty [25], adjacent digits are used to extend thumb length and, in doing so, deepen the first web (Fig. 1.2a, b). Distraction osteogenesis described by Matev IB [26] has been used in the past, but currently alternative options are preferable.

3. Total thumb amputations with preservation of the basal joint result in substantial impairment. Toe transfer is a good option for amputations distal to the carpometacarpal (CMC) joint and optimally where intrinsic thumb muscles are intact, providing the most reliable cosmetic and functional outcome. The procedure requires microsurgical expertise. A toe free transfer is usually performed as a delayed procedure to allow the patient time to appreciate the severity of the situation, although acute transfer has been described with equivalent

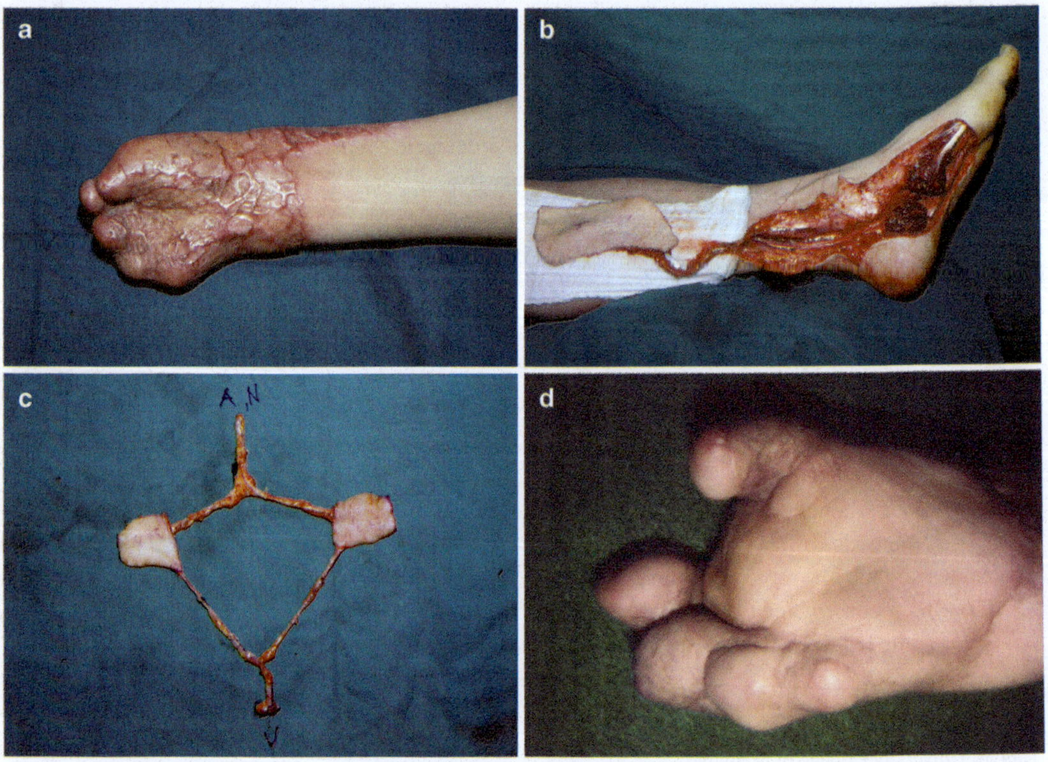


**Fig. 1.1** Phalangization of the thumb. (**a**) Mutilated hand after degloved injury. (**b**) Harvested medial plantar neurovascular flap. (**c**) Harvested twin digital neurovascular flaps from the ulnar side of the middle finger and radial side of the ring finger of opposite hand. (**d**) The first web and palm covered with medial plantar neurovascular free flap and insensate tips of the thumb and index finger covered with flow-through twin digital neurovascular free flaps

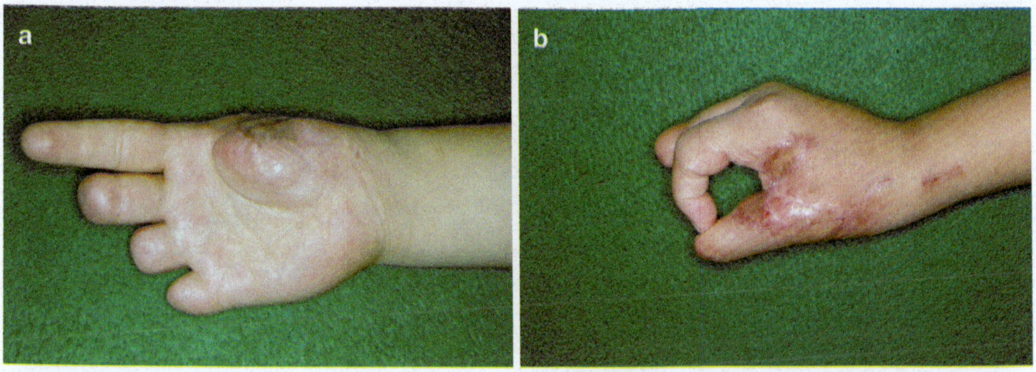


**Fig. 1.2** On-top plasty. (**a**) Thumb amputation with multiple fingers. (**b**) Postoperative result of neurovascular pedicle transfer of the distal segment of an amputated ring finger with ray amputation to lengthen the thumb

outcomes [27]. When a future toe transfer is likely, a local or regional flap is not advisable during the initial procedure because this may damage the critical vascular structures. A pedicled groin flap is an excellent option.

Trimmed toe transfer was described by Wei et al. [28] and involves a longitudinal osteotomy to thin the toe. This has the advantage of replicating the native thumb size and maintains some IP joint movement. Morrison et al. [29] described the wrap-around flap, which uses the great toe pulp and nail and a segment of the distal phalanx, which is transferred with an iliac crest bone graft. This procedure results in improved cosmesis of the donor and recipient sites. However, there is no IP joint movement, and the graft is subject to resorption. The second toe [30] is not critical during the gait cycle and allows the entire metatarsophalangeal joint to be harvested. This may be the only toe transfer possible for more proximal thumb amputations. Drawbacks include a poorer cosmetic appearance, the tendency to claw, and a short nail. Occasionally, because of anatomic or cultural reasons, free toe transfer is not a possibility. Alternatively, osteoplastic reconstruction, pollicization (Fig. 1.3a–c), or lengthening may be considered. Although possible, metacarpal lengthening via distraction as described by Matev [26] yields only osteogenesis approximately 3 cm. Although this is still beneficial, better alternatives usually exist. Other limitations include the prolonged length of treatment, poor cosmesis, and lack of movement. Two thirds of the metacarpal is required, along with good skin and a compliant patient.

Osteoplastic reconstruction involves a tricortical iliac crest bone graft (approximately 8 × 50 × 15 mm) that is inserted into the metacarpal medullary canal and secured, usually with Kirschner wires. This is then covered with a pedicled flap, most often a groin flap (McGregor [31]). (A) tubed pedicled skin flap and bone graft (osteoplastic) (Nicoladoni and independently by Noesske [32]); (B) Variations on category A are skin tube and bone graft in separate operations (Noesske [32] and Pierce [33]); skin tube and bone graft in the same operation; bone graft implanted subcutaneously awaiting its vascularization (Shepelmann [34]) before its transfer with skin investment to the thumb amputation stumps (Albee [35]). The author used free neurovascular medial plantar flap for skin investment [36] (Fig. 1.4a–c).

Eric Moberg [37] introduced the digital neurovascular pedicle skin island method for sensibility redistribution in the hand during a discussion of tactile-sense restoration. This perceptive innovation provided special coverage to critical areas of sensory deprivation. Not only were intact sensibility and peripheral circulation restored by this method but also coniferous skin for protective and more effective use of the hand. Tactile sense of traumatic thumb can be restored with free neurovascular digital flap [38]. Gosset [39] was perhaps the first to use the neurovascular pedicle finger transfer method.

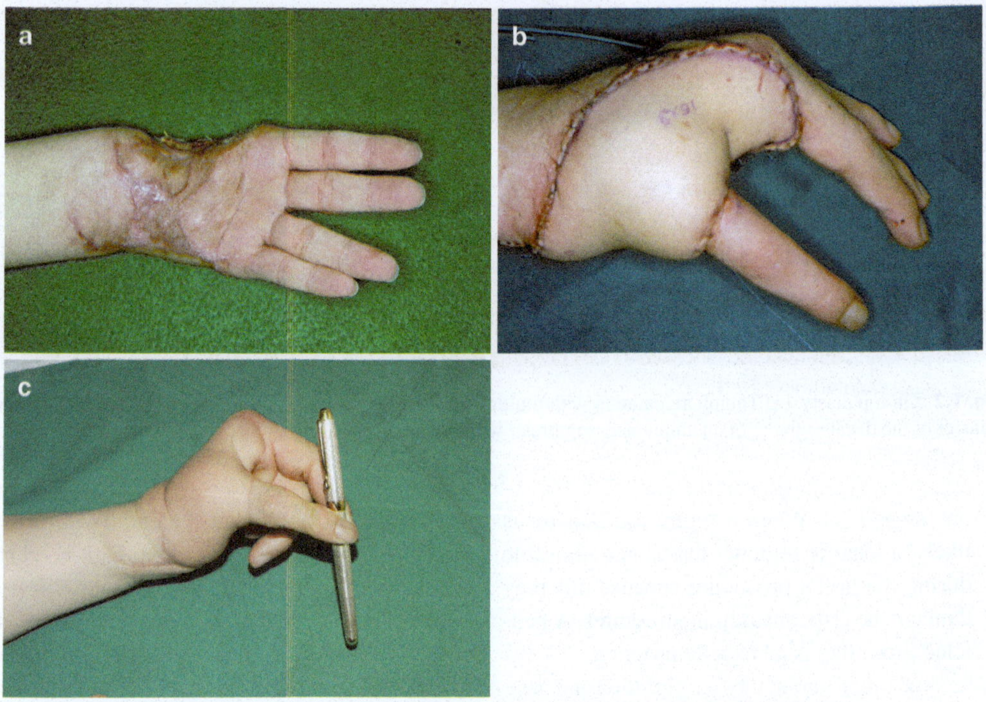


**Fig. 1.3** Index pollicization. (**a**) Total thumb amputation with exposed second metacarpal bone. (**b**) Index pollicization included with free radial forearm flap for the coverage soft tissue defect. (**c**) At 21-year follow-up, this patient used the well-pollicized thumb

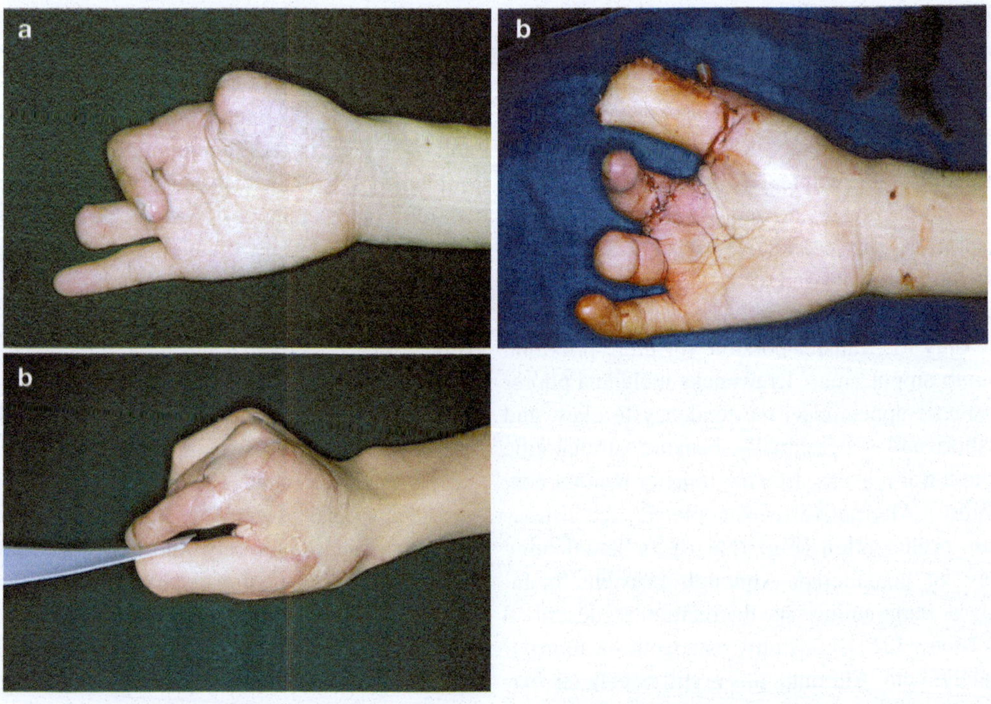


**Fig. 1.4** Osteoplastic sensate thumb. (**a**) Mutilated hand with malrotation deformity of the index. (**b**) Osteoplastic thumb reconstructed with a free neurovascular medial plantar flap and the second metacarpal bone graft. Deformed distal index finger transferred to the amputated stump on the third metacarpal head of the middle finger. (**c**) Patient achieved good pinch and grasp

His selection of the index finger was in keeping with Iselin's [40] concept of the ideal procedure for finger-to-thumb substitution. Hilgenfeldt's [41] middle finger-thumb formation method fulfills the essential requirements for thumb substitution. The finger was isolated on its neurovascular bundles with a narrow (unnecessary), longitudinal, pretendinous, palmar skin bridge. A phalangeal length sufficient to complement the thumb loss was determined precisely. The proximal retracted, scar-tethered end of the independent long extensor (EPL) was isolated and sutured to the combined extensor digitorum communis (EDC) and extensor indicis proprius (EIP) primarily; the FPL was transferred to the deep flexor of the transferred finger at a subsequent operation.

## Congenital Thumb Anomaly

Congenital thumb anomalies are common and have a major impact given the crucial functional role of the thumb. When surgery is needed to profoundly change the prehension apparatus, the main procedure must be performed early, at about 12 months of age, to coincide with the development of the cerebral pathways that control grasp. Congenital thumb anomalies may occur in isolation (e.g., duplication, hypoplasia, and aplasia) or in combination with other defects. The primary objective of surgery is to improve or restore function [42].

## Thumb Duplication

Recognizing and analyzing the duplication is the first step in management strategy. The classification developed by Wassel [43] distinguishes several types based on the level of the duplication. Although this classification is still in use, it is not sufficient to determine the principles of surgical management. Additional information required to that end is whether the duplication is symmetrical (with two digits of identical length and volume) or asymmetrical (with predominance of one digit, usually the ulnar-based digit) and whether there is malalignment in the coronal plane (clinodactyly) [44]. Simple excision of a small accessory digit is only very rarely performed. The main thumb is structurally normal, and its radial edge is attached by soft tissues to a floating thumb, which can easily be removed [45, 46]. Choosing between midline fusion of the two digits (Bilhaut [47]-Cloquet procedure) [48] and reconstruction based on one of the two digits is the next step in the management strategy. The choice is only theoretical, however, as midline fusion is now reserved for strictly symmetrical type I, II, or III duplication, which is rare. Reconstruction of a functioning thumb from one of the two digits is therefore the most widely used procedure and is performed in all cases of type IV duplication, which is by far the most common variant. In this complex technique, great care is given to a set of elementary procedures performed in combination with simple excision of the accessory digit.

## Thumb Hypoplasia

The therapeutic management of thumb hypoplasia follows a single guiding principle: major "irreparable" hypoplasia, in which removal of the thumb with pollicization of the index finger is the only valid strategy, must be distinguished from minor hypoplasia, in which the thumb may be improved or reconstructed. There are five types of thumb hypoplasia, originally described by Müller [49] in 1937. Blauth [50] refined Müller's concept, defining five grades of thumb hypoplasia in 1967. The Blauth classification identifies the variants of thumb hypoplasia and is extremely useful for planning treatment, yet it is only a general guideline. According to the severity of thumb hypoplasia, its reconstruction requires the release of the first web space [51], opponensplasty [52–55], and pollicization [56, 57].

## Thumb Agenesis

The work of Matthews [56] and Zancolli [57] made possible a high degree of surgical excellence in the transfer of the radial-most finger (preaxial, index) for thumb agenesis. Buck-Gramcko [58] reported a series of 100 consecutive pollicization operations for agenesis. Certain technical considerations of finger transfer in thumb agenesis, not encountered with traumatic thumb loss in the normal hand, demand special attention.

## References


1. Huguier PC. Du remplacement du pouce par son metacarpien, par l'agrandissement du premier espace interosseux. Arch Gen Med. 1874;1:78.
2. Littler JW. On making a thumb: one hundred years of surgical effort. J Hand Surg Am. 1976;1(1):35–51.
3. Nicoladoni C. Daumenplastik und organischer Ersatz der Fingerspitze (Anticheiroplastik und Daktyloplstik). Arch Klin Chir. 1900;61:606–14.
4. Buncke HJ Jr, Buncke CM, Schulz WP. Immediate Nicoladoni procedure in the Rhesus monkey, or hallux-to-hand transplantation, utilising micro-miniature vascular anastomoses. Br J Plast Surg. 1966;19(4):332–7.
5. Cobbett JR. Free digital transfer. Report of a case of transfer of a great toe to replace an amputated thumb. J Bone Joint Surg Br. 1969;51(4):677–9.
6. Graham DJ, Venkatramani H, Sabapathy SR. Current reconstruction options for traumatic thumb loss. J Hand Surg [Am]. 2016;41:1159–67.
7. Littler JW. Reconstruction of the thumb in traumatic loss. In: Converse JM, editor. Reconstructive plastic surgery. Philadelphia: Saunders; 1977. p. 3352.
8. Lister G. The choice of procedure following thumb amputation. Clin Orthop Relat Res. 1984;195:45–51.
9. Moberg E. Aspects of sensation in reconstructive surgery of the upper extremity. J Bone Joint Surg Am. 1964;46:817–25.
10. Littler JW. Neurovascular pedicle transfer of tissue in reconstructive surgery of the hand. J Bone Joint Surg. 1956;38A:917.
11. Woo SH, Lee GJ, Kim KC, et al. Immediate partial great toe transfer for the reconstruction of composite defects of the distal thumb. Plast Reconstr Surg. 2006;117(6):1906–15.
12. Piñal F, Moraleda E, de Piero HG, Ruas J, Galindo C. Onycho-osteo-cutaneous defects of the thumb reconstructed by partial hallux transfer. J Hand Surg [Am]. 2014;39(1):29–36.
13. Foucher G, Khouri RK. Digital reconstruction with island flaps. Clin Plast Surg. 1997;24(1):1–32.
14. Gurdin M, Pangman JW. The repair of surface defects of fingers by trans-digital flaps. Plast Reconstr Surg. 1950;5:368–71.
15. Hoskins DH. The versatile cross-finger pedicle flap. J Bone Joint Surg Am. 1960;42:261–77.
16. Costa H, Soutar DS. The distally based island posterior interosseous flap. Br J Plast Surg. 1988;41(3):221–7.
17. Groenevelt F, Schoorl R. The reversed forearm flap using scarred skin in hand reconstruction. Br J Plast Surg. 1985;38(3):398–402.
18. Harii K, Omori K, Torii S, Murakami F, Kasai Y. Free groin skin flaps. Br J Plast Surg. 1975;28(4):225–37.
19. Oh SJ, Koh SH, Chung CH. Wide thumb and the first web reconstruction using a neurovascularised instep free flap. J Plast Reconstr Aesthet Surg. 2010;63:1565–8.
20. Ivy RH. Who originated the Z-plasty? Plast Reconstr Surg. 1971;41(1):67–72.
21. Woolf RM, Broadbent TR. The four flap Z-plasty. Plast Reconstr Surg. 1972;49(1):48–51.
22. Marble K, Fudem G. First web space release with the dorsal hand rotation flap: closing the donor site. Ann Plast Surg. 1995;35(1):83–5.
23. Woo SH, Choi BC, Oh SJ, Seul JH. Classification of the first web space free flap of the foot and its applications in reconstruction of the hand. Plast Reconstr Surg. 1999;103:508–17.
24. McGregor IA, Jackson IT. The groin flaps. Br J Plast Surg. 1972;25(1):3–16.
25. Kelleher JC, Sullivan JG, Baibak GJ, Dean RK. "On-top plasty" for amputated fingers. Plast Reconstr Surg. 1968;42(3):242–8.
26. Matev IB. Thumb reconstruction through metacarpal bone lengthening. J Hand Surg [Am]. 1980;5(5):482–7.
27. Yim K, Wei FC, Lin C. A comparison between primary and secondary toe-to-hand transplantation. Plast Reconstr Surg. 2004;114(1):107–12.
28. Wei FC, Chen HC, Chuang CC, Noordhoff MS. Reconstruction of the thumb with a trimmed-toe transfer technique. Plast Reconstr Surg. 1988;82:506–15.
29. Morrison WA, O'Brien BM, MacLeod AM. Thumb reconstruction with a free neurovascular wrap-around flap from the big toe. J Hand Surg [Am]. 1980;5(6):575–83.
30. Biemer E. Thumb replacement by transplantation of the second toe. Handchirugie. 1981;13(1–2):31–5.
31. McGregor I, Simonetta C. Reconstruction of thumb by composite bone-skin flap. Br J Plast Surg. 1964;17:37.
32. Noesske K. Uber den plastischen ersatz von ganz oder teilweise verlorene fingern, insbesondere des daumens, und iiber handtellerplastik. Munch Med Wochenschr. 1909;56:1403.
33. Pierce GW. Reconstruction of thumb after total loss. Surg Gynecol Obstet. 1927;45:825.

34. Shepelmann: Plastischer ersatz bei totaldefekt des rechten daumens. Z Orthop Chir. 34:1914; 35:1916; 39:1919.
35. Albee F. Synthetic transplantation of tissue to form a new finger with restoration of the function of the hand. Ann Surg. 1919;69:379.
36. Eo SR, Kim YS, Kim JYS, Oh SJ. The Versatility of the dorsalis pedis compound free flap in hand reconstruction. Ann Plast Surg. 2008;61:157–63.
37. Moberg E. Discussion of paper, in Brooks, D.: Nerve grafting in orthopaedic surgery. J Bone Joint Surg [Am]. 1955;37:299–305.
38. Oh SJ, Koh SH, Chung CH. Twin digital and in-step neurovascularised free flap for reconstruction of the degloved mutilated hand. J Plast Reconstr Aesthet Surg. 2010;63:1853–9.
39. Gosset J. La Pollicisation de L'index (technique chirurgicale). J Chir (Paris). 1949;65:403–11.
40. Iselin M. Reconstruction of the thumb. Surgery. 1937;2:619.
41. Hilgenfeldt 0. Operativer daumenersatz, Stuttgart, 1950, F Management
42. Dautel G. Strategy for congenital thumb differences in paediatric patients. Orthop Traumatol Surg Res. 2017;103:125–33.
43. Wassel HD. The results of surgery for polydactyly of the thumb. A review. Clin Orthop Relat Res. 1969;64:175–93.
44. Dautel G, Barbary S. Duplications du pouce. Chir Main. 2008;27(Suppl. 1):S82–99.
45. Dobyns JH, Lipscomb PR, Cooney WP. Management of thumb duplication. Clin Orthop Relat Res. 1985;195:26–44.
46. Tada K, Yonenobu K, Tsuyuguchi Y, Kawai H, Egawa T. Duplication of the thumb. A retrospective review of two hundred and thirty-seven cases. J Bone Joint Surg [Am]. 1983;65:584–98.
47. Bilhaut M. Guerison d'un pouce bifide par un nouveau procede.operatoire. Congrés Francais de. Chirurgie. 1889;4:576–80.
48. Tonkin MA, Bulstrode NW. The Bilhaut-Cloquet procedure for Wassel types III, IV and VII thumb duplication. J Hand Surg Eur. 2007;32:684–93.
49. Müller W. Die angeborenen Fehlbildungen der menschlichen Hand. Leipzig: Thieme; 1937.
50. Blauth W. Der hypoplastische Daumen. Arch Orthop Unfallchir. 1967;62:225–46.
51. Strauch B. Dorsal thumb flap for release of adduction contracture of the first web space. Bull Hosp Joint Dis. 1975;36(1):34–9.
52. Camitz H. Über die beHandlung der Opposition-lähmung. Acta Chir Scand. 1929;65:77.
53. Royle NO. An operation for paralysis of the intrinsic muscles of the thumb. JAMA. 1938;111:612.
54. Huber E. Hilfsoperation bei Medianuslahmung. Dtsch Z Chir. 1921;162:271–5.
55. Lister G. The hand: diagnosis and indications. 2nd ed. London: Churchill Livingstone; 1984. p. 312–51.
56. Matthews D. Congenital absence of functioning thumb. Plast Reconstr Surg. 1960;26:487.
57. Zancolli E. Transplantation of the index finger in congenital absence of the thumb. J Bone Joint Surg Am. 1960;42:658.
58. Buck-Gramcko D. Pollicization of the index finger method and results in aplasia and hypoplasia of the thumb. J Bone Joint Surg Am. 1971;53:1605.

# 2 Anatomy and Biomechanics

Young Keun Lee

## Skin

The skin of the thumb on both dorsal and palmar aspect is the same as that of the fingers. The dorsal skin arises immediately from the thin skin of the dorsum of the hand. It has very different characteristics from that of the palmar aspect. It is thin and mobile over the proximal phalanx and has a few hairs in the proximal portion. At the interphalangeal (IP) joint, it creates several creases when the thumb is in extension (Fig. 2.1). The dorsal skin possesses a nail at the distal end of the thumb. It constitutes an external skeleton for the pulp of the thumb, thus improving precision handling.

The palmar skin of the thumb is very thick and hairless and is set off from the skin of the palm by two flexion creases of the metacarpophalangeal (MP) joint. In abduction of the thumb, proximal crease roughly continues the longitudinal line defined by the radial margin of the index finger. A deep IP joint crease marks off the skin over the proximal phalanx off from that of the tip (pulp) of the thumb (Fig. 2.1). It is firmly attached to deeper tissue layers by Grayson's ligaments, which lie proximal to the IP joint, and Cleland's ligaments, which arise from the tendon sheath near the bone and courses obliquely and distally, inserting into the skin on the radial and ulnar aspects of the thumb. These ligaments prevent the skin from bulging excessively during flexing of the thumb or the grasping of objects.

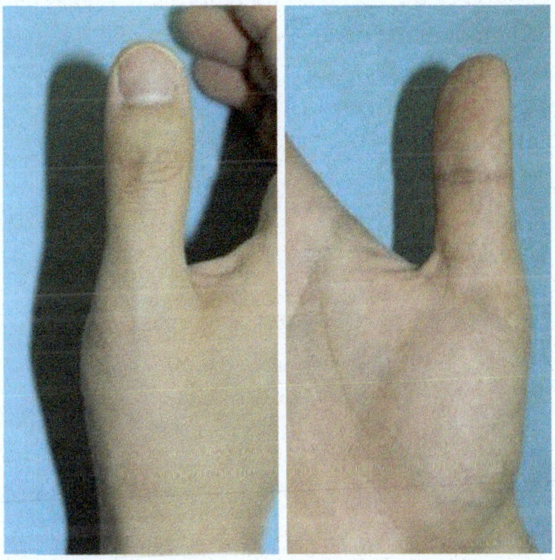

**Fig. 2.1** The right thumb. Dorsal and palmar aspect

The skin on the dorsal aspect of the thumb is supplied by fine branches of the superficial radial nerve. The palmar aspect is supplied by the proper palmar digital nerves from the median nerve. In contrast to the fingers, the palmar nerves of the thumb do not give off dorsal branches, but they normally each branch into three main branches just before entering the pulp to provide sensory supply to the palmar skin of the distal phalanx of the thumb, so the pulp is a true sen-

Y. K. Lee (✉)
Department of Orthopaedic Surgery, Research Institute of Clinical Medicine of Chonbuk National University-Biomedical Research Institute of Chonbuk National University Hospital, Jeonju, South Korea


S. H. Woo (ed.), *The Thumb*, https://doi.org/10.1007/978-981-10-4400-7_2

sory organ [1]. The normal value of two-point discrimination of the distal phalanx of the thumb is 2.5–5 mm.

## Vascular Structures

Though there are many variations, the blood supply of the thumb is mainly made up of the princeps pollicis artery, the first common palmar digital artery which is the terminal branch of the superficial palmar arch and the dorsal digital artery originating primarily from the terminal portion of the radial artery before it descents into the palm of the hand [2–4].

The princeps pollicis artery is considered to be a branch of the radial artery or deep palmar arch and is also called the first palmar metacarpal artery. It is located between the first dorsal interosseous and the adductor pollicis (ADP) muscles and passing deep to the flexor pollicis longus (FPL) tendon proximal to the MP joint. And then it divided into two radial and ulnar palmar digital arteries; the ulnar palmar digital artery is nearly twice as thick as the radial palmar digital artery (Fig. 2.2) [2].

Both palmar arteries of the thumb communicate via the digito-palmar arch and the arcade of the distal phalanx of the thumb. The digito-palmar arch gives off branches which supply the FPL tendon

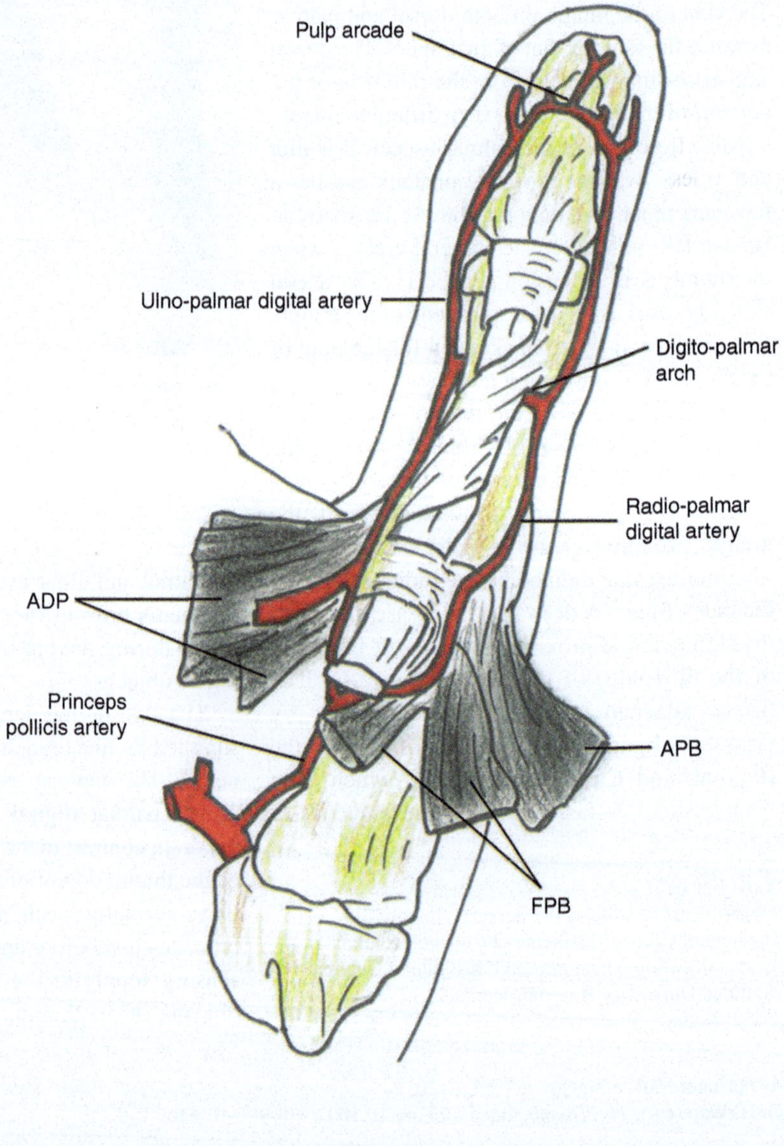


**Fig. 2.2** The arterial supply of the thumb. (*APB* abductor pollicis brevis; *FPB* flexor pollicis brevis; *ADP* adductor pollicis)

via a short vinculum. The distal arcade supplied the distal phalanx and the nailbed of the thumb.

The dorsal digital arteries of the thumb have a high variation in their origins and courses. There are few exceptions; these arteries usually arise from the first dorsal metacarpal artery, which itself arises into two or three branches from the terminal portion of the radial artery before it descends into the palm. Radio-dorsal arteries arise from the anatomical snuff box and course distally along the abductor pollicis brevis (APB), and they end in a dorsal arterial arcade at the level of the nail matrix. Ulno-dorsal arteries have various origins, such as the first dorsal metacarpal artery, the dorsal branch of the radial artery, and branches of the princeps pollicis artery, but they may be absent in 30% of the population [5, 6]. There are normally anastomoses between the dorsal and palmar arteries of the thumb at the level of the head of the proximal phalanx [7].

A well-developed ulno-dorsal venous network and a less well-developed radio-palmar venous network provide superficial venous drainage in the thumb. They drain into the cephalic vein.

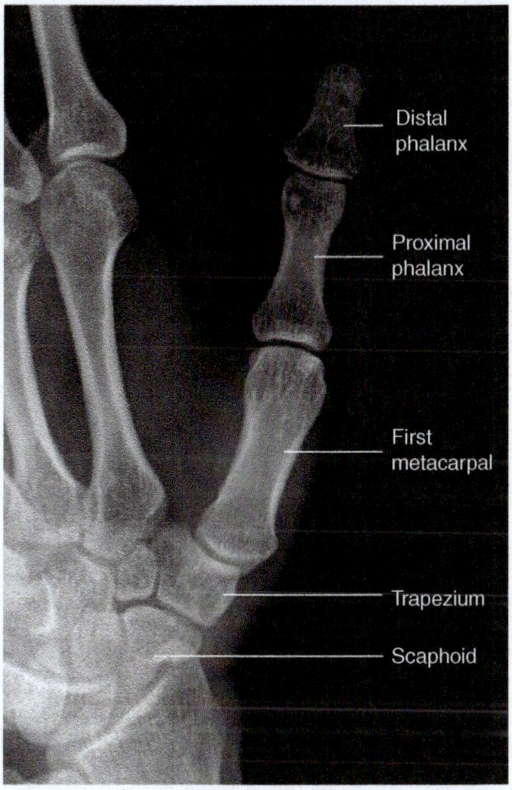


**Fig. 2.3** Osteoarticular column of the thumb

## Bones of the Thumb

The osteoarticular column of the thumb is formed from the whole of the lateral ray of the hand (Fig. 2.3). Therefore, it begins with the scaphoid, passing then to the trapezium. After this comes the first metacarpal, and finally it ends with only two phalanges. Thus, the thumb has an important characteristic that the column itself articulates with the rest of the hand at a point much more proximal than the other digits. Also it is clearly much shorter than they are, since the tip of the thumb reaches only the middle of the proximal phalanx of the index finger.

### Trapezium

Trapezium changes its shape from proximal to distal; owing to this characteristic, it was called a multiangular bone. The bone is situated at the radial column of the wrist between the scaphoid and first metacarpal [8]. The proximal surface is smooth and contains a small, slightly concave facet which articulates with the scaphoid. The distal surface is oval and saddle shaped and faced distolaterally. It articulates with the base of the first metacarpal. The dorsal surface is elongated and rough and rests in relationship to the radial artery. The palmar surface is narrow and rough. At its palmar part is a deep groove, which is medial and contains the flexor carpi radialis (FCR) tendon. The groove is bounded laterally by a tubercle. This surface gives origin to the opponens pollicis (OPP), flexor pollicis brevis (FPB), and APB and provides attachment to the two layers of the flexor retinaculum. The lateral surface is broad and rough for the attachment of the radial collateral ligament and capsular ligament of the carpometacarpal (CMC) joint of the thumb. The medial surface is large and presents two facets: a large, concave, proximal one, which articulates with the

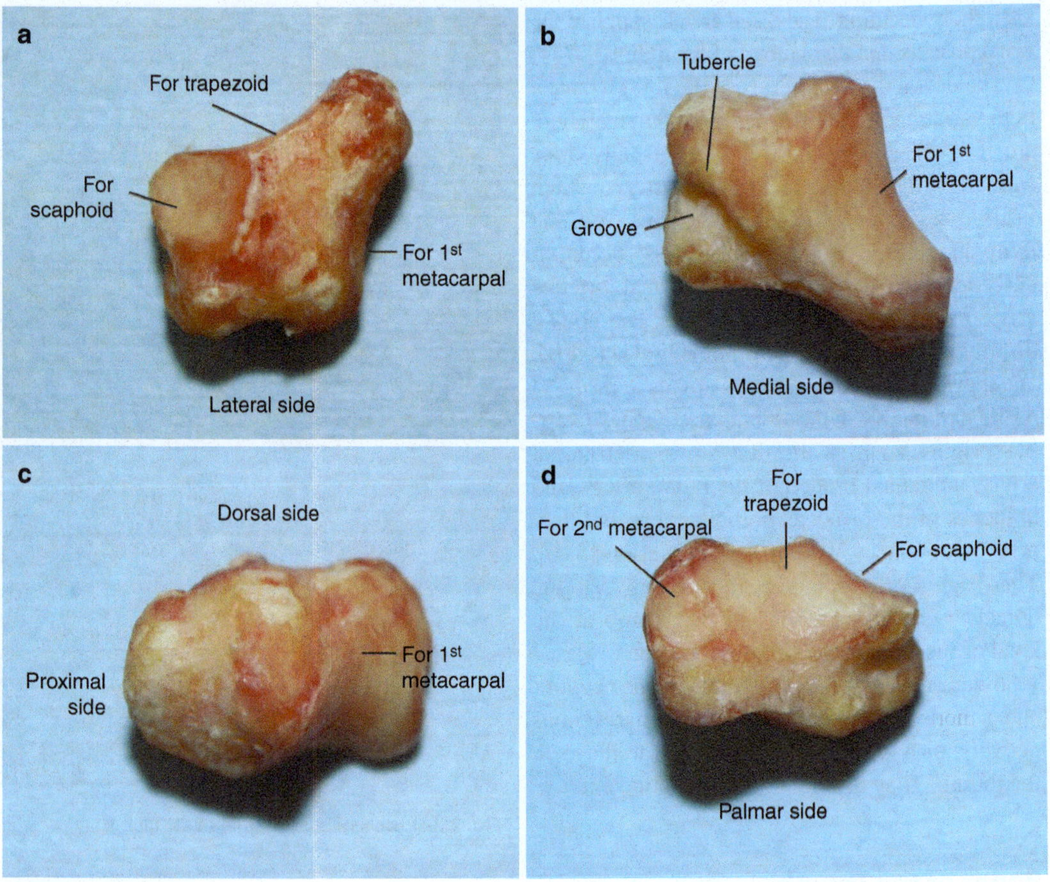


**Fig. 2.4** The left trapezium. (**a**) From the dorsal aspect, (**b**) from the palmar aspect, (**c**) from the radial aspect, (**d**) from the medial aspect

trapezoid, and a small, distal one, which articulates with the second metacarpal (Fig. 2.4).

## First Metacarpal

The first metacarpal bone is short and broad [9]. Its long axis diverges distolaterally from the other metacarpals. It is more anterior and rotated medially on its long axis through 90°, so that its palmar surface is directed medially toward the radial side of the second metacarpal and its dorsal surface is directed laterally. The shaft is flattened and broad, and its dorsal surface is slightly convex. Its palmar surface is concave and divided by a ridge into a larger lateral (anterior) part, which gives attachment of the OPP, and a smaller medial (posterior) part, which gives origin to the radial head of the first dorsal interosseous muscle. The base has a characteristic saddle-shaped articular surface for articulation with trapezium. It has a small tubercle on its lateral side for the insertion of the abductor pollicis longus (APL). The head is rounded and less convex than in other metacarpals and is transversely broad. Two articular eminences are on the palmar surface of the head for the sesamoid bones; the lateral is larger than the medial (Fig. 2.5).

## The Proximal Phalanx

The shaft of the proximal phalanx is short, tapers distally, and is convex dorsally. The base presents oval and concave articular surface. Further, it is transversely broad and articulate with the

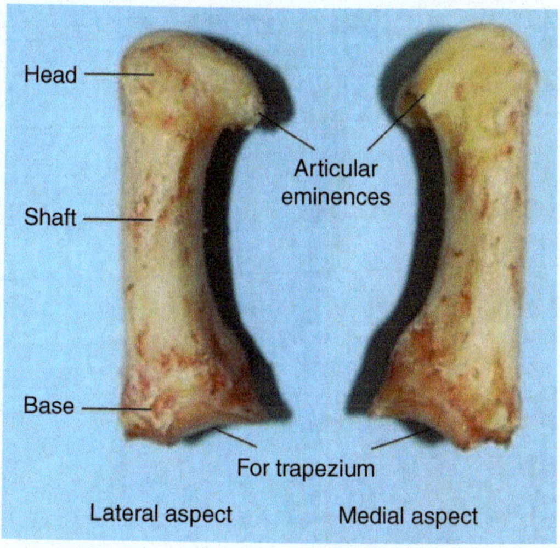


**Fig. 2.5** The left first metacarpal bone

rounded, smooth heads of the metacarpal bone. The head is smaller than the base and ends in two condyles, which are dissimilar, the medial one being more protruding and longer palmarly and medially than its lateral one.

### The Distal Phalanx

The distal phalanx is convex on dorsal and flat on palmar surfaces. The base is oval, concave articular surface and articulates with the head of the proximal phalanx. The head of the distal phalanx is nonarticular and carries a rough, horse-shaped palmar tuberosity, called the ungual tuberosity, to which the pulp of the thumb tip is attached.

## Joints of the Thumb

### Trapeziometacarpal Joint (TM Joint)

The TM joint of the thumb is a biconcave-convex or reciprocal saddle joint. The trapezial articular surface is in convex from dorsal to palmar and concave from radial to ulnar, and the midsagittal diameter is 11.96 ± 1.32 mm [10]. The joint surface is actually asymmetrical, and the articulating surface is located mainly on the volar aspect [11].

The articular surface of the first metacarpal is asymmetrical as well. In this surface a groove is present in the radio-ulnar direction. This groove forms the concavity of the joint surface. It is deepest in the center and becomes shallow at the radial and ulnar extremities. In the center the groove flares out, forming a widening of the joint surface in the palmar direction, and it has a triangular beak on its palmar surface. The midsagittal diameter is 16.03 ± 1.27 mm (Fig. 2.6).

The trapezium and first metacarpal articulate such that the concave surface of the trapezium opposes the convex surface of the first metacarpal. As a result, it configurates an interlocking appearance and two reciprocally opposed saddles, whose longitudinal axes are perpendicular. This configuration allows flexion and extension axis as well as an abduction and adduction axis [6, 12]. The discrepancy in the diameters of the articulating surfaces of trapezium and first metacarpal implicates the joint stability. As a result, the bony articular structures provide little inherent constraint for joint stability. Therefore, TM joint stability mainly relies on the joint capsule, the reinforced ligaments, and the tendons that pass the joint. This feature of this joint also allows for rotation.

The axis of the thumb at the TM joint rests in a pronated position, flexed approximately 80° relative to the plane of the other metacarpals. This optimizes thumb position for opposition to the pulp of one of the four fingers or all of them simultaneously.

The capsule of the TM joint of the thumb is broad and sufficiently lax to allow its wide range of motion including rotation. Several reinforcing ligaments are also necessary to provide stability of the joint through its range of motion. There are four basic ligaments (Fig. 2.7) [11–13]. Anterior oblique ligaments arise from the volar tubercle of the trapezium and extend to the volar beak of the first metacarpal base. It is under tension in thumb abduction, extension, and opposition positions. It is also referred to as the volar ligament of ulnar ligament. Posterior oblique ligament arises from a dorso-ulnar eminence of the trapezium and extends in a palmar spiral to insert with the anterior oblique ligament on the volar beak of the first

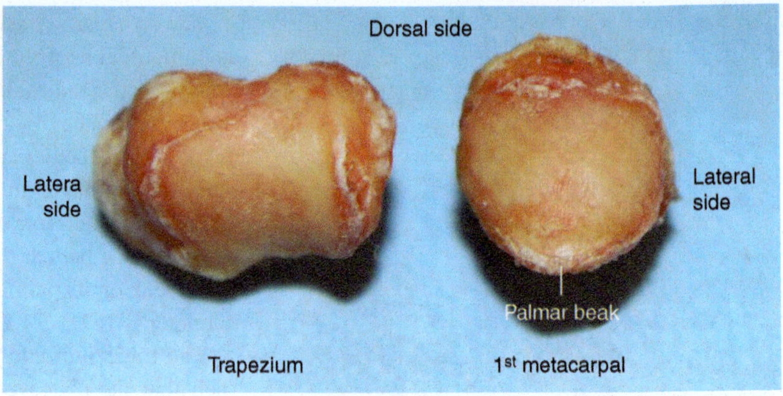


**Fig. 2.6** The articular surfaces in the trapeziometacarpal joint of the left thumb

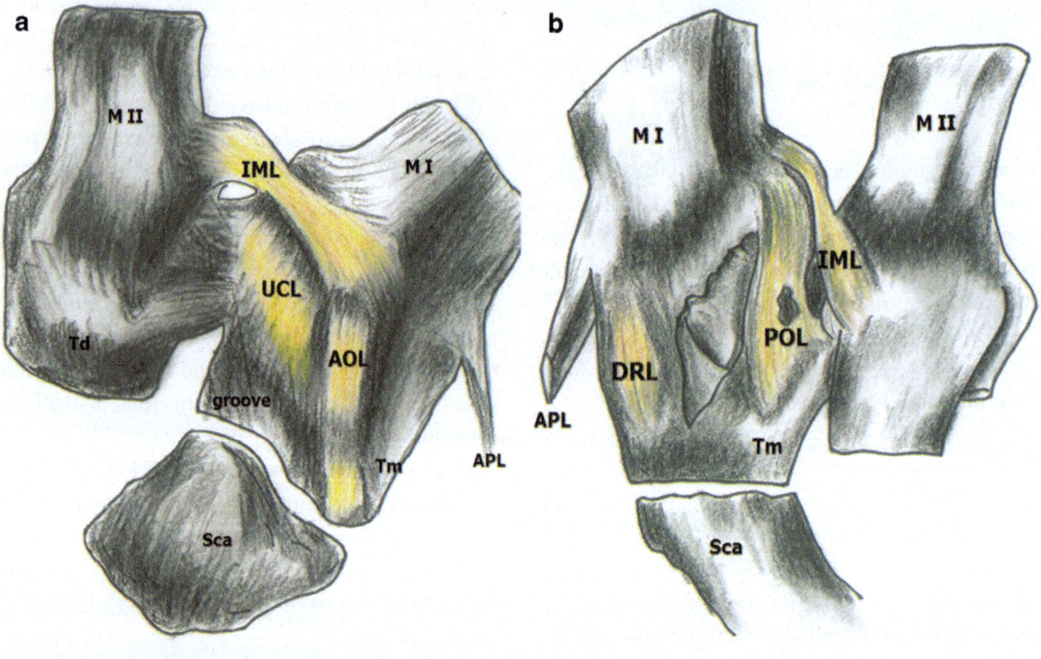


**Fig. 2.7** Volar view and dorsal view of the right trapeziometacarpal joint. (*M I* first metacarpal bone; *M II* second metacarpal bone; *Td* trapezoid; *Tm* trapezium; *IML* intermetacarpal ligament; *UCL* ulnar collateral ligament; *AOL* anterior oblique ligament; *APL* abductor pollicis longus; *DRL* dorsoradial ligament; *POL* posterior oblique ligament). Volar view (**a**) and dorsal view (**b**) of the right trapeziometacarpal joint

metacarpal. This ligament tightens with the thumb flexion, abduction, and opposition positions. The dorsoradial ligament arises from the dorsoradial eminence of the trapezium and inserts on the dorsal edge of the first metacarpal base. It is taut in adduction and flexion positions and also referred to as dorsal ligament or radial collateral ligament. The first intermetacarpal ligament traverses the first and second metacarpal bases, and it is taut in abduction positions. In addition, the fibers of the APL tendon close to their insertions also reinforce the dorsal capsule.

The TM joint provides approximately 60° of flexion and extension, 40° of abduction and adduction, and 10° rotation [12]. Flexion is produced by FPB and OPP and aided by FPL when the other joints of the thumb are flexed. Extension is produced by APL and extensor pollicis brevis (EPB) and longus (EPL). Abduction is produced by APB and APL. Adduction is produced by ADP. Opposition is produced by APB, OPP, and FPB that simultaneously flex and pronate the abducted thumb. Interpulpal pressure, or that generated by digital grasping, is increased by ADP and FPL [7]. Circumduction is produced by extensors, abductors, flexors, and adductors acting consecutively in this or reversed order [12].

## Metacarpophalangeal Joint (MP Joint)

The MP joint of the thumb is not a hinge but a condylar joint. This joint is different from the MP joint of the other fingers, because it has the following characteristics: (1) it has constant presence of sesamoids, (2) it has the vicinity of the insertions of the thenar muscles, and (3) it has lesser mobility, in the flexion-extension and in the abduction-adduction planes. These differences are related to the main role of this joint, namely, to stabilize the thumb in power grip, especially by locking the thumb in the grasping of large objects.

The articular surface configuration of the first metacarpal head is more quadrilateral and less sphenoidal than the other metacarpals. The medial condyle extends slightly more distally than the lateral condyle, which accounts for the small amount of pronation that occurs with joint flexion. The chief difference is that the surface spreads over the palmar tubercles which protrude condyle-like (especially the lateral one) to correspond to the sesamoids.

The articular surface of the base of the proximal phalanx is oval, shallow concave and transversely broad (Fig. 2.8). The difference in the area of contact between the two articular surfaces permits usually less flexion and extension (average 53° of flexion and 8° of extension), and there is limitation in abduction and adduction (average 10°) than in fingers. Rotation is restricted by its ligamentous structures.

The capsule of the MP joint of the thumb is reinforced radially and ulnarly by the collateral and accessory collateral ligament. Volarly it comprises the thick fibrocartilaginous volar plate, whereas dorsally, the capsule is very thin and inserts into the dorsal base of the proximal phalanx, along with the thumb sagittal band [12, 13]. The EPL and EPB tendons are intimately associated with the dorsal capsule and serve to reinforce it.

The collateral ligaments arise from the ulnar and radial side dorsolateral region of the metacarpal head and run distally and volarly to insert into the base of the proximal phalanx. The accessory collateral ligaments arise from more proximal and volar to the collateral ligaments at the metacarpal head. They run obliquely to insert into the volar plate and the sesamoids, which are also restrained on the radial side by the FPB tendon and APB tendon and on the ulnar side by the ADP tendon and by A1 pulley [14, 15]. The collateral ligaments are taught in flexion and relaxed in extension, whereas the accessory collateral ligaments are taught in extension and relaxed in flexion [14, 16].

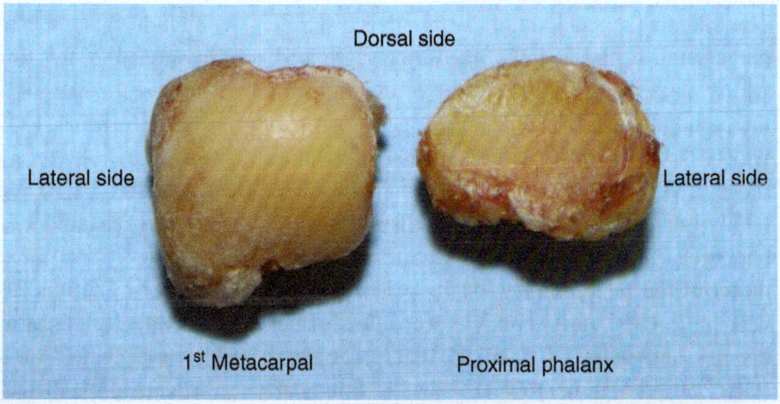


**Fig. 2.8** The articular surfaces in the metacarpophalangeal joint of the left thumb

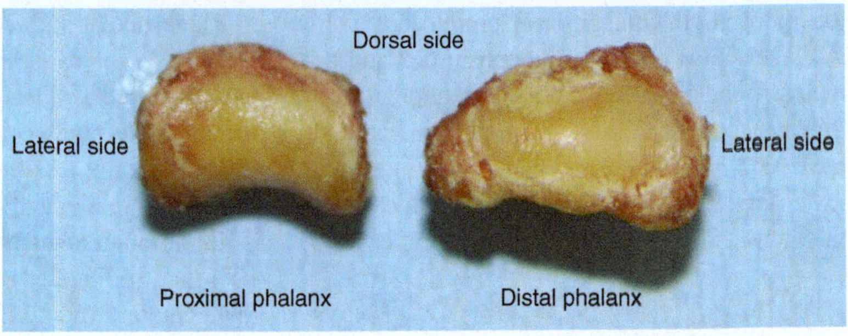


**Fig. 2.9** The articular surfaces in the interphalangeal joint of the left thumb

The volar plate is a thick, fibrocartilaginous capsule and resists MP joint hyperextension. The edges of the volar plate provide an attachment for the thenar muscles and collateral ligaments. It originates at the volar neck of the metacarpal and inserts into the base of the proximal phalanx. The proximal one third of the plate is thinner than the distal portion. The distal portion of the plate is thick and contains the two sesamoids. They move with the proximal phalanx during flexion and extension, and their articular surface matches a corresponding surface on the head of the metacarpal. The volar plate is additionally reinforced by the insertion of the intrinsic thumb muscles into the sesamoids.

Both sesamoids are connected by a stout transverse fibrous band that is part of the fibrous tunnel within which runs the FPL. Anatomically sesamoids also provide insertion points for the intrinsic muscles and mechanical advantage for these muscles by increasing their moment arm and stability to the FPL as it crosses the MP joint [15].

## Interphalangeal Joint (IP Joint)

The interphalangeal joint of the thumb is a simple hinge joint. It had a single fixed transverse axis, which passes through the center of curvature of the condyles of the phalangeal head, around which flexion-extension movement occurs in a range of 90°.

In practice, as it flexes, the distal phalanx undergoes 5–10° of pronation due to the asymmetry of the two condyles of the proximal phalanx [17]. The medial condyle protrudes further distally and palmarly than the lateral condyle (Fig. 2.9). Its ligamentous structure is similar to the IP joints of the fingers. However, the volar plate is significantly thicker and displaces the FPL tendon for palmarward from the joint space. A sesamoid is sometimes embedded in the volar plate.

# Functional Anatomy of the Muscles and Tendons of the Thumb

The nine motor muscles act on the thumb. Every joint can be moved by itself or together with others. All forces exerted by the muscles act as dynamic stabilizers of the thumb, facilitating pinch and grasp function.

It may be divided into two groups:

1. The intrinsic muscles, which are situated in the thenar eminence and work simultaneously on the TM, MP, and IP joints. Therefore, they are responsible for performing the different types of grip. These muscles include APB, FPB, OPP, and ADP.
2. The extrinsic muscles, whose muscle bellies are situated in the forearm. These muscles include APL, EPB, EPL and FPL. They are responsible for thumb motion and stability and are the ones used to release the grip except the FPL [8, 13, 18–20].

## Intrinsic Muscles

### Abductor Pollicis Brevis (APB)

It lies directly beneath the skin and radial to the FPB. It provides the shape and contour of the radial side of the thenar eminence. APB arises primarily from the flexor retinaculum. Accessory bundles of fibers may also arise from the scaphoid tubercle, the trapezium, and the tendons of palmaris longus (PL) and APL [6]. It inserts into the radial base of the proximal phalanx, the lateral side of the capsule of the MP joint, and the radial sesamoid at the MP joint and onto the dorsal aponeurosis of the extensor pollicis longus (Fig. 2.10a). The muscle is supplied by the recurrent branch of the median nerve (95%) or ulnar nerve (2.5%) or

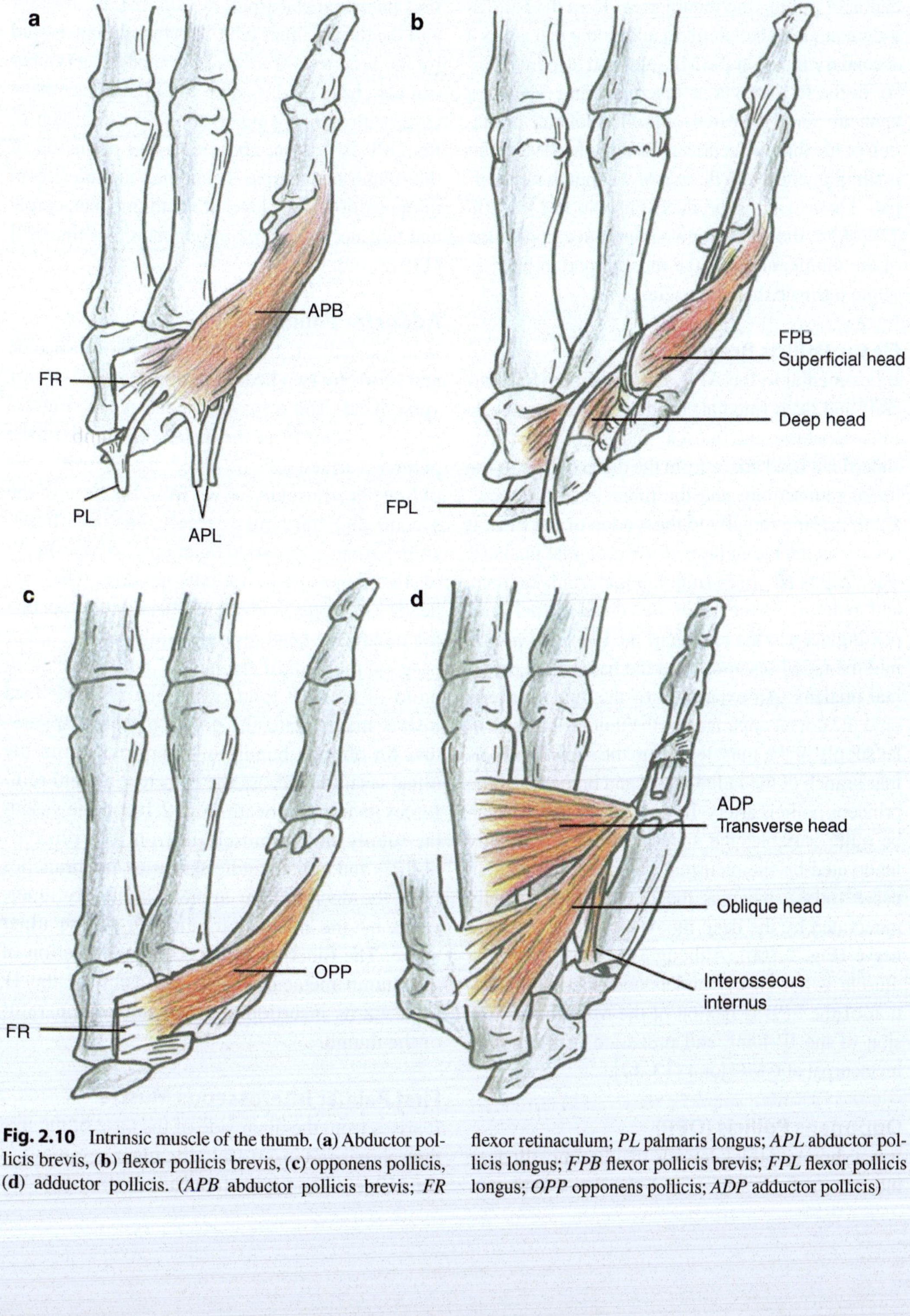


**Fig. 2.10** Intrinsic muscle of the thumb. (**a**) Abductor pollicis brevis, (**b**) flexor pollicis brevis, (**c**) opponens pollicis, (**d**) adductor pollicis. (*APB* abductor pollicis brevis; *FR* flexor retinaculum; *PL* palmaris longus; *APL* abductor pollicis longus; *FPB* flexor pollicis brevis; *FPL* flexor pollicis longus; *OPP* opponens pollicis; *ADP* adductor pollicis)

by dual innervation (2%) [13, 20]. The vascular supply of this muscle is from the superficial palmar branch of the radial artery and often by a separate branch arising directly from the radial artery. The main function of the APB is abduction and flexion of the thumb metacarpal, performing the action of pulling the thumb away from the palm at a right angle to the palm. In addition it can act as a secondary flexor in the MP joint and also in extensor in the IP joint via its insertions into the dorsal aponeurosis of the extensor pollicis longus: pronation of the thumb occurring through the CMC joint is simultaneous with flexion of the thumb metacarpal. These actions produce opposition [18, 20]. Therefore, the APB alone can produce opposition of the thumb, and it is the most important muscle of the intrinsic thenar muscle.

### Flexor Pollicis Brevis (FPB)

It lies medial to the APB and has superficial (lateral) and deep (medial) heads. The tendon of the FPL separates the muscle into two parts. The superficial head arises from the distal border of the flexor retinaculum and the tubercle of the trapezium, passing radially to the tendon of the FPL. It inserts on the radial base of the proximal phalanx. The deep head arises from the trapezoid, capitate, and palmar ligaments of the distal carpal row, passing deep to the tendon of the FPL, and inserts into the radial sesamoid and the base of the proximal phalanx. An expansion of the tendon inserts onto the dorsal apparatus of the thumb. The vascular supply of the muscle is from the superficial palmar branch of the radial artery and branches of the princeps pollicis artery. Innervation of the FPB can be quite variable; the superficial head is mainly innervated by the recurrent branch of the median nerve (60%), whereas the deep head is usually innervated by the deep motor branch of the ulnar nerve (Fig. 2.10b). Although the function of the muscle is not clearly understood, the main function of the FPB is flexion of the MP joint, extension of the IP joint, and pronation of the thumb metacarpal at CMC joint [13, 17].

### Opponens Pollicis (OPP)

It is a short and thick muscle that lies mostly deep into the APB. It arises from the flexor retinaculum, CMC joint capsule, and the tubercle of trapezium and fans out to insert on the whole-length volar radial aspect of the first metacarpal (Fig. 2.10c). The vascular supply of the muscle is from the superficial palmar branch of the radial artery and branches from the princeps pollicis, first palmar metacarpal, radialis indicis arteries, and the deep palmar arch. It is mainly innervated by the recurrent branch of the median nerve but can also have dual median and ulnar innervation or just ulnar nerve innervation. The function of the OPP is flexion, abduction, and pronation of the thumb metacarpal. It initiates the movement of opposition at the level of the thumb metacarpal and enhances the work of opposition of the APB [13, 18, 20].

### Adductor Pollicis (ADP)

It is the largest, most powerful thenar muscle and arises by two heads, an oblique and a transverse head. The transverse head is a triangular muscle arising from the distal two thirds of the palmar surface of the third metacarpal. The oblique head usually arises from the base of the second and third metacarpals, capitate, trapezoid, palmar intercarpal ligament, and the sheath of the flexor carpi radialis tendon. The two heads converge, and their fibers rotate so that the transverse head inserts mainly into the ulnar base of the proximal phalanx and ulnar sesamoid of the MP joint, while the oblique head inserts mainly into the dorsal extensor apparatus. An oblique bundle of fibers runs from the ulnar sesamoid across the FPL tendon and reinforces its fibrous sheath (Fig. 2.10d). The vascular supply of the muscle is from the princeps pollicis and radialis indicis arteries and branches from the deep palmar arch. It is mainly innervated by the deep motor branch of the ulnar nerve. The function of the ADP is adduction of the thumb metacarpal and extension of the IP joint via its insertion onto the dorsal apparatus of the thumb.

### First Palmar Interosseous Muscle

It arises from the ulnar side of the base of the first metacarpal and inserts into the ulnar sesamoid of the MP joint, and it is often rudimentary [8].

## Extrinsic Muscles

### Flexor Pollicis Longus (FPL)

The fibrous sheath for the FPL begins at the wrist approximately 2.0 cm proximal to the radial styloid and ends just distal to the IP joint [21]. The fibrous sheath is a double-walled hollow tube and lined by a thin synovial membrane that provides a sealed lubrication system containing synovial fluid. The fibrous wall layer is reinforced by ligamentous pulleys. There are three constant pulleys: two annular and one oblique (Fig. 2.11).

The A1 annular pulley is located at the MP joint. It is stronger, 7–9 mm wide, and about 0.5 mm thick. Its proximal two thirds fused with the volar plate of the MP joint, and its distal one third fused with the base of the proximal phalanx. The A2 annular pulley is located just proximal to the IP joint and is fused with volar plate of the IP joint. It is slightly wider (8–10 mm) but significantly thinner (0.25 mm). The oblique pulley begins at the ulnar aspect of the base of the proximal phalanx and continues in a distal and oblique direction to end on the radial aspect of the proximal phalanx near the IP joint. It is 9–10 mm wide and about 0.5–0.15 mm thick. The proximal end of the oblique pulley arises from one portion of the inserting tendons of the ADP. The oblique pulley is the most important pulley in the thumb for preserving normal flexion of the thumb [21–23].

The inserting tendon of the FPL passes through the carpal tunnel. At the thenar eminence, it is located between the OPP and the oblique head of the ADP. It inserts into the palmar surface of the base of the distal phalanx. During the course, it is accompanied by carpal, metacarpal, and phalangeal mesotendons that occur in the form of short and long vincula. The arterial supply of the tendon arises from the two digital arteries of the thumb, the princeps pollicis artery and the superficial palmar arch, and the accompanying artery of the median nerve [24]. It is innervated by the anterior interosseous branch of the median nerve, and the principal function is flexion of the phalanges. The excursion of the FPL tendon is 7.7 mm in the MP joint and 10.9 mm in the IP joint. Therefore, a total excursion over the first metacarpal is 19.6 mm.

### Extensor Pollicis Longus (EPL)

The tendon of the EPL is formed just proximal to the wrist and passes through the third extensor compartment. After it turns around the Lister's tubercle, it obliquely crossed the extensor carpi radial longus and brevis; with slight ulnar displacement, it then continues obliquely to the center of the MP joint and past the center of the

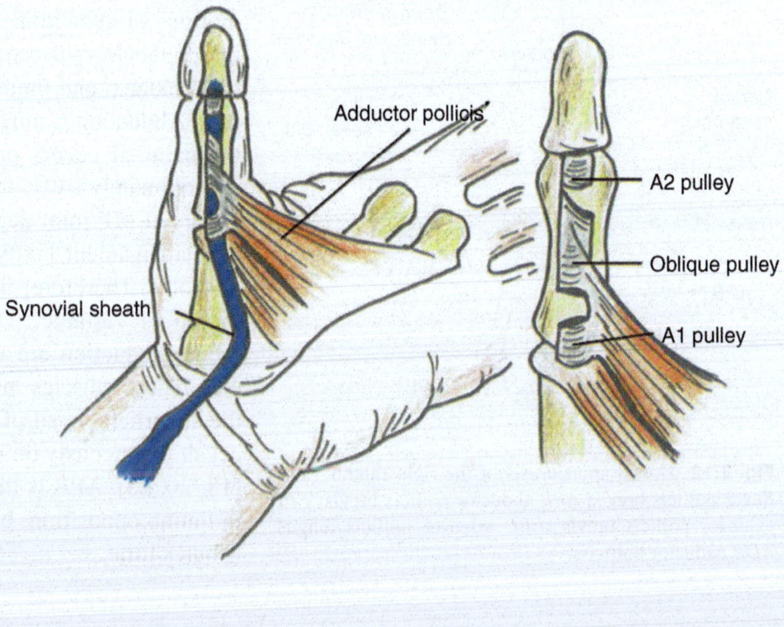


**Fig. 2.11** The left thumb flexor sheath

proximal phalanx and is attached to the dorsal base of the distal phalanx.

The transverse retinacular ligament is a thin membrane that arises from the flexor tendon sheath immediately distal to the MP joint. It inserts into the dorsal aponeurosis over the proximal phalanx. The oblique retinacular ligament arises from the lateral margin of the base of the proximal phalanx and from the tendon of the APB and ADP. It traverses the MP joint palmar to dorsal and reaches the EPL tendon at the distal half of the proximal phalanx and inserts the tendon into the distal phalanx (Fig. 2.12). Both retinacular ligaments control the dorsal aponeurosis of the thumb.

EPL is innervated by the posterior interosseous nerve. It extends the distal phalanx and also extends the metacarpal and proximal phalanx with the associated action of the EPB and APL. Due to the obliquity of its tendon, it adducts the extended thumb and rotates it laterally.

### Extensor Pollicis Brevis (EPB)

This tendon runs between APL and EPL and is inserted into the base of the proximal phalanx (Fig. 2.12). Because the EPB and the EPL tendon are two separate tendons, it is possible to extend the MP and IP joints independently of one another. It is innervated by the posterior interosseous nerve. It extends up to the proximal phalanx and first metacarpal.

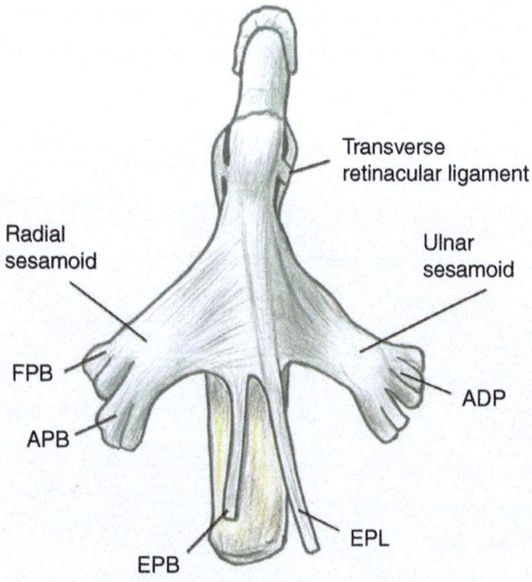


**Fig. 2.12** Dorsal aponeurosis of the right thumb. (*FPB* flexor pollicis brevis; *APB* abductor pollicis brevis; *EPB* extensor pollicis brevis; *EPL* extensor pollicis longus; *ADP* adductor pollicis)

### Abductor Pollicis Longus (APL)

This tendon is formed just proximal to the wrist and runs under the first extensor compartment, accompanied by the tendon of EPB. It usually splits into two slips: one is inserted into the base of the first metacarpal and the other is inserted into the trapezium. It is innervated by the posterior interosseous nerve. It is a pure extensor of the TM joint and abducts the first metacarpal.

## Dynamics of Opposition

In terms of biomechanical motion, there are seven maneuvers in the hand in order to perform most of the hand function [19]. For the hand function, the opposition is the most important function in the thumb. The axis of the thumb has its foundation at the TM joint and rests in a pronated and flexed position approximately 80° relative to the plane of the other metacarpals. This unique position allows opposition of the thumb to digits.

Thumb opposition involves the complex motions of abduction, flexion, pronation of the thumb metacarpal, radial deviation of the proximal phalanx, and thumb motion toward the fingers. Abduction is moving the thumb away from the palm. It occurs primarily at the TM joint approximately 40° to 50° and additionally occurs at MP joint depending on the degree of normal ligament laxity and the morphology of the joint. Therefore, the total abduction of the thumb is variable. The muscles involved in thumb abduction are the intrinsic thenar muscles. These muscles include the APB, OPP, and the superficial head of the FPB. These muscles act simultaneously on the TM and the MP joints [18, 20, 25]. APB is the most important muscle in thumb opposition, but the extrinsic APL contributes little.

The flexion component of opposition occurs all at three joints in the thumb. TM joint flexion permits positioning of the head of the thumb metacarpal in the same sagittal plane as that of the head of the middle finger metacarpal. MP and IP joint flexion facilitates the thumb toward the fingers, and it depends on the sizes of the objects and prehensile activity. The involved muscles are the intrinsic thumb muscles. For forceful flexion, there are important contributions from the ADP and from the FPL [24]. The pronation component of opposition occurs simultaneously with flexion and abduction of the TM joint caused by the configurations of its articular surfaces and ligaments [10–12].

## Summary

The thumb is a very unique portion in the human body and one of the sites with the most complex biomechanical system. The functional mobility of the thumb is the most important part of the function of the hand. Therefore, a careful understanding of the functional anatomy of the thumb will help physicians to provide the best nonsurgical or surgical treatment for the impaired hand function and thumb.

## References

1. Chow SP. Digital nerves in the terminal phalangeal region of the thumb. Hand. 1980;12(2):193–6.
2. Earley MJ. The arterial supply of the thumb, first web and index finger and its surgical application. J Hand Surg Br. 1986;11(2):163–74.
3. Brunelli F, Gilbert A. Vascularization of the thumb. Anatomy and surgical applications. Hand Clin. 2001;17(1):123–38.
4. Ikeda A, Ugawa A, Kazihara Y, Hamada N. Arterial patterns in the hand based on a three-dimensional analysis of 220 cadaver hands. J Hand Surg Am. 1988;13(4):501–9.
5. Parks BJ, Arbelaez J, Horner RL. Medical and surgical importance of the arterial blood supply of the thumb. J Hand Surg Am. 1978;3(4):383–5.
6. Schmidt HM, Lanz U. Thumb. In: Surgical anatomy of the hand. Stuttgart: Georg Thieme Verlag; 2004. p. 85–113.
7. Pistre V, Pelissier P, Martin D, Baudet J. Vascular blood supply of the dorsal side of the thumb, first web and index finger: anatomical study. J Hand Surg Br. 2001;26(2):98–104.
8. Ross AC. In: Standring S, editor. Wrist and hand. Gray's anatomy. 41st ed. Amsterdam: Elsevier; 2016. p. 862–894 e1.
9. McFadden D, Bracht MS. Sex and race differences in the relative lengths of metacarpals and metatarsals in human skeletons. Early Hum Dev. 2009;85(2): 117–24.
10. Bettinger PC, Berger RA. Functional ligamentous anatomy of the trapezium and trapeziometacarpal joint (gross and arthroscopic). Hand Clin. 2001;17(2):151–68.
11. Pieron. In: Tubina R, editor. The first carpometacarpal joint. The hand. Philadelphia: W. B. Saunders; 1981. p. 169–83.
12. Barmakian JT. Anatomy of the joints of the thumb. Hand Clin. 1992;8(4):683–91.
13. Leversedge FJ. Anatomy and pathomechanics of the thumb. Hand Clin. 2008;24(3):219–29.
14. Frank WE, Dobyns J. Surgical pathology of collateral ligamentous injuries of the thumb. Clin Orthop Relat Res. 1972;83:102–14.
15. Gibeault JD, Saba P, Hoenecke H, Graham A. The sesamoids of the metacarpo-phalangeal joint of the thumb: an anatomical and clinical study. J Hand Surg Br. 1989;14(2):244–7.
16. Aubriot JH. The metacarpophalangeal joint of the thumb. In: Tubiana R, editor. The hand, vol. 1. Philadelphia: WB Saunders; 1981. p. 184–7.
17. Kapanji IA. Biomechanics of the interphalangeal joint of the thumb. In: Tubiana R, editor. The hand, vol. 1. Philadelphia: WB Saunders; 1981. p. 188–90.
18. Kapandji IA. Biomechanics of the thumb. In: Tubiana R, editor. The hand, vol. 1. Philadelphia: WB Saunders; 1981. p. 404–22.
19. Duncan SF, Saracevic CE, Kakinoki R. Biomechanics of the hand. Hand Clin. 2013;29(4):483–92.
20. Gupta S, Michelsen-Jost H. Anatomy and function of the thenar muscles. Hand Clin. 2012;28(1):1–7.
21. Doyle JR, Blythe WF. Anatomy of the flexor tendon sheath and pulleys of the thumb. J Hand Surg Am. 1977;2(2):149–51.
22. Zissimos AG, Szabo RM, Yinger KE, Sharkey NA. Biomechanics of the thumb flexor pulley system. J Hand Surg Am. 1994;19(3):475–9.
23. Esplin VS, Tencer AF, Hanel DP, Cosio MQ. Restoration of function of the thumb flexor apparatus requires repair of the oblique and one adjacent flexor tendon pulley. J Orthop Res. 1996;14(1):152–6.
24. Zbrodowski A, Gajisin S, Bednarkiewicz M. Mesotendons of the flexor pollicis longus muscle. Acta Anat (Basel). 1994;151(2):131–7.
25. Posner MA, Kapila D. Restoration of opposition. Hand Clin. 2012;28(1):27–44.

# Part II

# Developmental Anomalies

# Duplicated Thumb and Secondary Deformity

# 3

Sang Hyun Woo and Young Seok Lee

## Introduction

Radial polydactyly of the hand is the second most common congenital hand disorder, and it ranges from a vestigial radial skin tag to varying degrees of splitting to complete duplication. It is believed to arise from excessive cell proliferation and disturbed cell necrosis of preaxial ectodermal and mesodermal tissues before the eighth week of embryonic life. It occurs sporadically and unilaterally. Hereditary influence has not been documented in isolated thumb polydactyly, although autosomal dominance has been reported in triphalangism and polysyndactyly. It is difficult to establish the true incidence of polydactyly because many minor cases are treated in the nursery by pedicle ligation shortly after birth. Region, race, and combined numbers of all polydactylies, or only radial- or ulnar-sided polydactyly, provide very different incidences in published series. The incidence of preaxial polydactyly is reported as 0.08 to 1.4 per 1000 live births [1, 2]. The IFSSH (International Federation of Societies for Surgery of the Hand) classifies these malformations in group III [3].

S. H. Woo (✉) · Y. S. Lee
W Institute for Hand and Reconstructive Microsurgery, W Hospital, Daegu, South Korea

## Classification

Since late 1960, Wassel's classification [4] is the most widely accepted and is very simple to understand and remember. It was based on the duplication level of the bone checked only by simple radiograph. Recently, nomenclature of this classification has been changed to "Flatt classification" [5] although 40% of duplicated thumbs could not be classified using this system [6]. This classification does not account for the anatomic complexity of congenital hand differences, including soft tissue deficiencies and redundancies, axial plane deformities, joint instability, and functionality. Simple X-ray shows only bone and soft tissue shadow with limitations in describing the concrete morphology of the duplication. Surgeons can imagine only the presence and shape of the cartilage and joint between bones. In 2013, Chung et al. suggested a new classification system of the radial polydactyly [7] based on the anatomic morphology of osseous or chondral connection of the joint and epiphysis. However, they did not show the true nature of the joint. Modern magnetic resonance imaging (MRI) techniques can show exquisite anatomic detail. Imaging with 3.0 tesla (T) MR units can show very small field-of-view imaging at high resolution, especially a baby's diminutive cartilage and joints (Fig. 3.1). It also can show tendons and vessels in three dimensions. In a certain type V or VI polydactyly by Flatt classification on the X-ray, the extra digit is connected to the main digit by soft tissue alone without any chondral connection. Because this type needs only soft tissue sur-


S. H. Woo (ed.), *The Thumb*, https://doi.org/10.1007/978-981-10-4400-7_3

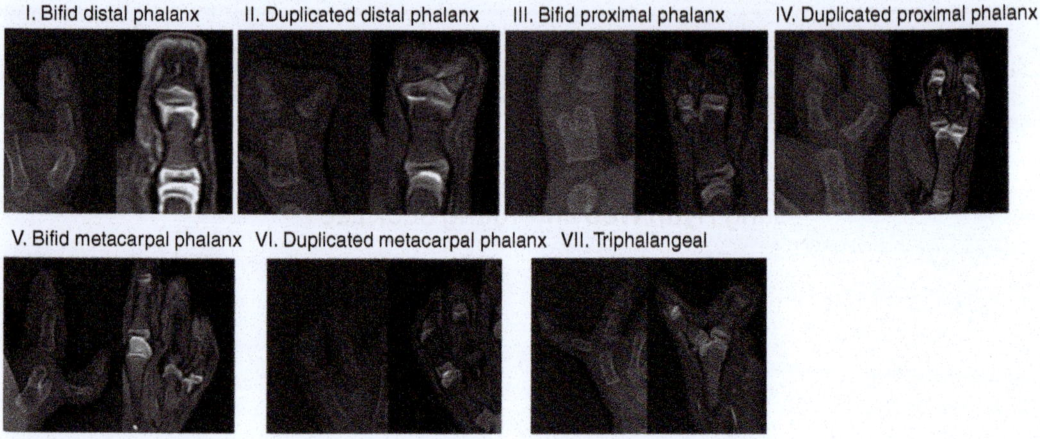


**Fig. 3.1** Flatt classification of radial polydactyly based on radiograph and coronal images using 3.0 T system (Achieva, Philips Medical Systems, Netherlands) magnetic resonance scanner

gery, both operation timing and surgical planning should be changed (Fig. 3.2).

Of the 1138 radial polydactyly cases of the senior author (SH Woo) during the last 20 years, the three most common Flatt types are, respectively, 495 cases of type IV (44.2%), 223 cases of type II (20%), and 188 cases of floating type (16.8%) (Table 3.1). In the author's cases, there were many cases of thumb duplications that defied classification, and there was no radial polydactyly involving carpal bone.

Among many proposed classifications, there is a new "Rotterdam classification" based on the triphalangeal components, triplication, hypoplasia or floating components, deviation, and symphalangism [8]. This classification includes designations for complex osseous, and soft tissue elements may prove more useful in conveying the full extent of the radial-sided hand deformity and for informing surgical technique (Fig. 3.3).

## Preoperative Considerations: Operation Timing and Anesthesia

The initial operation for radial polydactyly should be determined based on the child's age and overall health including tolerance for anesthesiology and the surgeon's experience or preference. Informed consent should be dealt on advantages and disadvantages of the surgery as well as the possibility of secondary surgery. Preoperative discussion with the parents allows for physical examination and clarification of the expected surgical steps necessary for reconstruction of the new thumb. The potential need for secondary revision, which can include scar revision, joint capsule plication, tendon transfer, and osteotomy with or without joint fusion, is also informed at the time of initial operation.

The timing and methods of anesthesia of the initial surgery are very different between cases. According to the anatomical variation checked by MRI, complexity of the surgical procedure, method of anesthesia, and operation timing will be determined. In addition to MRI, ultrasonography can show the dynamic images of joint and tendons as well as location of the flexor or extensor tendons.

Generally, parents want the period of hiding the baby's hand with polydactyly to be shortened. The thumb and index finger function develops at 10–12 months, and coordinated function of the thumb does not appear until a child is 2–3 years of age. Developmentally, waiting until the patient is 3 years of age will not alter the function of the reconstructed thumb when the extra digit is connected to the main digit by soft tissue alone without any chondral connection, the operation can be performed under local anesthesia with or without oral sedatives around 100 days after birth. Floating thumb can be ligated or resected before 1 month at the outpatient clinic. In Flatt type IV cases, timing of the operation is recommended at around 8–10 months under general anesthesia. Frequent surgical procedures include extra digit resection,

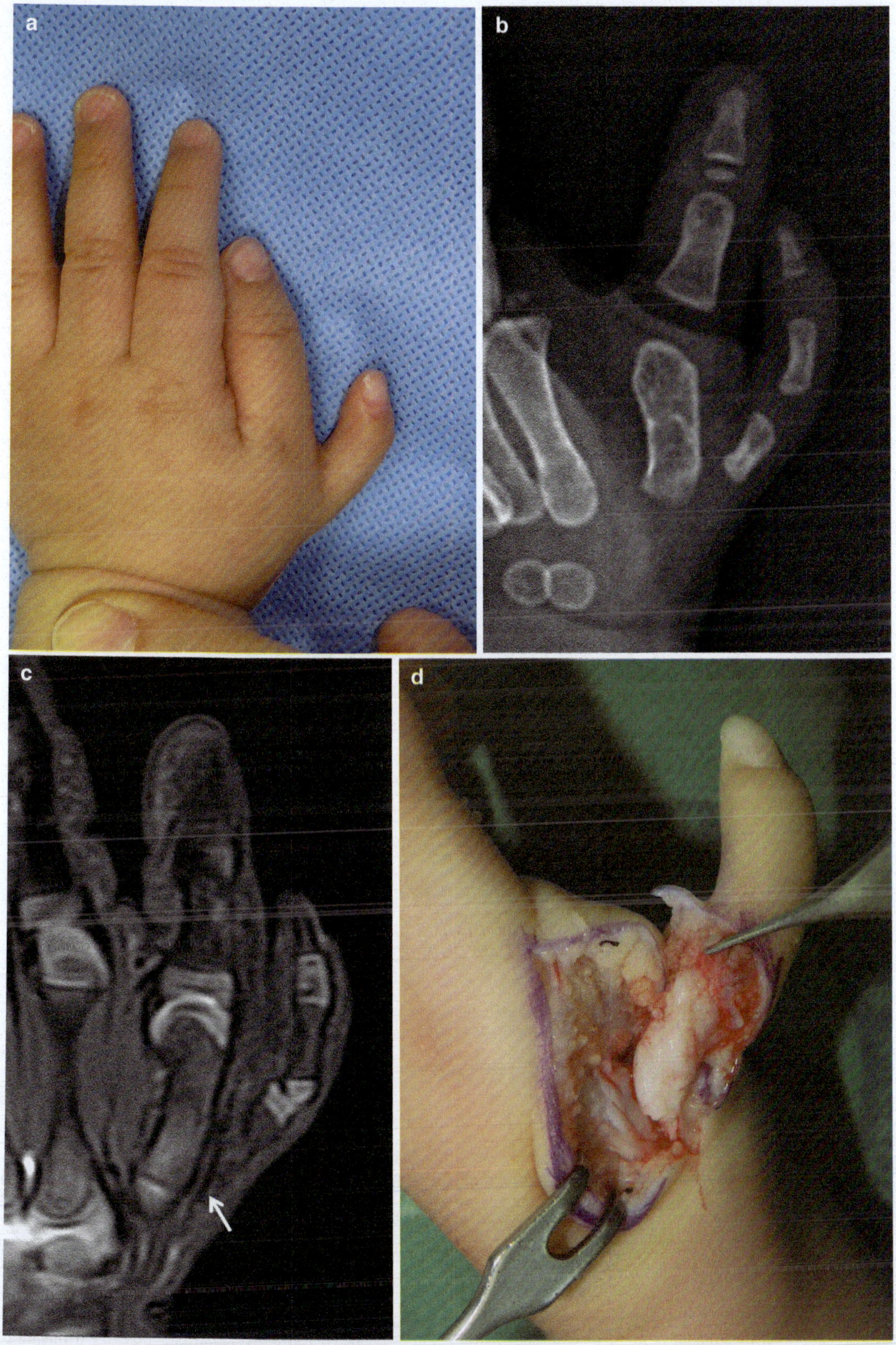


**Fig. 3.2** (**a** and **b**) Radial polydactyly looks like type V. (**c** and **d**) MR scan (white arrow) and intraoperative view show no chondral connection between two metacarpal bases

resection of the radial head of metacarpal bone, and ligament and muscle repair with or without extensor tendon transfer. Because all these procedures take less than 1 hour under a tourniquet, intravenous sedation with fentanyl and combined injection of local anesthesia during the procedure are preferred. This also provides a comfortable situation for the surgeon as this anesthesia works especially well where the parents refuse or are averse to endotracheal intubation.

**Table 3.1** Flatt classification of the author's 1138 cases of radial polydactyly

| Type | I | II | III | IV | V | VI | VII |
|---|---|---|---|---|---|---|---|
| No. | 37 | 223 | 55 | 495 | 76 | 26 | 19 |
| % | 3 | 20 | 4.9 | 44.2 | 6.7 | 2.3 | 1.6 |
| Floating type: 188 (16.8%) | | | | | | | |

In cases of required osteotomy and bone fixation and more proximal radial polydactyly than type V, surgical procedures may be more complicated. For this reason, initial surgery is usually delayed until the child is at least 1 year of age and should be done under general anesthesia. This minimizes anesthetic risks and allows time for the thumb growth.

## Operative Principles

Except with very simple polydactyly, the surgeon always reflects upon or regrets the previously adapted operation method or surgical technique when the patients having residual deformities in shape or limited range on the long-term follow-up irrespective of the initial type. Therefore, the strategy for the initial operation should be ingenious

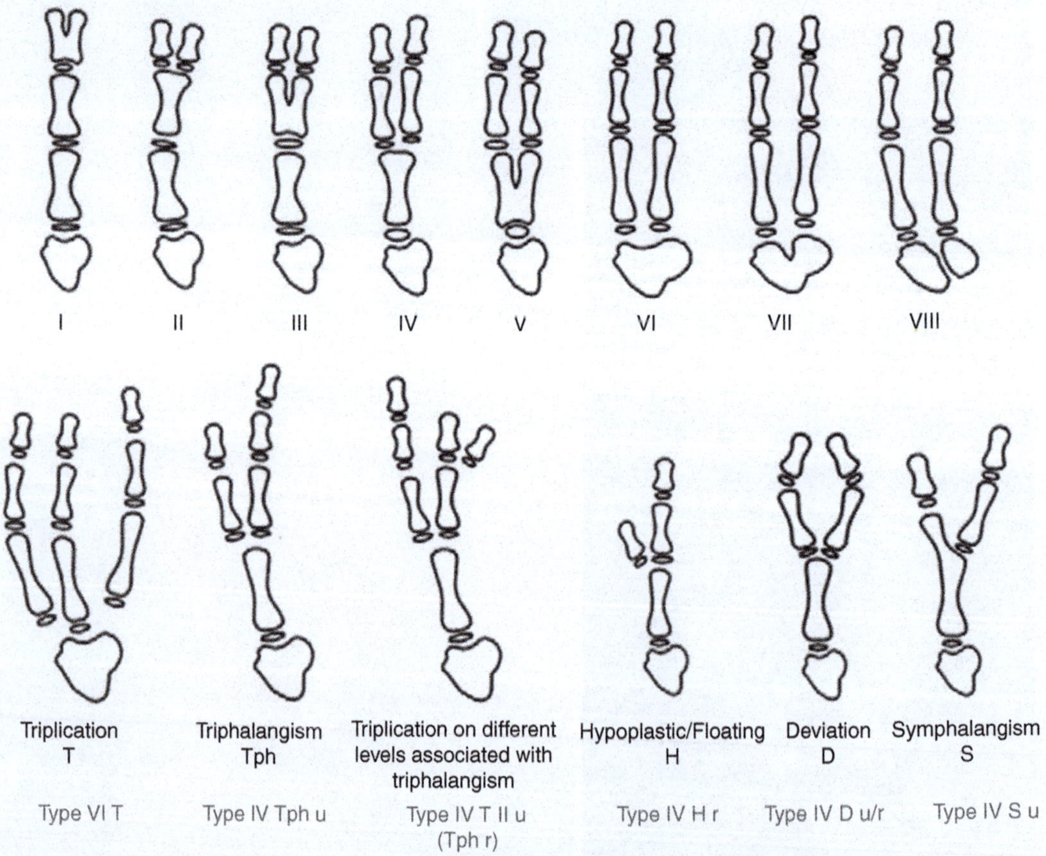


**Fig. 3.3** The Rotterdam classification of radial polydactyly as described by Zuidam et al. cited with permission from Zuidam JM, Selles RW, Ananta M, Runia J, Hovius SE. A classification system of radial polydactyly: inclusion of triphalangeal thumb and triplication. J Hand Surg Am. 2008;33:373–377. Abbreviations can be used for the different associated deformities: *Tph* triphalangeal, *T* triplication, *S* symphalangism, *D* deviation, *H* hypoplastic or floating positions of the duplicated parts or deformities are assigned by the abbreviations u (ulnar), m (middle), and r (radial)

and creative, not conservative. The surgeon should apply the "best part" doctrine, in which the most complete anatomic parts from all duplicated parts are used to construct a new thumb as normal as possible [9]. Operation for the radial polydactyly does not involve the removal of extra digit but reconstruction of the new thumb with proper function of the joint and tendons as well as achieving acceptable aesthetic outcome in length, axis of the phalangeal bone, and bulkiness of the soft tissue.

## Flatt Types I and II

In this type, the deformity is divided into two types according to appearance. One involves equal components for both the radial and ulnar side which share a common epiphysis or where there are two epiphyses. The other involves a larger ulnar and smaller radial component of the distal phalanx. Selection of the operation method between resection of smaller or radial component and combination of the two components is always debated.

The "rule of 70 or 80%" will be the guide to choose operation technique. If the nail width at nail fold of the larger component is over 70–80% of the contralateral thumb, resection of the smaller component is reasonable [10]. To excise the smaller thumb, the incision can be made laterally in an elliptical shape to result in a straight scar. More lateral incision leaves less conspicuous scars. Surgical procedure includes ablation of the smaller component and shaving of the articular cartilage of the proximal phalanx. If possible, centralization of the extrinsic tendons on the distal phalanx and reattachment and reeling of the capsule of the distal IP joint should be done. At the lateral side distal to the IP joint, the collateral ligament with periosteal flap is preserved proximally. If the articular cartilage was trimmed to produce a flat joint surface, the joint capsule should be strongly repaired (Fig. 3.4). Where the longitudinal axis through IP joint is not

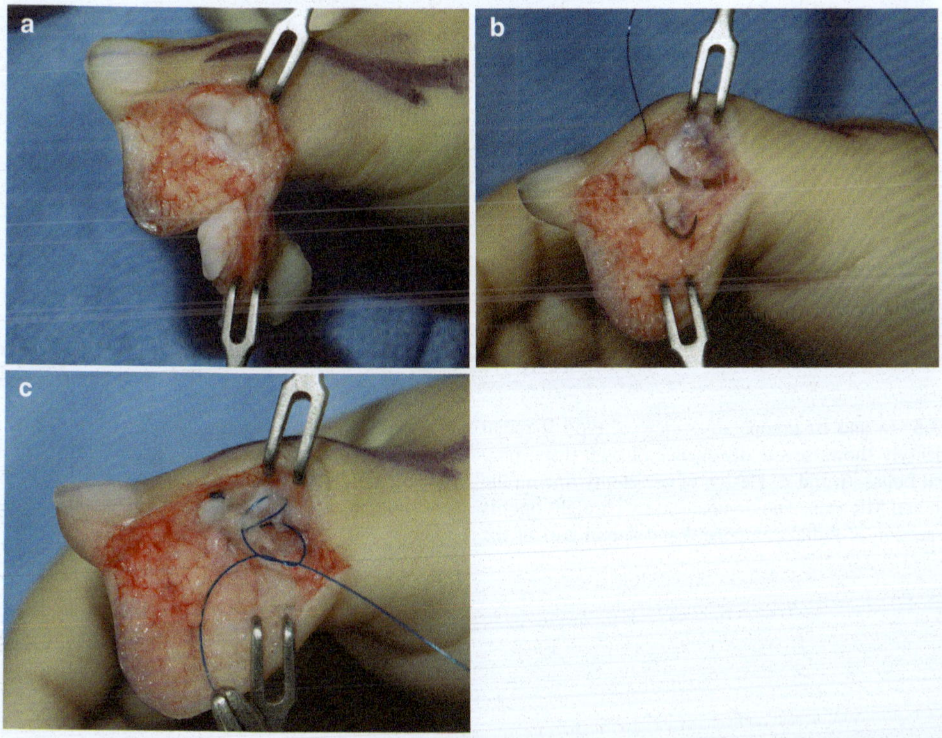

**Fig. 3.4** (**a**) The radial component is resected in type II radial polydactyly. At the lateral side distal to the IP joint, the collateral ligament with periosteal flap is preserved proximally. (**b** and **c**) Suture needle passes the radial cartilage of the distal phalangeal bone, and the strong repair is performed at the joint capsule and collateral ligament with periosteal flap with nonabsorbable suture

straight with an oblique joint surface, primary corrective osteotomy is very useful to correct angulation. This procedure involves closing wedge ostectomy at the neck of proximal phalanx and one 0.7 mm Kirschner wire fixation under C-arm (Fig. 3.5). In many cases, the proximal nail fold is not horizontal but slanted, and so simultaneous eponychial fold plasty helps improve the aesthetic outcome. The longitudinal incision is made on the short side of the proximal nail fold in the same length as the opposite side. The incised eponychium is proximally folded and fixed with half-buried horizontal mattress sutures (Fig. 3.6).

In cases where the nail width at nail fold of the larger component is the same size or less than 70% of the contralateral thumb, treatment is more

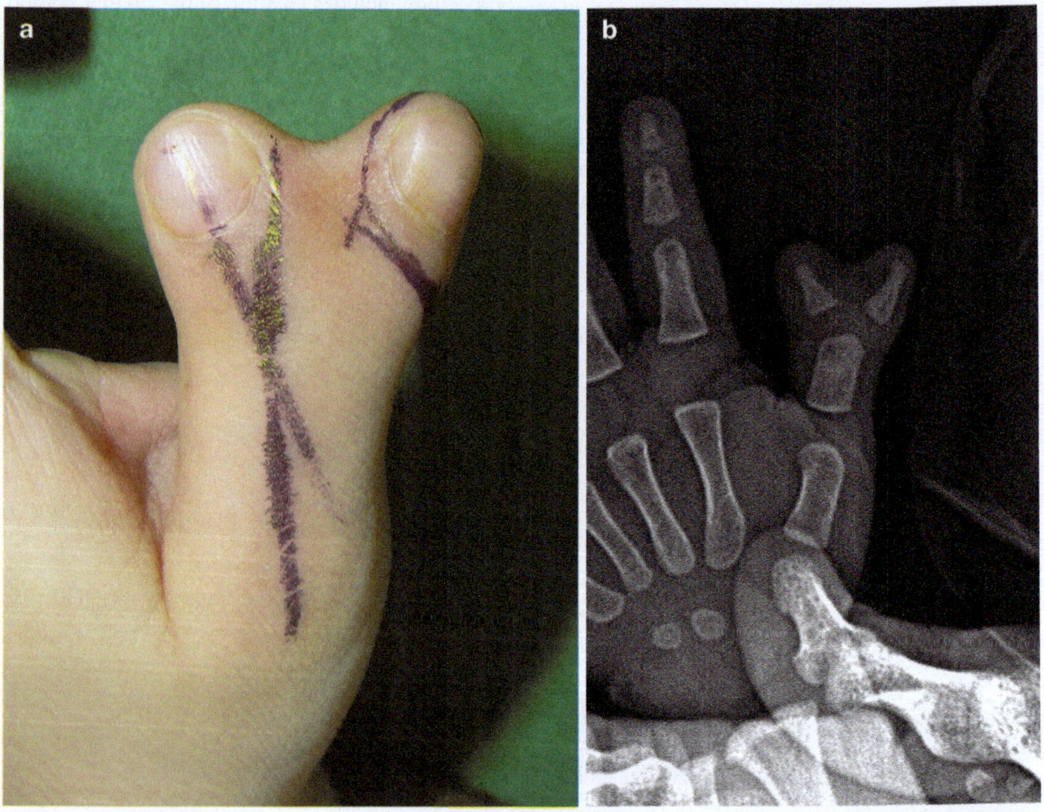


**Fig. 3.5** (**a** and **b**) Preoperative view of type II radial polydactyly shows severe divergence of both distal phalangeal bones. (**c** and **d**) Design of ostectomy line on the thumb and MR scan. The first ostectomy (straight line) is for resection of radial component and lateral part of the proximal phalanx. Closing wedge ostectomy (broken line) is made at the neck of proximal phalanx. (**e**) Fixation with two 0.7 mm Kirschner wires under C-arm. (**f**) Immediate post-operation. (**g** and **h**) Postoperative view and radiograph

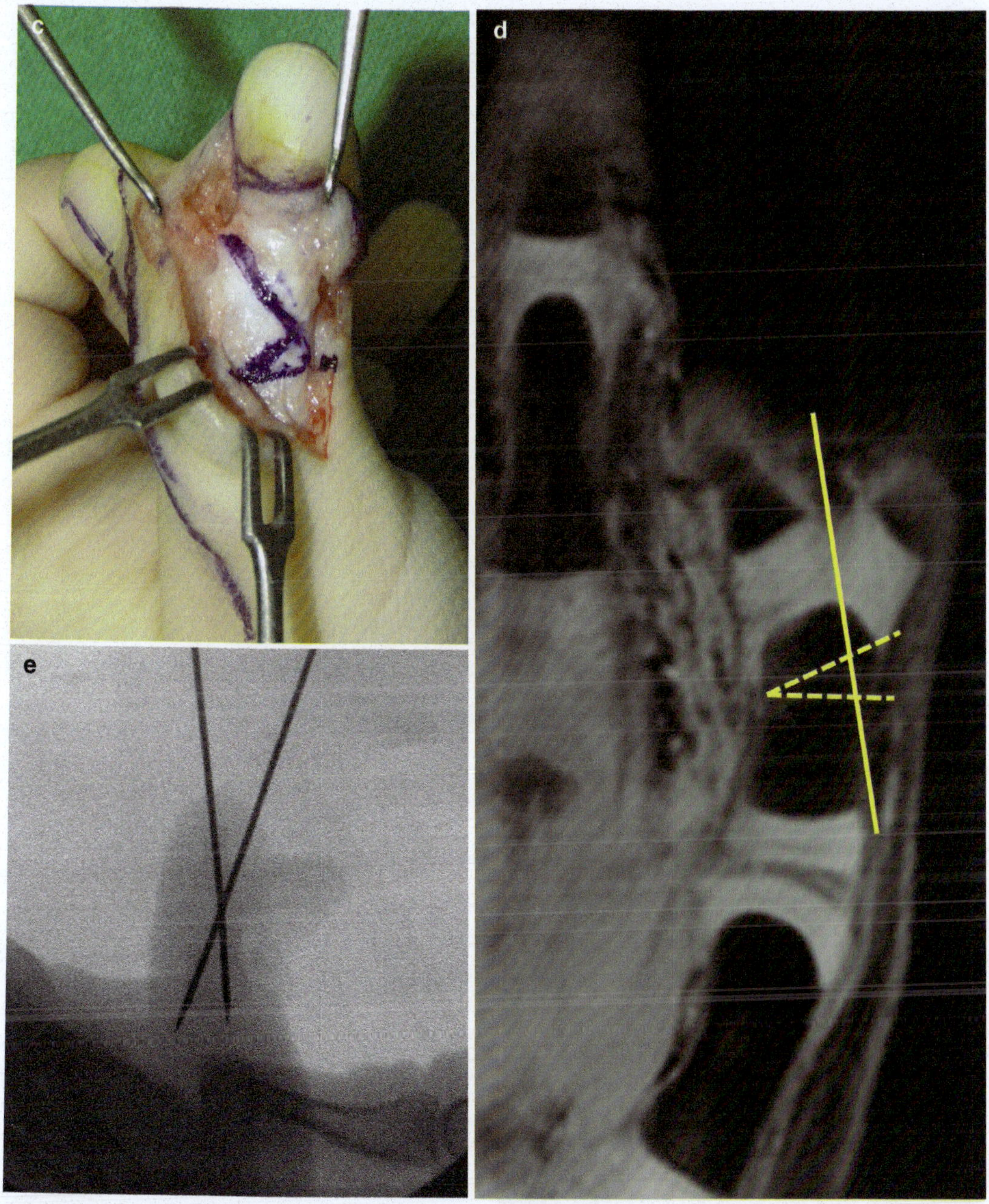


**Fig. 3.5** (continued)

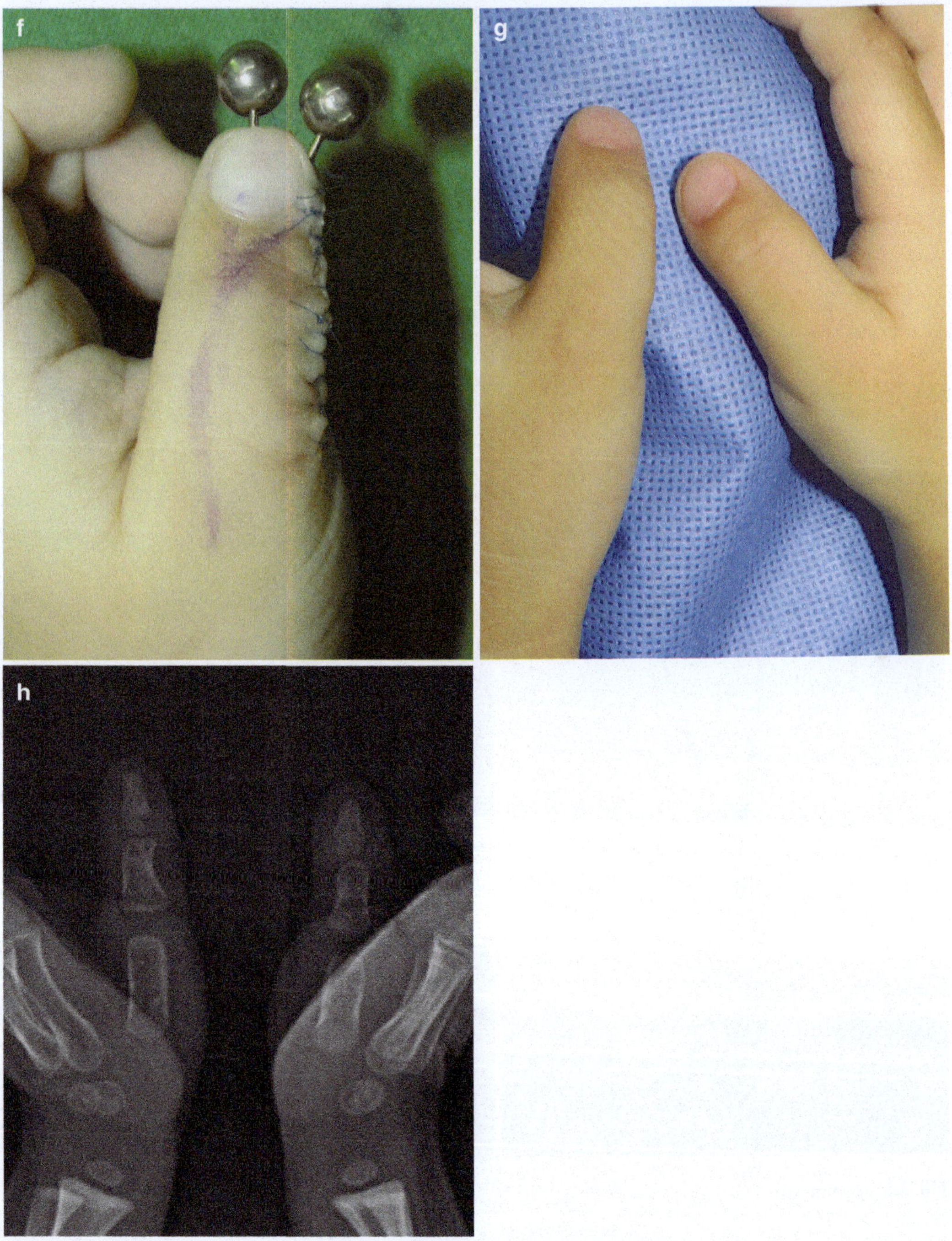

**Fig. 3.5** (continued)

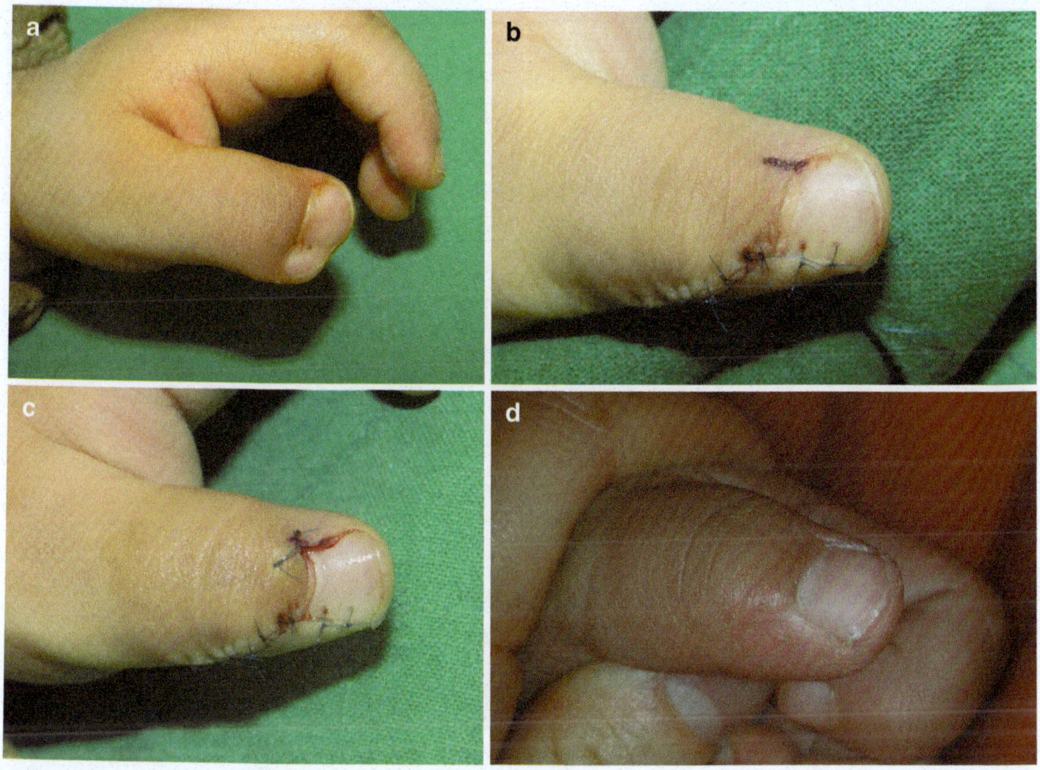

**Fig. 3.6** (**a**) Preoperative view of type II radial polydactyly. (**b**) Slant proximal nail fold after resection of radial component. Design of nail fold plasty at the junction between ulnar and proximal nail folds. (**c**) Nail fold is retracted and sutured proximally and ulnarly. (**d**) Postoperative view

complex. The Bilhaut-Cloquet operation of central wedge resection is reserved for only Flatt type I or II thumbs so that not more than one growth plate is violated (Fig. 3.7). Commonly this procedure makes an uneven nail bed, a central split ridge, and an uneven eponychial nail fold.

## Flatt Type III

In this type of radial polydactyly, there are many factors that should be considered preoperatively, such as divergence angles of the MP joint, convergence angle of the IP joint, and shape and longitudinal axis of proximal phalanx and metacarpal bone based on simple radiology. The status of epiphyseal sharing at the base of the proximal phalanx as well as eccentric insertion of extrinsic tendons can be identified with MR scanning. The shape and width of nail and bulkiness of the pulp should also be examined.

Postoperative thumb length, girth, and nail width may influence the aesthetic outcome. The most common reason for lower satisfaction is angulation; thus, the goal of surgical reconstruction of radial polydactyly is to create a thumb that is well-aligned, stable, and of normal size with appropriate range of motion [11].

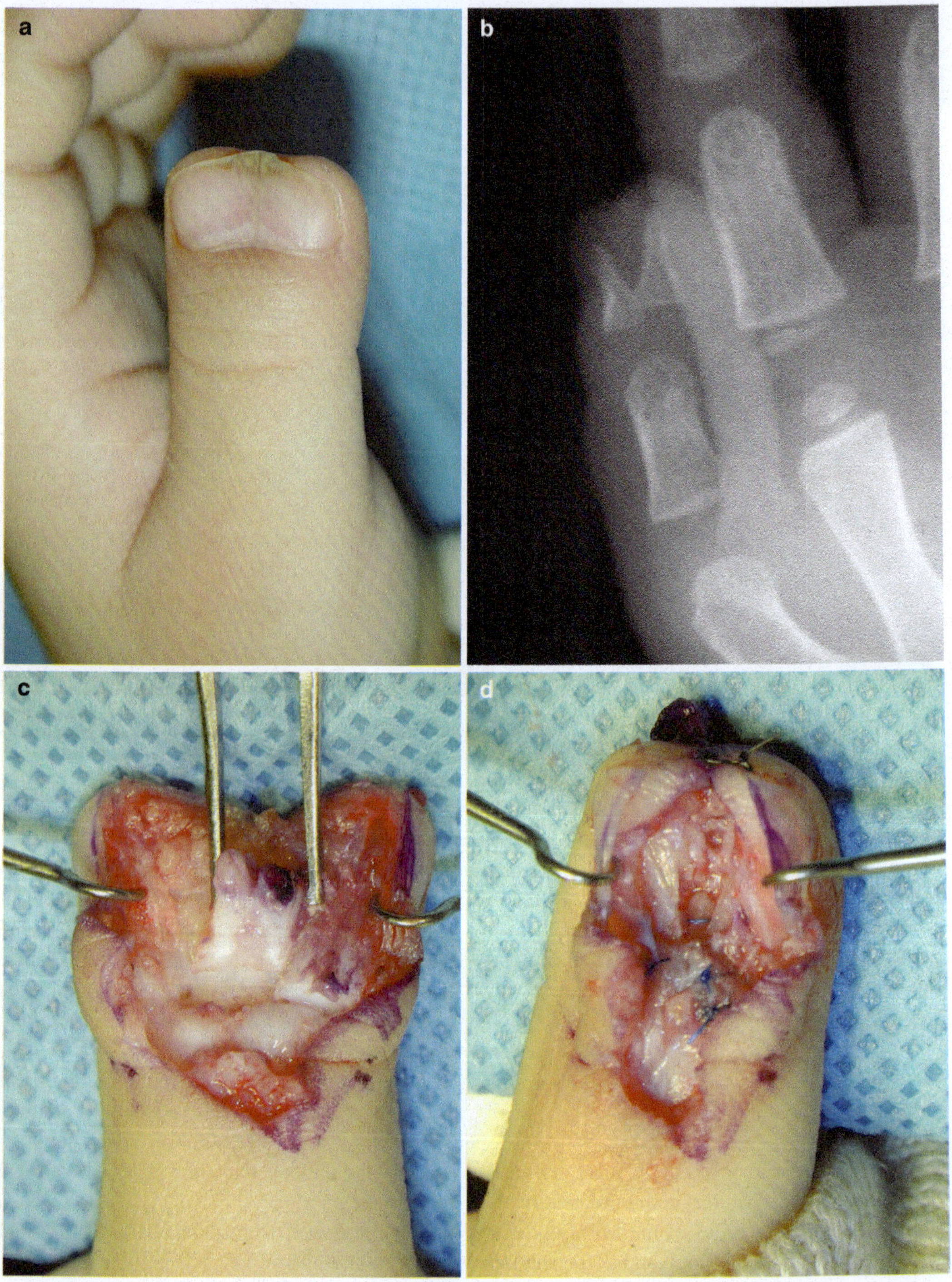


**Fig. 3.7** (**a** and **b**) Type II polydactyly with very symmetrical nail plate and similar size of distal phalangeal bone on the radiograph. (**c**) Longitudinal ostectomy of the distal phalangeal bone according to the Bilhaut-Cloquet procedure. (**d**) Intraosseous wiring of the bone and extensor tendon repair. (**e**) Immediately after operation, nail plate and skin closure. (**f–h**) Post-operation, 10 years later plus radiograph

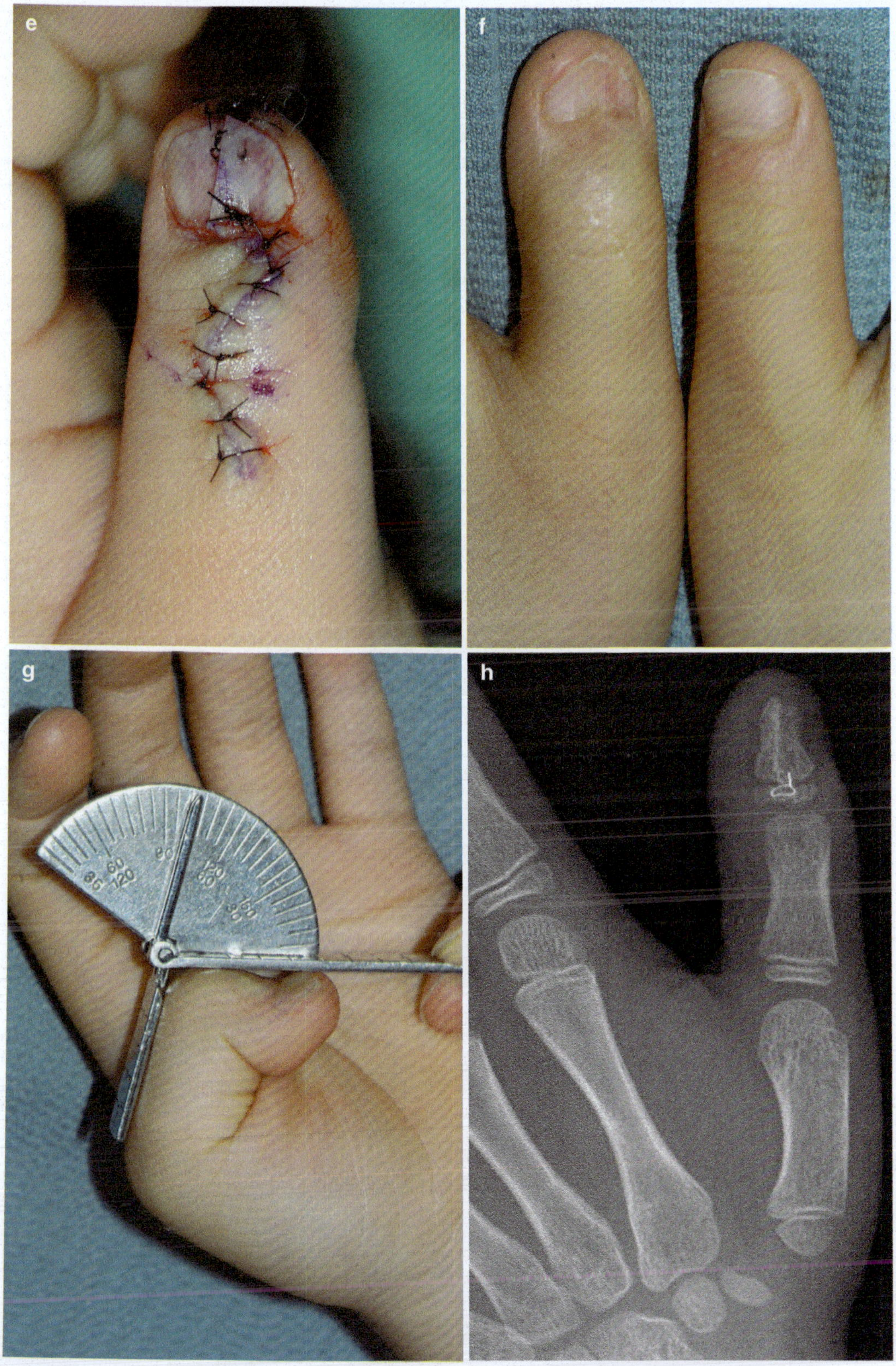


**Fig. 3.7** (continued)

In type III polydactyly with equal or almost equal size, even though modified Bilhaut-Cloquet procedures have been introduced [11, 12], complicated surgical technique and unpromising outcomes are frequently the results (Fig. 3.8). With the modified technique of Manske [13] for type II, instead of narrowing the distal articular surface, distal and radial portion of proximal phalangeal bone should be preserved to prevent radial angulation of the distal phalanx [14] (Figs. 3.9 and 3.10). The radial collateral ligament along with the cartilage is sutured to the ulnar distal phalanx. The EPL tendon of the retained thumb is augmented by the EPL tendon of the excised thumb. Fillet flap from the radial thumb can provide additional coverage of the radial pulp. The radial paronychium is also reconstructed with soft tissue from the excised thumb. The IP joint is temporarily fixed by K-wire.

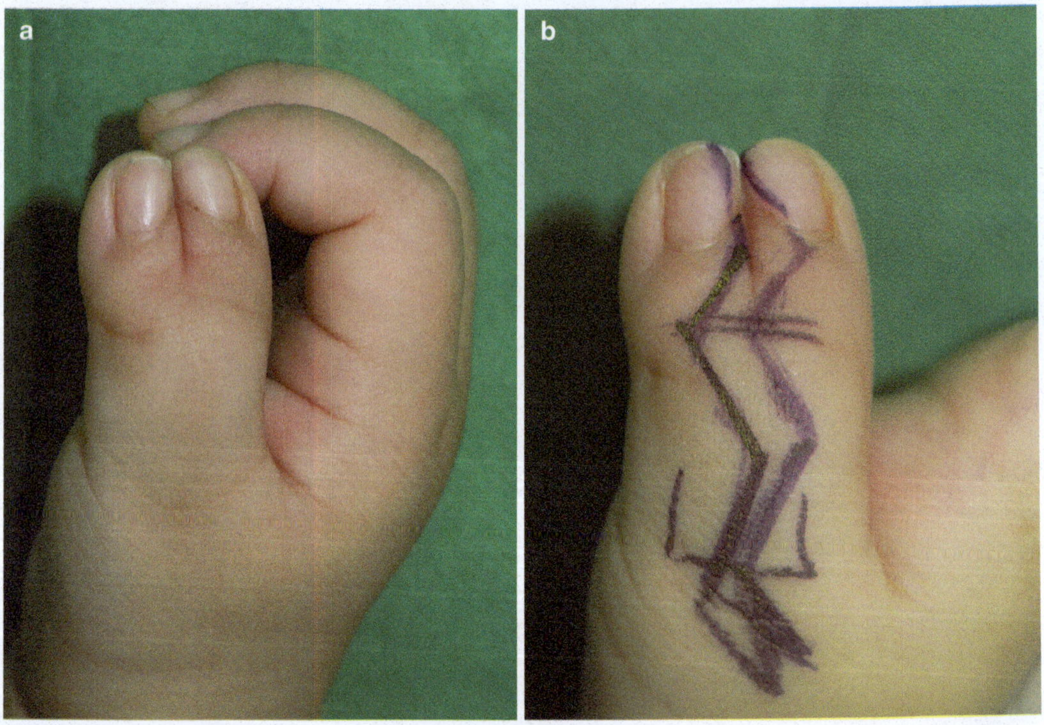


**Fig. 3.8** (**a**) Type III polydactyly with very symmetrical nail plate and similar size of distal phalangeal bone on the radiograph. (**b–d**) A zigzag incision matching volar and dorsal surfaces is made. Small Z-plasty is designed on the pulp tip. (**e**) The required width of bone is then excised from the proximal and distal phalanges, using a fine osteotome, to complete the longitudinal osteotomies. (**f**) Transverse bone fixation with multiple 0.7 mm Kirschner wires. (**g** and **h**) After key sutures on the hyponychium, the nail bed is repaired using an 8.0 Vicryl suture. The extensor and flexor tendons are repaired using a 5.0 Prolene suture. (**i–k**) The skin is closed with 6.0 Vicryl Rapide sutures. One nail is firmly replaced between two nail folds. (**l**) Post-operation. (**m–o**) Radiograph of the thumb preoperative, immediate post-operation, and post-operation

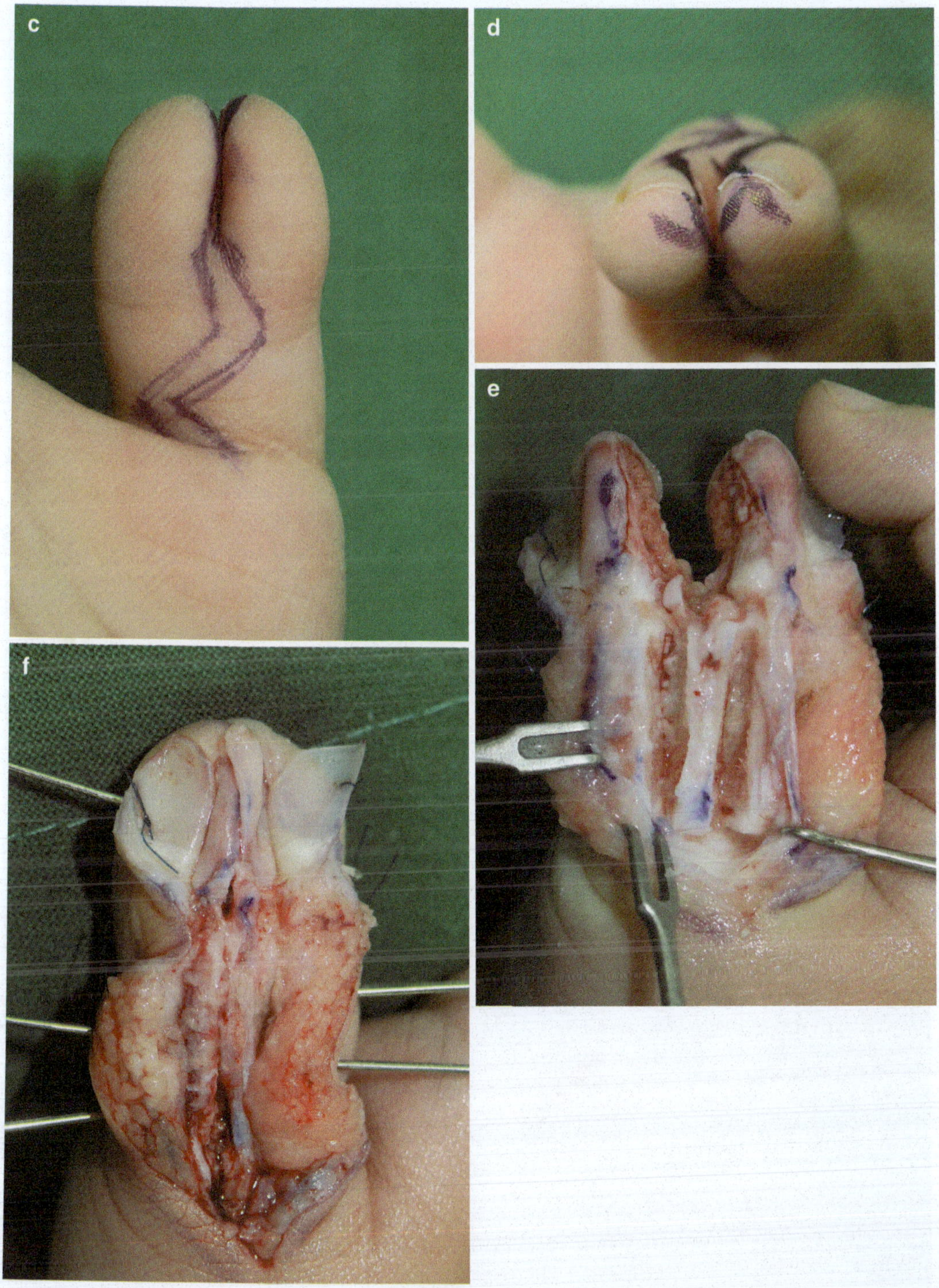


**Fig. 3.8** (continued)

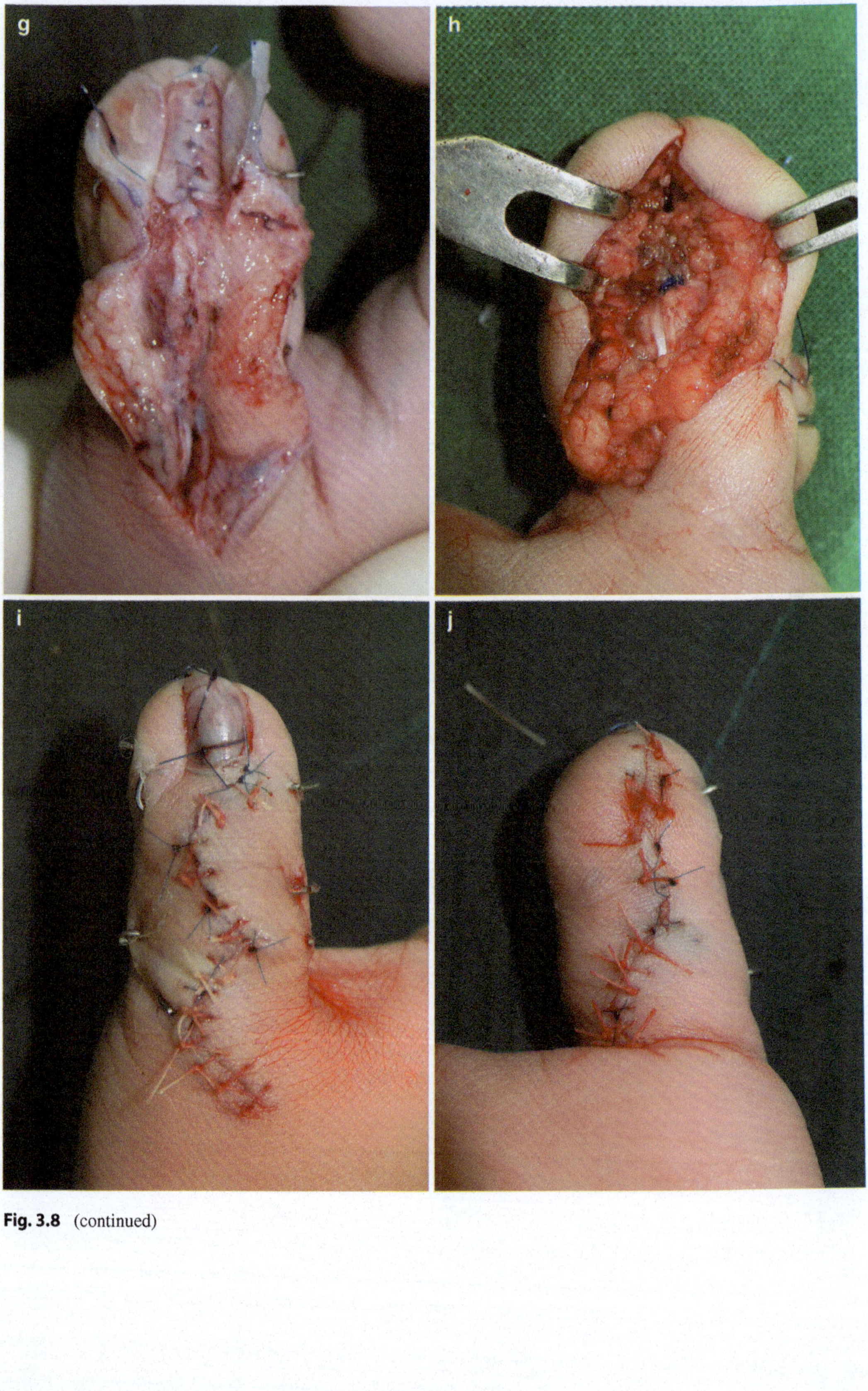


**Fig. 3.8** (continued)

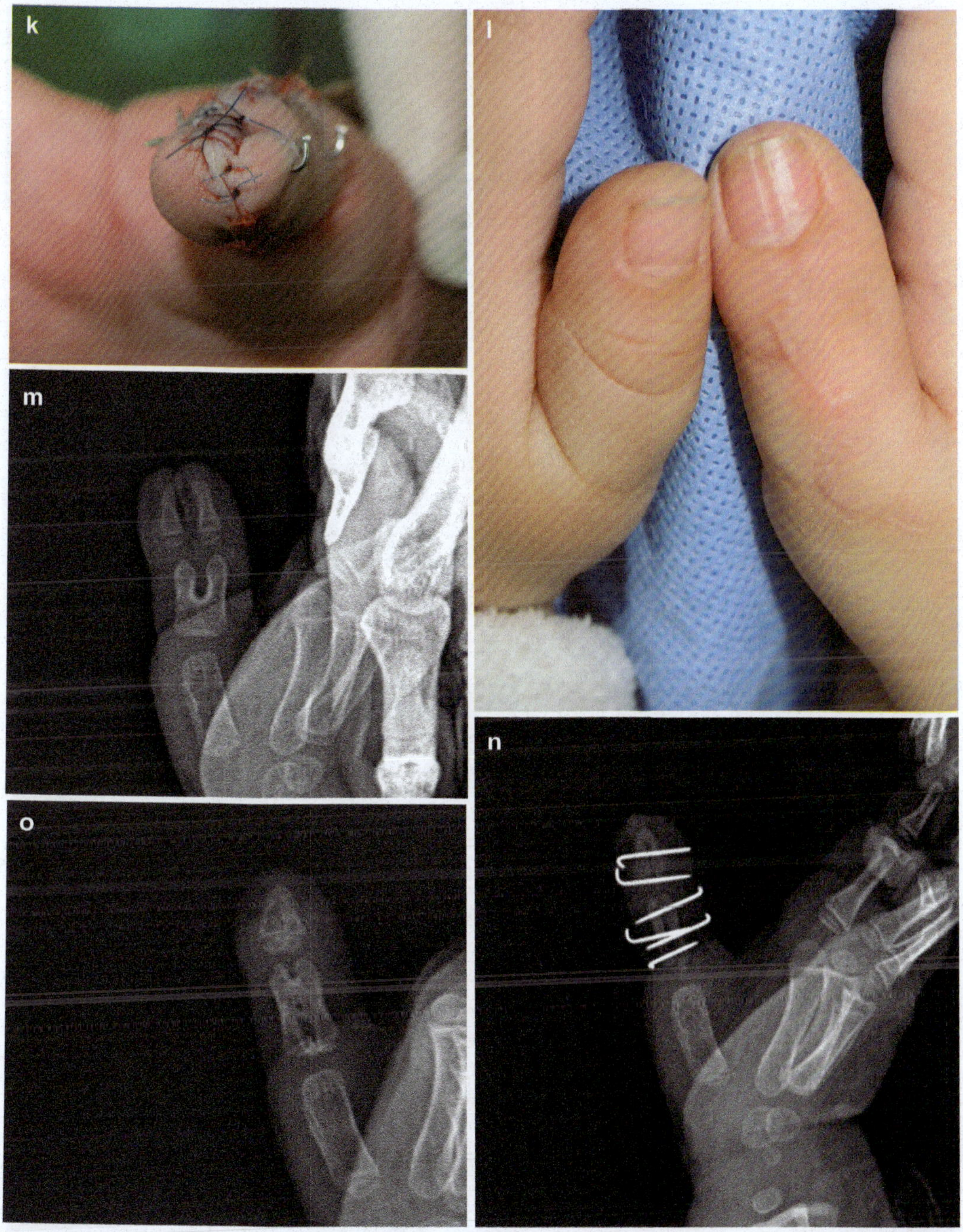


**Fig. 3.8** (continued)

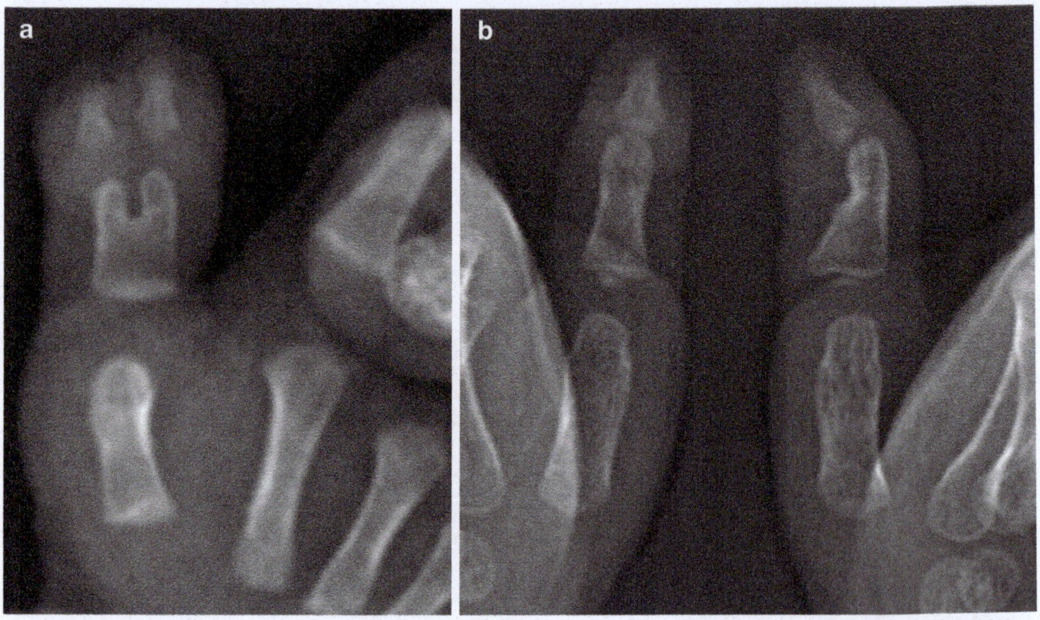


**Fig. 3.9** (**a**) Preoperative view of type III radial polydactyly. (**b**) Severe radial deviation of the ulnar distal phalangeal bone after simple ablation of the radial digit

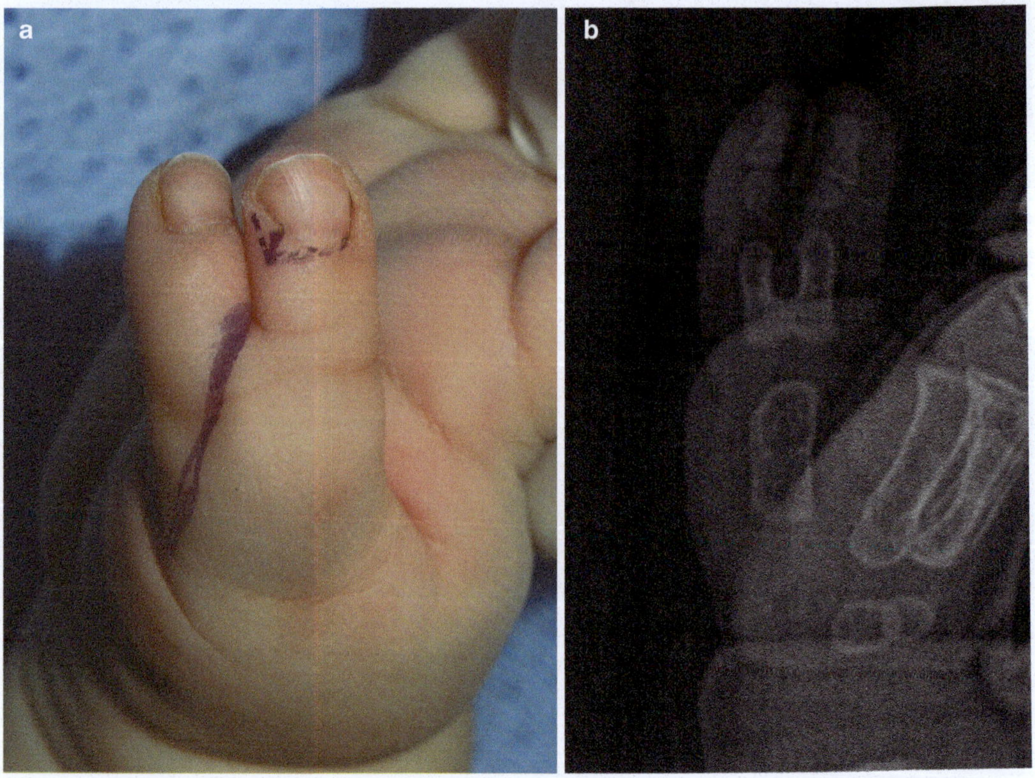


**Fig. 3.10** (**a** and **b**) Preoperative view of type III radial polydactyly. (**c** and **d**) The radial proximal phalangeal bone is preserved to prevent radial deviation of the ulnar distal phalangeal bone after simple ablation of the radial digit

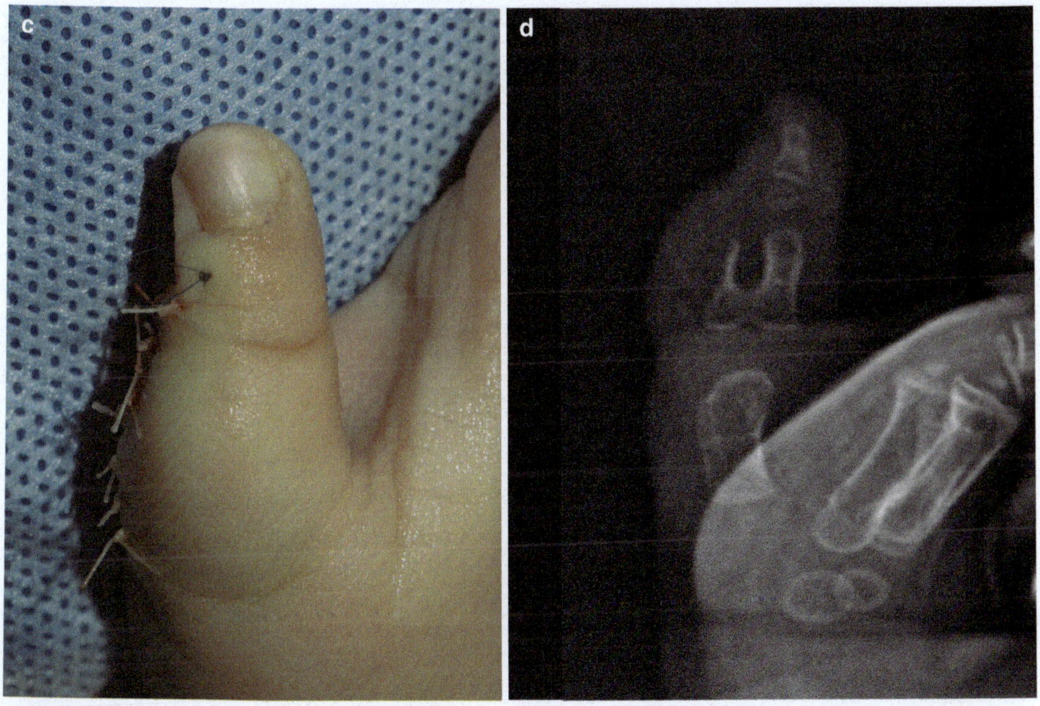


**Fig. 3.10** (continued)

## Flatt Type IV

From personal data of cases operated by the senior author (SH Woo) for the radial polydactyly, type IV duplication is the most common. There are many variations of type IV duplications. When the ulnar component is straight in axis and relatively similar in nail size, the radial component should be excised without undue concern. In Rotterdam type IV D with severe divergence at MP joint and convergence of IP joint, there may be a high incidence of Z-deformity postoperatively. That's the reason why modification of Bilhaut techniques with longitudinal combination procedures is still useful to achieve a straight and large thumb (Fig. 3.11). Even revision surgery in Z-deformity requires more technical consideration for reconstruction, but the postoperative result is not always promising. According to the divergence and convergence of the joints, shape of the P1 and metacarpal bone, and volume of soft tissue and nail shape, different operation options should be adopted.

The ulnar thumb should always be preserved because it maintains the critical ulnar collateral ligament at the MP joint, which is important for stability during pinch. In easy cases of type IV, the ulnar thumb is usually bigger than the radial side in size, and the longitudinal axis of the ulnar thumb is almost straight (Fig. 3.12). An elliptical incision is made on the radial thumb extended proximally in a curvilinear fashion along the junction between dorsal and volar aspect. The radial thumb is amputated through the MP joint preserving EPL and FPL tendon as well as elevated periosteal flap from the base of the radial side of the proximal phalanx and proximally in continuity with the collateral ligament. The widened metacarpal head has two facets, of which the radial facet is removed in an oblique fashion by scalpel, preserving the peri-

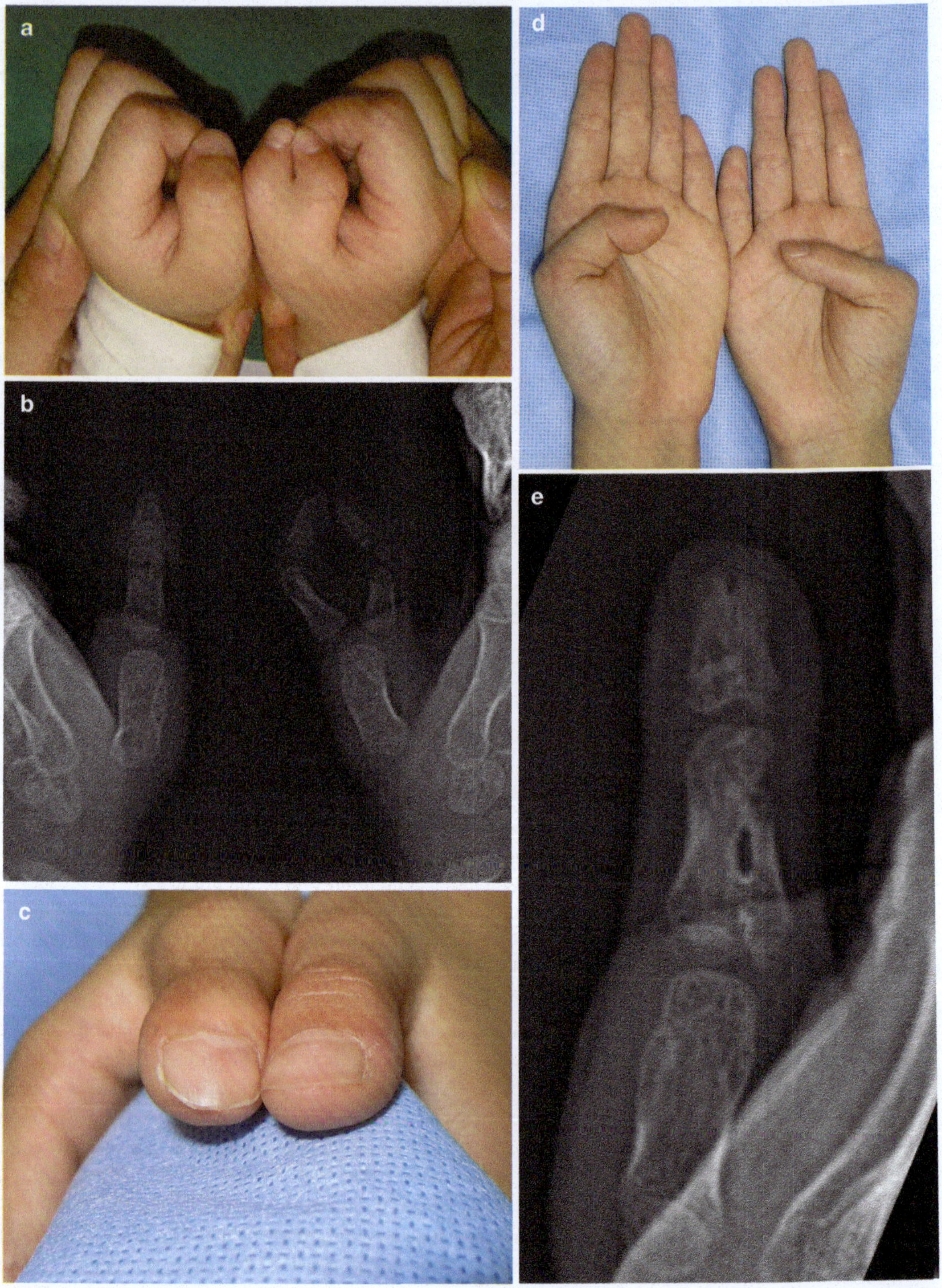


**Fig. 3.11** (**a** and **b**) In Rotterdam type IV D radial polydactyly. Preoperative view. (**c** and **d**) Postoperative view, 11 years later. Normal range of motion at the MP joint with 15° of active motion at the IP joint. (**e**) Complete bone union of the distal phalangeal bone is mandatory to achieve aesthetically acceptable nail shape

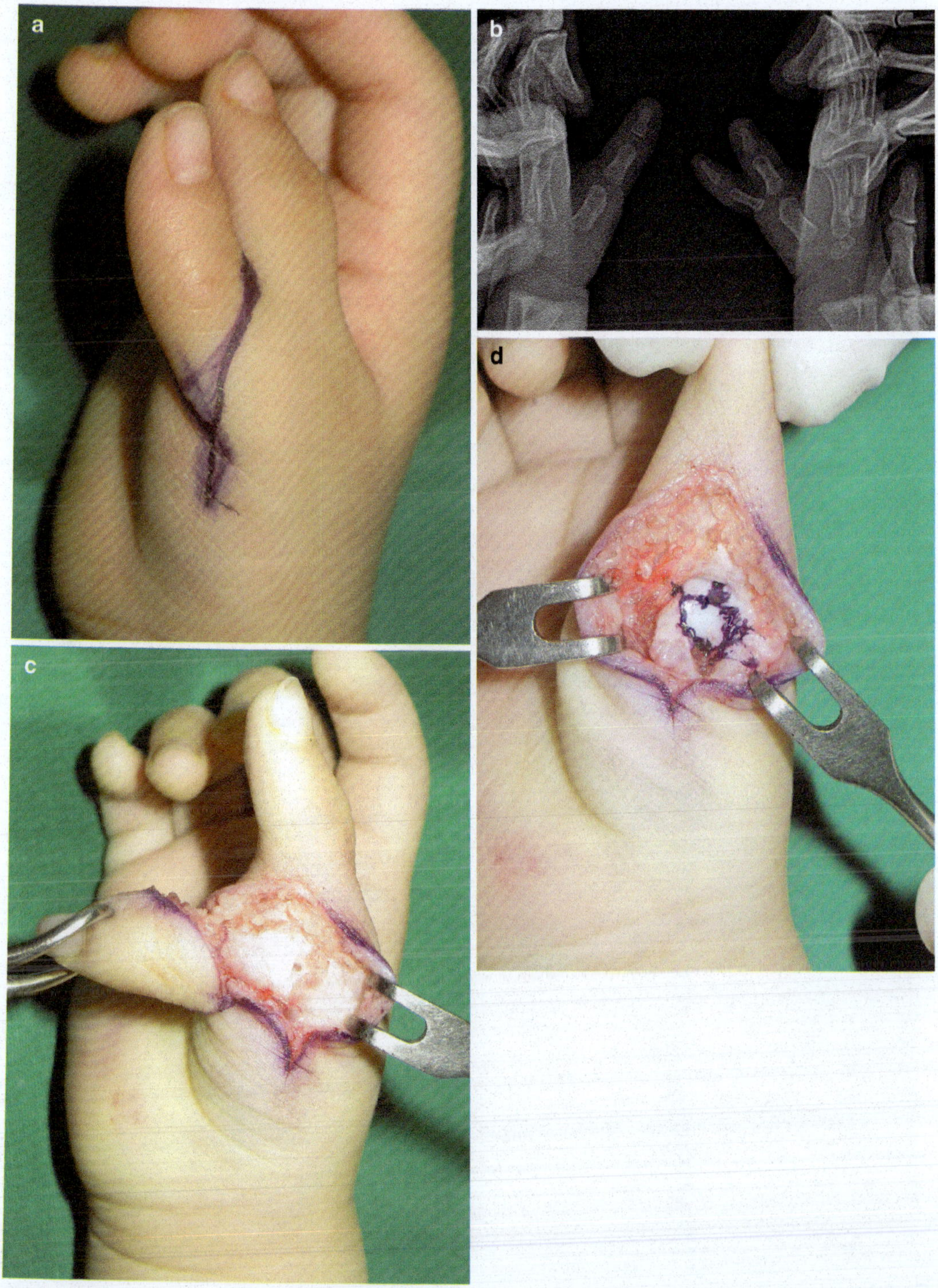


**Fig. 3.12** (**a** and **b**) Type IV radial polydactyly. Preoperative view shows straight and bigger ulnar components. (**c**) During elliptical excision of the radial thumb, care is taken to preserve the radial collateral ligament, and it is then detached in a distal to proximal fashion, preserving a periosteal sleeve. (**d** and **e**) The radial part of the metacarpal cartilage should be shaved. (**f**) The elevated abductor pollicis brevis muscle is fixed to the dorsal capsule of the MP joint. (**g**–**i**) Postoperative view and radiograph

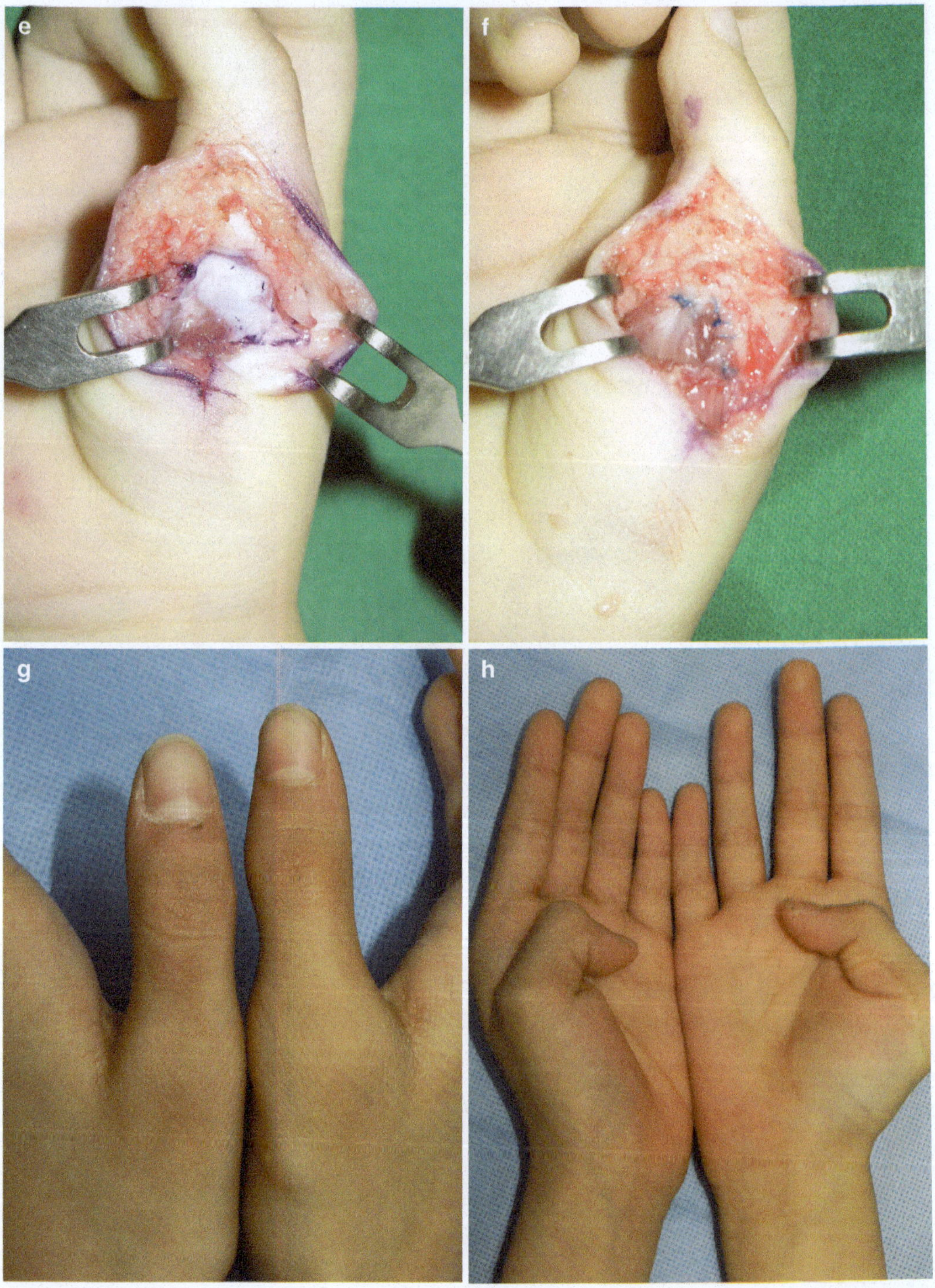


**Fig. 3.12** (continued)

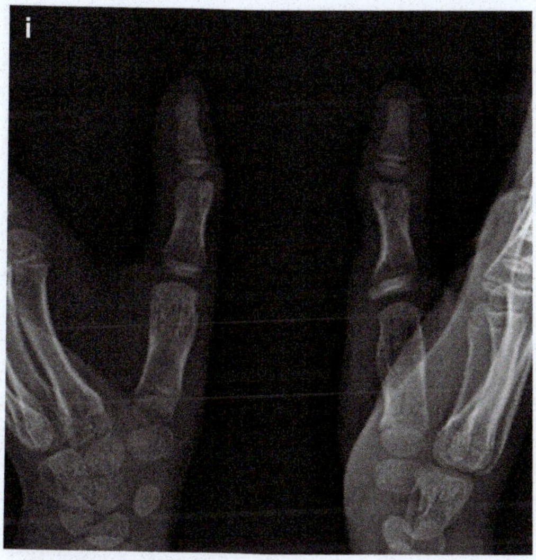

**Fig. 3.12** (continued)

osteal flap. The abductor pollicis brevis that is inserted on the bone remnant is transferred to the proximal phalanx of the preserved portion of the digit, and the capsule of the MP joint is reconstructed. Even in wide divergence of the proximal phalanx in type IV, this procedure alone is sufficient to prevent secondary angulation deformity (Fig. 3.13).

Regarding correction of convergence of the IP joint, there are three options. In a mild case, V-Y advanced plication of ulnar collateral ligament and release of radial collateral ligament are enough. Additional longitudinal K-wire fixation is necessary for 3 weeks. In moderate to severe cases or where the parents are resistant to bone surgery, tendon transfer of the radial half of EPL tendon only (Fig. 3.14) or combined with FPL tendon (Fig. 3.15) is a good option. Harvested tendons from radial component are passed under the dorsal or volar skin around IP joint and then fixed at the ulnar collateral ligament. In severe convergence, closing wedge ostectomy and internal fixation at the P1 shaft (Fig. 3.16) or sometimes at the distal shaft of metacarpal bone (Fig. 3.17) are mandatory. Fixation with one or two Kirschner wires is enough to maintain the straightened position of the joints. There is no risk of scar contracture even with a straight closure of the incision on the radial aspect of the thenar area.

## Flatt Types V and VI

The radial polydactyly has three bones including the metacarpal remnant. If there is no connection of cartilage or joint capsules between the metacarpal bones, this is not metacarpal polydactyly but floating type. In type V, the radial thumb is crooked and small on the distal end with a near-normal ulnar component. Compared with normal extrinsic tendons of the ulnar thumb, a part of thenar muscle is shared with the radial thumb. When the ostectomy of the radial prominence of the metacarpal bone is performed, thenar muscle should be preserved and repaired to metacarpal bone again. The first web space is sometimes narrow, which should be released with flap or Z-plasty (Fig. 3.18).

In type VI, the development of the metacarpal bone is very different. One component has a better proximal portion of nearly normal metacarpal bone with good and stable carpometacarpal joint, and the distal portion is usually hypoplastic and angulated interphalangeal joint. The other component has poor or absent carpometacarpal joint but better morphology of distal portion with a near-normal nail. Hypoplastic metacarpal bone shows a tendency of under- or no development of extrinsic tendons. Transposition of the relatively well-aligned ulnar digit to the radial ray is named as "on-top-plasty" technique [15, 16]. Preoperatively, the surgeon should check the shape and size of the nail, bulkiness of the pulp, length and axis of phalangeal and metacarpal bone, and presence of instability

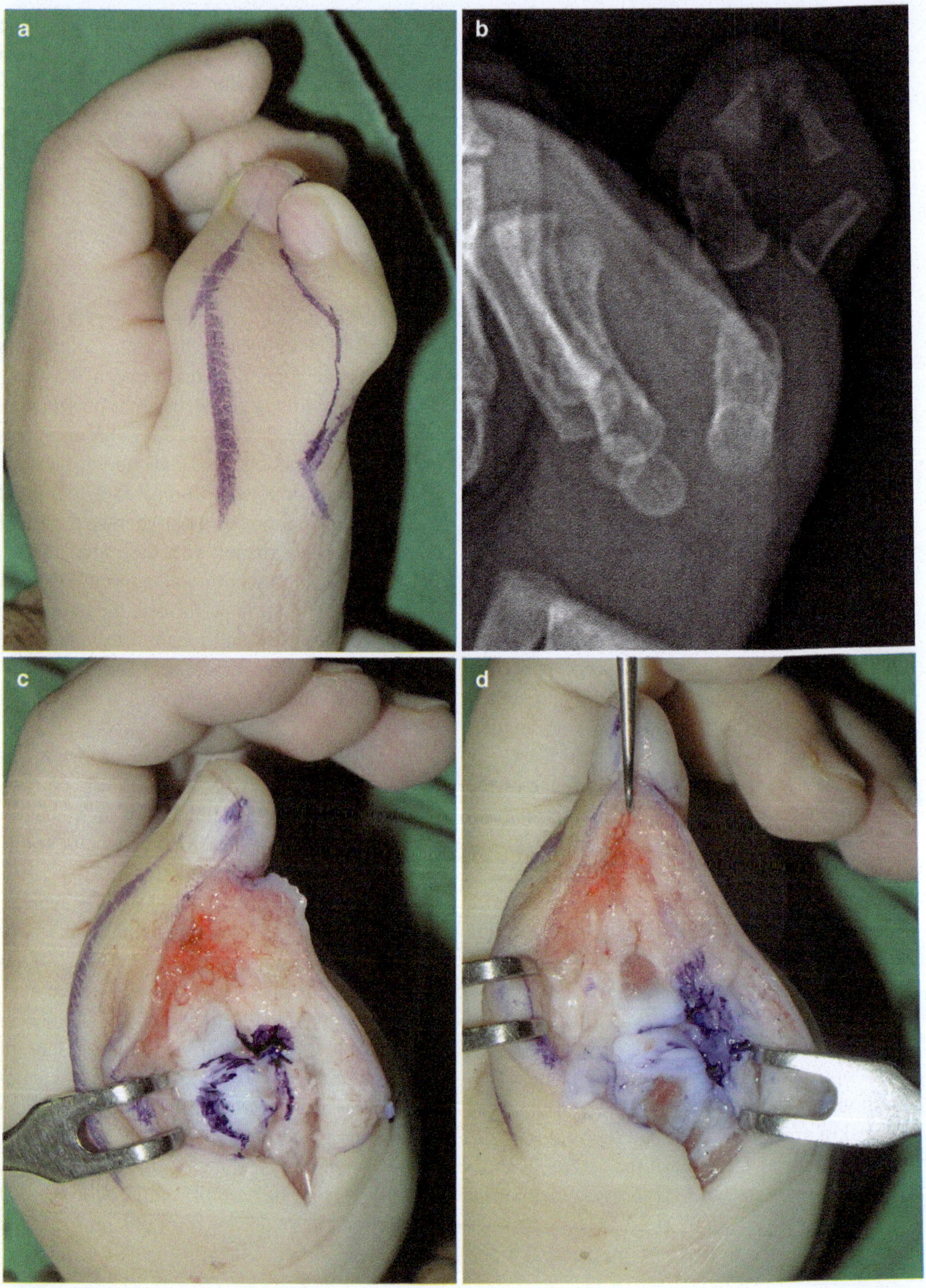


**Fig. 3.13** (**a** and **b**) In Rotterdam type IV D radial polydactyly. Preoperative view demonstrates bigger ulnar components. (**c–e**) Routine procedure of excision of the radial thumb, bone shaving of the radial part of the metacarpal cartilage, and abductor pollicis brevis muscle suturing to the dorsal capsule of the MP joint. (**f**) Additional K-wire fixation for 3 weeks and custom-made thumb brace for 3 weeks more. (**g–i**) Postoperative view and radiograph

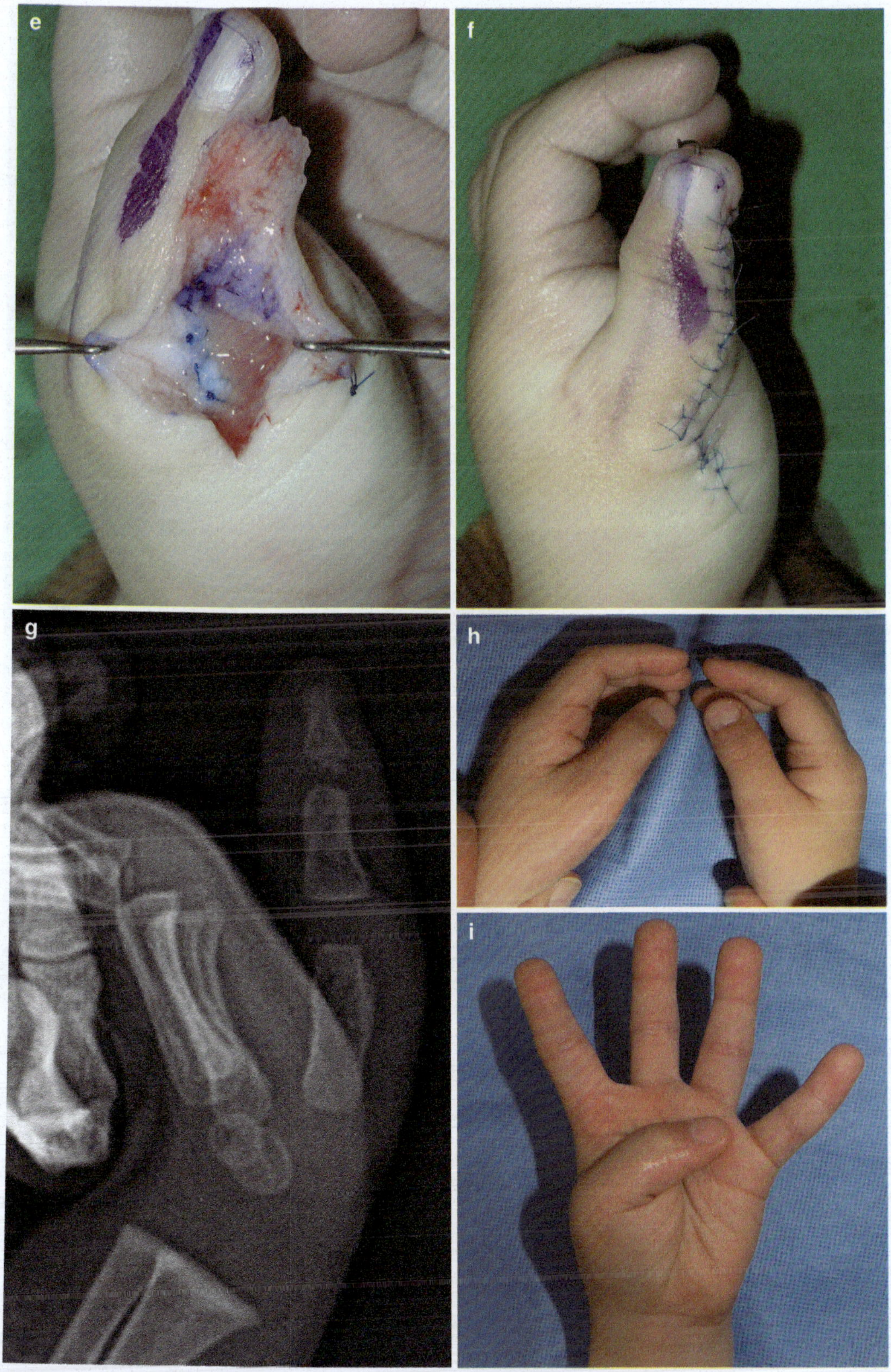

**Fig. 3.13** (continued)

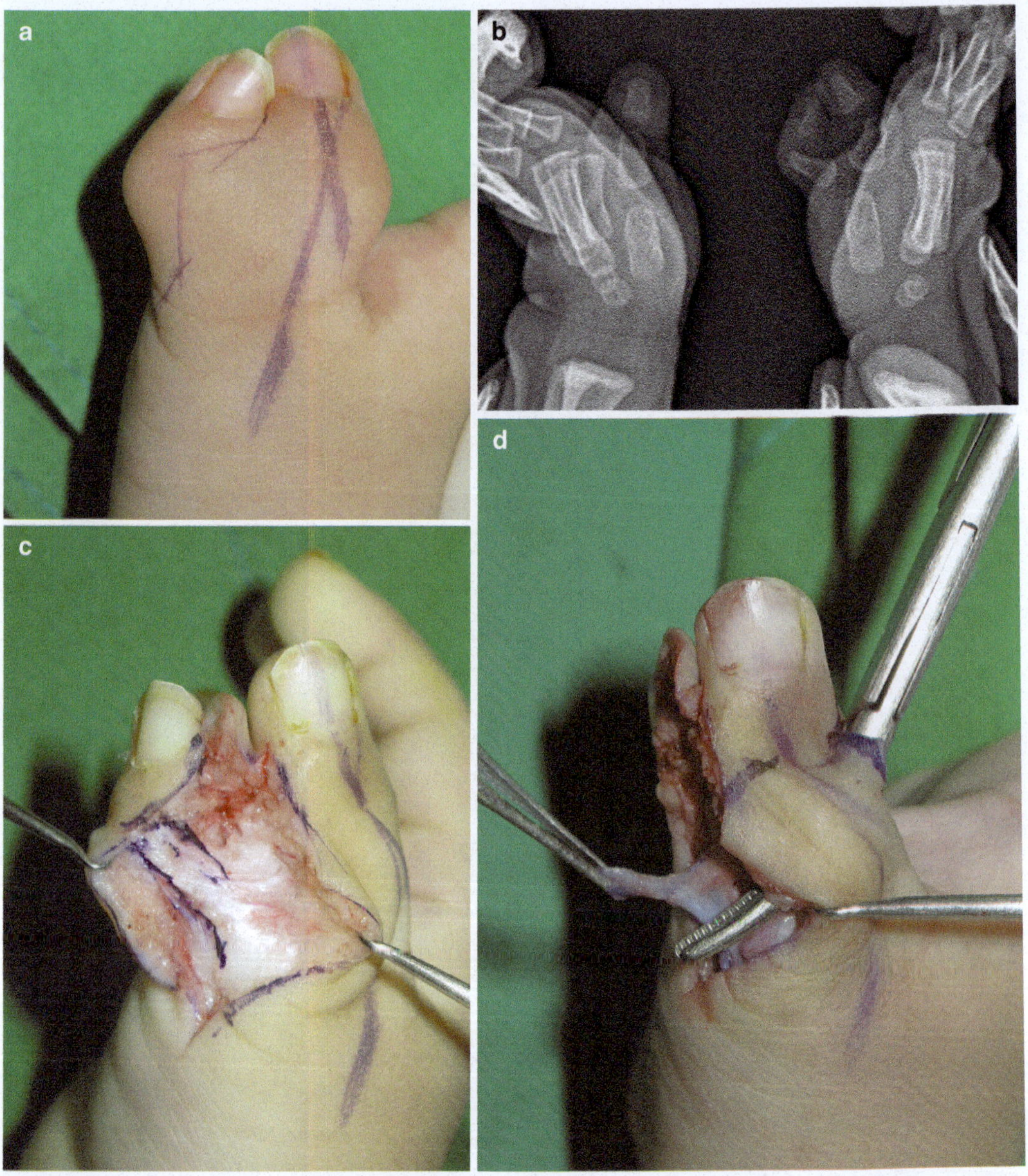


**Fig. 3.14** (**a** and **b**) Preoperative view of Rotterdam type IV D radial polydactyly. (**c**) Extensor pollicis longus tendon is harvested from the radial polydactyly. (**d** and **e**) Harvested extensor tendon is passed subcutaneously under the dorsum to the ulnar collateral ligament. (**f** and **g**) Postoperative view and radiograph

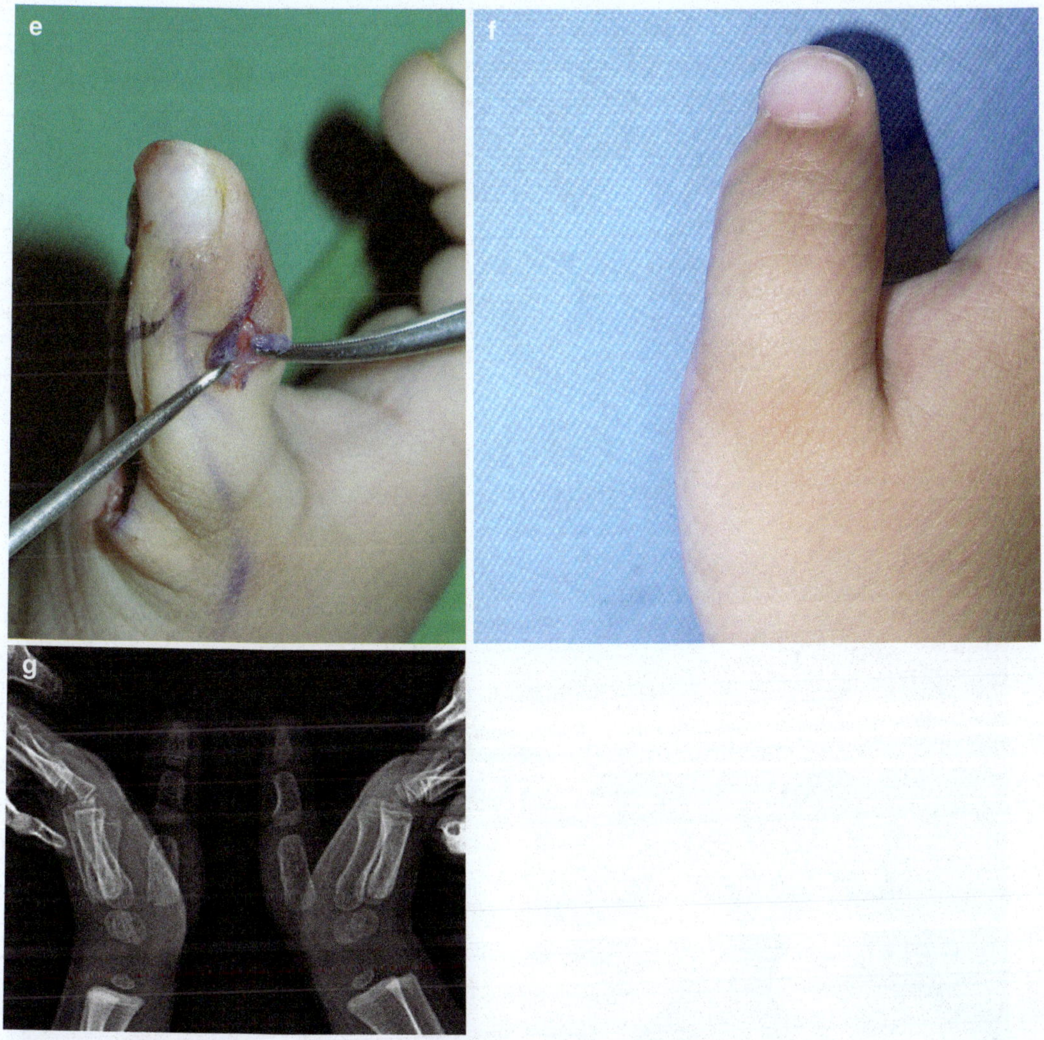


**Fig. 3.14** (continued)

of the joints. According to this, abnormality and malposition of the intrinsic and extrinsic muscles should be identified before surgery. Three-dimensional ultrasound technique [17] or 3.0 T MR image can be a great help to plan strategies in radial polydactyly if intrinsic muscular anomalies are suspected to be involved. If so, the operation should be delayed until the active motion of the baby's ulnar thumb is observed. The appropriate age

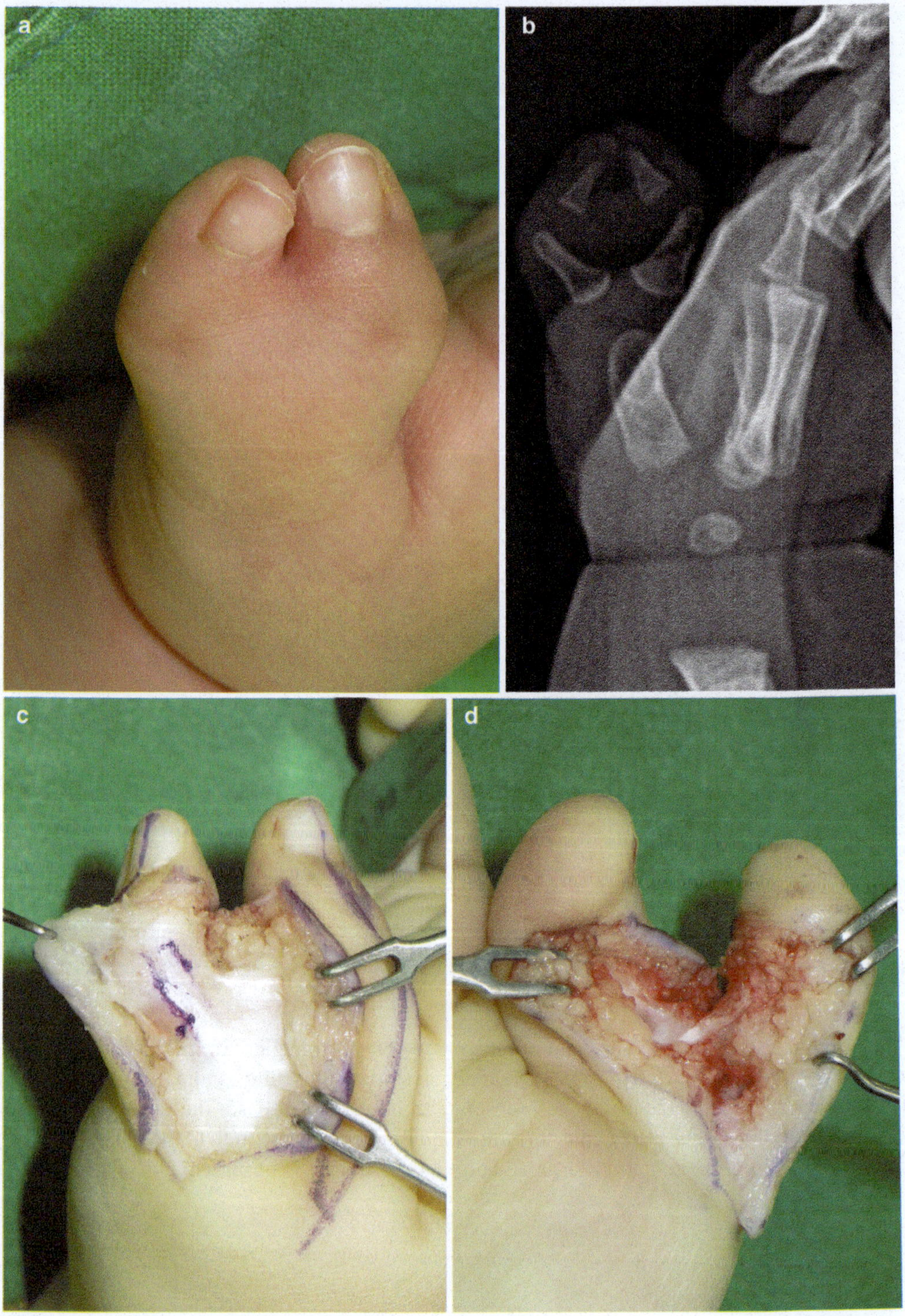


**Fig. 3.15** (**a** and **b**) Preoperative view of Rotterdam type IV D radial polydactyly. (**c** and **d**) Extensor pollicis longus tendon and flexor pollicis longus tendon are harvested from the insertion portion of distal phalangeal bone of the radial polydactyly. (**e**) The lateral collateral ligament of the MP joint and the medial collateral ligament of the IP joint were tightened to correct the alignment. The radial collateral ligament is then proximally pulled as Y-V advancement pattern. (**f** and **g**) Harvested two tendons are passed subcutaneously in both dorsum and volar aspect. Two tendons are sutured to the proximally advanced ulnar collateral ligament of the IP joint. (**h**) Post-operation after K-wire fixation. (**i–k**) Postoperative view and radiograph

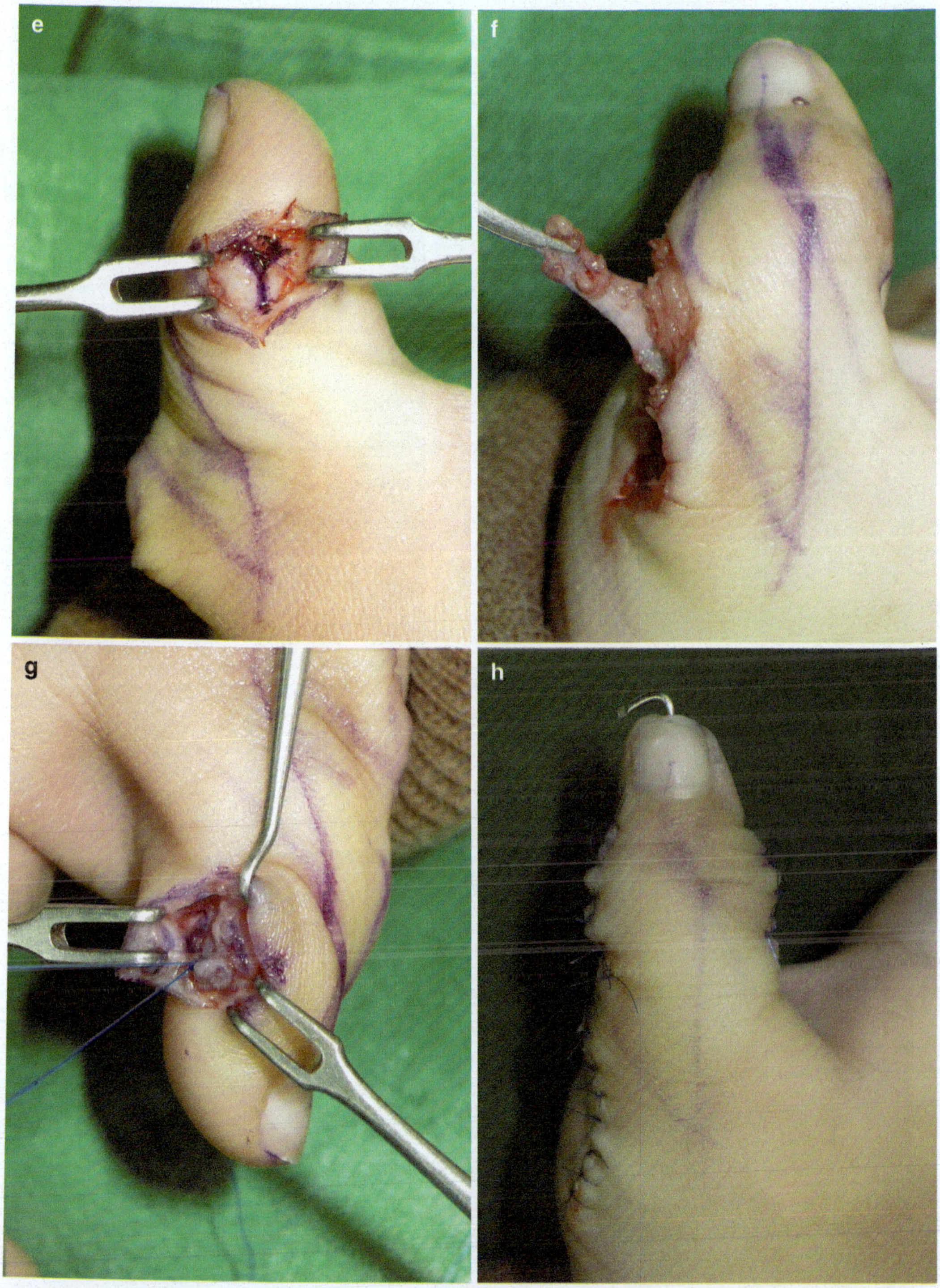


**Fig. 3.15** (continued)

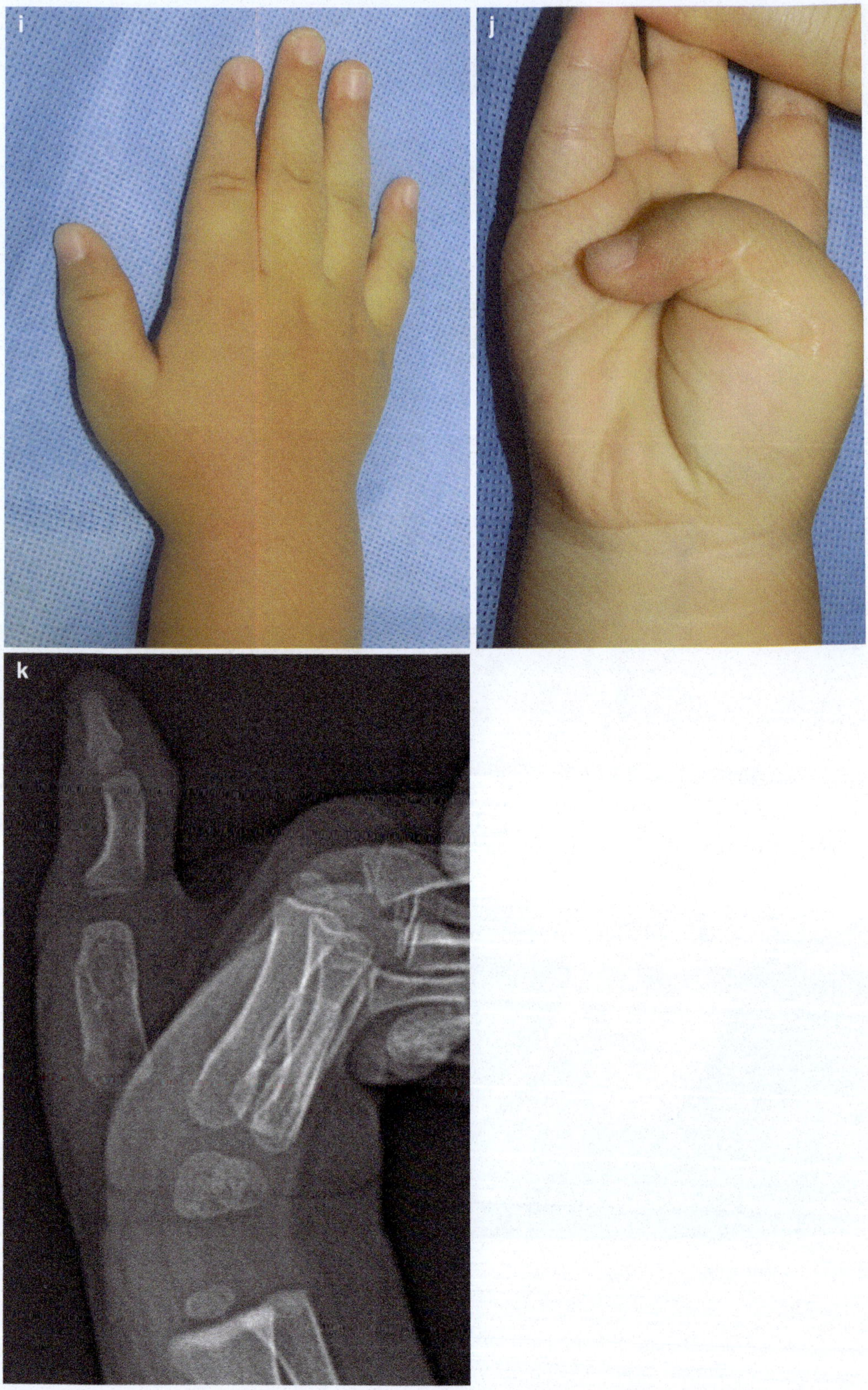


**Fig. 3.15** (continued)

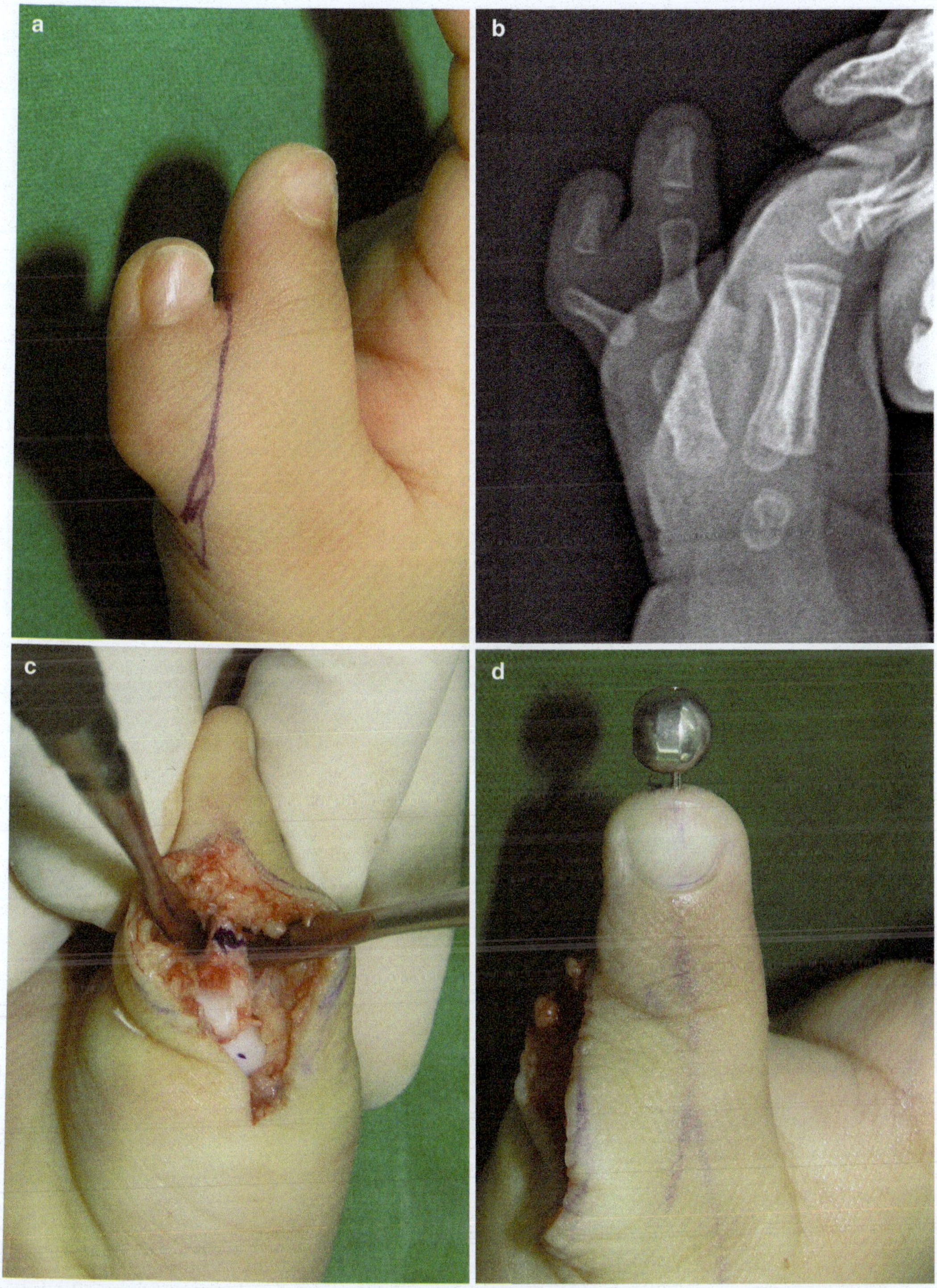


**Fig. 3.16** (**a** and **b**) Preoperative view of type IV radial polydactyly. It shows supination deformity of the nail and ulnar angulation of the ulnar thumb. (**c**) After resection of radial polydactyly, ulnar deviation of the proximal phalanx is corrected by closing wedge ostectomy at the radial proximal phalangeal bone. (**d** and **e**) Immediate after operation with two K-wire fixation. (**f** and **g**) Postoperative view and radiograph

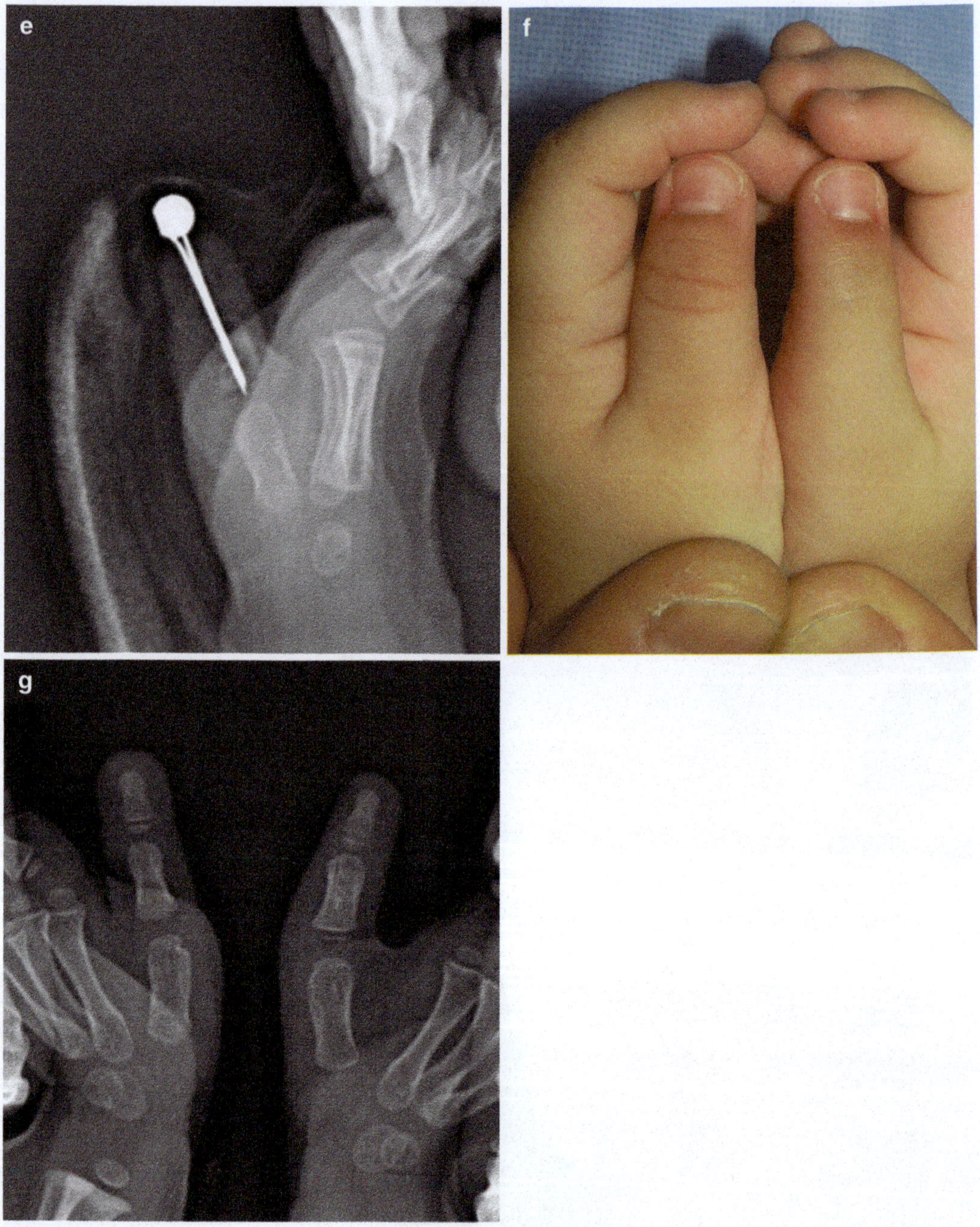


**Fig. 3.16** (continued)

for complex operative procedures is from around 2 years old. In most cases, parents prefer to preserve the apparently dominant thumb even with reduced functionality. The strategy of this complex procedure is very important to achieve not only an aesthetically pleasing appearance but adequate function of the reconstructed thumb by using osteotomy and tendon transfer.

After confirmation of the presence of extrinsic FPL/EPL tendon, resection of hypoplastic soft tissues and bones as well as level of oste-

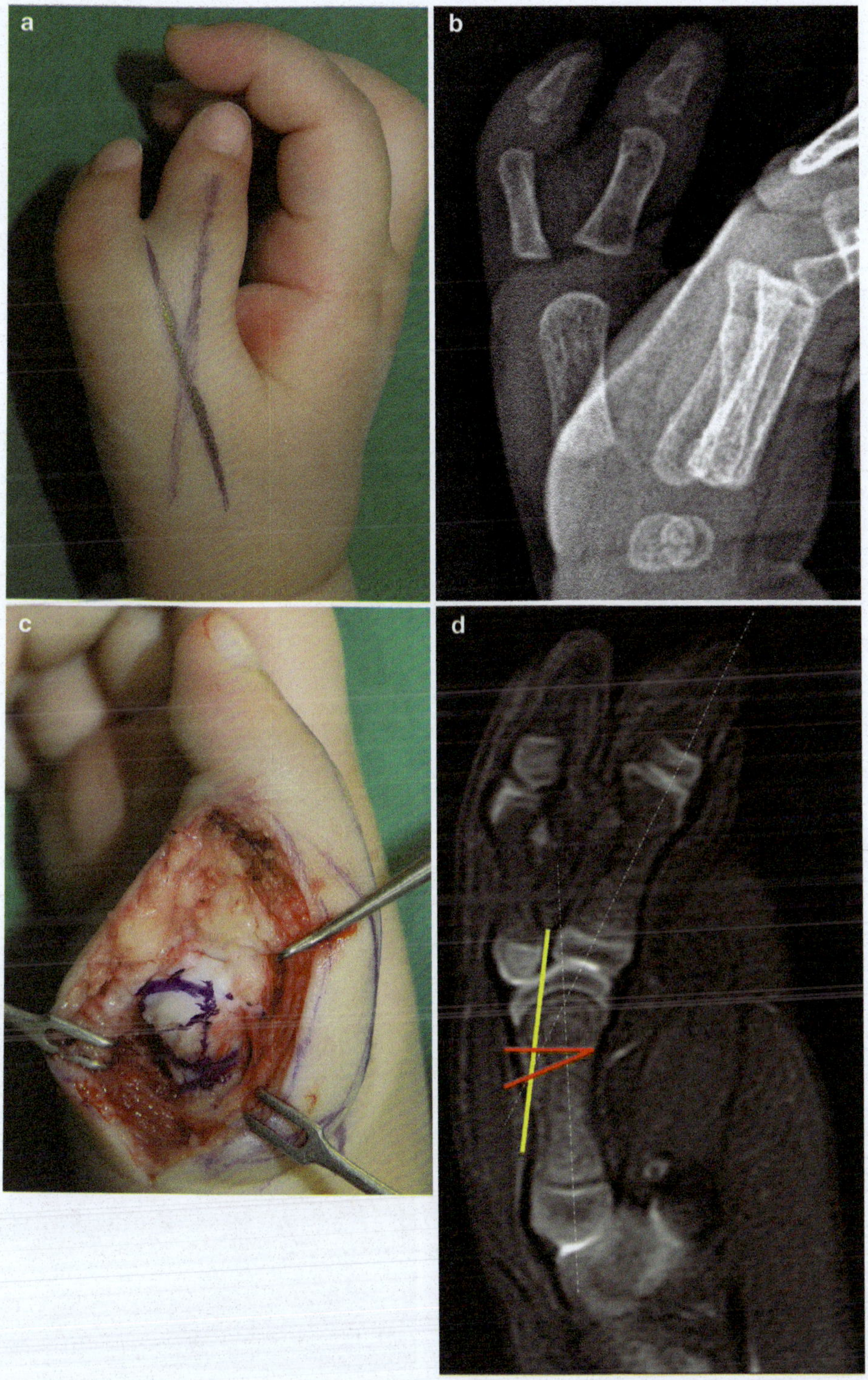


**Fig. 3.17** (**a** and **b**) Preoperative view of type IV radial polydactyly. It shows ulnar angulation of the ulnar thumb at the MP joint. (**c**) After resection of radial polydactyly, the radial cartilage of the metacarpal bone is ostectomized first. (**d**) Longitudinal axis of IP joint and MP joint (dashed line) and the first (yellow) and second (red line) ostectomy line on the magnetic resonance image. (**e**) Bone fixation with longitudinal K-wire on the metacarpal bone. (**f**) Immediate after operation. (**g** and **h**) Postoperative view and radiograph

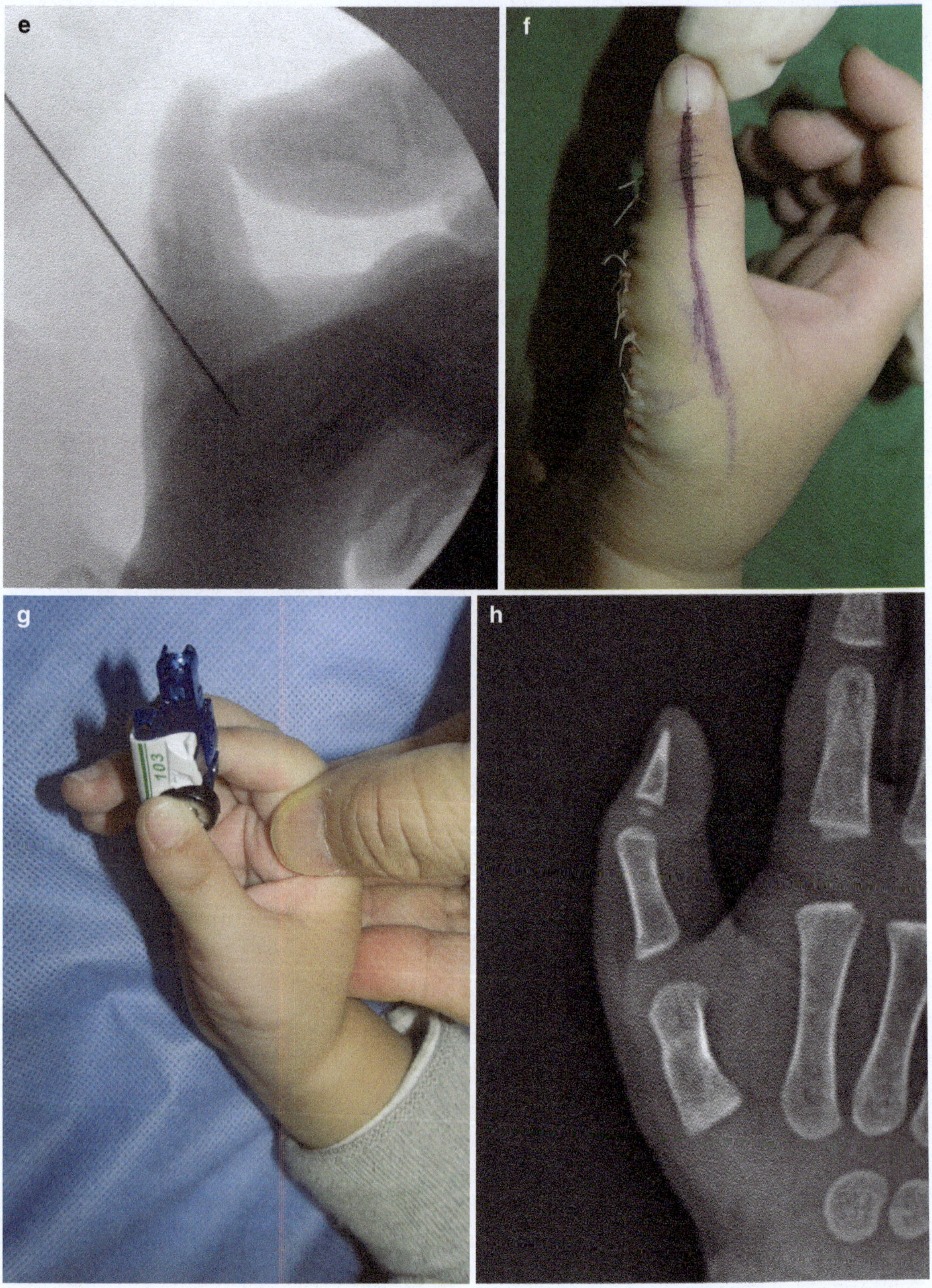


**Fig. 3.17** (continued)

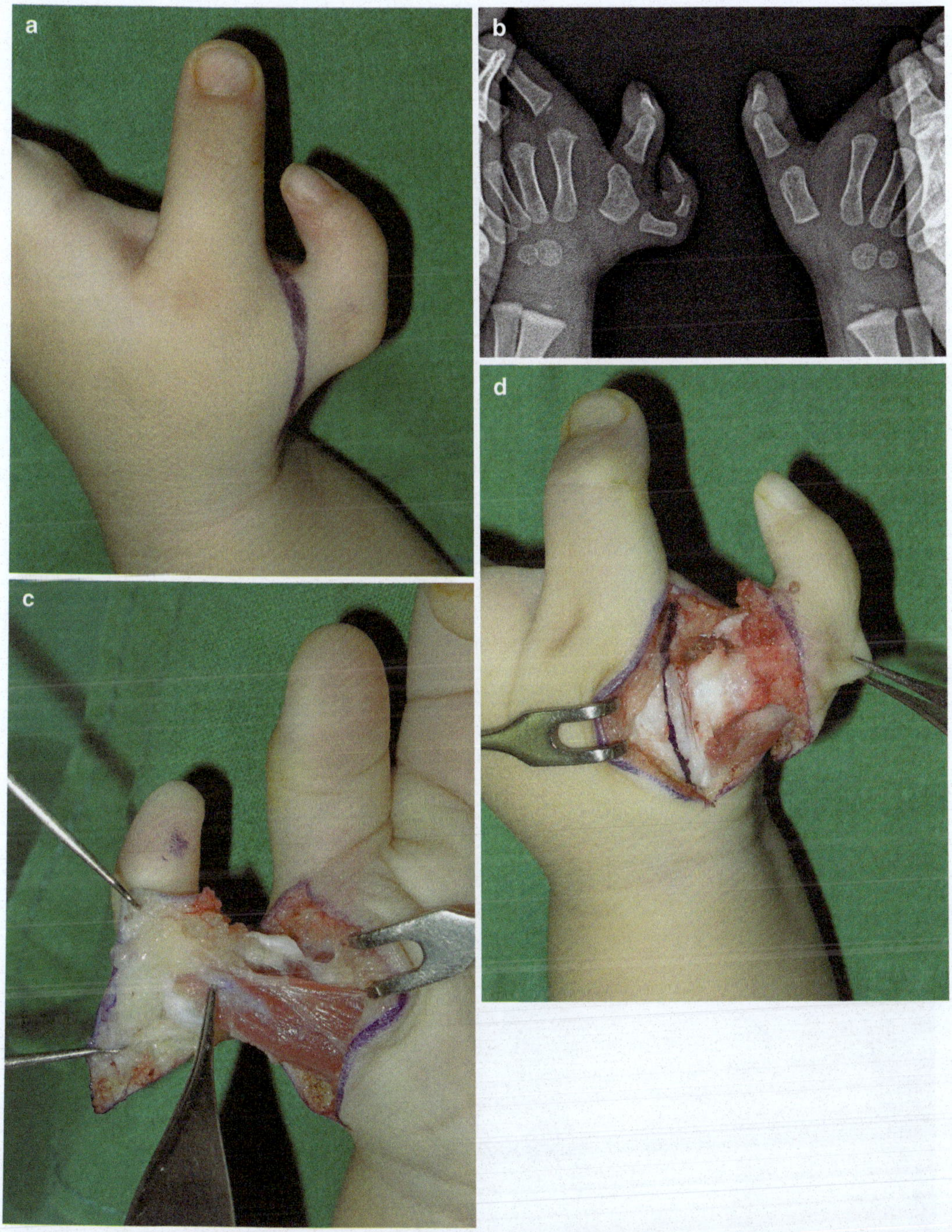


**Fig. 3.18** (**a** and **b**) Preoperative view of type V radial polydactyly. (**c**) Thenar muscle inserted on radial polydactyly is preserved to reconstruct thenar portion of the ulnar thumb. (**d** and **e**) Ostectomy is made at the radial part of the metacarpal bone, and then the bone is covered with preserved thenar muscle. (**f** and **g**) The narrow first web space is released with simple Z-plasty. (**h**–**j**) Postoperative view and radiograph

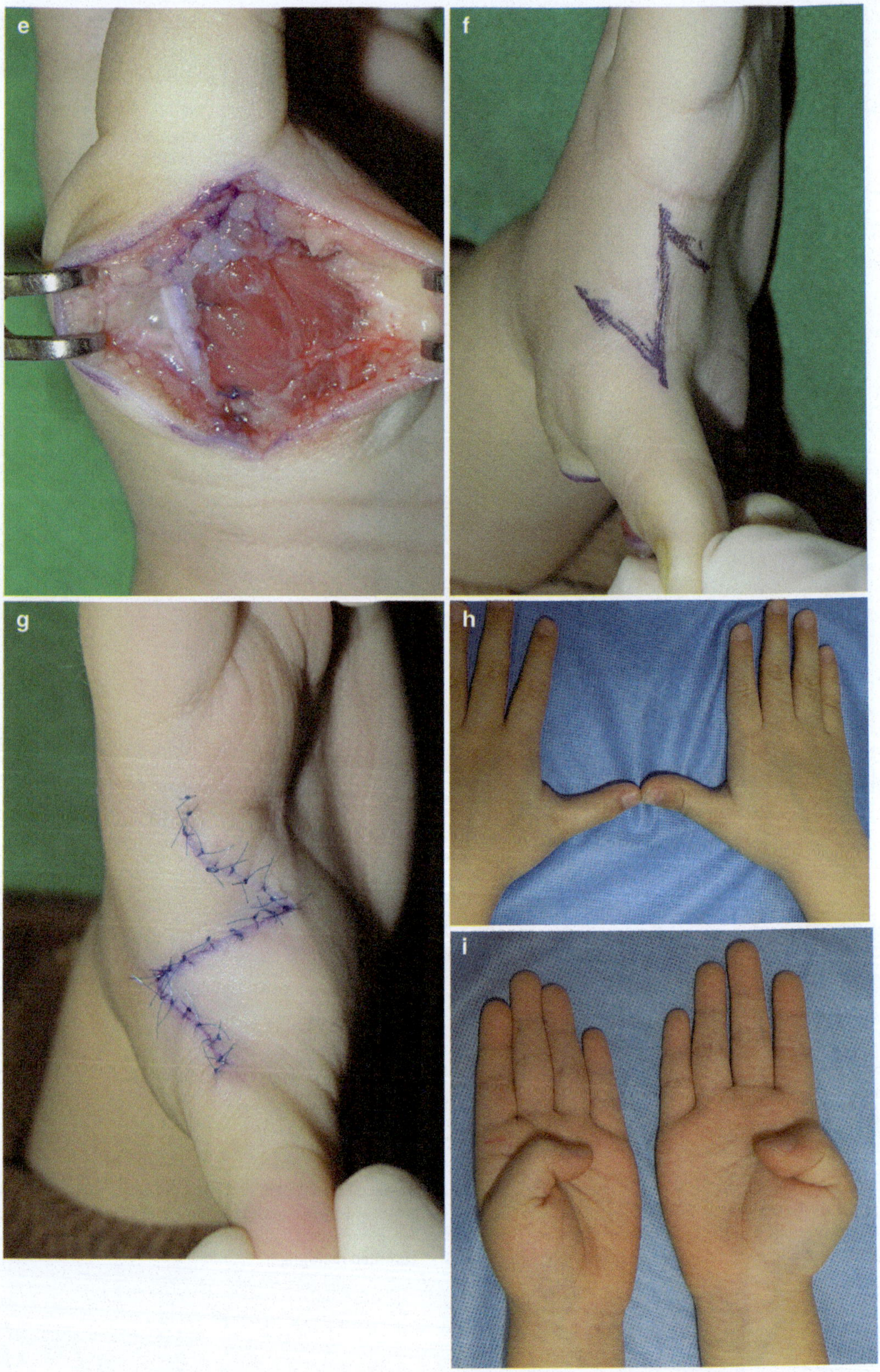


**Fig. 3.18** (continued)

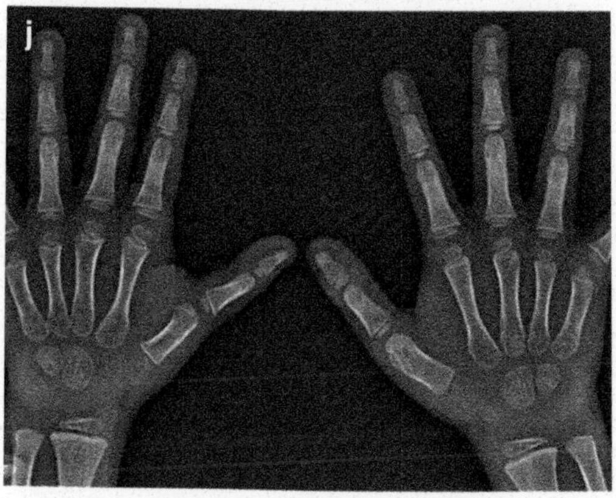


**Fig. 3.18** (continued)

otomy should be predetermined preoperatively. Under tourniquet application, a Y-shaped incision is placed at the midline of the dorsum between both thumbs. The skin flaps are elevated with intact neurovascular pedicle and venous channel. After marking the osteotomy site, the flexor and extensor tendons are elevated with periosteal flap, which will be sutured to the proximal parts of FPL/EPL. According to the better distal portion, the level of osteotomy varies at distal phalangeal bone (Fig. 3.19), proximal phalangeal bone (Fig. 3.20), or metacarpal bone (Fig. 3.21). Depending on the location of the osteotomy, detachment and reattachment of the thenar muscle insertion may be necessary. Length as well as proper rotation and angulation are carefully evaluated prior to final fixation with Kirschner wire under C-arm. Long-arm splint is applied for 2 weeks, and then a custom-made thumb brace is kept for 6 weeks (Fig. 3.22). K-wire is removed about 3–4 weeks after the operation, and a gentle range of motion exercises are begun.

## Secondary Deformity and Its Reconstruction

As children grow, the need for reoperation increases. Concern for cosmetic issues supersedes the lack of function of the joints or pain issues. Residual deformities occurring after correction of radial polydactyly involves the soft tissue, joint, and bone separately or combined [18, 19]. Instability is mainly caused by hyperlaxity or hypoplasia of supportive tissues of the joint and by abnormal insertion of a tendon. Angulation is the result of an incorrect axis of a bone, an excessively large cartilaginous head, imbalance and abnormal insertion of a tendon, an interposed delta phalanx, and scarring. The joint problem is stiffness, deviation and instability, bone abnormality including angled bone growth, and presence of a delta bone. The soft tissue abnormality shows nail deformity, narrowing of the first web space, hypoplasia of thenar muscles, and anomalous insertion of the flexor and extensor tendons. These outcomes can be avoidable or not, and surgical results are largely dependent on the severity of the initial deformity. These are usually associated with incomplete correction at the time of initial operation or with failure of the patient to return for subsequent steps of reconstruction.

Evaluation of long-term outcomes following radial polydactyly reconstruction was made by Tada et al. in 1983 [20] and by Stutz et al. in 2014 [21]. In spite of a 30-year time interval, the results are very similar, 76 vs. 79% good, 20 vs. 21% fair, and 4% vs. no poor outcomes using the same evaluation scales based on range of motion, instability, and malalignment. Reoperation rate varies by 12% [22], 19%, [21] and 26% [23] of cases. However, reoperation rate is not significantly meaningful because it does not always mean poor function of the reconstructed thumb. Often the reason for reoperation arises from cosmetic desire and sometimes pain. The greatest deformity occurs with significant angular deformity of the IPJ in Rotterdam type IV D [19, 24].

Before the reoperation, the secondary deformities should be analyzed in detail involving the structures. Regarding joints, it may involve IP joint or MP joint only or together. In the case of IP joint angulation deformity only, closing wedge ostectomy and internal fixation at

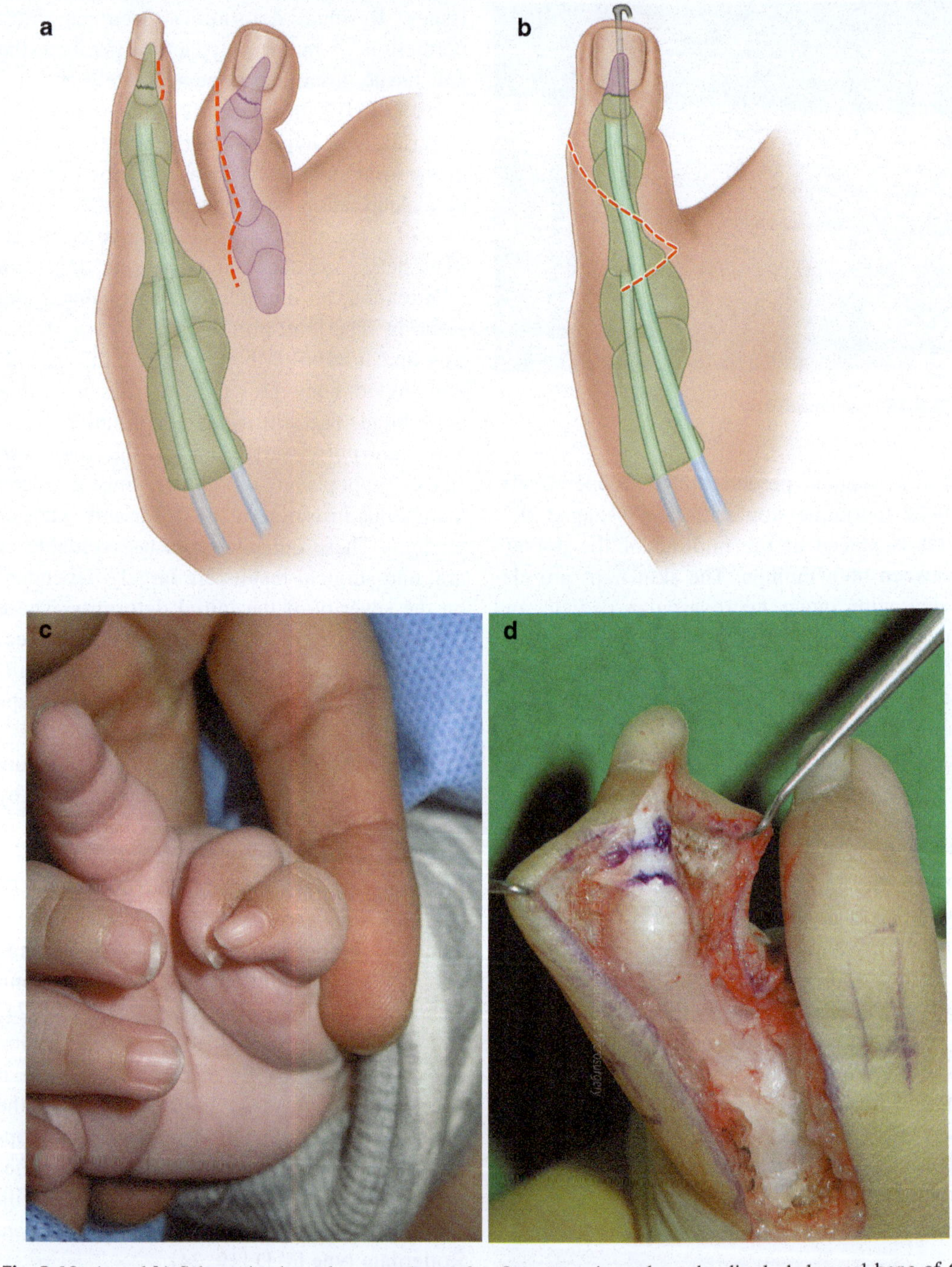


**Fig. 3.19** (**a** and **b**) Schematic view of on-top plasty of the type VI radial polydactyly. (**c**) The ulnar component has good nail but weak tendons and small remnant metacarpal bone. The radial polydactyly had very narrow and slender nail with strong proximal bone. (**d** and **e**) Ostectomy is made at the distal phalangeal bone of the both radial and ulnar components. (**f** and **g**) Postoperative view shows transposition of the distal portion of the ulnar digit to proximal radial digit. (**h** and **i**) Pre- and postoperative radiograph

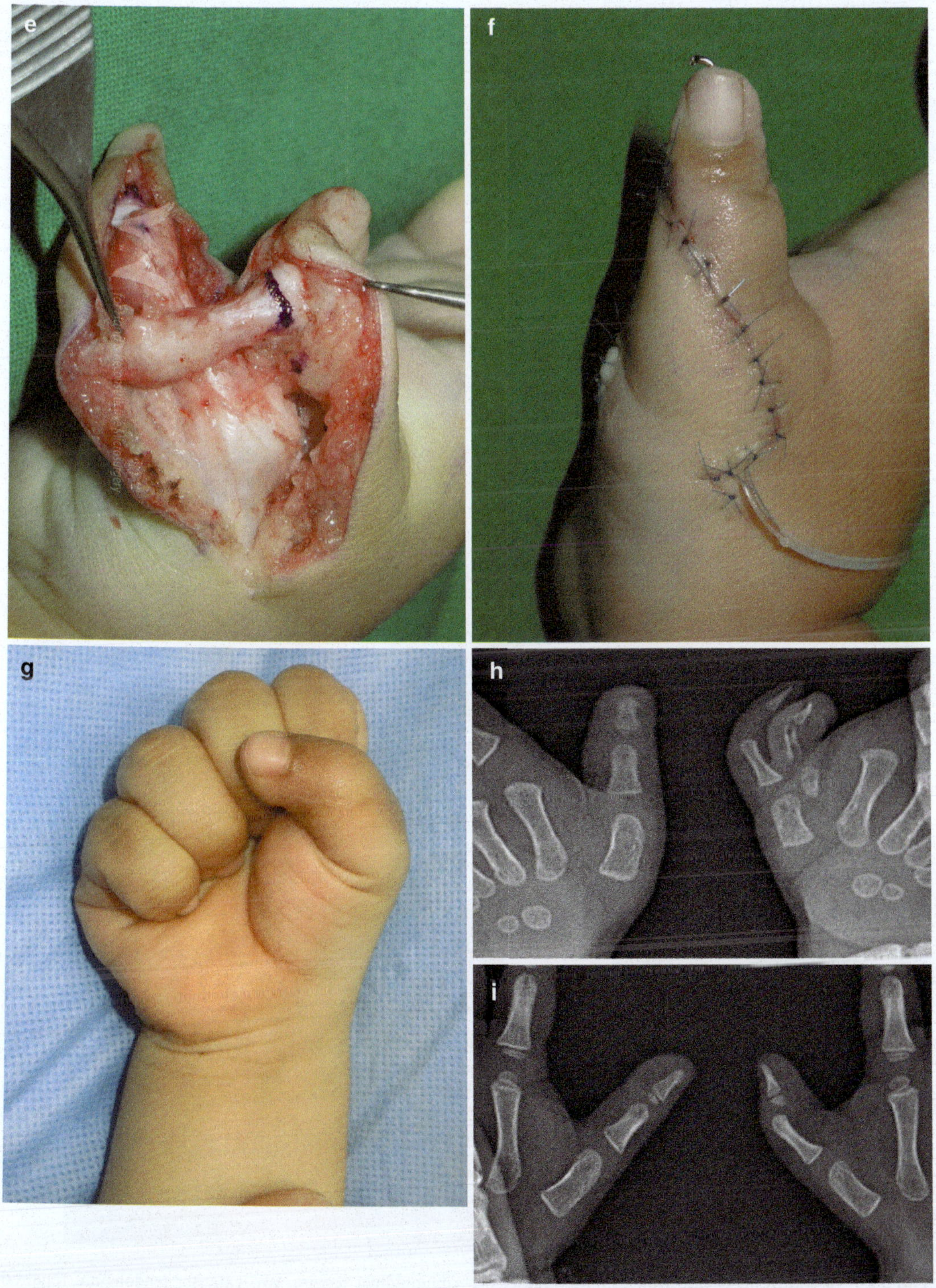


**Fig. 3.19** (continued)

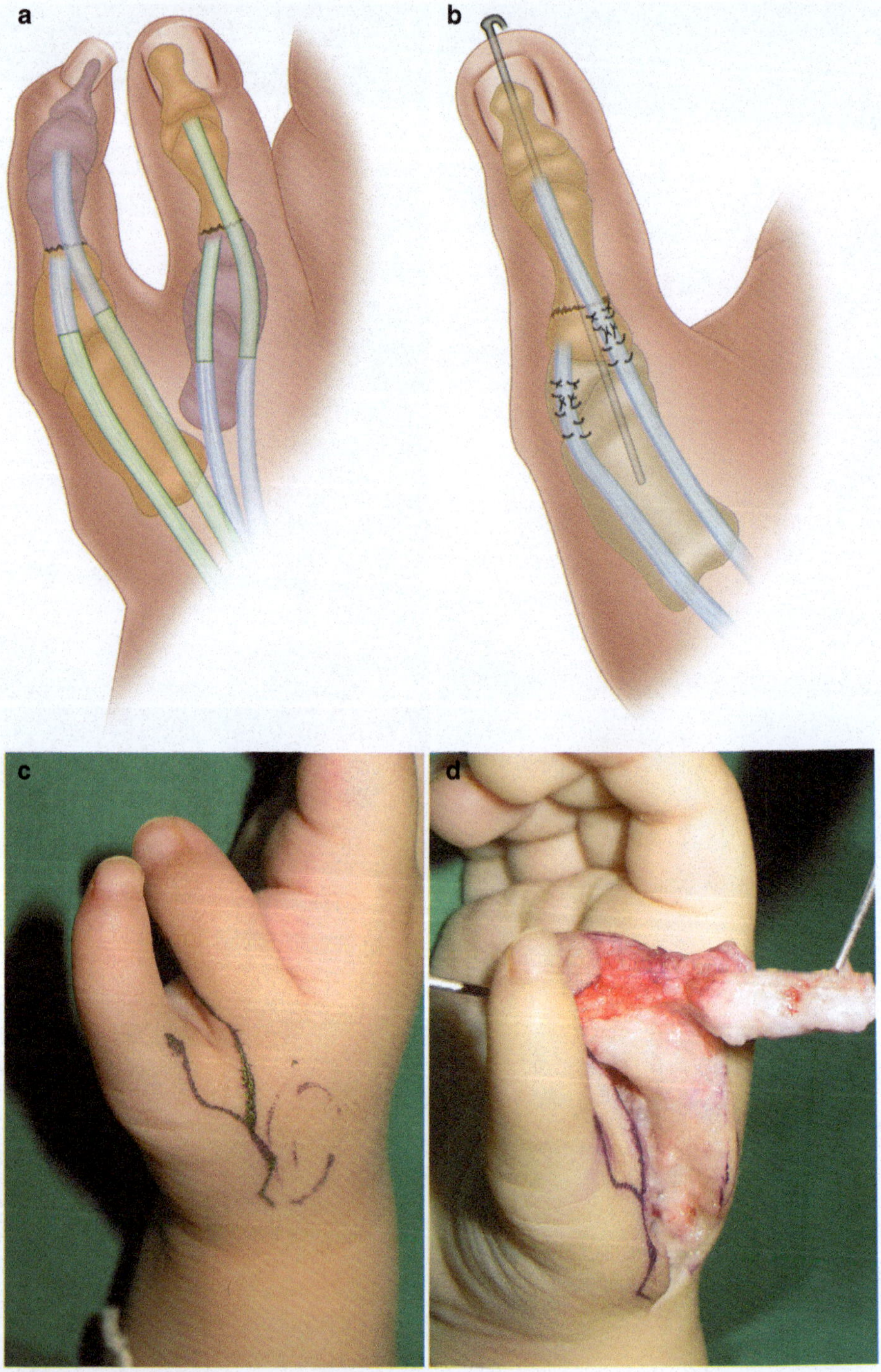


**Fig. 3.20** (**a** and **b**) Schematic view of on-top plasty of the type VI radial polydactyly. (**c**) Preoperative Y-shaped design on the dorsum of both components. (**d** and **e**) Transverse ostectomy is performed at the base of proximal phalangeal bone of ulnar components, and remnant metacarpal bone is removed. (**f**) After bone fixation with a longitudinal K-wire, two extensor tendons are repaired. (**g**) Immediate postoperative view shows transposition of the distal portion of the ulnar digit on the proximal radial digit. (**h** and **i**) Postoperative view. (**j** and **k**) Pre- and postoperative radiograph

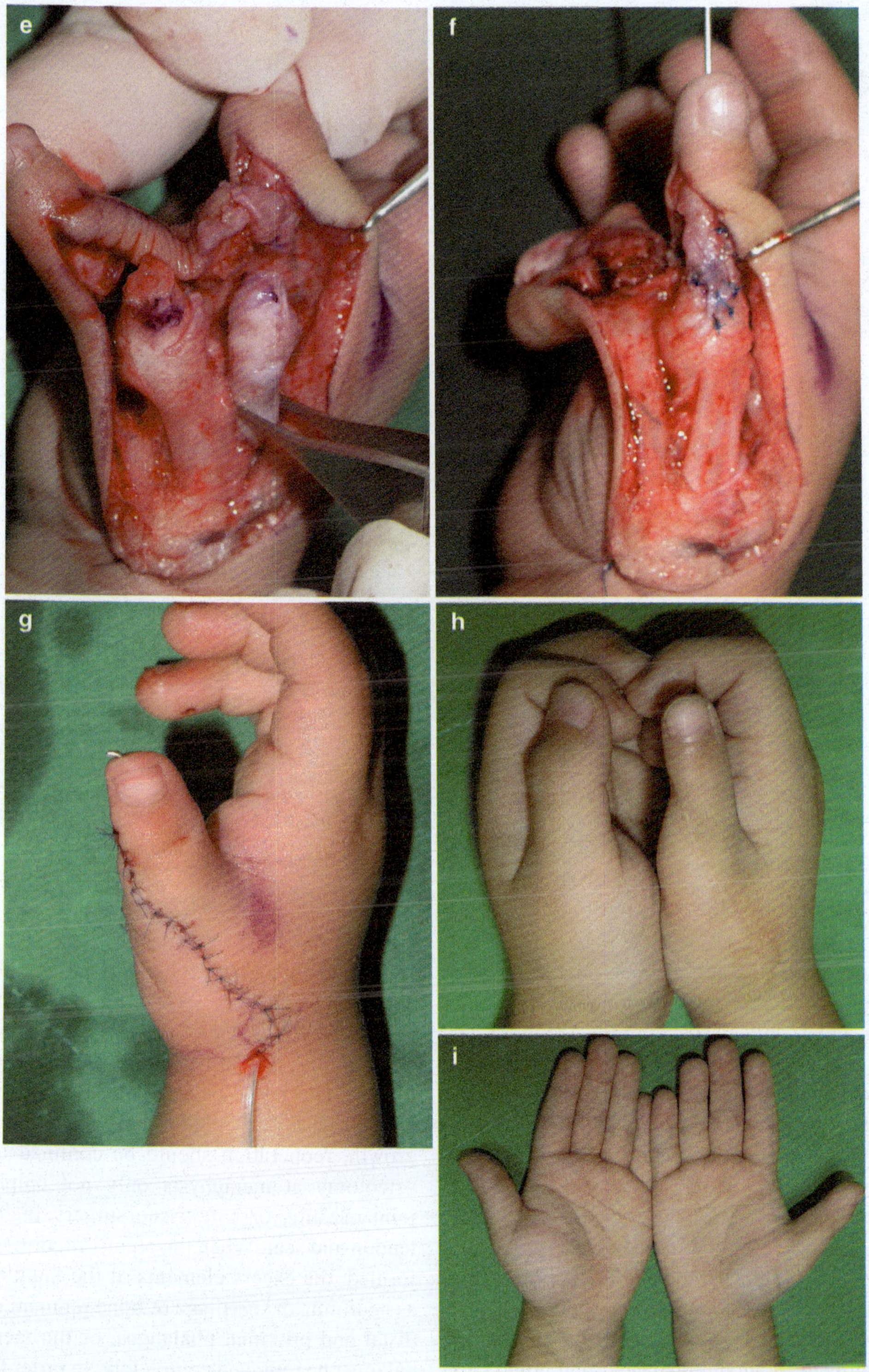


**Fig. 3.20** (continued)

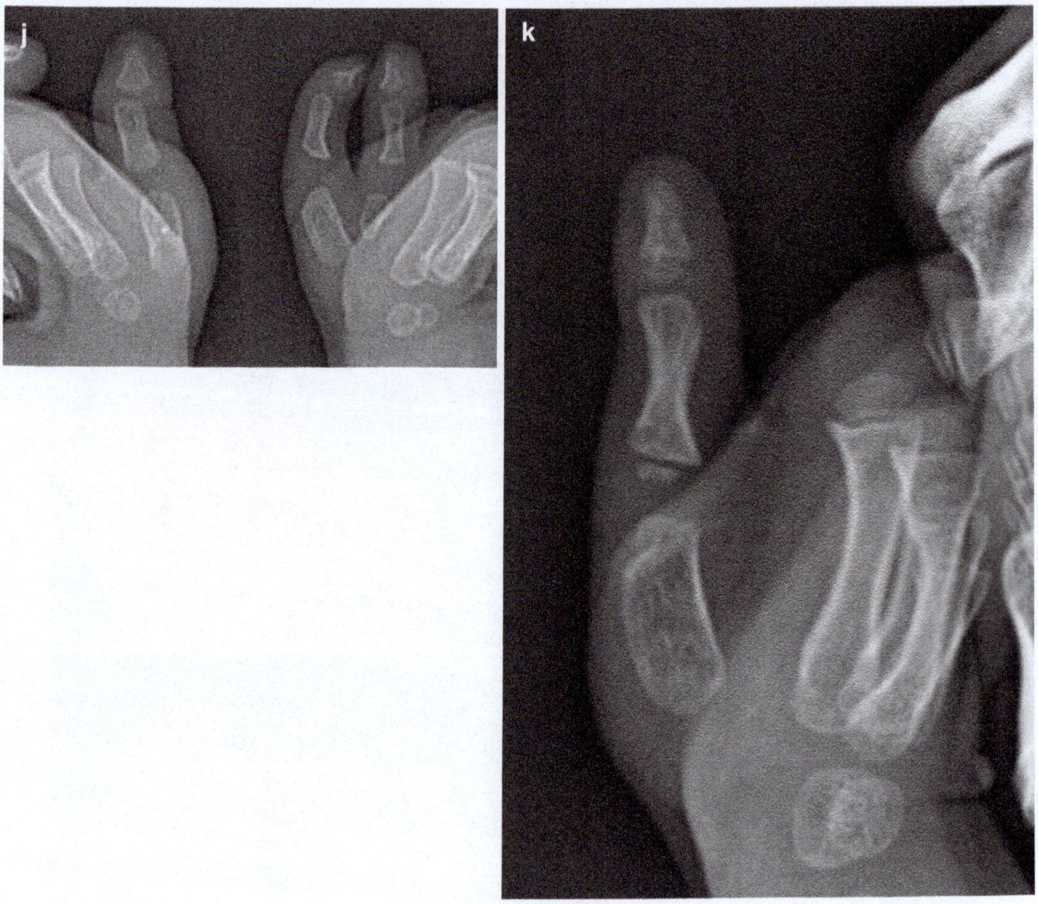


**Fig. 3.20** (continued)

the proximal phalangeal bone guarantee much better functional and cosmetic results rather than other soft tissue surgeries (Fig. 3.23). Centralization, ulnarization, or radialization of the tendons and/or plication or release of the joint capsule cannot support straight axis of the thumb. To prevent recurrence of the angulation deformity of the joint, overcorrection is indispensable.

The most severe deformity is a zigzag deformity, either angulated radially at the IP joint and ulnarly at the MP joint or the reverse [25]. With growth, secondary problems may include bony overgrowth, tendon imbalance, and joint stiffness. Surgeons must be aware of these potential complications when the performance of initial surgery and long-term follow-up of the child are necessary.

Regarding the age of the patients and operation options, performing an osteotomy at the joint should be suspended after closure of the epiphyseal growth plate. During the period of growth, reoperation should be confined to the osteotomy at metaphysis only not epiphysis, joint capsule, or soft tissue surgery including tendon and scar. When the reconstruction is performed, the excess elements of the thumb such as neuroma, the cartilage or bone remnant of the distal and proximal phalanges, or the metacarpal must be removed completely. In order to stabilize the joint, the distal insertion of the collateral ligament is elevated while preserving

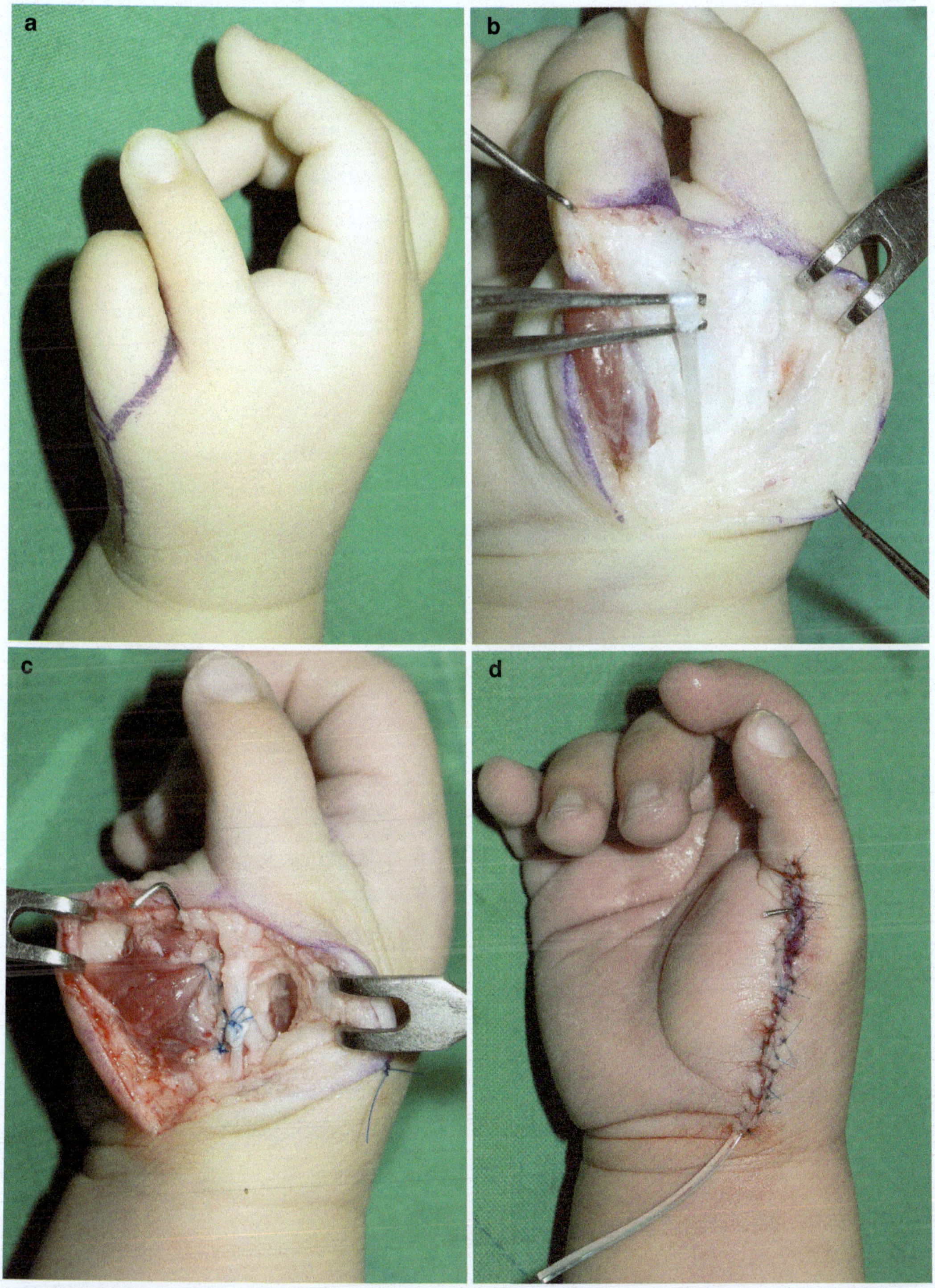


**Fig. 3.21** (**a**) Preoperative hockey stick design for on-top plasty of the type VI radial polydactyly. (**b**) Flexor and extensor tendons are preserved to be repaired. Y-shaped design on the dorsum of both components. (**c**) After oblique ostectomy at the base of proximal metacarpal bone on both components, one K-wire is fixed. Extensor tendon is strengthened and abductor pollicis brevis muscle is sutured. (**d**) Immediate postoperative view. (**e** and **f**) Postoperative view. (**g** and **h**) Pre- and post-operative radiograph

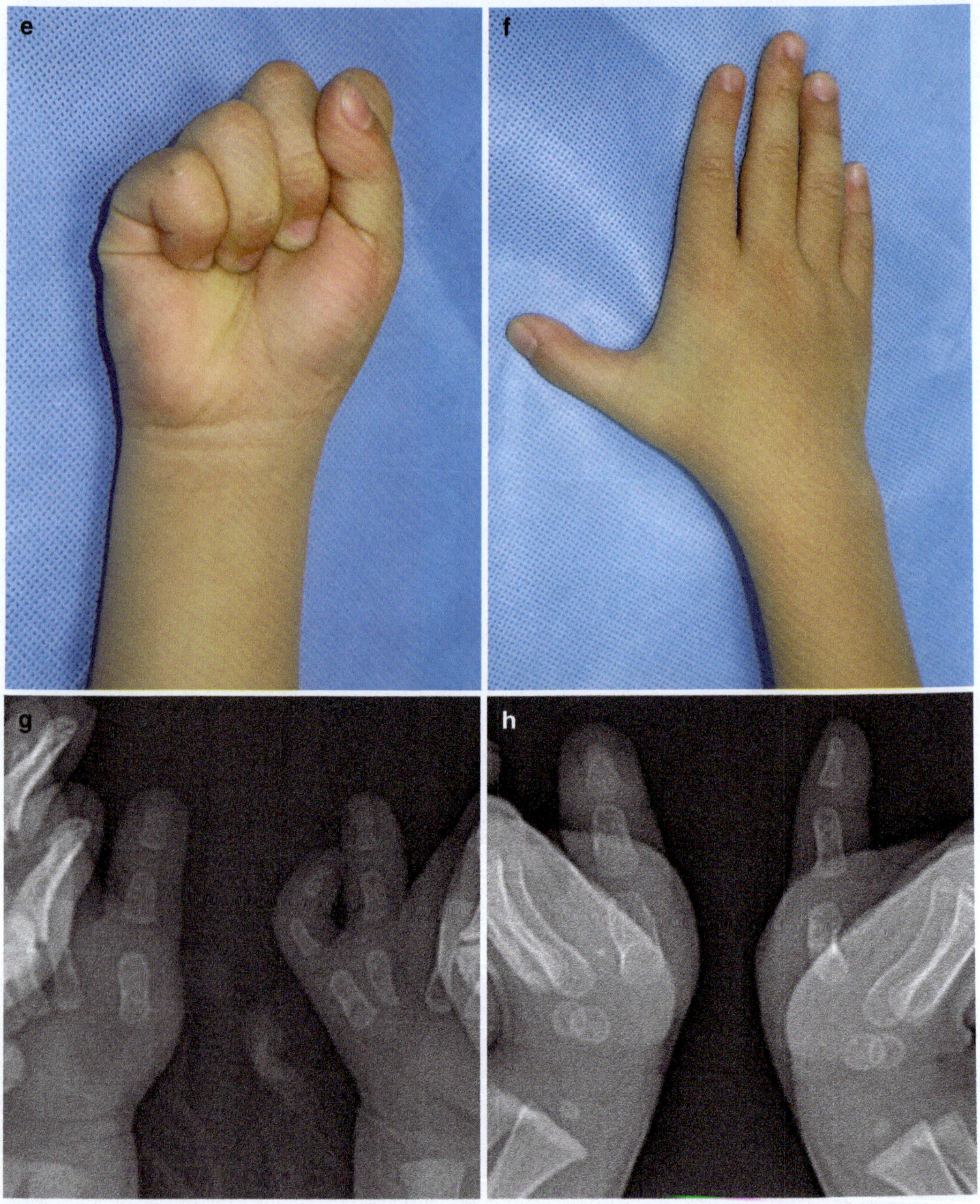


**Fig. 3.21** (continued)

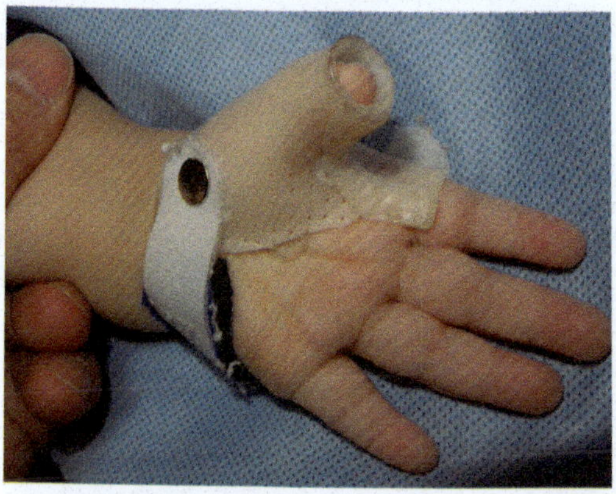

**Fig. 3.22** Custom-made brace for the thumb is applied for 3 weeks all day after stitches removed and then each night for 3 weeks

a slip of the subperiosteal tissue for reattachment together with the distal insertion of the collateral ligament, or if this is not possible, a new ligament should be created with part of the ablated tendon (Fig. 3.24).

Regarding correction of alignment of the joint, joint space should be transverse by the osteotomy or shaving of articular cartilage first. Tendon rebalancing is then very important to prevent dynamic instability. If a previous operative scar or a skin contracture is suspected to cause angulation, employ soft tissue release with local flap or Z-plasty (Fig. 3.25). Bulky soft tissue should certainly be excised, and fat or dermo-fat graft is sometimes necessary to replace the depressed area.

In cases of a MP joint deformity, the remaining base of the proximal phalanx is removed preserving the subperiosteal insertion of the abductor pollicis brevis and the radial collateral ligament. However, excision of soft tissue is also important to prevent prominence at the joint. The abductor pollicis brevis is reinserted into the radial base of the proximal phalanx.

In angulated deformity of the joint, almost all extrinsic tendons are hypoplastic and have eccentric abnormal insertion. Successful reconstruction can be achieved with combined closing wedge osteotomy at the metacarpal neck with reduction of its widened head, reconstruction of the radial collateral ligament of the MP joint with a periosteal capsular sleeve, and centralization of the FPL with relocation of its insertion in a more ulnar position. Even weak FPL and EPL tendon should be centralized or reinserted to the opposite direction. If it is insufficient, extension lag or radial angulation at IP joint can be corrected with EIP tendon transfer which provides force to correct dynamic instability [26]. In a severe zigzag deformity, double osteotomy at the phalangeal bone or double arthrodesis of the IP joint and the MP joint is the final salvage procedure in adults (Fig. 3.26).

Correction of any angulation deformity and any instability should result in as little sacrifice of the arc of motion as possible. Alignment and size of the thumb, the shape of the nail, and even the circumference of the thumb are more important than the function of the thumb. Alignment can be corrected in the secondary operation, but deformities of the nail, such as hypoplasia, splitting, and distortion, are too difficult to treat properly.

To prevent secondary deformity of the radial polydactyly, the radial nail should be removed, preserving part of the radial distal phalanx to provide breadth for distal duplication in types I and II. Though this exposes the proximal and distal

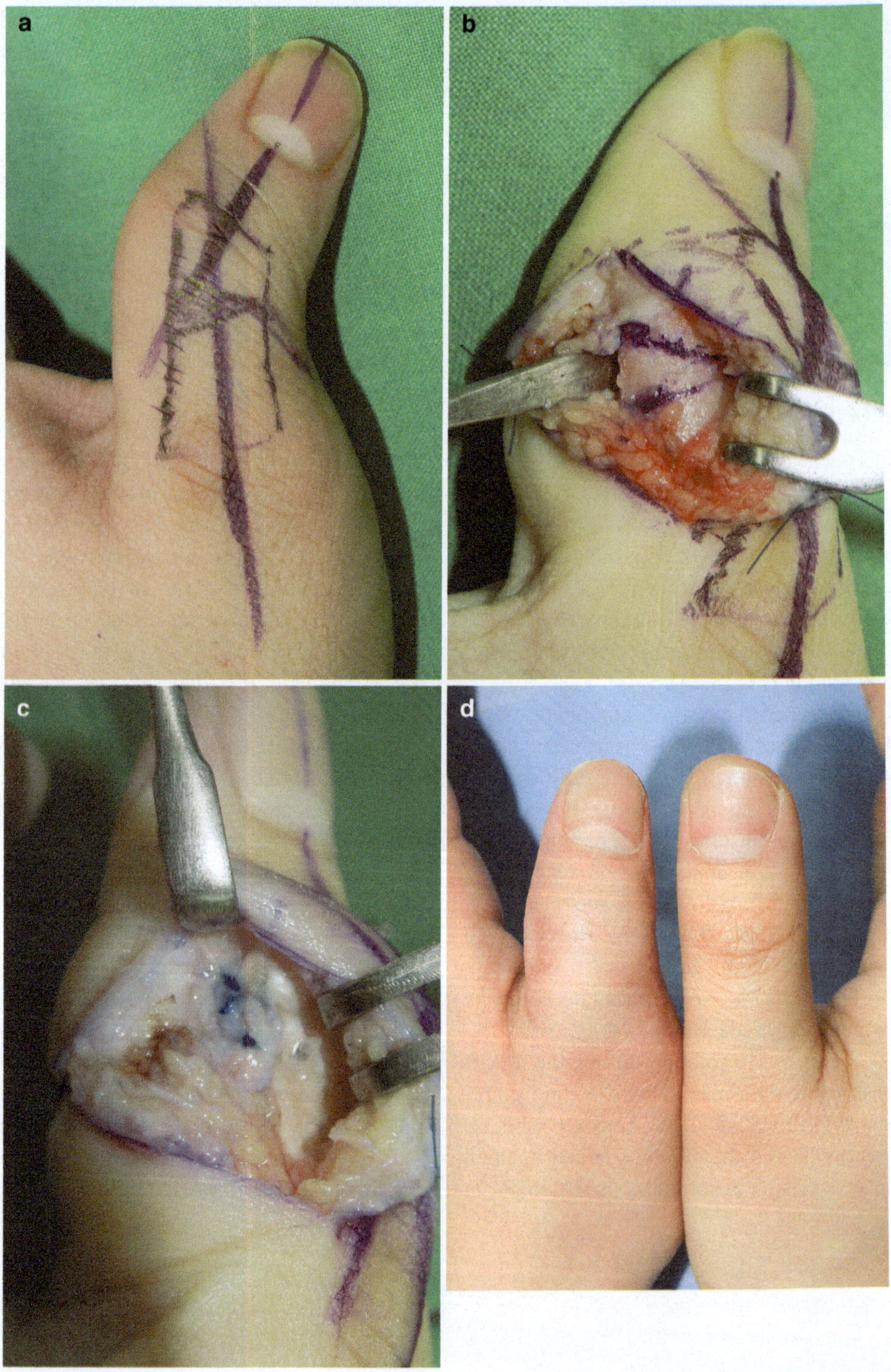


**Fig. 3.23** (**a**) Radial angulation deformity of the left thumb after resection of radial polydactyly. (**b**) Closing wedge ostectomy at the ulnar side of the proximal phalanx. (**c**) Plication of the extensor tendon and ulnar collateral ligament of the IP joint. (**d**) Postoperative view. (**e–g**) Preoperative radiograph, bone fixation with 3 K-wire, and postoperative radiograph

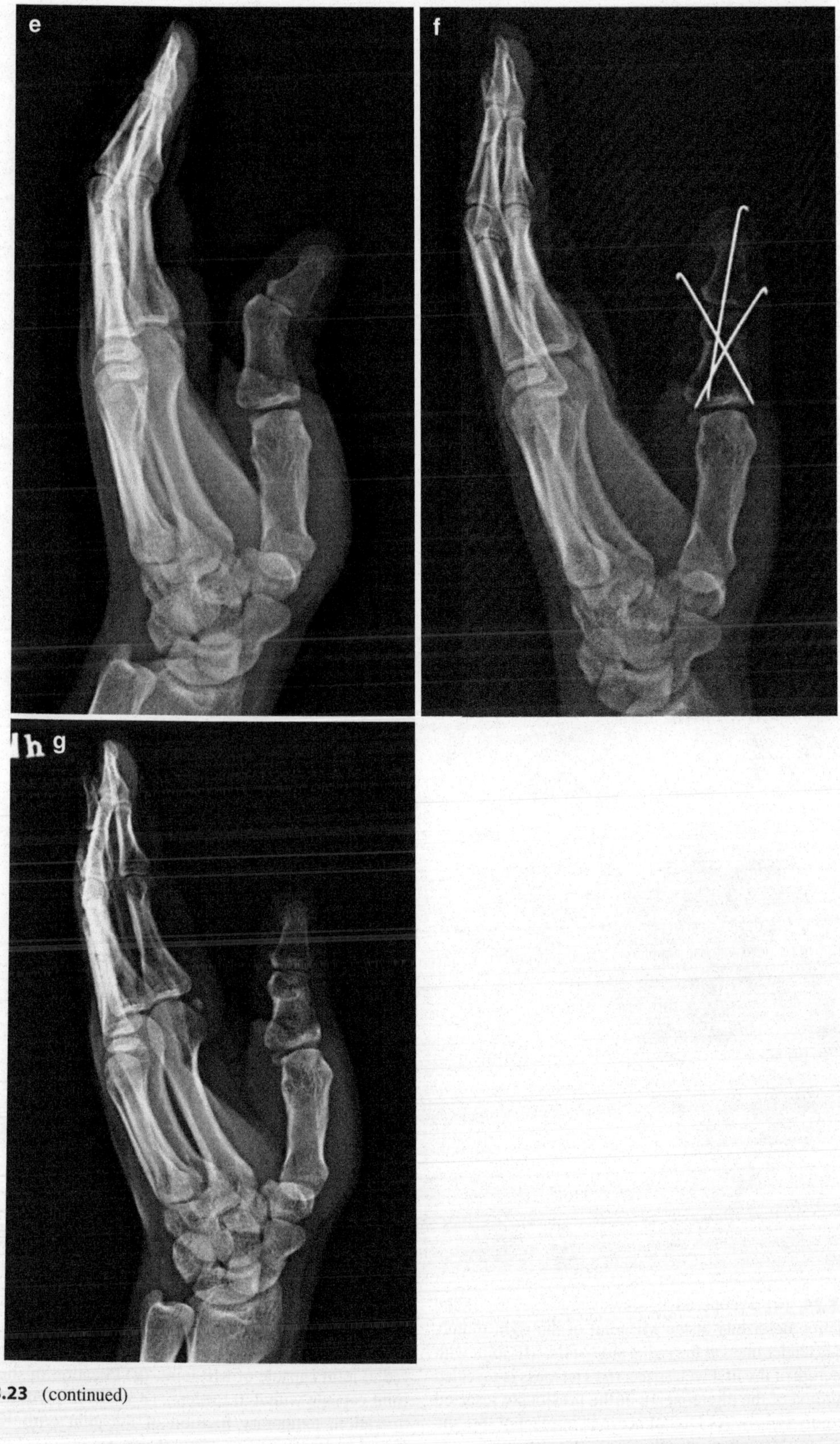


**Fig. 3.23** (continued)

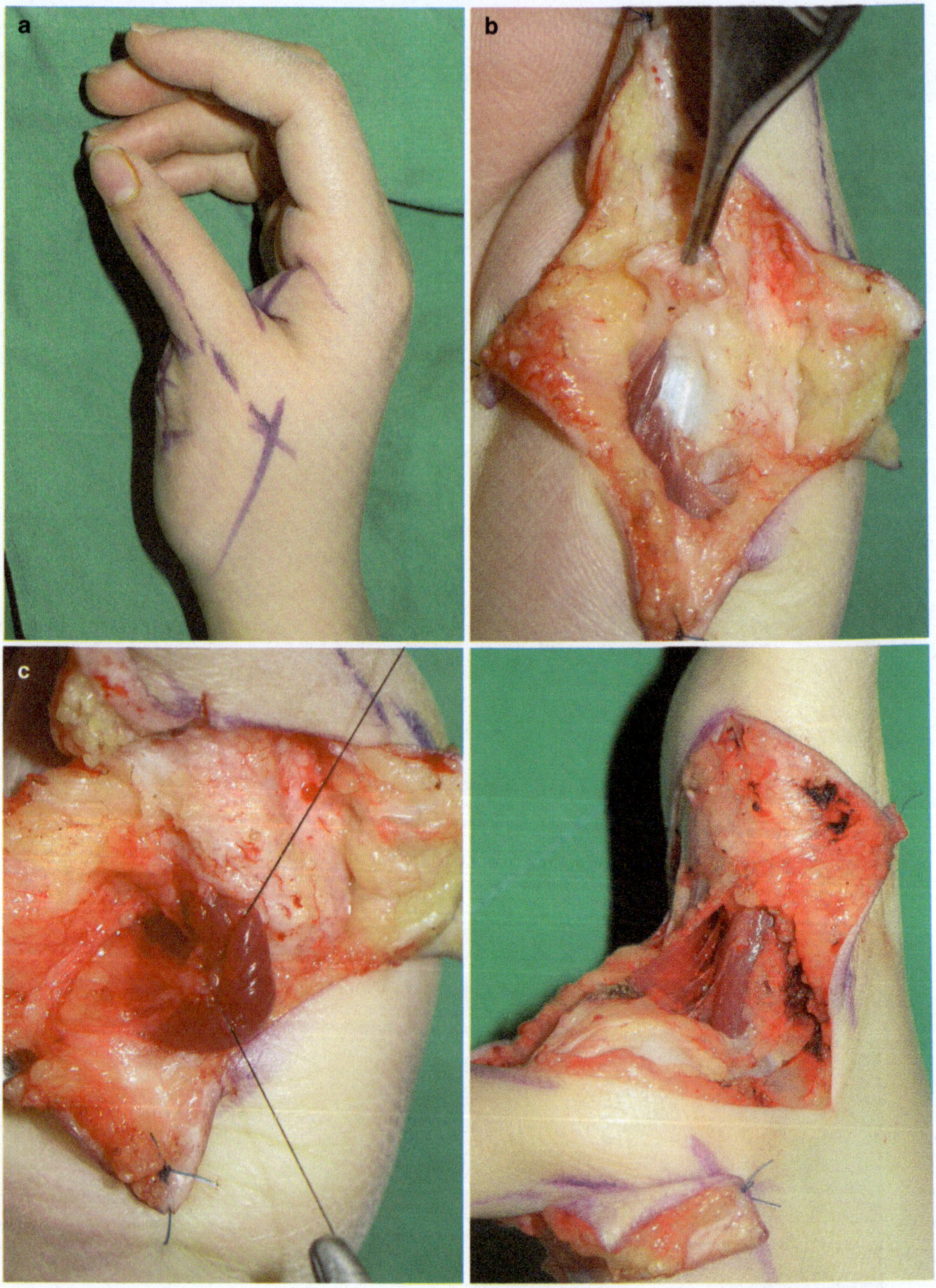


**Fig. 3.24** (**a**) Preoperative view shows severe radial angulation deformity at the MP joint of the right thumb. There is tender mass at the radial side of the MP joint with contracture of the first web space. (**b**) The mass is revealed as neuroma of the digital nerve of the previously resected radial polydactyly. (**c**) Digital nerve is implanted into the thenar muscle after resection of the neuroma. (**d**) Myotomy of the adductor pollicis muscle is made for release of the first web space. (**e**) Joint capsulotomy is made on the ulnar side of the MP joint for plication. (**f**) Open capsulotomy is performed to release the contracted radial joint capsule of MP joint. (**g**) Plication of the ulnar joint capsule with 4–0 Prolene. (**h** and **i**) Immediate post-operation, temporary fixation of the joint with K-wire. (**j** and **k**) Postoperative view. (**l** and **m**) Pre- and postoperative radiograph

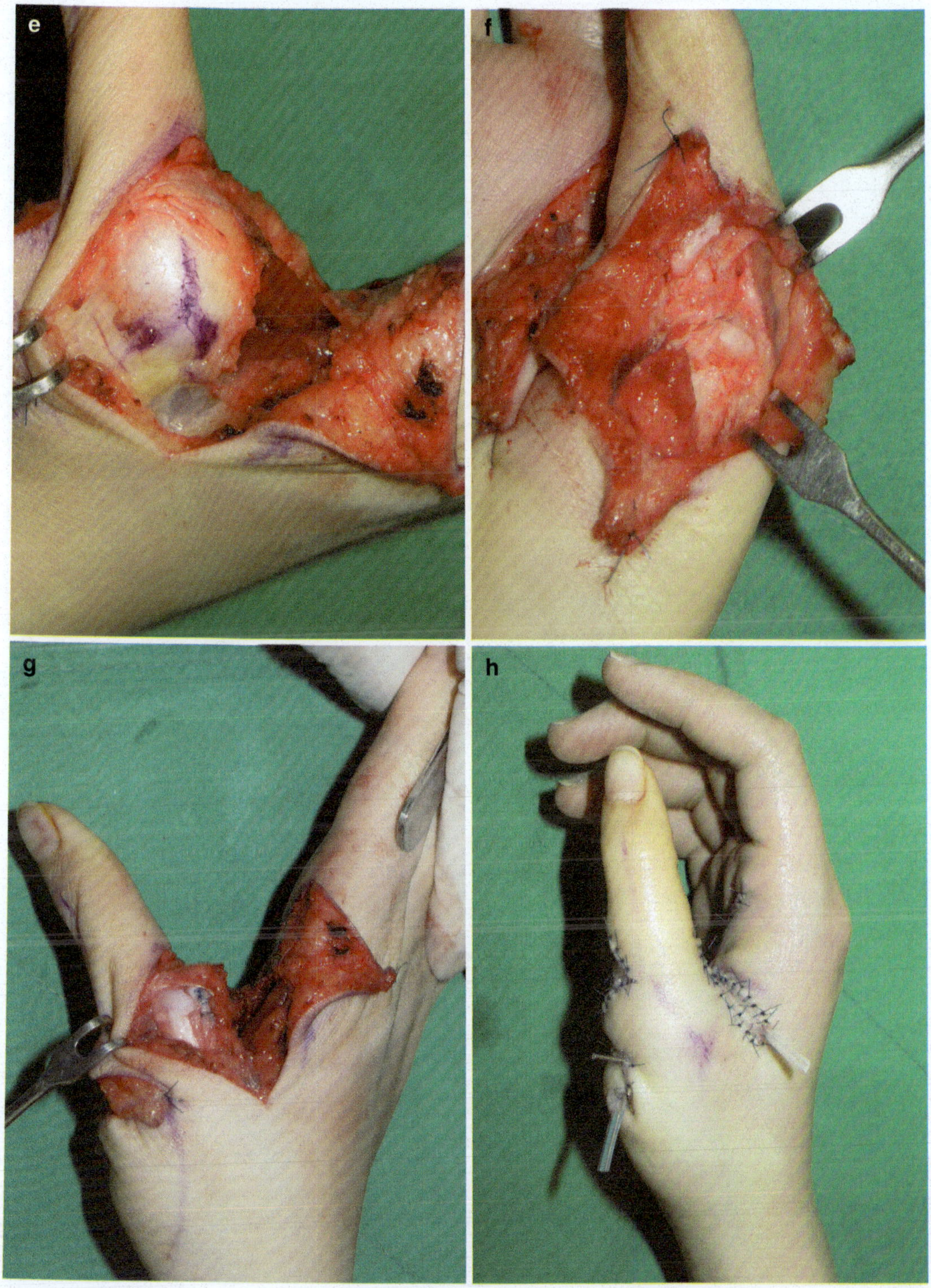


**Fig. 3.24** (continued)

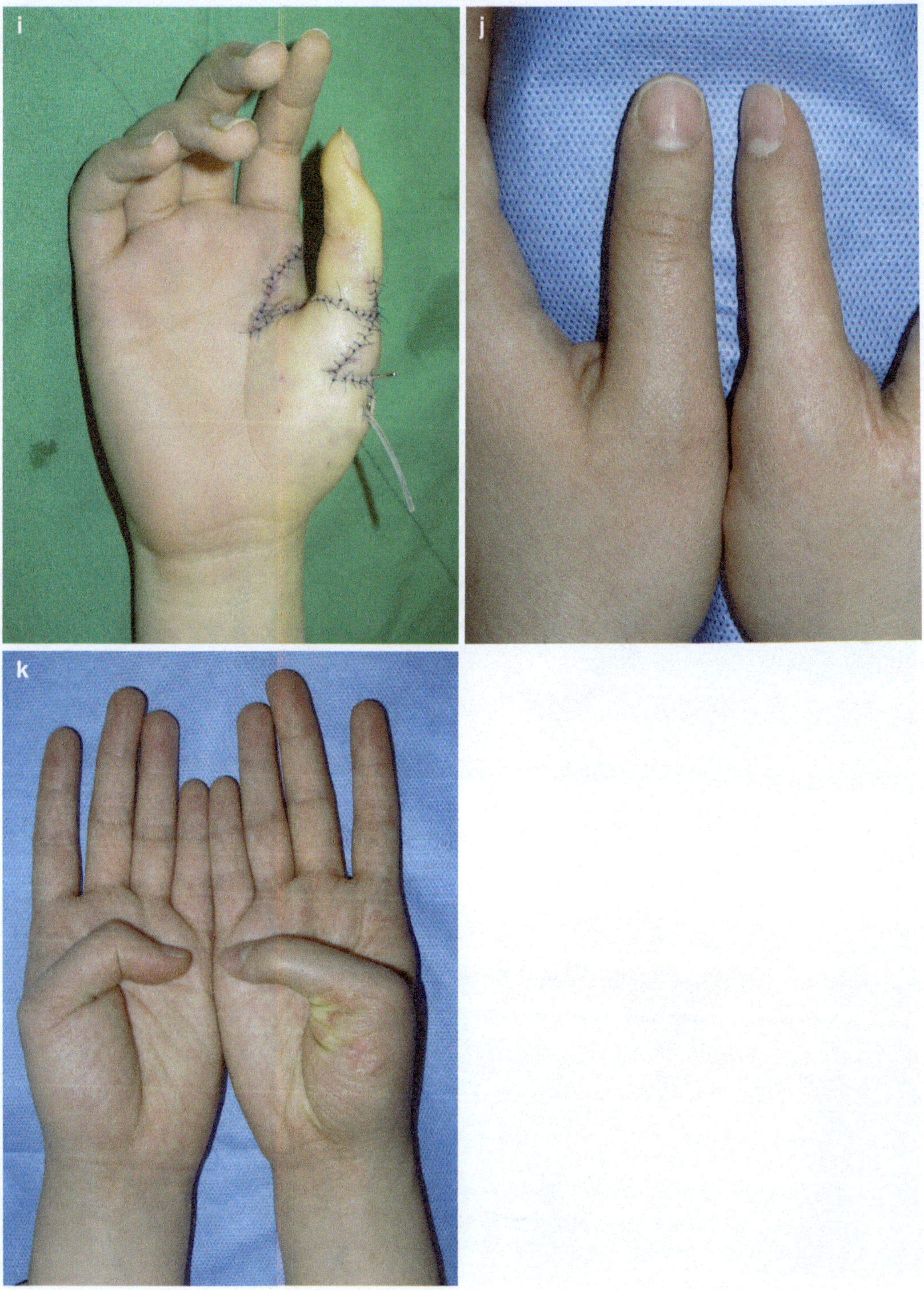

**Fig. 3.24** (continued)

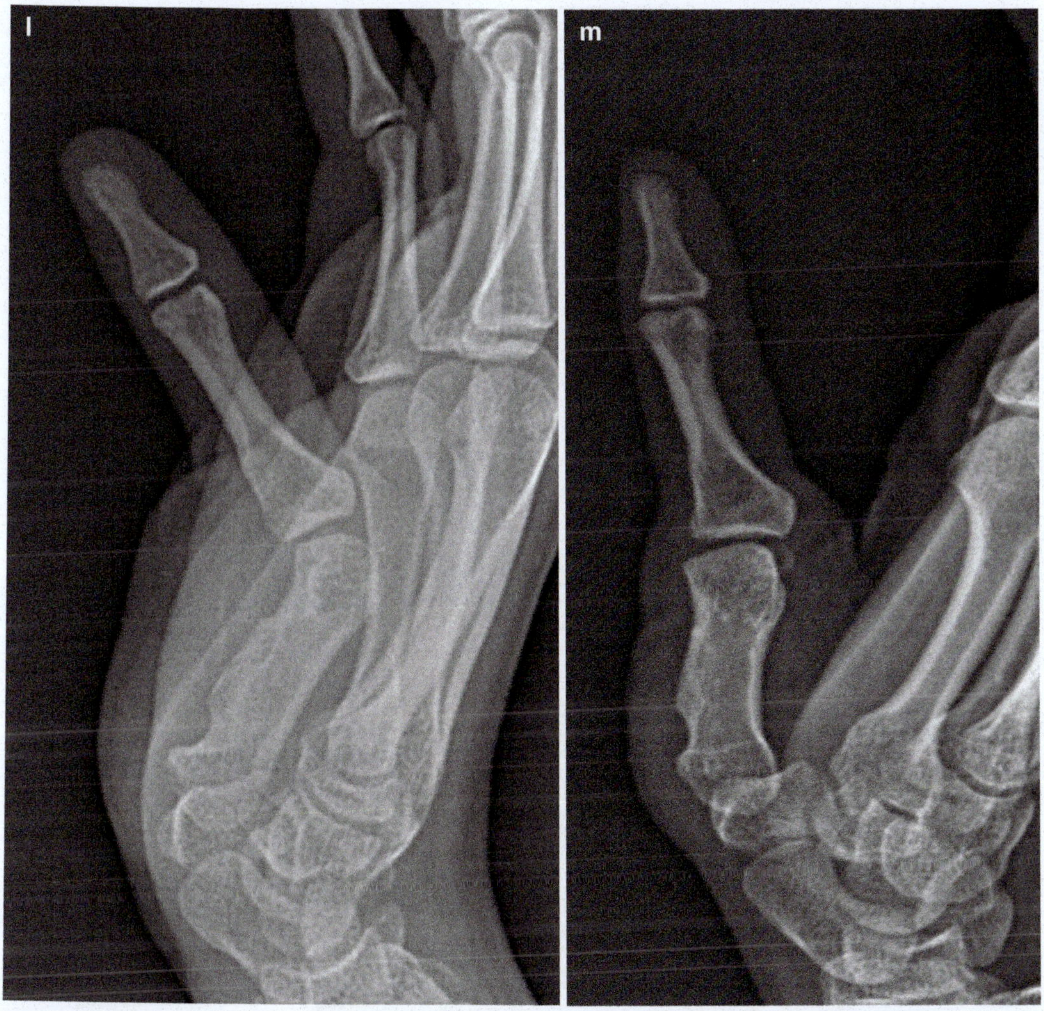


**Fig. 3.24** (continued)

deforming structures, conjoint EPL/FPL tendons can be identified. In the first operation, secure stabilization of joints with collateral ligament advancement is mandatory. Primary corrective osteotomy and internal fixation may guarantee prevention of severe secondary deformity, where corrected tendon and joint stabilization cannot be achieved. In excision of the radial component, the surgeon should carefully consider how to use the resected bone, tendon, and even soft tissue or nail.

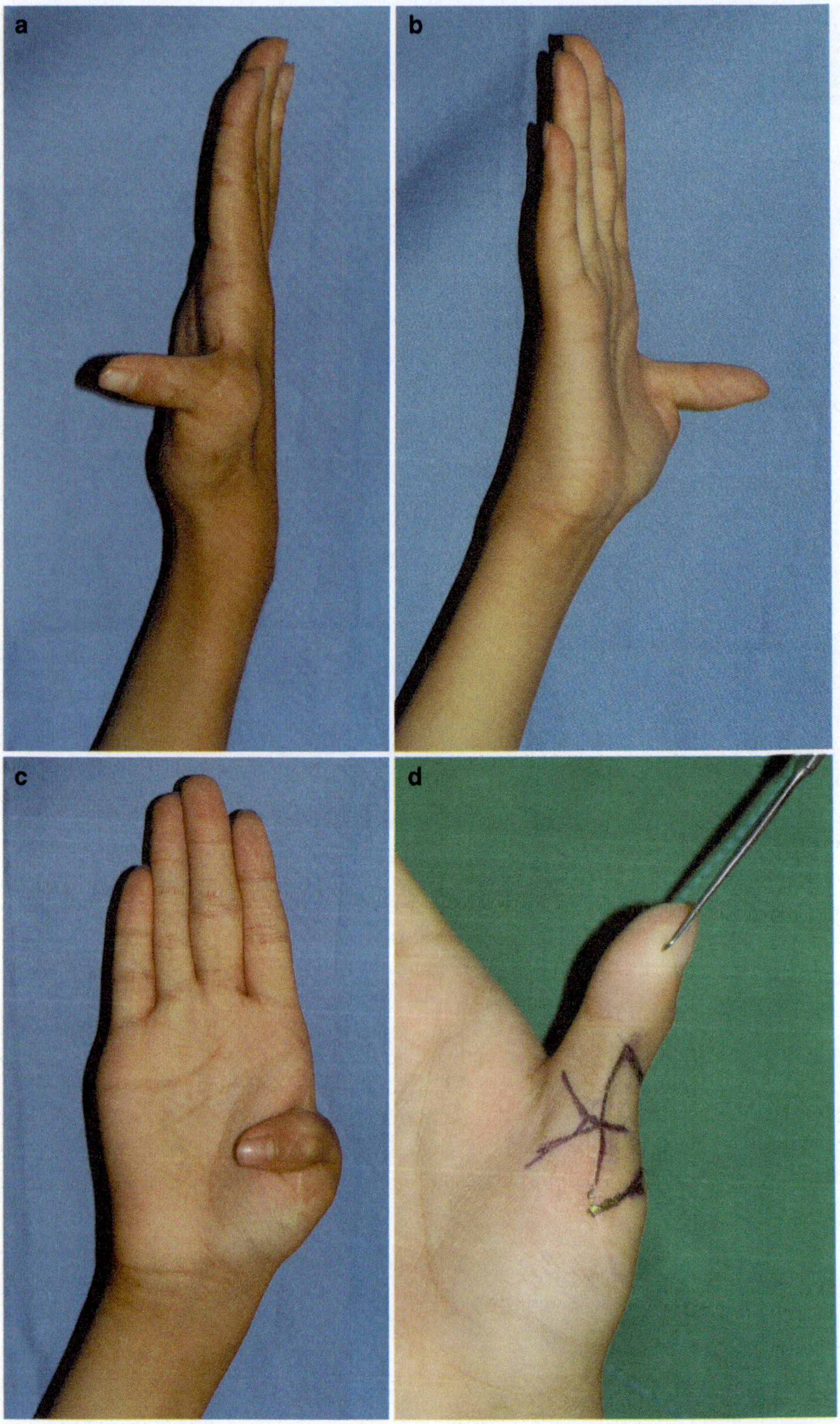


**Fig. 3.25** (**a–c**) Preoperative view shows severe radial angulation deformity at the MP joint of the right thumb. (**d**) Incision is made on the radial side of MPJ as double opposing Z-plasty with Y-V advancement flap. (**e**) Ulnarization of the extensor tendon is made after release of the ulnar collateral ligament and plication of the radial collateral ligament. Closing wedge ostectomy and internal fixation are performed at the proximal phalanx. (**f**) Immediate after operation. (**g–i**). Postoperative view. (**j** and **k**) Pre- and postoperative radiograph

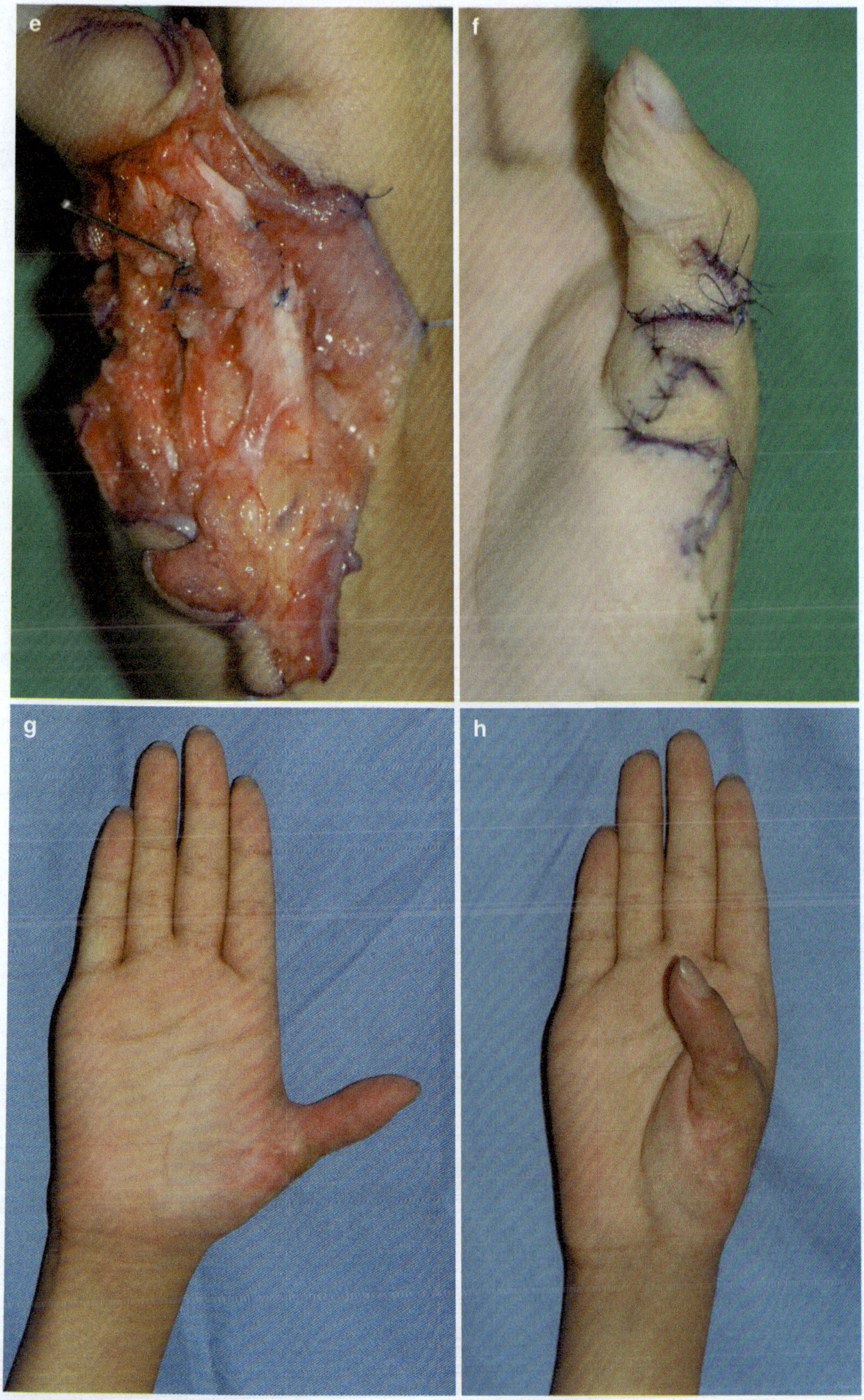


**Fig. 3.25** (continued)

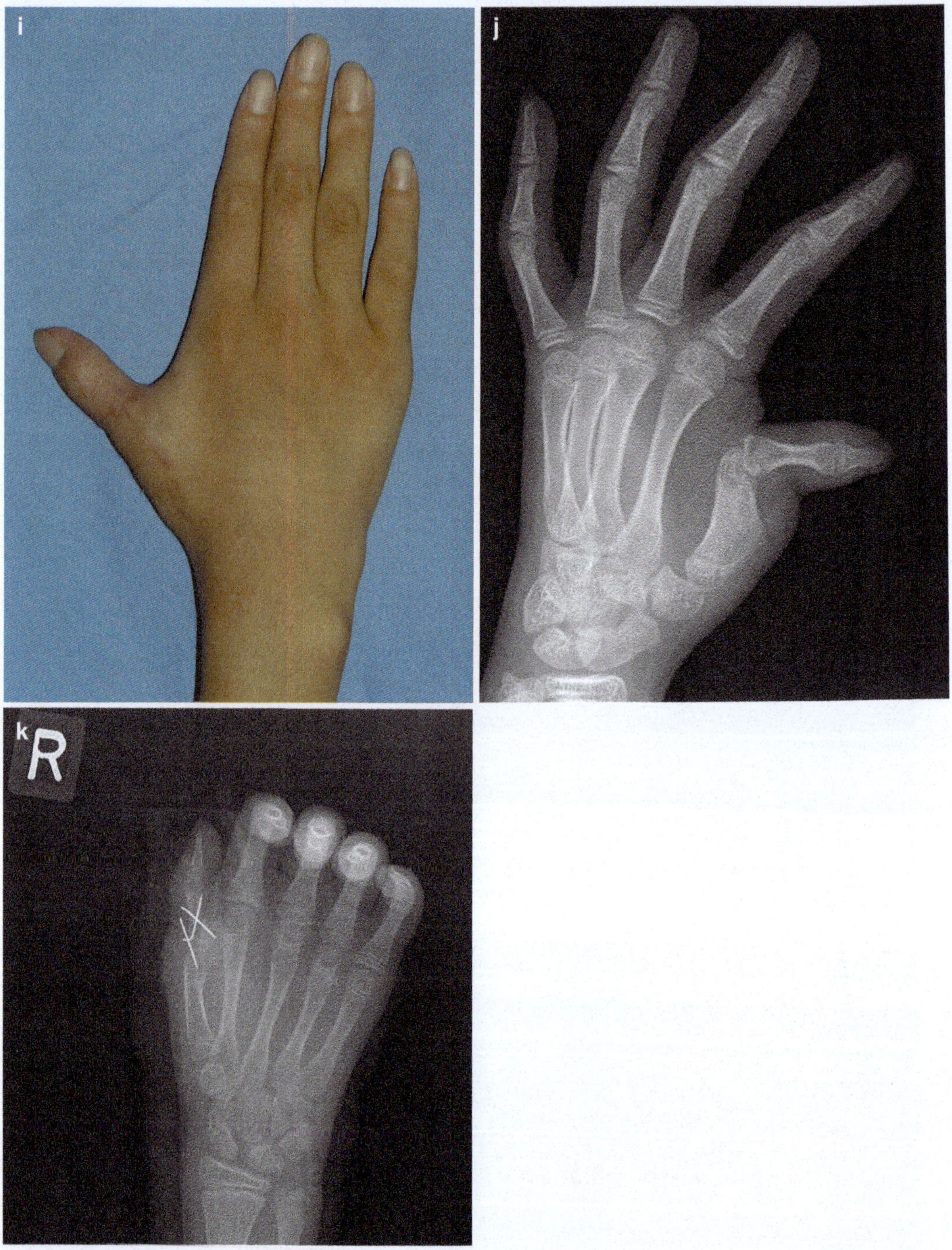


**Fig. 3.25** (continued)

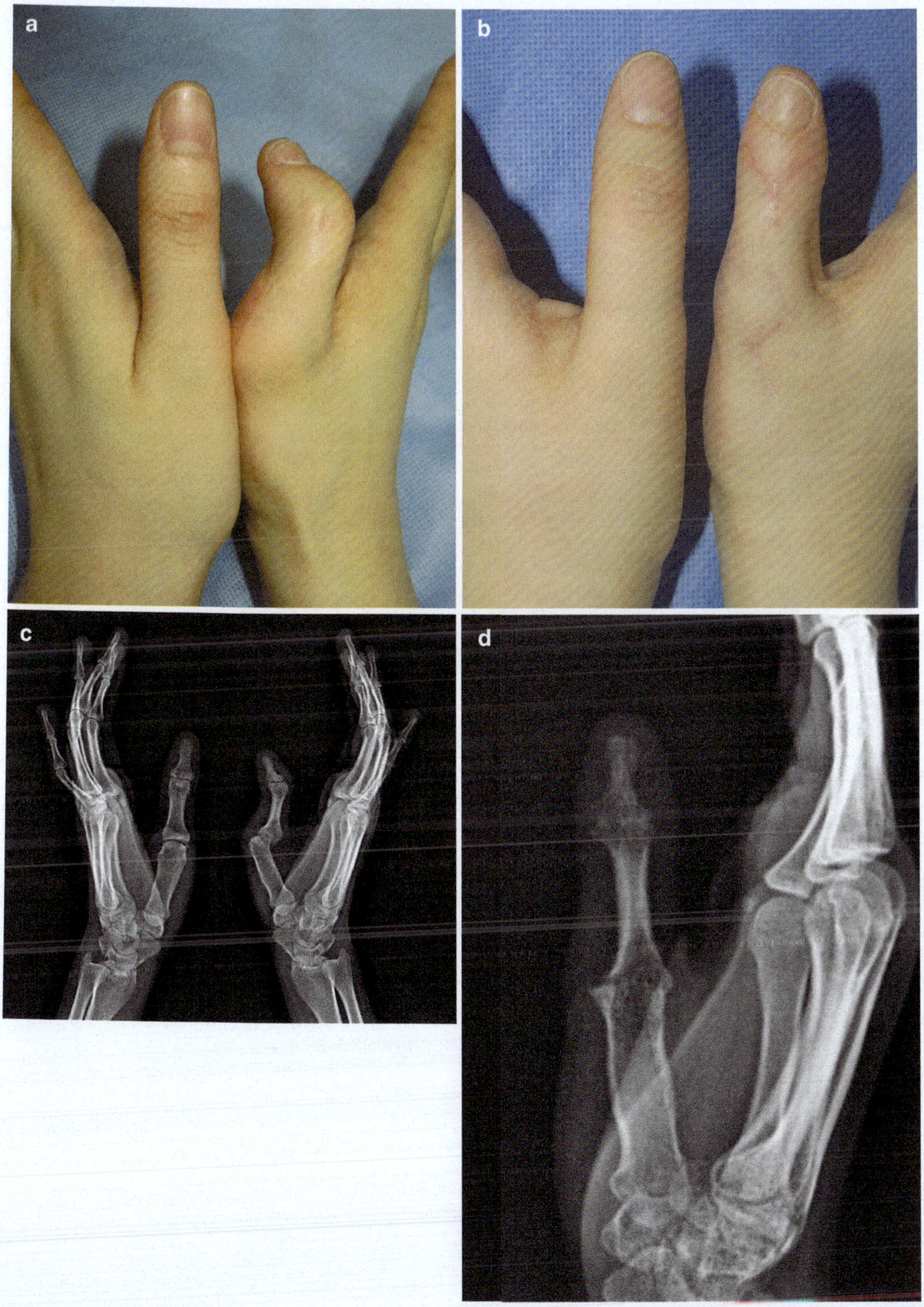


**Fig. 3.26** (**a**) Severe Z-deformity of the right thumb, preoperative view. (**b**) Postoperative view. (**c** and **d**) Pre- and postoperative radiograph after double arthrodesis of the IP joint and MPJ

## References


1. Jobe MT. Congenital anomalies of the hand. In: Canale ST, Beaty JH, editors. Campbell's operative orthopaedics. 11th ed. Philadelphia: Mosby; 2008. p. 4367–449.
2. Goldfarb CA, Wall LB, Bohn DC, Moen BA, Van Heest AE. Epidemiology of congenital upper limb anomalies in a Midwest United States population: an assessment using the Oberg, Manske, and Tonkin classification. J Hand Surg Am. 2015;40:127–32.
3. Swanson AB, Swanson GD, Tada K. A classification for congenital limb malformation. J Hand Surg Am. 1983;8:693–702.
4. Wassel HD. The results of surgery for polydactyly of the thumb. Clin Orthop Relat Res. 1969;64:175–93.
5. Manske MC, Kennedy CD, Huang JI. Classifications in brief: the Wassel classification for radial polydactyly. Clin Orthop Relat Res. 2017;475:1740–6.
6. Dijkman RR, van Nieuwenhoven CA, Selles RW, et al. A multicenter comparative study of two classification system for radial polydactyly. Plast Reconstr Surg. 2014;134:991–1001.
7. Chung MS, Baek GH, Gong HS, Lee HJ, Kim J, Rhee SH. Radial polydactyly: proposal for a new classification system based on the 159 duplicated thumbs. J Pediatr Orthop. 2013;33:190–6.
8. Zuidam JM, Selles RW, Ananta M, Runia J, Hovius SE. A classification system of radial polydactyly: inclusion of triphalangeal thumb and triplication. J Hand Surg Am. 2008;33:373–7.
9. Upton J, Hergrueter C. Congenital anomalies of the hand. In: Cohen M, editor. Mastery of plastic and reconstructive surgery, vol. 3. Boston/New York: Little, Brown; 1994. p. 1424–53.
10. Dobyns JH, Lipscomb PR, Cooney WP. Management of thumb duplication. Clin Orthop Relat Res. 1985;195:26–44.
11. Tonkin MA, Bulstrode NW. The Bilhaut-Cloquet procedure for Wassel types III, IV and VII thumb duplication. J Hand Surg. 2007;32B:684–93.
12. Baek GH, Gong HS, Chung MS, Oh JH, Lee YH, Lee SK. Modified Bilhaut-Cloquet procedure for Wassel type-II and III polydactyly of the thumb. J Bone Joint Surg. 2007;89A:534–41.
13. Manske PR. Treatment of duplicated thumb using a ligamentous/periosteal flap. J Hand Surg. 1989;14A:728–33.
14. Horii E, Hattori T, Koh S, Majima M. Reconstruction for Wassel type III radial polydactyly with two digits equal in size. J Hand Surg Am. 2009;34:1802–7.
15. Shen K, Wang Z, Xu Y. Reconstruction of Wassel type VI radial polydactyly with Triphalangeal thumb using an on-top osteotomy. Plast Reconstr Surg Glob Open. 2017;5:e1216–22.
16. Bell B, Butler L, Mills J, Stutz C, Ezaki M, Oishi S. "On-Top Plasty" for radial polydactyly reconstruction. J Hand Surg Am. 2017;42:753.e1–753.
17. Saito S, Ueda M, Takahashi N, Kawakatsu M, Suzuki S. Three-dimensional ultrasonography for visualization of muscular anomalies in type VI and VII radial polydactyly. Skelet Radiol. 2016;45:541–7.
18. Cohen MS. Thumb duplication. Hand Clin. 1998;14:17–27.
19. Mih AD. Complications of duplicate thumb reconstruction. Hand Clin. 1998;14:143–9.
20. Tada K, Yonenobu K, Tsuyuguchi Y, et al. Duplication of the thumb. A retrospective review of two hundred and thirty-seven cases. J Bone Joint Surg Am. 1983;65:584–98.
21. Stutz C, Mills J, Wheeler L, et al. Long-term outcomes following radial polydactyly reconstruction. J Hand Surg. 2014;39:1549–52.
22. Ogino T, Ishii S, Takahata S, Kato H. Long-term results of surgical treatment of thumb polydactyly. J Hand Surg. 1996;21A:478–86.
23. Larsen M, Nicolai JP. Long-term follow-up of surgical treatment for thumb duplication. J Hand Surg Br. 2005;30:276–81.
24. Goldfarb CA, Patterson JM, Maender A, et al. Thumb size and appearance following reconstruction of radial polydactyly. J Hand Surg. 2008;33:1348–53.
25. Kawabata H, Tada K, Masada K, Kawai H, Ono K. Revision of residual deformities after operations for duplication of the thumb. J Bone Joint Surg Am. 1990;72:988–98.
26. Kawabata H, Masatomi T, Shimada K, Kawai H, Tada K. Treatment of residual instability and extensor lag in polydactyly of the thumb. J Hand Surg Br. 1993;18:5–8.

# Thumb Hypoplasia

4

Luis R. Scheker

The thumb represents 40% of the hand function. When the thumb is missing in its entirety, many activities are limited, such as turning a door knob, buttoning a shirt, or holding a drinking glass with one hand among others. Congenital anomalies are the main cause of thumb deficiencies in children. These congenital thumb anomalies include hypoplasia and aplasia, constriction ring syndrome, brachydactylic, and true transverse absence. Congenital thumb anomalies account for approximately 11.2% of all birth deformities of the hand. Of these deformities, 6.6% are radial polydactyly; the rest are divided between hypoplasia and aplasia (total absence) of the thumb [1].

Thumb hypoplasia is found in longitudinal deficiencies or in underdevelopment of the preaxial ray. In radial clubhand, the thumb can be absent or just hypoplastic. Hypoplasia is encountered in cases of thumb duplication in which the tissue that is supposed to form a single thumb is divided into two small thumbs that share the tendons, intrinsic muscles, and ligaments (Fig. 4.1). These duplicated thumbs frequently have unstable unicondylar joints. Partial aplasia arises because of transverse absence, symbrachydactyly, and constriction ring syndrome (Fig. 4.2). In constriction ring syndrome, the proximal part of the thumb is frequently normal. In brachydactyly and symbrachydactyly, the whole ray is underdeveloped, but, in contrast to constriction ring syndrome, there is a remnant nail. An uncommon form of hypoplasia of the thumb can be seen in patient s with Du Pan syndrome in which the thumb has a constriction band at its base (Fig. 4.3). In 1937, Muller [2] initially classified hypoplasia/aplasia of the thumb into four categories per degree of deficiency. Blauth, in 1967, later expanded this classification into five categories [3]:

## Blauth Classification

### Type I

Minor hypoplasia in which the thumb, though smaller than the contralateral thumb, functions quite normally.

### Type II

The thumb is smaller and less stable than normal (Fig. 4.4). The hypoplasia in type II has three elements: (1) adduction contracture of the first web space apparent because of (2) the lack of thenar muscles, and the hand compensates by exhibiting (3) laxity of the ulnar collateral ligament that allows abduction of the metacarpo phalangeal (MCP) joint. The skeleton is small, and the metacarpophalangeal joint ulnar collateral ligament is incompetent (Fig. 4.5).

L. R. Scheker (✉)
Division of Hand Surgery, Department of Plastic and Reconstructive Surgery, Kleinert Institute for Hand and Microsurgery, University of Louisville School of Medicine, Louisville, KY, USA


S. H. Woo (ed.), *The Thumb*, https://doi.org/10.1007/978-981-10-4400-7_4

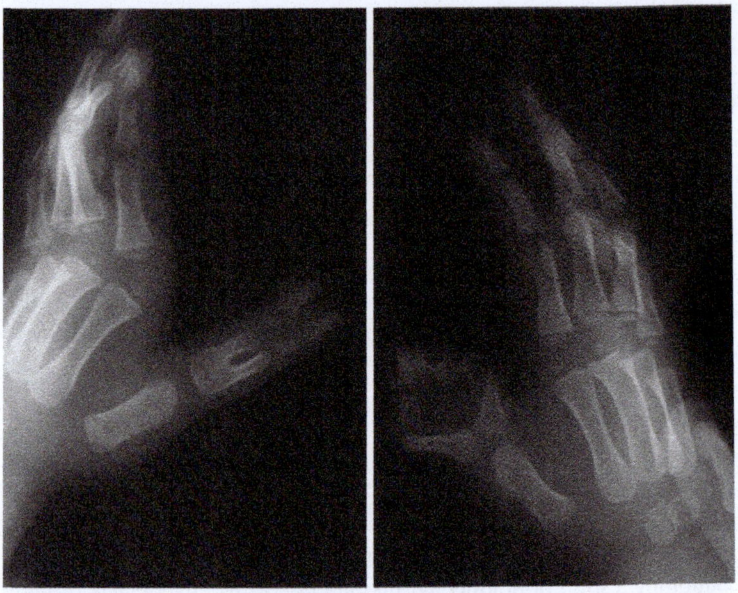

**Fig. 4.1** Duplicated thumb types III and IV both have instability at the IPJ; the type IV can also have problems at the MCP joint. The tissue of the thumb has been divided; therefore joints tend to be unicondylar and unstable

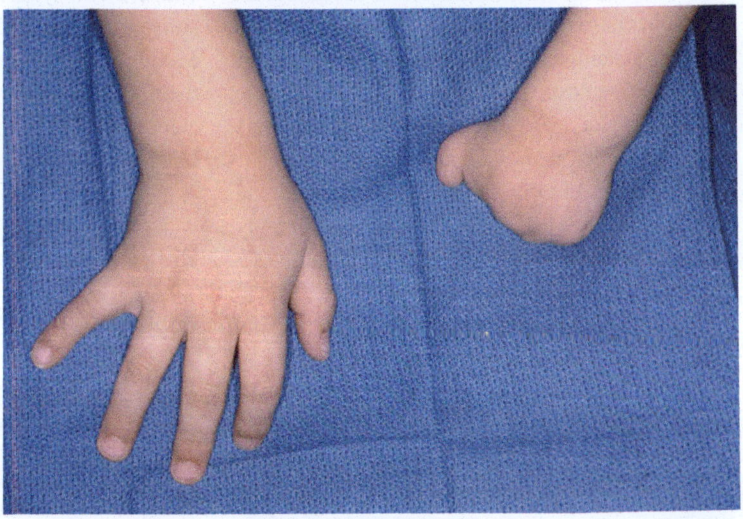

**Fig. 4.2** The thumb can be absent with the other digits in peromelic symbrachydactyly, also in cases of constriction ring, where the proximal part is normal and amenable to toe-to-hand transfer

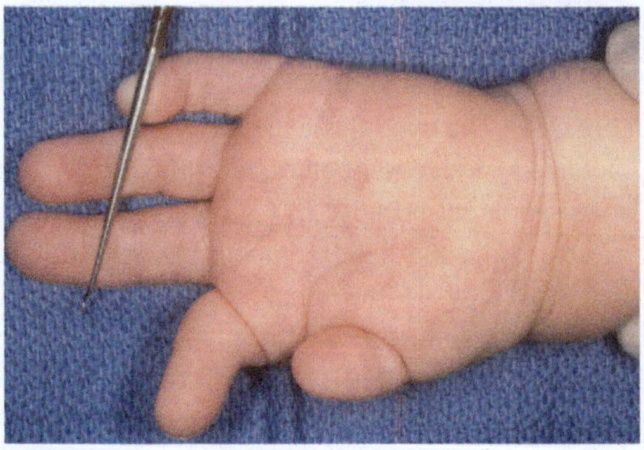

**Fig. 4.3** Incompetent thumbs can be found in deformities like the Du Pan syndrome in which the index finger is short and radially deviated. The thumb has a constriction band at its base and lacks bone support

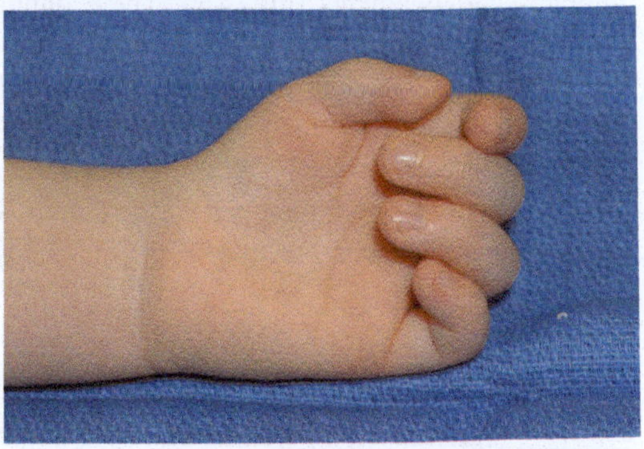

**Fig. 4.4** In type II hypoplasia of the Blauth classification, the thenar eminence is absent, and as a consequence the web space is narrow

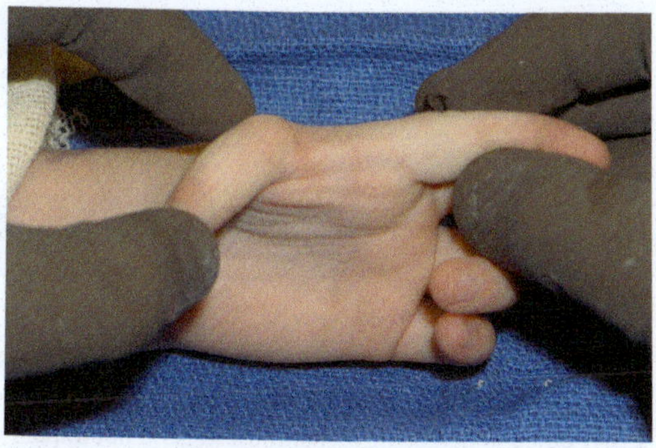

**Fig. 4.5** The narrow web space is compensated by having an incompetent ulnar collateral ligament to the ulnar side of the metacarpophalangeal joint of the thumb

## Type III

This progression includes type II plus skeletal hypoplasia in which the carpometacarpal (CMC) joint is vestigial, the intrinsic muscles are absent, and the extrinsic muscles, when present, are rudimentary and anomalous (Fig. 4.6).

Manske and McCarroll proposed a modification of the Blauth classification by dividing type III into two subcategories, type III-A and type III-B [4]:

### Type III-A

This subdivision comprises extensive extrinsic and intrinsic musculotendinous deficiencies with intact carpometacarpal joint.

### Type III-B

This second subdivision comprises extensive extrinsic and intrinsic musculotendinous deficiencies with basal metacarpal aplasia.

## Type IV

This comprises the floating thumb (*pouce flottant*, Fig. 4.7).

## Type V

Total absence of the thumb (Fig. 4.8).

Despite attempts to classify all cases accurately for correct treatment, there are many varia-

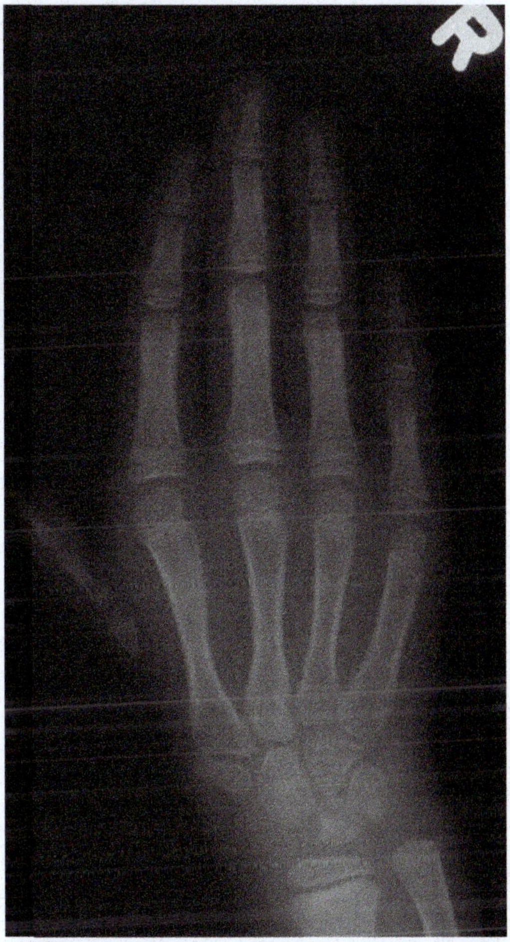

**Fig. 4.6** Type III has been subdivided into III-A and III-B. The original classification of Blauth mentioned that there is no carpometacarpal joint. If the joint is present, it is a type II

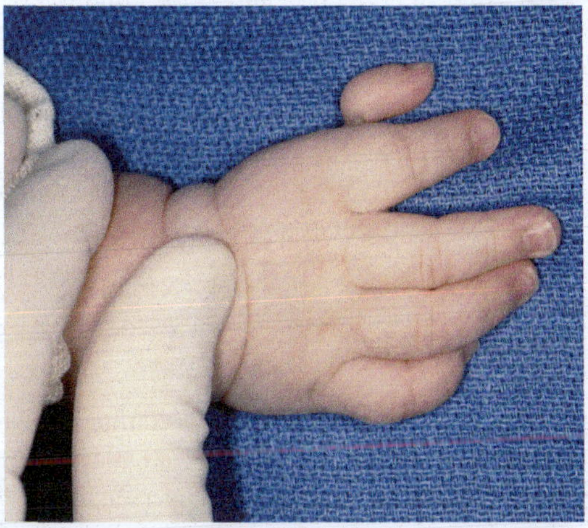

**Fig. 4.7** Type IV has mainly a very small and rudimentary thumb. The French called it "pouce flottant" meaning floating thumb

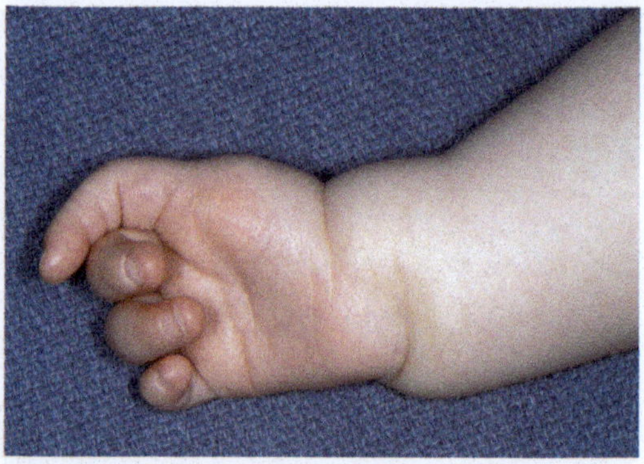

**Fig. 4.8** Type V is a complete absence of the thumb

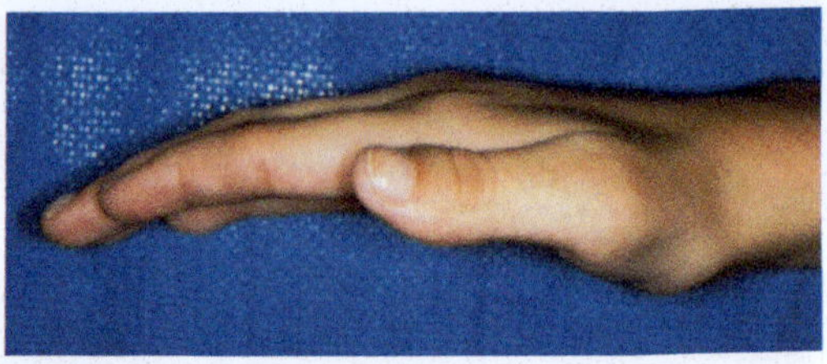

**Fig. 4.9** The distal phalanx thumb is relatively short; there is no thenar eminence in her hands. She was treated in another unit for severe bilateral carpal tunnel, as the EMG failed to detect the thenar muscles. Did not improve with surgery because what she has is a condition called trichorhinophalangeal syndrome

tions in these deformities and in the severity of the manifested underdevelopment. Occasionally, the deformities are even more severe. It is important, therefore, to treat patients according to their needs and not with a rigid approach based solely upon these types.

## Surgical Approaches to the Hypoplastic Thumb

I believe that congenital reconstruction should be performed as soon as the child is immunologically mature. This is achieved at the 6 months of life. The only thing to take into account is that the hospital has good pediatric anesthesiologists and good pediatric recovery room. Children start organizing manipulation schemes very early. Early surgical correction allows the child to create those patterns without interruption and having to restart once healed. Early surgery has been advocated on psychological grounds, because it may be beneficial if the child considers the scarring and deformity to be the result of an operation rather than the result of a personal deficiency.

## Blauth Type I

Treatment must be approached according to the deformity present. Most patients with Blauth type I deficiency do not need surgical intervention. The affected thumb tends to be smaller than the contralateral thumb in patients with unilateral underdevelopment. In cases of bilateral hypoplasia, the patients have no reference and may not notice the deformity. The Blauth classification is extremely useful for planning treatment, yet it is only a general guideline. We must understand that some variations can occur.

A good example is the 16-year-old girl shown in Fig. 4.9 who suffers from trichorhinophalangeal syndrome that affected her mother and her younger sister (Fig. 4.10). Thin hair, a pear-shaped nose, and short phalanges of the thumb characterize this syndrome. In her case, both thumbs were hypoplastic with a stable MCP joint and a wide first web space but without the thenar muscles. We considered this case a variation of type I in the Blauth classification. Others will consider this case an intermediate between types I and II, while still others will consider it a mild case of type II.

## Opponensplasty

For opposition, it is possible to use the Camitz palmaris longus transfer [5], the ring finger flexor digitorum superficialis transfer as described by Royle [6], or the hypothenar transfer as described by Huber [7]. In this same young female patient, an opponensplasty utilizing the abductor digiti minimi was required to improve function. This technique is known as Huber's transfer because he first described it to restore opposition after median nerve injuries [7]. The abductor digiti minimi is used to reconstruct thumb opposition and to give better cosmetic appearance to the thumb by reshaping the thenar eminence.

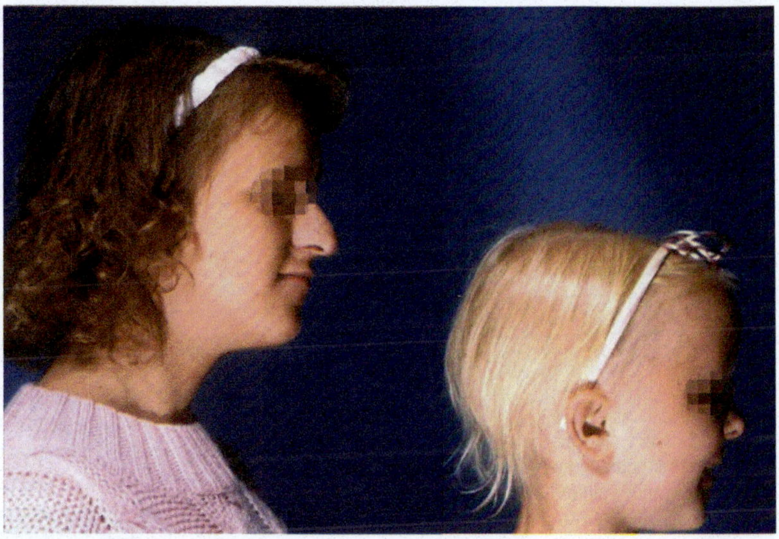

**Fig. 4.10** Sparse hair as seen in the younger sister and pear-shape nose as seen in the patient are features of this condition. This group of features were missed by the original treating physician

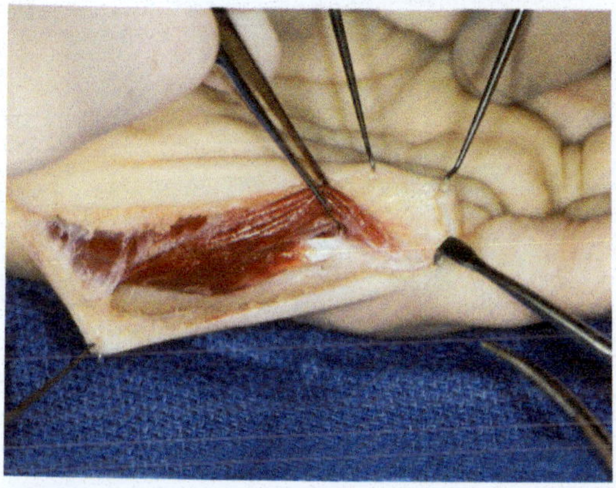

**Fig. 4.11** The approach to Huber's transfer starts with a longitudinal incision at the junction between the dorsal and palmar skin on the hypothenar region, extending from the pisiform to the proximal finger crease; this will provide an excellent view to protect the vital structures

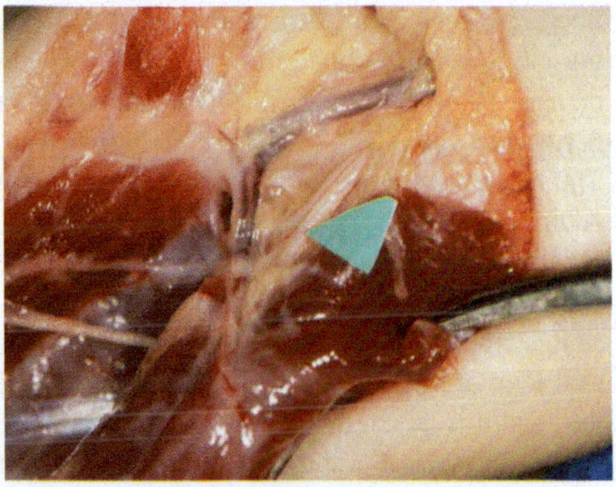

**Fig. 4.12** Marked with a green piece of plastic is the common branch to the hypothenar muscles; care should be taken to separate the branch to the abductor digiti minimi from that of the flexor digiti minimi. Keeping the attachment/origin of the ADM to the pisiform prevents damage to the vascular pedicle that originates from the deep branch of the ulnar artery

This demanding surgical technique begins with the first incision made at the midportion of the ulnar aspect of the proximal phalanx of the small finger (Fig. 4.11). The incision extends slightly curved radially to a point distal from the pisiform and ends at the wrist crease in line with the ring finger. The membrane that covers the abductor digiti minimi (ADM) is incised, and the muscle and its two tendon insertions are exposed. The distal tendon insertion is detached, keeping as much tendon length as possible. The proximal insertion lies at the MCP joint capsule, and it should be detached carefully to preserve the capsule. The ADM muscle is dissected proximally. Care should be taken to identify and protect the divisions of the minor pedicles from the common digital artery to the fourth metacarpal space as well as the proper digital nerve. The neurovascular structures at their entrance at the radial aspect should also be protected (Fig. 4.12). The flexor digiti minimi lies adjacent to the ADM on its radial aspect, and, in some instances, some of its

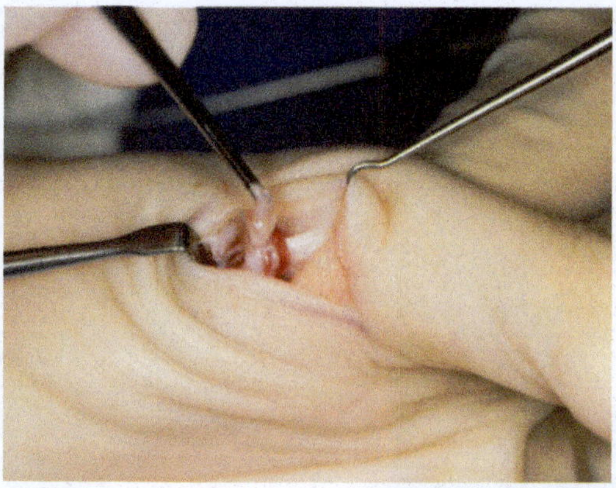

**Fig. 4.13** After passing the ADM through the wide tunnel created subcutaneously from the pisiform to the base of the proximal phalanx of the thumb on the radial side, the tendon is weaved to the insertion of the fibrous remnant of the APB

fibers are dissected along with the ADM. The muscle is never detached from its origin to avoid damage to its blood supply. Once this has been performed, the ADM is ready to be transferred. The extensor digiti minimi takes over from the ADM and provides small finger abduction.

A subcutaneous tunnel is made, connecting the hypothenar area to the thumb, and a second incision is made at the level of the metacarpophalangeal joint of the thumb. The ADM is then rotated 90°, and it is transferred from the pisiform to the second incision at the dorsum of the thumb through the tunnel. It is important to widen the tunnel so that the ADM lies freely through it. The distal insertion is sutured to the extensor hood and to the ulnar capsule of the MCP joint. The proximal insertion is sutured to the radial capsule (Fig. 4.13). We feel that the appropriate name for this procedure is abductorplasty, as we cannot make the thumb to rotate to oppose the other digits. This procedure is also a good indication for Blauth type II even though there are many other steps necessary that are not corrected by the Huber's transfer.

## Blauth Type II

A type II thumb is characterized by a hypoplastic thenar eminence that is responsible for a narrow first web space. An aberrant muscle often runs

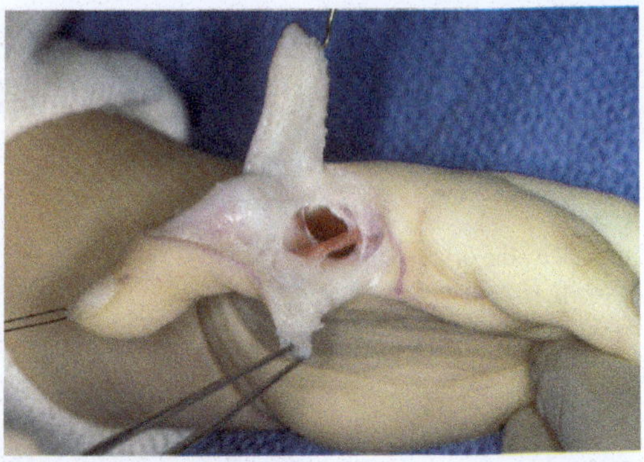

**Fig. 4.14** This little aberrant muscle between the thumb and the index metacarpophalangeal joints, even small, aggravates the contracture of the first web space

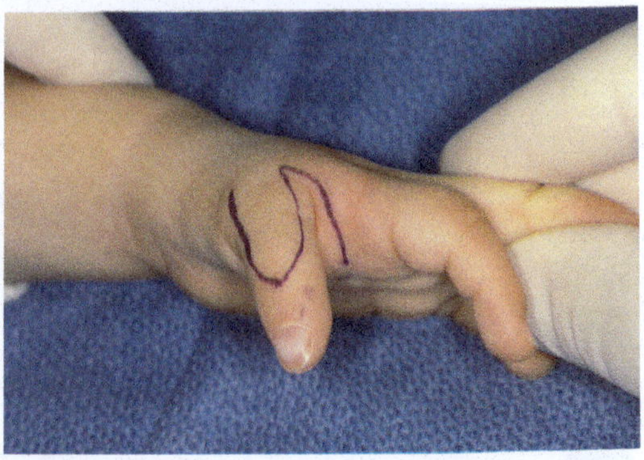

**Fig. 4.15** The dorsal thumb flap described by Strauch must be drawn passing the interphalangeal joint by up to 3 mm in order the right point in the palm of the hand to release the first web contracture

between the thumb and index finger, thus exacerbating the contracture (Fig. 4.14). To allow for a grasp with some span in the first web space, the metacarpophalangeal joint is lax at the ulnar collateral ligament. Treatment of this condition requires release of the first web space, reconstruction of the ulnar collateral ligament, and an opponensplasty. A flap is needed to widen the first web space and can be obtained either from the dorsum of the index finger or from the dorsum of the thumb, as described by Strauch in 1975 (Fig. 4.15) [8]. The Strauch flap should be raised up to 3–4 mm distal from the interphalangeal (IP) joint of the thumb. Radial and ulnar mid-axial lines are marked. The radial mid-axial line extends proximally to the basilar crease of the thumb. The ulnar mid-axial line widens at the

MCP joint to the middorsal aspect of the first web space, and it extends over the palmar aspect between the thumb and index finger to open the web space. The palmar incision extends from the free border of the web space to the connection point of the first and second metacarpals.

The flap can then be elevated to expose the fascia, the superficial veins, and the branches of the radial nerve. We then expose the adductor brevis, the insertion of the palmar thenar intrinsic muscles, and the whole ulnar aspect of the thumb. Once the soft tissues have been released and the aberrant muscle is divided, the thumb can be totally abducted, and the previously elevated flap lies over the dorsal aspect of the web space. This flap is then slid to the palmar surface, closing the previous incision. To close the donor defect on the thumb, the radial-palmar aspect of the divided web is rotated dorsally to the mid-axial line. The remaining area on the dorsal aspect of the thumb is closed with a full thickness skin graft.

A technique described by Lister [9] reconstructs the ulnar collateral ligament and creates an opponensplasty with the use of the flexor digitorum superficialis (FDS) of the ring finger, while the first web space is widened with a dorsal flap from the thumb. For cosmetic purposes, however, the best opponensplasty uses the ADM muscle. Sometimes a combination of both techniques is necessary to obtain desired function. Royle first described the opponensplasty using the FDS of the ring finger [6]. Lister added the reconstruction of the ulnar collateral ligament to this technique and also combined it with the flap from the dorsum of the thumb described by Strauch.

This technique is as follows. Incisions are marked at the proximal crease of the ring finger, toward the ulnar side at the distal wrist crease and in the middle of the first web space (Fig. 4.16). The first incision is made at the base of the ring finger. Through this incision, the flexor tendon sheath is opened between the A1 and the A2 pulleys. At this point, the superficialis tendon is still superficial to the profundus, so the decussation of the FDS tendon and the palmar aspect of the proximal interphalangeal (PIP) joint are avoided. A second incision is made proximally and ulnarly from the carpal tunnel to retract the palmar fascia

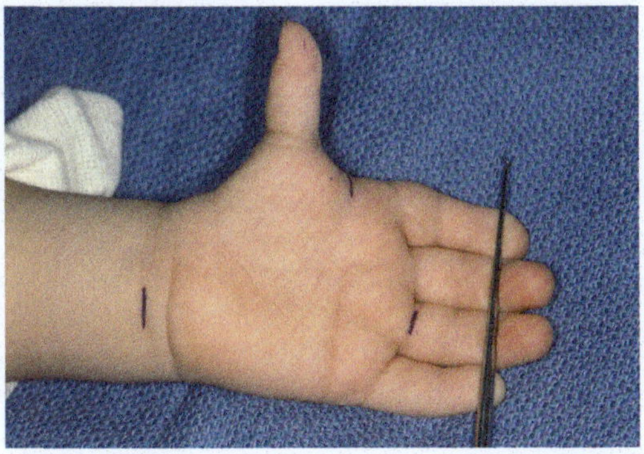

**Fig. 4.16** The three incisions needed to do the reconstruction of the Blauth type II thumb hypoplasia using Lister technique. The incision of the first web space is adjusted according to the length of the dorsal thumb flap

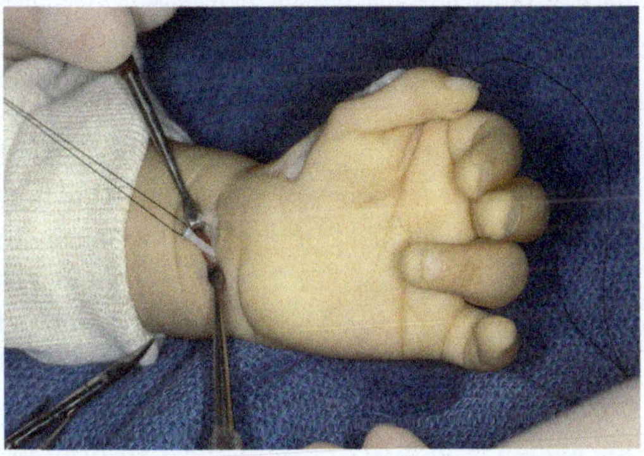

**Fig. 4.17** The FDS to the ring finger is identified and tested before it is divided

radially. Through this incision, the flexor digitorum superficialis to the ring finger is identified (Fig. 4.17). An incision is made over the dorsal aspect of the thumb at the level of the MCP joint. A subcutaneous tunnel is made between the last two incisions. It is important to create the tunnel wide enough so that the tendon runs freely. A hole is created at the head of the first metacarpal from ulnar to radial, that will allow the FDS tendon to be inserted once it has been passed through the tunnel created between the wrist crease and the first metacarpal head. A second tunnel is drilled from anterior to posterior aspects at the ulnar side of the first proximal phalanx, distal from the epiphysis. The flexor digitorum superficialis that was divided at the base of the ring finger is then transported from the ring finger into the palmar incision and through the tunnel previ-

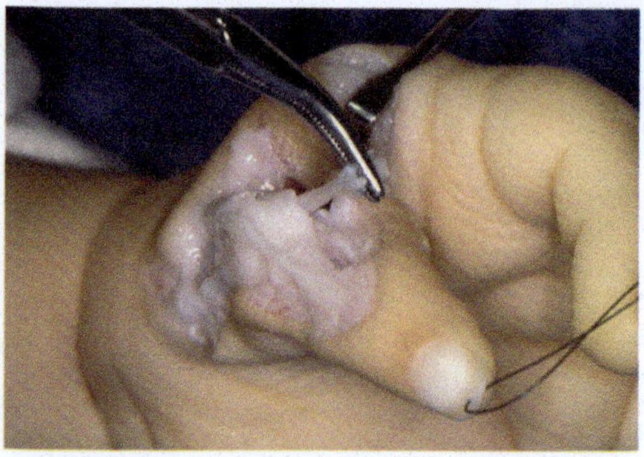

**Fig. 4.18** Once the FDS tendon has been passed in the subcutaneous tunnel between the wrist crease and the radial aspect of the thumb. The tendon is passed from radial to ulnar at the first metacarpal head. Tighten as much as required to abduct the thumb; then it is passed at the base of the proximal phalanx to reconstruct the ulnar collateral ligament of the MCP joint

ously made to the incision at the dorsal aspect of the thumb. The tendon is passed through the hole at the metacarpal head from radial to ulnar with the use of a 12-gauge needle to create the opponensplasty (Fig. 4.18). The tendon is then passed through the holes at the base of the first proximal phalanx. Appropriate tension is applied, and then the tendon is sutured to itself at the exit from the phalanx. In this manner, we achieve the reconstruction of the ulnar collateral ligament as anatomically accurate as possible. The incisions are then closed.

## Blauth Type III

Type III represents a further deficiency in the development of the thumb. Here we have instability of the metacarpophalangeal joint and, in some cases, a rudimentary or even absent basal joint of the thumb. Reconstruction of type III-B, as described by Manske, requires, in many cases, transposing a joint to stabilize or fuse the MCP joint. This procedure, however, creates a thumb in a position of reduced mobility and strength. These children have little cortical representation of the thumb, and, for this reason, they will continue to use the prehension between the index and middle fingers.

Many surgeons disagree about the possibility of reconstruction of type III thumbs in the Blauth classification. Manske and others have subclassified these thumbs into types III-A and III-B. The Japanese group headed by Minoru Shibata [10] has performed extensive reconstruction in these cases. They reported on four patients with reconstruction of a Blauth type III-B hypoplastic thumb with the use of a free vascularized metatarsophalangeal joint. Several tendon transfers also were performed, either primarily or secondarily, to mobilize the reconstructed thumb. Three patients (three hands) were followed for at least 2 years after the reconstruction; the results for these three patients were compared with those for four patients (six hands) who had been managed with pollicization of the index finger because of a similar deformity of the thumb. The patients were evaluated with regard to grip strength, key pinch strength, and the range of motion of the joints of the thumb in the operatively treated and contralateral hands as well as with regard to skill in performing activities of daily living as assessed with the use of the Kobe hand function test. Although the appearance of the thumb was closer to normal in the group that had had the pollicization procedure, total function of the hand and grip strength were greater in the group that had had the transfer procedure. Guy Foucher et al. [11] reported their finding, and it was different from those of Shibata. Foucher et al. said that they felt that pollicization is the solution for subtype III-B where the basal joint is absent. They had reviewed 14 cases of thumb hypoplasia type III, 4 of them being type III-B. After performing a first step with a free vascularized second metatarsophalangeal joint transfer, the secondary steps were identical in both subgroups. After a mean follow-up of 5 years, no great difference was found in the two subgroups, and basal stability was even better in type III-B. However, the results were functionally and cosmetically inferior to the ones observed after pollicization. He said that when the relatives refuse pollicization or the patient consults late for functional improvement, reconstruction remains worthwhile. In some countries, cultural reasons require that people have a thumb and four fingers; thus, the surgeon may have no alternative but to perform this reconstruction.

## Pollicization

Some surgeons believe that type III should be reconstructed by joint transfer or by another type of joint stabilization that will maintain a hand with all four fingers and a thumb. But as Littler and Riordan [12–15] assert, a reconstructed thumb with better mobility, tactile sensibility, and joint stability will provide a much better thumb for type III children. Therefore, we feel that types III, IV, and V should be treated by pollicization of the index finger for the best possible hand function. Because most apparatus used in activities of daily life are designed for people with the thumb on the radial side of the hand, pollicization of the index finger is preferred to pollicization of the little finger. Pollicization of the index finger will provide the best hand function, even in severe cases of radial clubhand where the hypoplastic phenomenon takes place from radial to ulnar, the index finger has a reduced range of motion at the PIP and distal interphalangeal (DIP) joints, and the flexor digitorum profundus (FDP) and flexor digitorum superficialis (FDS) tendons are conjoined. In children with severe aplasia of the index finger, however, pollicization is still performed even though the little finger will be used for handling small objects. The newly created thumb will be used as an opposing post to the other digits for handling larger objects.

The pollicization technique was described initially by Gosset in 1949 [16] and has been modified over the years. The first pollicization of the index finger in a child was performed by Zancolli [17] in 10-year-old boy. Buck-Gramcko [18] deserves special credit for improving and popularizing the index pollicization technique based on his work with many children who were affected by the mother's use of thalidomide. Many of the changes he implemented continue to be the norm for pollicization today. This technique is universally accepted for thumb reconstruction in congenital aplasia or hypoplasia.

The pollicization technique includes flap transposition to create a web space, removal of the shaft of the second metacarpal to provide three bones of the correct length equivalent to that of a normal thumb, and the use of the intrinsic muscles for stabilizing the new thumb. The first dorsal interosseous for thumb abduction and the first palmar interosseous for thumb adduction are especially important.

Basing our work on Buck-Gramcko and Lister, we have adapted the technique as follows. An acute angle is marked with its vertex located proximally over the most prominent point of the MCP joint of the index finger. The limbs of this angle face distally toward the neutral lines on the radial and ulnar sides of the index finger corresponding to the level of the web fold. The acute angle on the dorsum of the index finger is bisected by a line that is marked from the MCP joint to the PIP joint on the dorsum of the index finger (Fig. 4.19). The limbs are extended along the neutral line and meet at a transverse line drawn 2–3 mm proximal to the crease of the PIP joint at its palmar aspect (Fig. 4.20). In effect, we have

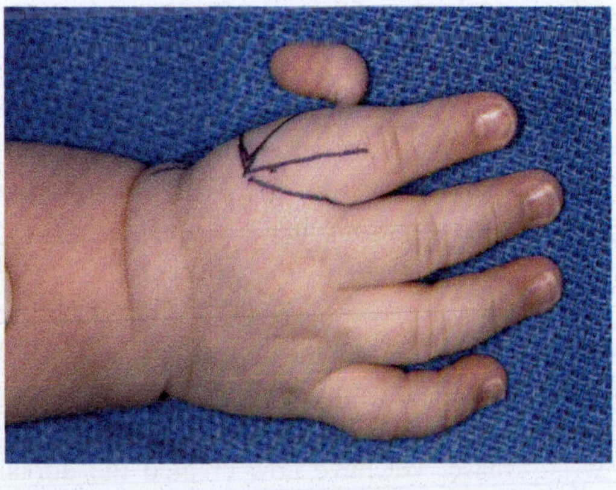

**Fig. 4.19** The markings on the dorsum of the index finger include an angle which vertex in resting on top of the proximal end of the metacarpal head. The limbs of the angle are directed to the mid-axial line of the index radially and ulnarly to the middle of the proximal phalanx. A line running from the PIPJ to MPJ bisects the angle

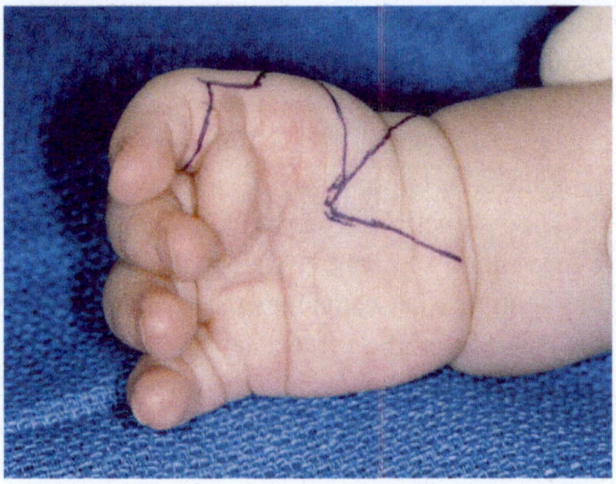

**Fig. 4.20** The proximal flap is triangular shape and oriented toward the volar midline of the long finger which will become the radial-most digit of the hand

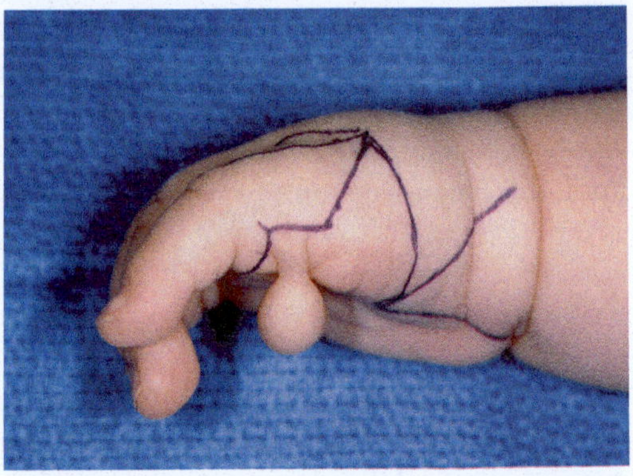

**Fig. 4.21** The markings are finished by connecting the dorsal incision on the index finger to a palmar line 2–3 mm proximal to the PIP joint crease on the volar aspect by a line running on the mid-axial line of the index finger. A line connects the vertex of dorsal angle to the vertex of the proximal flap in the radio-palmar aspect of the hand

now planned the dorsal flaps. The position of the new thumb is planned in relation to the middle finger that will become the radial-most finger.

A flap that will interdigitate with the dorsal flaps of the index finger is now created in the junction of the palmar and dorsal skin on the radial side, where the new thenar eminence will be. The palmar marking is created by first imagining a line extending from the center of the middle finger to a point in the distal wrist crease. We then make an actual marking that starts at the distal wrist crease and continues at an angle toward the metacarpal head of the index finger. This palmar marking must be the same length as the previous dorsal marking extending from the PIP to the MCP joint on the dorsum of the index finger. We then extend the neutral line from the base of the index finger to a point at the wrist (dorsal). From this starting point at the wrist, we make a second marking drawn proximal to distal to meet the distal edge of the previous palmar marking. In other words, the palmar marking and this second marking now join to form the vertex of a second acute angle whose limbs aim toward the wrist crease. We have now created the dorsal flap (Fig. 4.21). A line connecting both angles completes the surgical markings needed before we incise the skin.

Before we incise the skin, we slightly exsanguinate the forearm and set the tourniquet at 100 mmHg above the systolic pressure. Keeping

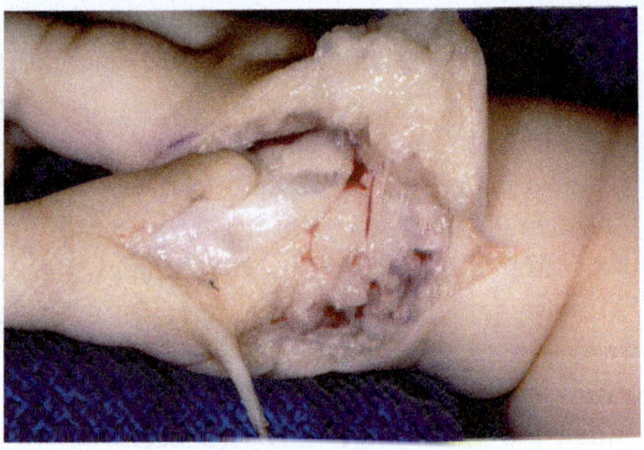

**Fig. 4.22** The skin and subcutaneous tissue are elevated from the venous system as far as the wrist. Here is where you notice the need not to exsanguinate completely the hand as the veins are visual with a little blood in them

some blood in the veins will help us to protect them once we start the dissection. The operation proceeds by incising the limbs of the acute angle on the dorsum of the hand. The skin is then elevated, and the venous system is identified, making sure that it is freed from the dorsa l skin to provide mobility (Fig. 4.22). The line that bisects the acute angle and extends from the MCP joint to the PIP joint of the index finger is now incised. We raise the skin flaps from the dorsum of the index finger, thus creating two dorsal flaps. The key point of pollicization is to avoid kinking of the blood vessels, especially the venous drainage. Once the dorsum of the hand has been incised and the veins have been identified and freed, the two flaps from the index finger have been created. One of these flaps will go toward the palmar aspect of the hand, while the other will stay at the dorsal aspect. Next, the extensor tendon mechanism is identified. The extensor indicis proprius is going to become the extensor pollicis longus. The extensor digitorum communis is used as an adductor in many cases. When elevating these tendons, it is important to identify them by different-colored sutures. Adhesions may exist between them and should be freed so that they can glide independently. In the dorsum of the index finger between the metacarpal head and the PIP joint, three slips of the extensor mechanism are created (Fig. 4.23). The radial slip will be woven to the first dorsal interosseous to create the abductor of the thumb forming the new thenar eminence muscle, and the ulnar slip will be woven to the first palmar interosseous. The central slip will be sutured to the extensor indicis proprius that will work as an extensor pollicis longus (Fig. 4.24).

Now that the dorsal aspect has been prepared and we are happy that the veins will be free from kinking, the palmar aspect is approached by elevating the palmar skin from the web space toward the middle finger, including the palmar skin over the proximal phalanx of the index finger (Fig. 4.25). Then we identify the neurovascular bundle and flexor tendon sheath of the index finger.

In a few cases, the radial digital artery is present in the index finger. When present, the radial digital artery should be preserved, together with the common digital artery between the long and the index fingers. If the radial digital artery is not present, then before we divide the branch that goes to the middle finger, we must check that a good blood supply is present to the middle finger through its ulnar digital artery. Before this vessel is divided, we apply clamps and deflate the tourniquet to check for blood supply. The proper digital artery to the middle finger is divided between ties of 8-0 nylon (Fig. 4.26). The common digital nerve is then separated longitudinally with scissors from distal to proximal up to the carpal ligament, avoiding damage to the fascicles going to either digit (Fig. 4.27).

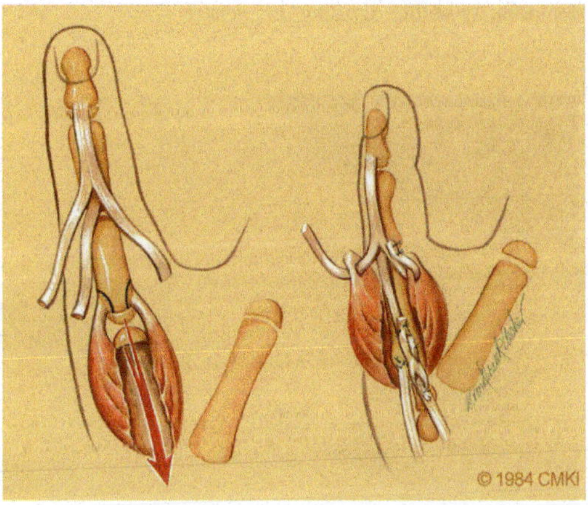


**Fig. 4.24** As depicted in the illustration, the central slip is weaved to the extensor indicis proprius (EIP) to become the extensor pollicis longus (EPL); the tension required is that which keeps the new thumb extended at the end of the procedure. The radial slip is woven to the first dorsal interosseous and the ulnar slip to the first palmar interosseous

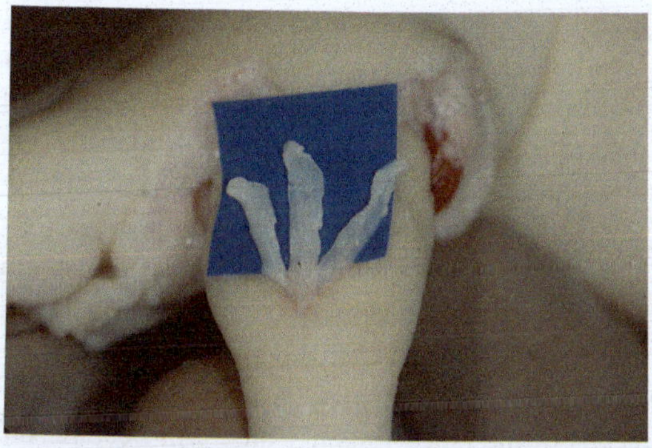

**Fig. 4.23** The three slips of the extensor apparatus must be dissected to the PIP joint. Enough length is required to weave them through the end of the intrinsic muscles

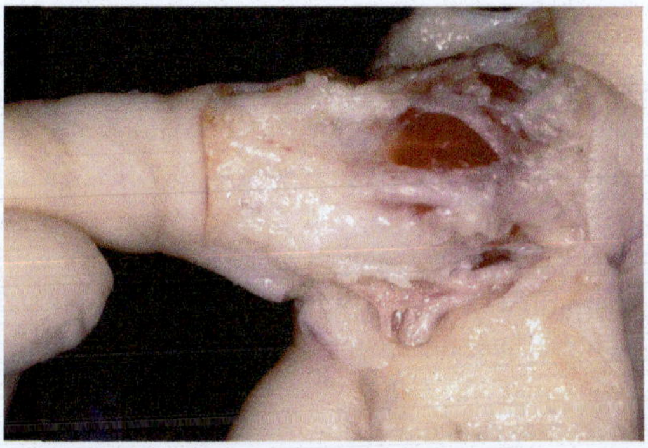

**Fig. 4.25** The palmar skin is elevated from the tendon sheath; care should be taken to avoid damage to the radial digital nerve and the vascular pedicle when it is present like in this case

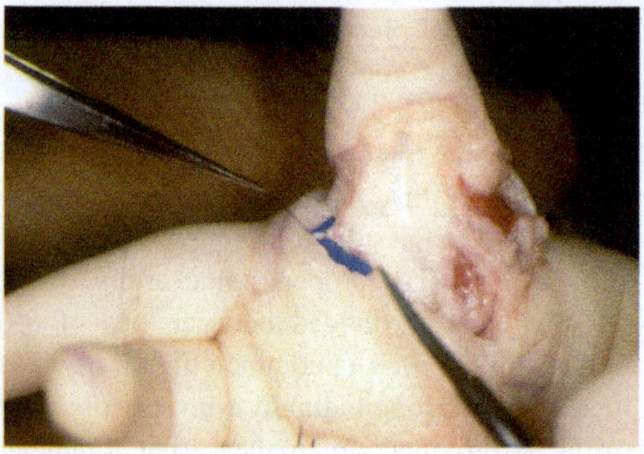

**Fig. 4.26** The proper radial digital artery to the long finger is divided between 8-0 nylon sutures in order to identify this vessel if circumstances arise. In cases of severe hypoplasia, we clamp the vessel and release the tourniquet temporarily before dividing this vessel

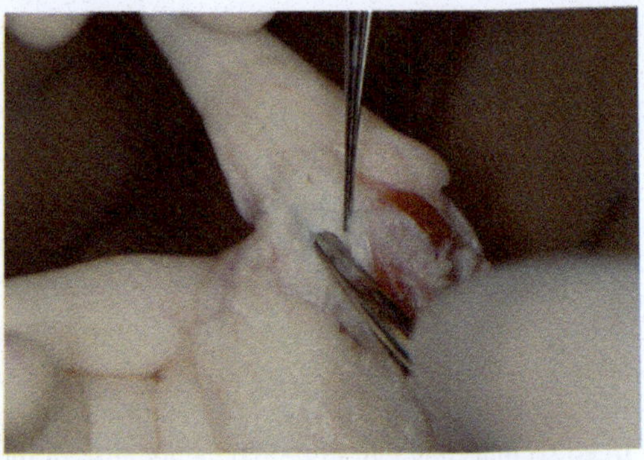

**Fig. 4.28** After we examine the flexor tendons to be sure they are free from adhesions and able to flex the new thumb, the tendon sheath is opened up to the proximal border of the A3 pulley; this will become the A1 pulley of the new thumb

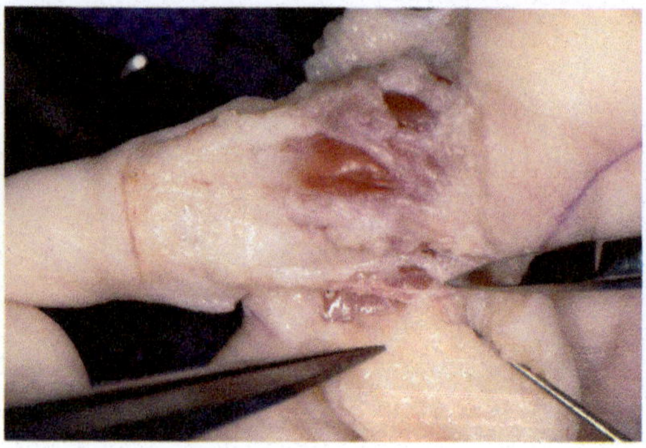

**Fig. 4.27** The common digital nerve between the index and long fingers is separated with micro instruments to avoid damage to the fascicles

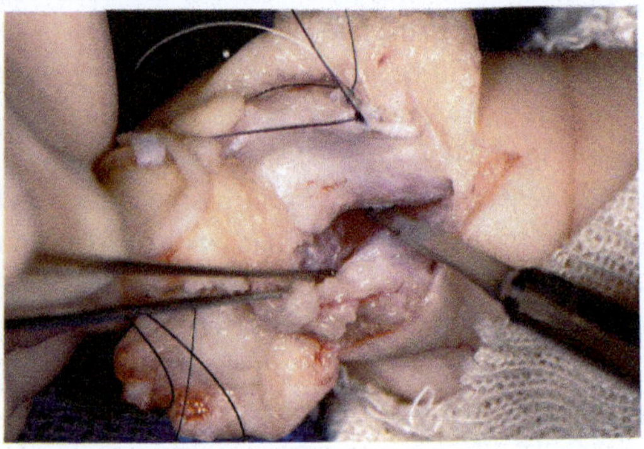

**Fig. 4.29** The intrinsic muscles are elevated from the periosteum of the second metacarpal with sharp dissection, keeping the periosteum intact in the second metacarpal. This will prevent the formation of unwanted bone in the future

The flexor tendons are then identified and mobilized to check that we have independent function between the superficialis and the profundus. The tendon sheath needs to be opened. We divide the A1 and A2 pulleys and stop at the level of the A3 pulley. This A3 pulley now becomes the A1 pulley of the new thumb (Fig. 4.28). The radial intrinsic muscle, the first dorsal interosseous, is then elevated from the second metacarpal with sharp dissection, avoiding damage to its innervation. Because the tendon of the first dorsal interosseous and the radial collateral ligament of the index finger blend together at the MCP joint, we are careful to separate the tendon of the muscle from the radial collateral ligament by sharp dissection. We must be sure that there is enough of the tendon to suture a slip of the dorsum of the extensor tendon to this muscle. We also maintain the stability of the MCP joint by preserving some of this radial collateral ligament. The muscle is then detached all the way to the base of the second metacarpal. At this point, the joint between the trapezoid and the second metacarpal is identified. The dissection of the first dorsal interosseous muscle should be done sharply, leaving the periosteum intact with the second metacarpal bone, which will be removed to avoid unwanted new bone formation in these areas (Fig. 4.29). The palmar interosseous of the index finger, which will become the thumb adductor, is also elevated and freed in a similar manner as the first interosseous. Small blood vessels will be present in the palmar aspect

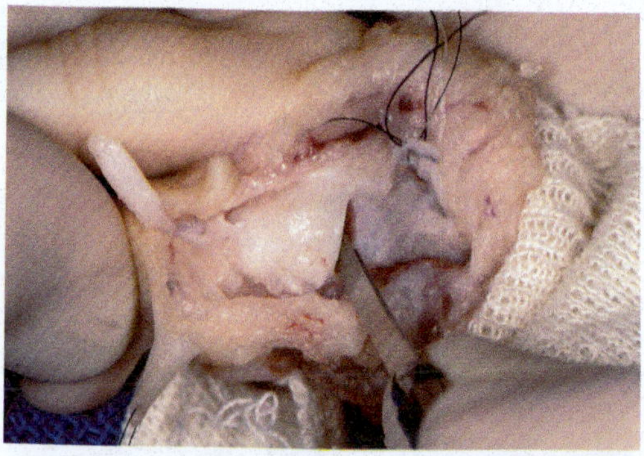

**Fig. 4.30** It is necessary to damage the growth plate at the proximal end of the metacarpal head. Failing to do that will allow further growth of bone in this area which produces zigzag deformity of the new thumb as the child grows

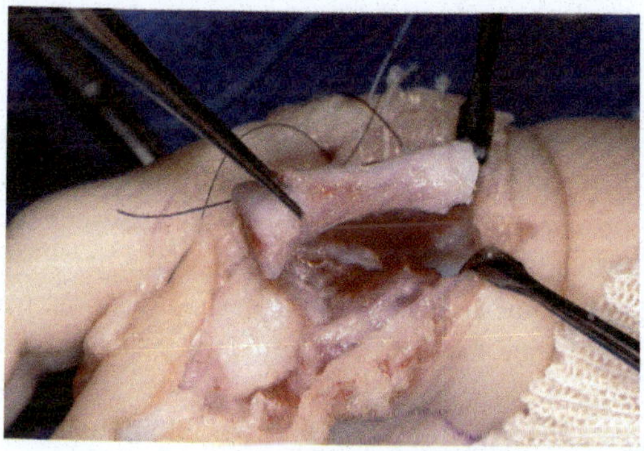

**Fig. 4.31** The shaft of the second metacarpal is removed from the distal epiphysis to the second carpometacarpal joint

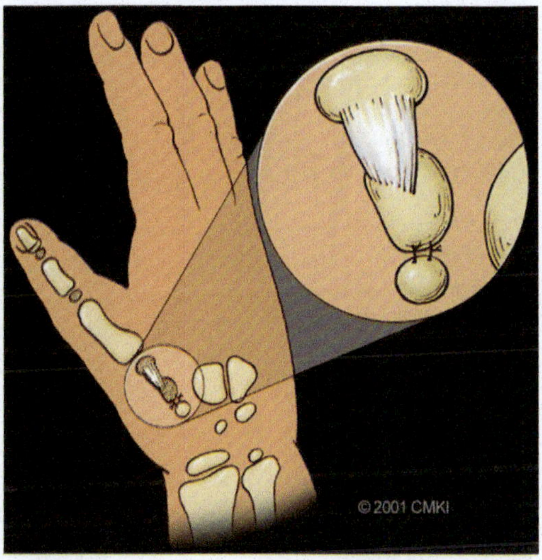


**Fig. 4.32** Hyperextending the metacarpophalangeal joint which becomes the new carpometacarpal joint of the new thumb will allow excellent flexion and prevent hyperextension of the new thumb, which affects the results both functionally and cosmetically

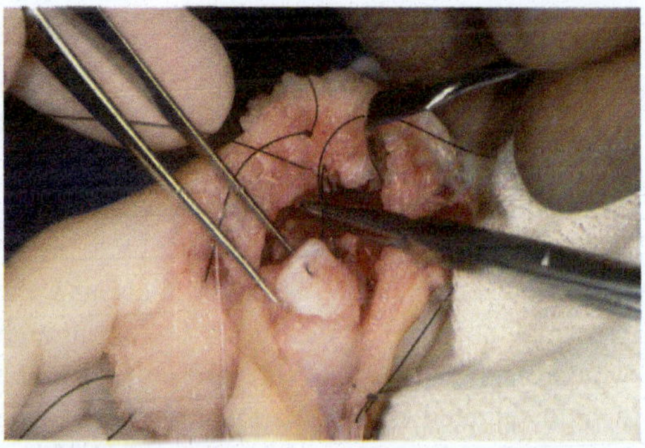

**Fig. 4.33** The head of the metacarpal is secured with nonabsorbable sutures to the area of the second carpometacarpal joint. This is the only need to fix the new thumb to the carpus; the rest is achieved by dynamic stabilization

of the metacarpal and must be coagulated carefully to prevent hematoma formation. The metacarpal is removed by utilizing a 69-beaver blade and penetrating the growth plate at the metacarpal head (Fig. 4.30). Destroying the growth plate is extremely important to avoid continuous bone growth in this area that eventually creates a zigzag deformity of the thumb. Once the metacarpal has been discarded (Fig. 4.31), we check to see if the index finger can move proximally without kinking any structures, especially the vessels.

As described by Buck-Gramcko [18], the metacarpal head now needs to be rotated into hyperextension before it is placed into position (Fig. 4.32), flexing proximally at the MCP joint that is now creating the CMC joint. Now the thumb will not hyperextend to create an ugly deformity in the hand. The metacarpal head is sutured by passing a nonabsorbable suture, preferably monofilament, through its most palmar aspect (Fig. 4.33). The index finger is then rotated 140° to oppose the middle finger (Fig. 4.34). The two sutures are placed into the trapezoid or in the remnant of the second metacarpal. This will be the only fixation for the base of the thumb.

The rest is a matter of balancing forces. The extensor indicis proprius is now woven to the central slip of the new thumb and will become the extensor pollicis longus.

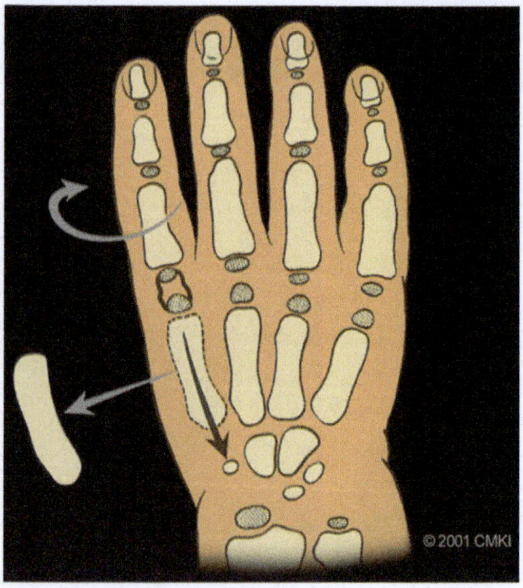


**Fig. 4.34** As suggested by Buck-Gramcko, the new thumb needs to be rotated 140° to oppose the rest of the digits. This is done when suturing the head of the metacarpal and maintained by the tension with the skin flaps

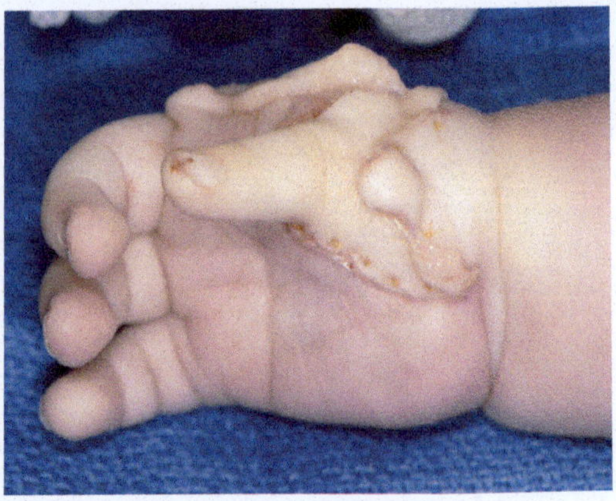

**Fig. 4.35** The position of the thumb depends on a good planning of the incision at the beginning of the case. Once the tendons have been secured, the final stability is given by the tension of the skin flaps. We need to make sure that we don't put too much tension as to create necrosis and infection but enough to obtain the best result

Enough tension is created, and the new thumb is fully extended on the operating table. The danger is that if the thumb is not fully extended, it will be flexed postoperatively. The abductor muscle should be as tight as possible to create opposition of the thumb. Care should be taken to create a window between the digital vessels and the proximal phalanx of the index finger through which we pass the tendon slip that is woven to the first dorsal interosseous. A similar weave is made between the ulnar slip and the first palmar interosseous. The interosseous muscles should not compress the neurovascular bundles on either side of the index finger, to assure the viability of the transposed digit.

Now we have all the muscle reconstruction needed. If desired, the extensor digitorum communis slip to the index finger is sutured at the base of the proximal phalanx of the transposed digit to create an adductor for this digit. Then we position the skin to create a good web space and properly extend and rotate the thumb into the desired position (Fig. 4.35). This is done by suturing the palmar aspect of the new thumb to the palm of the hand in the desired position. Both flaps on the dorsum of the index finger help to extend and to position the digit optimally. One flap will go between the palm of the hand and the proximal flap, while the other will go between the proximal flap and the dorsal skin of the hand. By tightening these flaps in the desired position, we can create the right cosmetic look of the thumb (Fig. 4.36). Equally important, the web space can be created so that no scar is placed immediately within the web space but rather dorsally. The scar should be a zigzag to avoid contraction in the future. It is important to note that the flexor tendons are not tightened. The flexor tendons can be free to avoid scarring while the child grows. The flexor tendons become competent approximately 6 months after pollicization.

Once all these steps have been completed, the tourniquet is released. We must check for good perfusion of the thumb. The skin should be trimmed to give the thumb a good cosmetic appearance. Before the dressing is applied, we should observe that the capillary refill is not too fast, which will mean that some venous obstruction is present. The dressing should be applied in a non-constrictive manner by avoiding circumferential dressing on the thumb. The elbow should be placed at 90°. The wrist is placed in neutral position. The tip of the thumb and the other digits should be visible so that the viability of these digits is maintained.

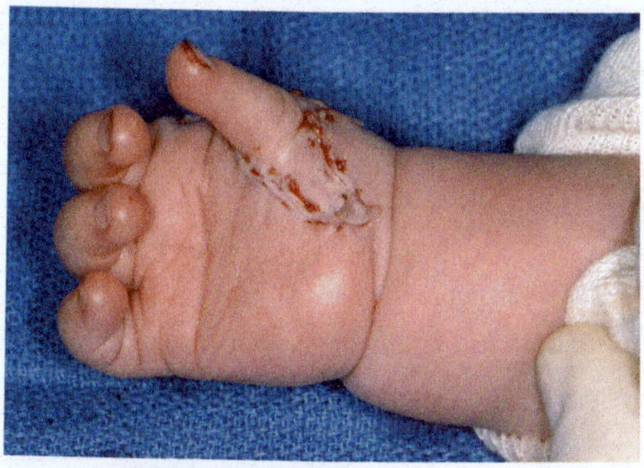

**Fig. 4.36** As the new thumb will have no opponens pollicis, the final position should have the new thumb touching the radio-palmar aspect of the tip of the long finger when they are flexed. After the tourniquet has been released for not less than 10 min, we check the speed of capillary refill; if too fast, we need to release some of the dorsal stiches to avoid congestion

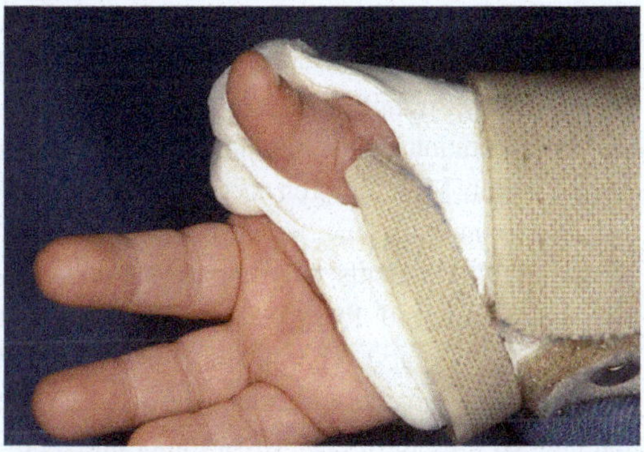

**Fig. 4.37** When the patient returns to the clinic for the above elbow cast to be removed, a plastic brace made to measure for the child is applied and used until the thumb flexor tendons are competent. This brace is only removed for bathing

Postoperative immobilization is essential. The arm must be elevated in a long arm cast that is maintained for 4 weeks. While applying the long arm cast, make sure that the assistant is not extending and bending the elbow as this will create constriction dressing bands.

The cast is then replaced with a properly made static brace that will maintain the thumb in a palmarly abducted position until the flexor tendons become competent, in approximately 6 months (Fig. 4.37). The patient's parent (or guardian) is given instructions for range-of-motion exercises that could include the use of the child's toys.

Pollicization is perhaps the most technically demanding procedure that a hand surgeon performs. To perform pollicization, the surgeon must know anatomy, biomechanics, and microsurgery. Technically, the surgeon must know how to plan and to manipulate skin flaps three dimensionally: to elevate and then rotate the flaps. The surgeon's microsurgical skill must also be highly developed just in case, at the end of the surgery, there is no blood supply either to the elevated index finger or to the middle finger left in place.

The results of pollicization depend upon the initial anatomic anomalies: when only the thumb is missing and the rest of the forearm muscles are normal, the results are very good. The more severe the anomaly, the less mobility can be expected, especially in a radial clubhand. In a child with severe radial clubhand, good results are not achieved as easily as in a patient with only a missing thumb but a normal hand and forearm. In severe cases of radial clubhand, the index is hypoplastic, the PIP joint is contracted, and there is little mobility of the flexor and extensor tendons. However, even in severe cases, the patients benefit from pollicization because they will be able to use the new thumb to grasp and to hold large objects and will continue to use the ring finger and small finger to grasp and hold small objects.

Variables in achieving good results include timing and the experience and skill of the hand surgeon. Timing is crucial: the earlier the better. A young child will be better able to adapt mentally to the new thumb. However, the child should be at least 6 months old so that the immune system is fully functional. Complications can arise from errors in the surgical procedure. For example, insufficient resection of the second metacarpal will make the thumb too long. Failure to destroy the epiphyseal plate will cause a flexion deformity. A lack of hyperextension of the MCP joint of the index finger at the time of pollicization, or incorrect rotation, will cause inappropriate opposition. Further complications can arise from accidental injuries to nerves or vessels or from inappropriate skin flap planning and excessive tension of skin flaps that may cause postoperative necrosis or infection. Of course, one disadvantage of pollicization is that we reduce the number of digits.

The advantages outweigh any disadvantage, however, because pollicization gives a child a hand with mobility, strength, sensitivity, and good cortical representation that is not present in the hypoplastic thumb. Most children accept this new thumb and use it naturally (Fig. 4.38). In fact, in a long-term study, 11 patients who underwent pollicization were followed for an average of 27 years (range, 20–38 years). The patients obtained good functional and cosmetic results. The results were maintained long-term [19]. Most importantly, pollicization gives the patient a new radial thumb that functions better than a stiff or ulnar-side thumb. Pollicization is also the most personally fulfilling procedure because the surgeon restores the function and usefulness of the hand to a child (Fig. 4.39a–d).

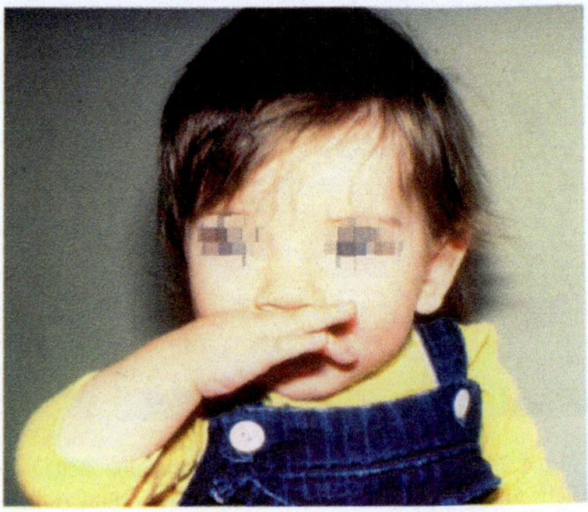

**Fig. 4.38** We know that the child has accepted the operation when he starts to suck his new thumb. At this point, nothing is needed; the child will use the hand with no limitations

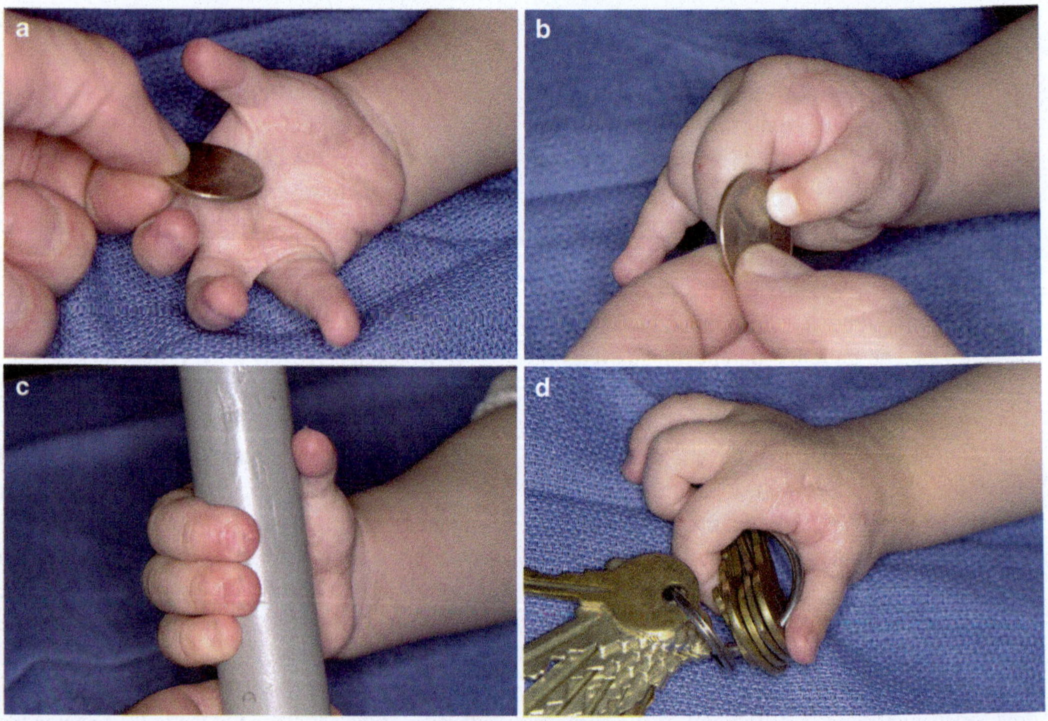


**Fig. 4.39** (**a, b, c, d**) The child should be able to open the hand with a good span; this is achieved only if the thumb can extend properly. Flexing the IPJ allows for a good and strong pinch. He should be able to hold big objects without the need for bilateral handling. Finally, he should be able to manipulate objects at will

## References


1. Lister G. Pollex abductus in hypoplasia and duplication of the thumb. J Hand Surg. 1991;16A(4):626–33.
2. Muller W. Die Angeboren en Fehlbildungen der menschlichen Hand. Leipzig: George Thieme; 1937.
3. Blauth W. Der hypoplastische daumen. Arch Orthop Unfallchir. 1967;62:225–46.
4. Manske PR, McCarroll HR Jr. Reconstruction of the congenitally deficient thumb. Hand Clin. 1992;8(1):177–96.
5. Camitz H. Über die beHandlung der Opposition-lähmung. Acta Chir Scand. 1929;65:77.
6. Royle NO. An operation for paralysis of the intrinsic muscles of the thumb. JAMA. 1938;111:612.
7. Huber E. Hilfsoperation bei Medianuslahmung. Dtsch Z Chir. 1921;162:271–5.
8. Strauch B. Dorsal thumb flap for release of adduction contracture of the first web space. Bull Hosp Joint Dis. 1975;36(1):34–9.
9. Lister G. The hand: diagnosis and indications. 2nd ed. London: Churchill Livingstone; 1984. p. 312–51.
10. Shibata M, Yoshizu T, Seki T, Goto M, Saito H, Tajima T. Reconstruction of a congenital hypoplastic thumb with use of a free vascularized metatarsophalangeal joint. J Bone Joint Surg Am. 1998;80(10):1469–76.
11. Foucher G, Gazarian A, Pajardi G. Reconstructive surgery of Blauth type III hypoplasia of the thumb. Chir Main. 1999;18(3):191–6.
12. Riordan DC. Congenital absence of the radius. J Bone Joint Surg. 1955;37A(6):1129–40.
13. Littler JW. The neurovascular pedicle method of digital transposition for reconstruction of the thumb. Plast Reconstr Surg. 1953;12:303–19.
14. Littler JW. Digital transposition. Curr Pract Orthop Surg. 1966;3:157–72.
15. Littler JW. On making a thumb: one hundred years of surgical effort. J Hand Surg. 1976;1A(l):35–51.
16. Gosset J. La Pollicisation de L'index (technique chirurgicale). J Chir (Paris). 1949;65:403–11.
17. Zancolli E. Transplantation of the index finger in congenital absence of the thumb. J Bone Joint Surg Am. 1960 Jun;42-A:658–60.
18. Buck-Gramcko D. Pollicization of the index finger. Method and results in aplasia and hypoplasia of the thumb. J Bone Joint Surg. 1971;53A(8):1605–17.
19. Clark D, Chell J, Davis TR. Pollicization of the index finger. A 27 year follow-up study. J Bone Joint Surg. 1998;80(8):631–5.

# Other Developmental Anomalies

# 5

Hyun Dae Shin and Soo Min Cha

## Clasped Thumb

Congenital clasped thumb may present with a number of findings including joint contracture [1–6], tendon [1, 6], and ligament insufficiency [4], intrinsic muscle abnormality [1, 2, 4], and thumb index web space contracture [1, 2, 4]. This deformity is usually associated with other generalized musculoskeletal malformations, including arthrogryposis, digitotalar dysmorphism, and Freeman–Sheldon syndrome. The initial classifications have not been useful in the clinical setting. Thus, a more practical approach has been proposed by McCarroll [4] and expanded by Mih [7] (Table 5.1).

**Table 5.1** The classification of clasped thumb by McCarroll and Mih

| Type | Features |
|---|---|
| I | Supple thumb<br>Absent or hypoplastic extensor mechanism |
| II | – Joint contracture<br>– Collateral ligament abnormality<br>– First web space contracture<br>– Thenar muscle abnormality |
| III | – Associated with arthrogryposis or its associated syndromes (mental retardation, aphasia, shuffling gait, and adducted thumbs)<br>– Extensor mechanism may have minimal or no abnormality |

H. D. Shin · S. M. Cha (✉)
Department of Orthopaedic Surgery,
Chungnam National University, Daejeon, South Korea
e-mail: hyunsd@cnu.ac.kr

## Clinical Features

Extension lag is present only at the metacarpophalangeal (MCP) joint, suggesting hypoplasia of the extensor pollicis brevis muscle tendon unit [5, 6]. Additional extensor pollicis longus and/or abductor pollicis longus anomalies have also been reported [7]. The diagnosis of clasped thumb is often delayed because an infant frequently holds the thumb within the palm for the first 3–4 months. The male-to-female ratio is reportedly 2.5:1 by Lin et al. [8] or 1:1 by Tsuyuguchi et al. [9]. This difference can be attributed to the wide variety of syndromes associated with clasped thumb and their different modes of inheritance, as well as the small number of reports in the literature that have documented the sex ratio of affected cases.

## Treatment

The generally established treatment methods follow Weckesser et al. [10], Lipskeir and Weizenbluth [1], and McCarroll [4], who divided clasped thumb into two types (supple and complex) and treated the supple type with splinting and tendon transfer if splinting failed, while the complex type was treated by correcting the fixed contractures, reconstructing the lax ligaments, and tightening the skin as appropriate. Tsuyuguchi et al. [9] treated types I and II cases by splinting and operative treatment for type III



S. H. Woo (ed.), *The Thumb*, https://doi.org/10.1007/978-981-10-4400-7_5

and type II cases that did not respond to conservative management. The results of splinting are excellent for cases of type I clasped thumb [8, 9]. The small number of patients who were followed with a nonoperative treatment in this study was attributed to the delayed presentation of the patients, which was after the age of 1 year. Surgery is indicated for children who have failed splinting or present after 2 years of age. However, the degree of impairment must be considered during establishment of a treatment plan. Mild MCP joint extension lag does not hinder hand function and does not always require treatment (Fig. 5.1). Some deficiency of thumb extension that prevents grasp warrants treatment. Any associated thumb MCP joint or thumb/index finger web space contracture also requires treatment (Figs. 5.2 and 5.3). Initially, serial casting or splinting may be tried to release the taut skin and correct the contracture. Residual contracture correction must be managed surgically. In a type I clasped thumb, release of skin and subcutaneous tissue is usually sufficient to correct the contracture. Thumb/index finger space deficiency is treated with standard techniques of four-flap "Z"-plasty or dorsal rotation advancement flap [11]. A palmar skin deficiency requires a rotational flap in the palmar aspect of the thumb MCP joint. A modified dorsal rotation advancement flap [12] provides a long wide flap that

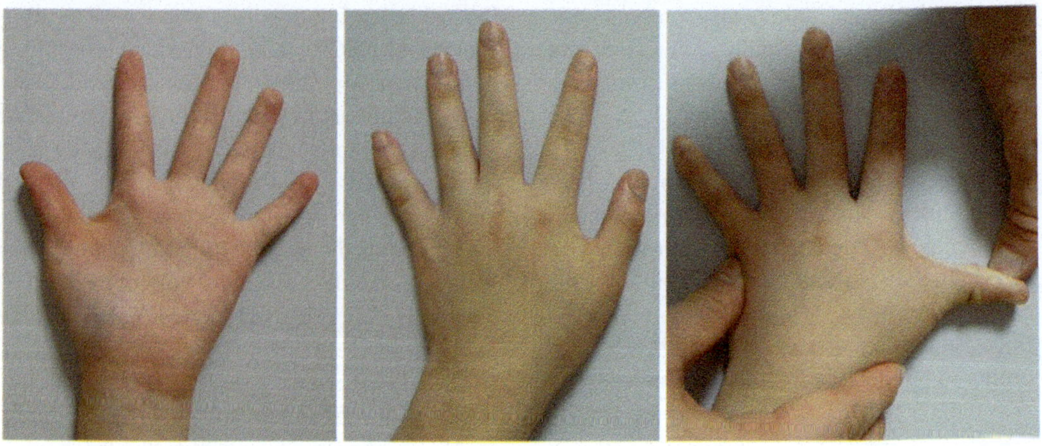

**Fig. 5.1** A type I clasped thumb with mild web contractures

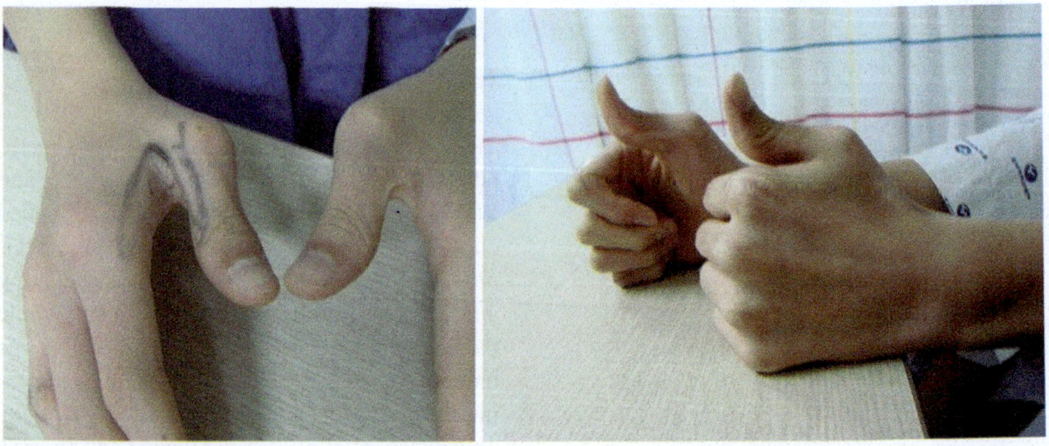

**Fig. 5.2** A type II bilateral clasped thumb with web contractures

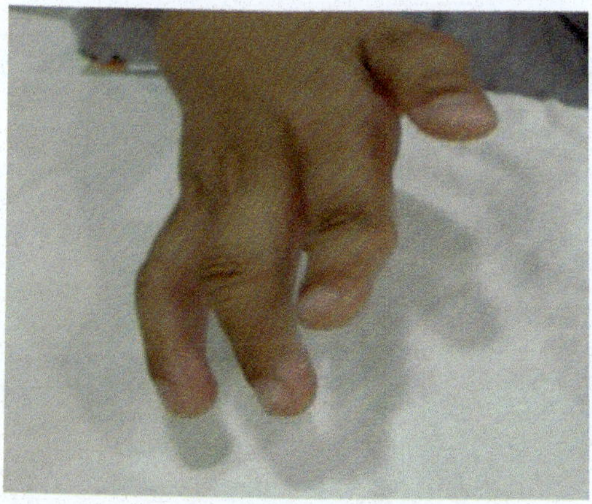

**Fig. 5.3** Clasped thumb in arthrogryposis

releases the thumb index web space with suture lines far beyond the web. In addition, it releases the palmar skin, even when very tight in cases of severe narrowing of the web. A second incision is made over the dorsum of the thumb metacarpal and proximal phalanx. The extensor apparatus is explored. The extensor pollicis brevis tendon is usually present but is small and attenuated. A tendon transfer is performed to reinforce thumb extensor function. The extensor indicis proprius tendon is the first choice, but it may or may not be present [6, 7]. Absence of the extensor indicis proprius requires selecting an alternative donor tendon. Options are the flexor digitorum superficialis and the abductor digiti minimi muscle [7]. The tendon transfer is secured into the attenuated tendon and/or the base of the proximal phalanx (Fig. 5.4). Tendon transfer was done as an original method using the bone tunnel of Broadbent [5] or suturing the extensor indicis to the weak extensor tendon of extensor pollicis brevis, as introduced by Mih [7].

## Treatment Considerations in Cases of Arthrogryposis

Hand function is highly variable, with intrinsic thumb flexion usually preserved even in the absence of other digital motion. There are several different patterns of hand deformities, some more commonly seen in specific arthrogryposis subtypes (Table 5.2). As with the general corrections for other deformities, fixed contractures need arthrodesis, whereas passively correctable contractures can be treated with a tendon transfer. In type 1, the CMC status remains an extension and the metacarpophalangeal (MP) shows a flexion contracture that is not flexible, and MP joint fusion (chondrodesis) is ideal. However, the more common thumb position is type 2 (flexed CMC, extended MP). In type 2, thumb opposition may vary from opposition to one or several fingers or to only the palm. If FPL motion is preserved despite the absence of other functions, reorientation of the thumb would be the more beneficial option for absence of proper prehension due to improper orientation of the thumb. The first web release is employed according to the degree of contracture. Traditional four-flap Z-plasty, dorsal rotational advance flap [12], and index rotational flap (Fig. 5.5) [13] are performed concurrently during surgery for chondrodesis/reorientation types 1 and 2. Modified new flaps have been introduced to cover a previous flap. Mahmoud et al. [14] designed a new flap to widen the web space further and correct the palmar contracture. They emphasized that the index rotational flap of Ezaki [13] provides insufficient skin at its apex, with the possibility of an incomplete correction and the frequent need for a thenar release incision. Abdel-Ghani et al. reported 4 years of follow-up outcomes in 39 patients with distal arthrogryposis [15]. They performed a modified rotational advance flap for the first web, an *a la carte* release of tight structures of the first web (intermetacarpal fascia, adductor pollicis muscle, first dorsal interosseous muscle, and capsule of the carpometacarpal joint of the thumb) to achieve full palmar abduction of the thumb, and finally stabilized the MP joint in extension by chondrodesis. They explained the importance of chondrodesis, as the presence of abnormal articular surfaces, poor inefficient muscles for transfer, and global instability of the MP joints making other reconstructions unpredictable. Chondrodesis also shortens the thumb ray, so it alleviates the need for release of deficient skin on the flexor aspect of the thumb

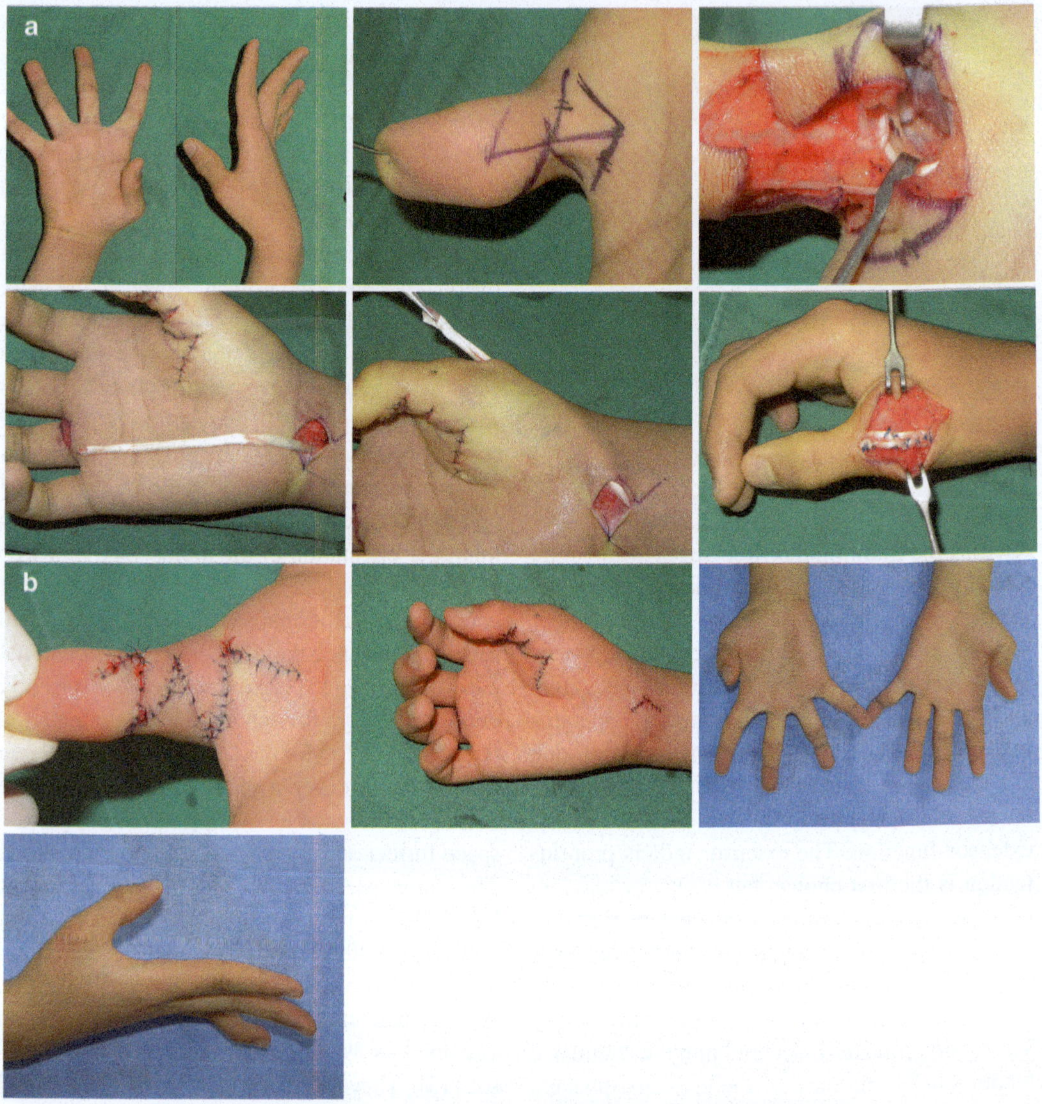


**Fig. 5.4** A type II clasped thumb with web contractures. (**a**) First, volar contracture was released by multiple Z-plasty and advanced local flap. Capsulotomy and adductor pollicis/volar plate release were performed. Instead of extensor indicis proprius, fourth FDS was harvested and transferred to extensor pollicis brevis (modified Becker's method). (**b**) After 53 months after surgery, abduction and extension of the thumb were all satisfactory. Images courtesy of Dr. Woo SH, with original copyright holder's permission

**Table 5.2** Classification of thumb contracture in children with arthrogryposis

| | Joint status | |
|---|---|---|
| Classification | CMC | MP |
| Type 1 | Extended | Flexed |
| Type 2 | Flexed | Extended |
| Type 3 | Flexed | Flexed |

and may also alleviate the need for lengthening the flexor pollicis longus muscle. In addition, they recommend waiting until radiological appearance of the ossific nucleus of the proximal epiphysis of the proximal phalanx of the thumb. This allows exposure of subcortical bone without injuring the physis and ensures good bone-to-bone union.

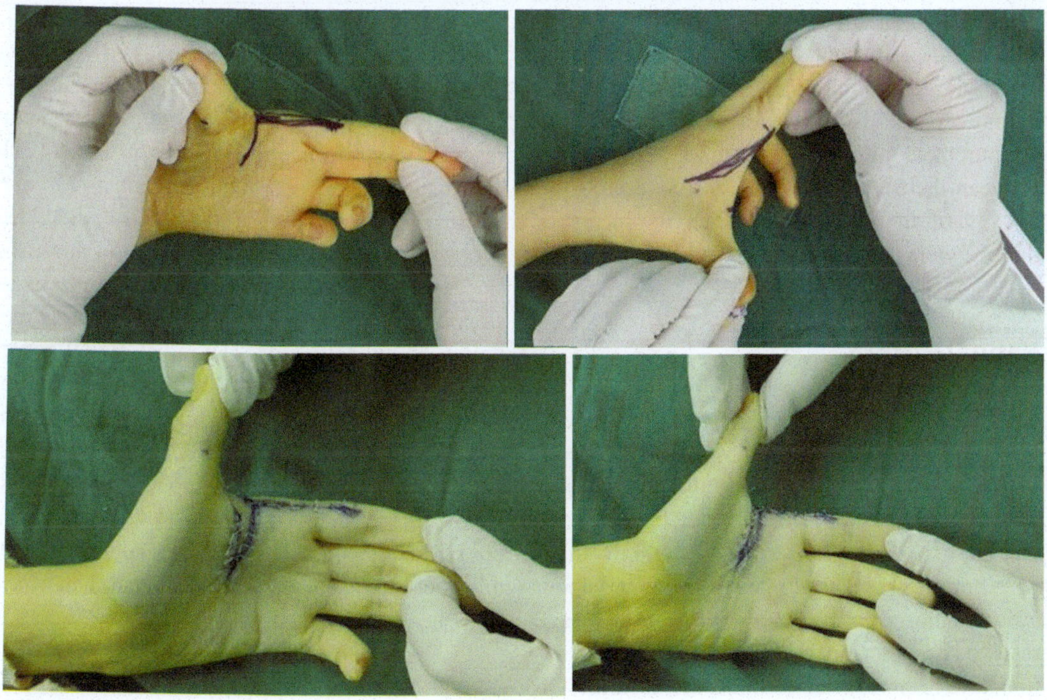

**Fig. 5.5** Index rotational flap

## Trigger Thumb

### Incidence and Etiological Findings

It is controversial whether pediatric trigger thumb is a congenital or acquired condition. However, several neonatal studies support the idea that it is an acquired condition. Initially, Get et al. reported an incidence of one patient per 2000 live births, based on a somewhat small sample size. The term "congenital" is now being abandoned because widespread evaluations of newborns have failed to discover trigger thumb. Rodgers and Waters [16] examined 1046 newborns, and Slakey and Hennrikus [17] examined 4719 newborns to determine the congenital incidence of this condition; however, no infants with trigger digits were identified by either study. After those reports, Moon [18] examined 7700 neonates within the first few days of life, and Kikuchi and Ogino [19] examined 1116 babies within 14 days after birth and noted no trigger thumbs. Furthermore, this condition of postnatal growth would come to be regarded not as "trigger thumb" but as "fixed flexion deformities" of the interphalangeal joint. The pathogenesis of trigger thumb was explained by two interesting ultrasonographic studies. First, Verna et al. [20] prospectively analyzed the FPL tendon and A1 pulley using dynamic ultrasonography in patients with pediatric trigger thumb. They explained that triggering always occurred at the A1 pulley and that there was focal enlargement of the FPL without abnormalities in the A1 pulley. They suggested that the initial inciting event is developmental enlargement of the FPL tendon. A second study by Kim et al. [21] clarified the anteroposterior and radioulnar diameter of the FPL just under the A1 and normal A1 pulleys. They found that the radioulnar distance of the FPL tendon increased to a greater extent than did the anteroposterior distance of the FPL tendon in cases of trigger thumb. However, they postulated that the developmental mismatch between the FPL tendon and the area under the A1 pulley is an important etiology of trigger thumb because the anteroposterior to radioulnar measurement ratio of the FPL tendon was similar between the trigger and contralateral thumbs; in this regard, the size of the FPL tendon in trigger thumbs seems to proportionately increase.

### Natural History

It is controversial whether pediatric trigger thumb is a congenital or acquired condition. However, several neonatal studies support the idea that it is an acquired condition. Dinham et al. [22] reported that approximately 30% of trigger thumbs diagnosed prior to 1 year of age resolved, and about 10% diagnosed from 6 months to 1 year of age resolved spontaneously. Higher rates of resolution have been reported from the serial studies on Asian populations [23, 24]. In particular, Baek et al. [25, 26] reported resolution of 63% of thumbs at an average of 48 months follow-up and 75.9% of thumbs (an additional 12.9%) at an average of 87 months follow-up. They emphasized that pediatric trigger thumb has the potential to spontaneously resolve after a sufficient observation period of more than 4 years, without developing residual deformities.

### Treatment

Nonsurgical management, including passive extension exercises as well as extension splinting, has been attempted but often results in persistently abnormal motion in 39–59% of patients [27]. Although steroid injections are commonly used to treat adult trigger fingers and are effective, they are not used in children and would be difficult to perform in an outpatient setting. Outcomes of splint therapy have been reported for a series of 40 trigger digits that were treated by applying a splint to hyperextend the interphalangeal (IP) joint during naptime and at night [28]. Twenty-three thumbs were relieved completely, and three patients required surgery. Slakey et al. [17] suggested that delaying surgery for up to 3 years would not be detrimental with regard to motion contracture. Kozin et al. [29] established their own guidelines, such as >1 year of age, with the need for stage IV surgery. The surgical procedure consisted of general anesthesia and loupe magnification. A transverse incision is made over the A1 pulley at the base of the thumb on the palm side. The radial digital nerve is identified and retracted. The A1 pulley is then identified and released. No further manipulation for a thickened nodule is needed. The wound is closed, and a soft dressing is applied with 1-week follow-up instructions. Percutaneous release [29, 30] of the A1 pulley has also been suggested, but this does not negate the need for general anesthesia (Figs. 5.6, 5.7, and 5.8).

## Triphalangeal Thumb

Several classification systems have been used, but the simplest and most often used is the Wood classification, which is based on the shape of the extra phalanx [31] (Table 5.3).

The incidence of triphalangeal thumb is about 1 in 25,000, representing about 3% of upper extremity congenital anomalies. It can occur sporadically, be inherited as an autosomal dominant trait, or appear as part of a syndrome (Holt–Oram syndrome).

### Treatment

There is no consensus on how this condition should be treated; thus, the definitive treatment depends on the type of triphalangeal thumb. The goal has been to reconstruct the thumb with adequate function prior to the development of oppositional pinch, which occurs between 12 and 18 months of age. Treatment of a minor length discrepancy or angulation can be delayed until later in life.

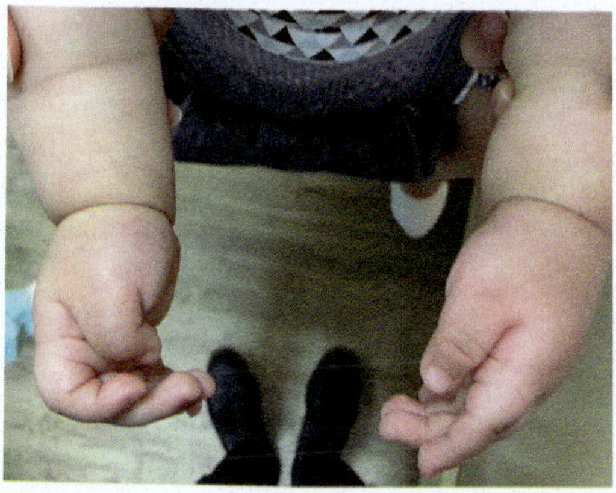

**Fig. 5.6** Trigger thumbs diagnosed at postnatal 9 months were relieved by conservative treatment at 4 years

- Type I: In an earlier presented case, excision of the extra ossicle, with or without reconstruction of the collateral ligament, and with or without pinning was recommended to allow for joint remodeling of the new IP joint with time [32]. Usually, a dorsal approach is preferred, with a longitudinal incision through the extensor mechanism. The extra phalanx is isolated and its size delineated. Osteoperiosteal sleeves are elevated from each side including the collateral ligaments. The extra phalanx is removed, and the collaterals are reattached (Fig. 5.9). Wang and Hutchinson reported good long-lasting results with acceptable

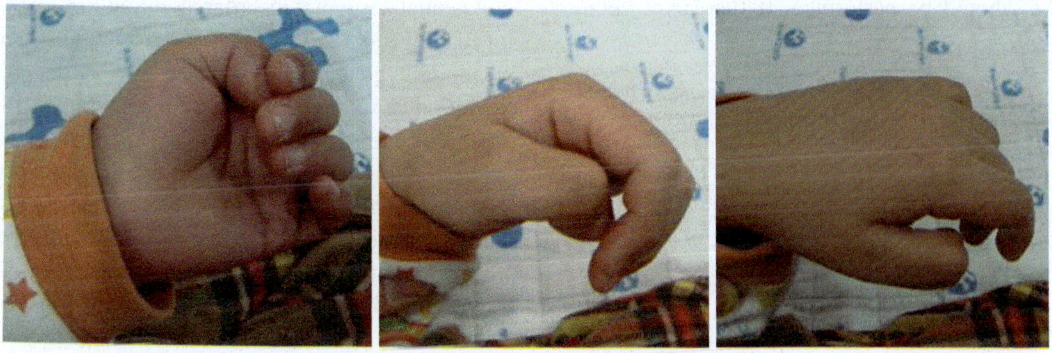

**Fig. 5.7** Trigger thumb diagnosed at postnatal 6 months was not relieved by conservative treatment until 5 years old

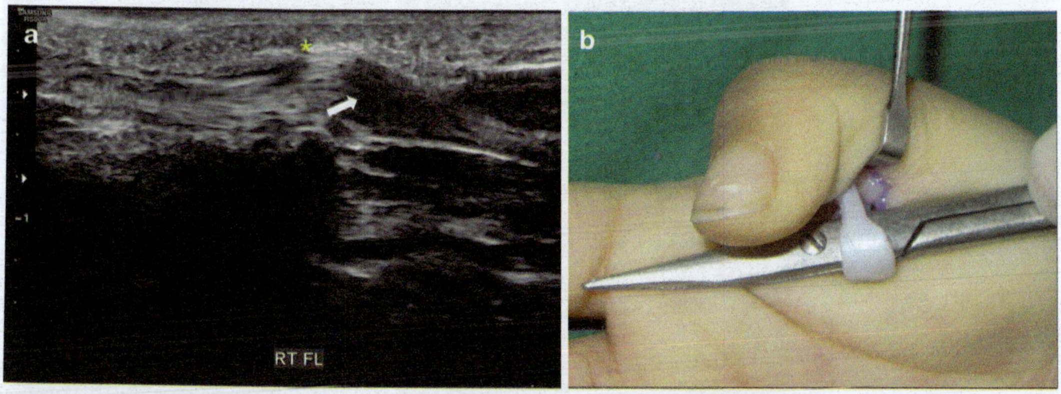


**Fig. 5.8** (**a**) A sagittal sonographic view of a trigger thumb showing thickening of the tendon (white arrows) just proximal A1 pulley (yellow asterisk). The thumb was passively extended during sonographic inspections with no more passage of the thickened area under the A1 pulley. (**b**) After surgery, the thickened flexor pollicis longus was identified with free movement. Images courtesy of Dr. Woo SH, with original copyright holder's permission

thumb IP range of motion (ROM) and no pain after excision for 21 thumbs with average ages of 22 months [33]. For cases that are older, a closing wedge osteotomy through the delta and distal phalanges with angular correction and resection of the extra joint is suggested for bony growth and further visualization of the bone and joint cartilage [34].

- Types II and III: The principle is that the joint with the greatest motion is preserved and the joint with the least movement is fused. A large, wedge-shaped extra phalanx has sufficient length; thus, a simple excision would commonly evoke subsequent instability. Proper bone resections, from the extra-phalangeal and adjacent joint side, to shorten and realign, should be performed. If there is a definitive angulatory deformity, an asymmetric osteotomy could correct the deformity [35].
- Duplicated thumb: The dominant part of a duplicated thumb should be preserved. If the triphalangeal component is determined to be the dominant part, the procedure for the extra phalanx is based on the above explanation [29].

**Table 5.3** The classification of triphalangeal thumb

| Type | Clinical features |
|---|---|
| Type I | The extra phalanx is triangularly shaped, often also called a delta phalanx |
| Type II | Rectangular- or trapezoid-shaped extra phalanx, which is not as developed as a full phalanx |
| Type III | Full extra phalanx |

## Symphalangism

Symphalangism is a rare condition in which the IP joint presents as congenital ankyloses in the thumb. The radial component in cases of thumb duplication has been reported as symphlagism in a few studies [36, 37]. It was used to describe an autosomal dominant disorder affecting PIP joints of the fingers [38, 39]. These are related to NOG or noggin gene mutations [40, 41]. However, many other studies considered congenitally stiff DIP and MP joints to be symphalangism. The nonhereditary symphalangism often seen with symbrachydactyly has a sporadic pattern. Baek and Lee graded three degrees, according to the clinical manifestations and radiological findings [42] (Table 5.4).

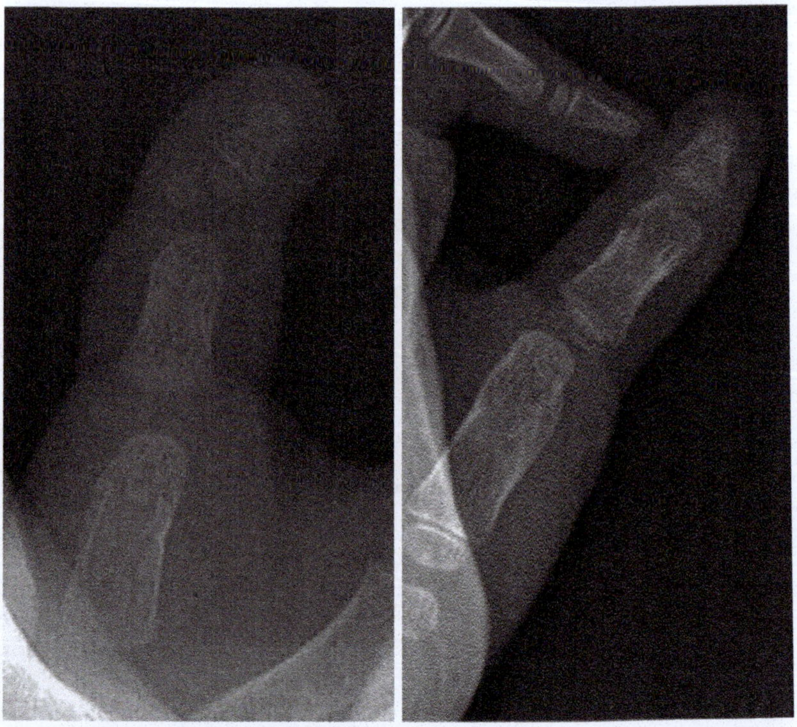

**Fig. 5.9** Delta phalanx was excised at 18 months and remained satisfactory until 5 years

**Table 5.4** Classification of symphalangism

| | Grade I (fibrous symphalangism) | Grade II (cartilaginous symphalangism) | Grade III |
|---|---|---|---|
| Volar skin crease | Faint or absent | Absent | Absent |
| Active motion | Absent | Absent | Absent |
| Passive motion | 10–20 | Only jerk | Absent or jerk motion |
| Joint space in simple radiographs | Mild narrowing | Definite narrowing | Joint space absent |
| Phalangeal head in lateral view | Round | Flat | Fused to adjacent bone |

Baek et al. [42] suggested grade I or early grade II thumb IP joint symphalangism before the age of 7 years could be an appropriate surgical indication. They explained that the thumb usually presents a slower progression than the fingers. Takagi et al. [43] resected all radial components of symphalangism and reported inevitable restricted motion at the IP joint type symphlagism (three cases) than at the MPJ joint type symphalangism (three cases). The dorsal capsule and dorsal halves of bilateral collateral ligaments divide after a Y-shaped dorsal incision. Gentle passive ROM exercises are initiated, with assistance, 2 days after surgery. Baek et al. explained that brain education may be needed to actively flex the joints, probably because the brain motor cortex for affected fingers has not yet formed.

## References


1. Lipskeir E, Weizenbluth M. Surgical treatment of the clasped thumb. J Hand Surg Br. 1989;14(1):72–9.
2. HR MC Jr, Manske PR. The windblown hand: correction of the complex clasped thumb deformity. Hand Clin. 1992;8(1):147–59.
3. Weckesser EC. Congenital flexion-adduction deformity of the thumb (congenital clasped thumb). J Bone Joint Surg Am. 1955;37(5):977–83; discussion 983–984.
4. McCarroll HR Jr. Congenital flexion deformities of the thumb. Hand Clin. 1985;1(3):567–75.
5. Broadbent TR, Woolf RM. Flexion-adduction deformity of the thumb: congenital clasped thumb. Plast Reconstr Surg. 1964;34:612–6.
6. White JW, Jensen WE. The infant's persistent thumb-clutched hand. J Bone Joint Surg Am. 1952;24(3):680–8.
7. Mih AD. Congenital clasped thumb. Hand Clin. 1998;14:77–84.
8. Lin SC, Hung TH, Hsu HY, Lin CG, Chiu HY. A simple splinting method for correction of supple congenital clasped thumbs in infants. J Hand Surg Br. 1999;24:612–4.
9. Tsuyuguchi Y, Masda K, Kawabata H, Kawai H, Ono K. Congenital clasped thumb: a review of forty-three cases. J Hand Surg Am. 1985;10:613–8.
10. Weckesser EC, Reed JR, Heiple KG. Congenital clasped thumb (congenital flexion-adduction deformity of the thumb). J Bone Joint Surg Am. 1968;50:1417–28.
11. Buck-Gramcko D. Syndactyly between the thumb and index finger. In: Buck-Gramcko D, editor. Congenital malformation of the hand and forearm. New York: Churchill Livingstone; 1998. p. 141–7.
12. Ghani HA. Modified dorsal rotation advancement flap for release of the thumb web space. J Hand Surg Br. 2006;31:226–9.
13. Ezaki MB, Oishi SN. Index rotation flap for palmar thumb release in arthrogryposis. Tech Hand Up Extrem Surg. 2010;14(1):38–40.
14. Mahmoud M, Abdel-Ghani H, Elfar JC. New flap for widening of the web space and correction of palmar contracture in complex clasped thumb. J Hand Surg Am. 2013;38(11):2251–6. https://doi.org/10.1016/j.jhsa.2013.08.107.
15. Abdel Ghani H, Mahmoud M, Shaheen A, Abdel-Wahed M. Treatment of congenital clasped thumb in arthrogryposis. J Hand Surg Eur Vol. 2017;42(8):794–8. https://doi.org/10.1177/1753193417712863. Epub 2017 Jun.
16. Rodgers WB, Waters PM. Incidence of trigger digits in newborns. J Hand Surg Am. 1994;19(3):364–8.
17. Slakey JB, Hennrikus WL. Acquired thumb flexion contracture in children: congenital trigger thumb. J Bone Joint Surg Br. 1996;78(3):481–3.
18. Moon WN, Suh SW, Kim IC. Trigger digits in children. J Hand Surg Br. 2001;26(1):11e12.
19. Kikuchi N, Ogino T. Incidence and development of trigger thumb in children. J Hand Surg Am. 2006;31(4):541–3.
20. Verma M, Craig CL, DiPietro MA, Crawford J, VanderHave KL, Farley FA, Caird MS. Serial ultrasound evaluation of pediatric trigger thumb. J Pediatr Orthop. 2013;33:309–13.

21. Kim J, Gong HS, Seok HS, Choi YH, Oh S, Baek GH. Quantitative measurements of the cross-sectional configuration of the flexor pollicis longus tendon using ultrasonography in patients with pediatric trigger thumb. J Hand Surg Am. 2018;43(3):e1–284.e7. https://doi.org/10.1016/j.jhsa.2017.08.011. pii: S0363-5023(16)31116-9. [Epub ahead of print].
22. Dinham JM, Meggitt BF. Trigger thumbs in children. A review of the natural history and indications for treatment in 105 patients. J Bone Joint Surg Br. 1974;56(1):153–5.
23. Michifuri Y, Murakami T, Kumagai S, et al. Natural history of the trigger finger in children. Seikei Geka. 1978;29:1648.
24. Sugimoto Y. Treatment of trigger finger digit in children. Seikei Geka. 1991;23:1047.
25. Baek GH, Lee HJ. The natural history of pediatric trigger thumb: a study with a minimum of five years follow-up. Clin Orthop Surg. 2011;3(2):157–9. https://doi.org/10.4055/cios.2011.3.2.157. Epub 2011 May 12.
26. Baek GH, Kim JH, Chung MS, Kang SB, Lee YH, Gong HS. The natural history of pediatric trigger thumb. J Bone Joint Surg Am. 2008;90(5):980–5. https://doi.org/10.2106/JBJS.G.00296.
27. Shah AS, Bae DS. Management of pediatric trigger thumb and trigger finger. J Am Acad Orthop Surg. 2012;20:206–13.
28. Nemoto K, Nemoto T, Terada N, Amako M, Kawaguchi M. Splint therapy for trigger thumb and finger in children. J Hand Surg Br. 1996;21(3):416–8.
29. Kozin SH. Deformities of the thumb. In: Wolfe SW, Pederson WC, editors. Green's operative hand surgery. 6th ed. Philadelphia: Elsevier; 2011. p. 1371–403.
30. Wang HC, Lin GT. Retrospective study of open versus percutaneous surgery for trigger thumb in children. Plast Recontr Surg. 2005;115:1963–70.
31. Wood VE. Treatment of the triphalangeal thumb. Clin Orthop. 1976;1120:188–200.
32. Horii E, Nakamura R, Makino H. Triphalangeal thumb with associated abnormalities: clinical characteristics and surgical outcomes. Plast Reconstr Surg. 2001;108:902–7.
33. Wang AA, Hutchinson DT. Results of treatment of delta triphalangeal thumbs by excision of the extra phalanx. J Pediatr Orthop. 2015;35(5):474–7. https://doi.org/10.1097/BPO.0000000000000319.
34. Jennings JF, Peimer CA, Sherwin FS. Reduction osteotomy for triphalangeal thumb: an 11-year review. J Hand Surg. 1992;17A:8–14.
35. Gousheh J, Arasteh E. Isolated bilateral triphalangeal thumb with delta phalanx: a case report. World J Plast Surg. 2013;2(2):111–4.
36. Flatt AE. The care of congenital hand anomalies. St. Louis: Mosby; 1977. p. 146–70.
37. Ogino T, Minami A, Fukuda K, Kato H. Congenital anomalies of the upper limb among the Japanese in Sapporo. J Hand Surg Br. 1986;11(3):364–71.
38. Cushing H. Hereditary anchylosis of the proximal phalangeal joints (symphalangism). Proc Natl Acad Sci U S A. 1915;1(12):621–2. No abstract available
39. Drinkwater H. Phalangeal anarthrosis (Synostosis, Ankylosis) transmitted through Fourteen Generations. Proc R Soc Med. 1917;10(Pathol Sect):60–8. No abstract available.
40. Takahashi T, Takahashi I, Komatsu M, Sawaishi Y, Higashi K, Nishimura G, Saito H, Takada G. Mutations of the NOG gene in individuals with proximal symphalangism and multiple synostosis syndrome. Clin Genet. 2001;60(6):447–51.
41. Takano K, Ogasawara N, Matsunaga T, Mutai H, Sakurai A, Ishikawa A, Himi T. A novel nonsense mutation in the NOG gene causes familial NOG-related symphalangism spectrum disorder. Hum Genome Var. 2016;3:16023. https://doi.org/10.1038/hgv.2016.23. eCollection 2016.
42. Baek GH, Lee HJ. Classification and surgical treatment of symphalangism in interphalangeal joints of the hand. Clin Orthop Surg. 2012;4(1):58–65. https://doi.org/10.4055/cios.2012.4.1.58. Epub 2012 Feb 20.
43. Takagi R, Kawabata H, Matsui Y. Thumb polydactyly with symphalangism in young children. J Hand Surg Eur Vol. 2009;34(6):800–4. https://doi.org/10.1177/1753193408092254. Epub 2009 Jul 10.

# Part III

# Bone and Joint Problems

# Fractures and Dislocations

# 6

Yun-Rak Choi

## Basic Anatomy of the Thumb

The thumb consists of only two phalanges, the proximal and distal, and one metacarpal, but it has greater movement than the other fingers, and it also has three plane motions from the trapeziometacarpal joint like flexion, extension, abduction, adduction, opposition, and retropulsion. The thumb interphalangeal (IP) and metacarpophalangeal (MCP) joints are hinge joints stabilized by proper and accessory collateral ligaments and volar plate. At the MCP joint, the proper collateral ligament arises from the lateral condyles and inserts on the volar aspect of the proximal phalanx. The accessory collateral ligaments arise more volarly and insert on the volar plate and sesamoids. The trapeziometacarpal joint, the key joint of the thumb, gives movements in three planes like sagittal, coronal, and axial planes with the unique anatomy, so-called the saddle joint. This joint consists of the concavo-convex articular surfaces of the thumb metacarpal base and the trapezium oriented in opposition to one another with perpendicular axes similar to two reciprocally opposed saddles. The joint is stabilized by its capsule and the palmar oblique, intermetacarpal, dorsoradial, and dorsal oblique ligaments. The primary restraints to dorsal subluxation and dislocation are the palmar oblique ligament and dorsoradial ligament [1].

All these three planar movements are controlled by extrinsic and intrinsic muscles like the flexor pollicis longus, the abductor pollicis longus, the extensor pollicis brevis, the thenar muscles (the adductor pollicis brevis, flexor pollicis brevis, and opponens pollicis), and the adductor pollicis muscle. The median nerve innervates most thumb muscles except the adductor pollicis and the deep head of the flexor pollicis brevis, which are innervated by the ulnar nerve. The blood supply is mainly from the princeps pollicis artery. Because of the thumb's unique, oblique orientation with respect to the palm, radiographs need to be taken orthogonally to the thumb, the lateral with the thumbnail perpendicular to the X-ray film, and either the posteroanterior or the anteroposterior (Robert) view with the thumbnail parallel to the cassette. The thumb carpometacarpal joint is best evaluated with a Robert view in which the forearm is fully pronated with the dorsum of the thumb on the cassette and the X-ray beam angled 15° from distal to proximal. (Fig. 6.1).

Y.-R. Choi (✉)
Department of Orthopaedic Surgery, Yonsei University College of Medicine, Yonsei University Health System, Seoul, South Korea
e-mail: yrchoi@yuhs.ac





S. H. Woo (ed.), *The Thumb*, https://doi.org/10.1007/978-981-10-4400-7_6

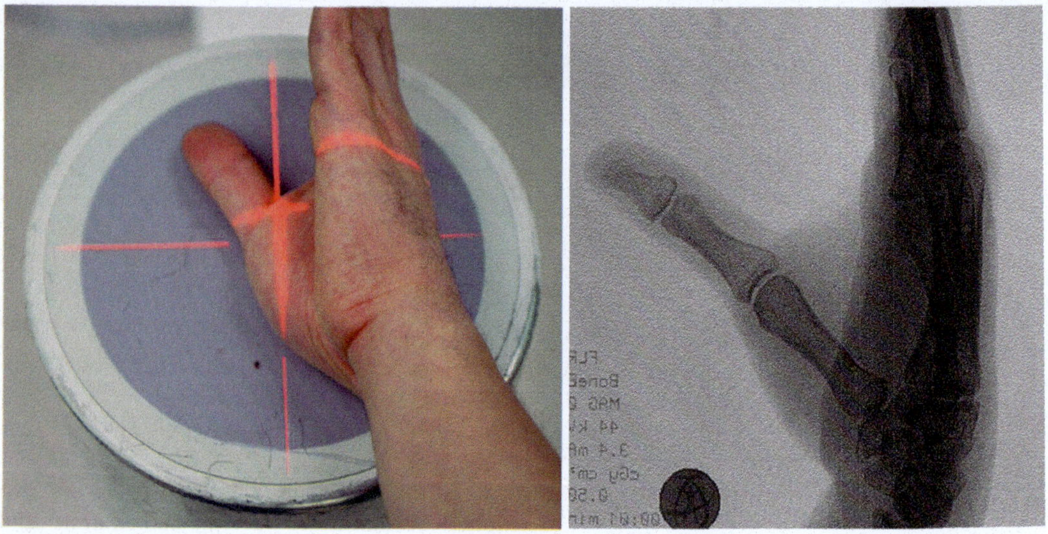

**Fig. 6.1** The thumb carpometacarpal joint is best evaluated with a Robert view in which the forearm is fully pronated with the dorsum of the thumb on the cassette and the X-ray beam angled 15° from distal to proximal

## Thumb Phalangeal Fractures

### Distal Phalanx Fractures

#### Extra-articular Fractures

Distal phalanx fractures are common sport- and work-related injuries and account for around 50% of all hand fractures [2]. These fractures are commonly from direct trauma or crush injuries, and the nail matrix and nail plate are often injured together because the nail bed adheres closely to the dorsum of the phalanx. Sometimes severe soft tissue injuries combine with distal phalangeal fractures. Deep laceration, hyperextension, hyperflexion, rotation, and, uncommonly, axial load can produce these fractures. The most common types of distal phalanx fractures are comminuted distal tuft fractures, longitudinal fractures, transverse fractures, avulsion fractures, and intra-articular fractures of the base.

A fracture of the fine cancellous bone at the distal tip of the phalanx is termed a tuft fracture. Tuft fractures are usually caused by a crush injury and comminuted in nature and are almost always associated with damage to the nail matrix or pulp or both. The tuft fractures are generally stable due to the adherence of the fibrous septa. Splint immobilization including the IP joint for 3–4 weeks is usually indicated without reduction or fixation. When there is painful subungual hematoma, it should be evacuated. Dermal and nail matrix lacerations should be repaired when indicated. Follow-up radiographs often do not show full osseous union, but it does not mean the need of operative treatment. Stable fibrous union is usually asymptomatic.

Transverse shaft fractures of distal phalanx tend to be quite unstable and often presented with a pseudomallet appearance as the fracture line is often just distal to the insertion of the extensor pollicis longus tendon. Transverse fractures should be evaluated for angulation as these are at greater risk of displacement. Widening of the fracture line may indicate entrapment of the nail bed within a transverse distal phalanx fracture (Fig. 6.2). If the fractures are minimally displaced or stable after reduction, they can be immobilized with an extension splint and care of soft tissue injury. If avulsed, the nail plate should be reduced beneath the nail fold to reapproximate the nail matrix and stabilize the fracture. However, in case reduction cannot be held in a splint, it necessitates an insertion of a longitudinal Kirschner wire driven in a retrograde fashion from the distal hyponychium just under the nail plate across the fracture and into the head of the proximal phalanx (Fig. 6.2). The Kirschner wire is removed after achieving clinical bone union usually around 4 weeks after surgery.

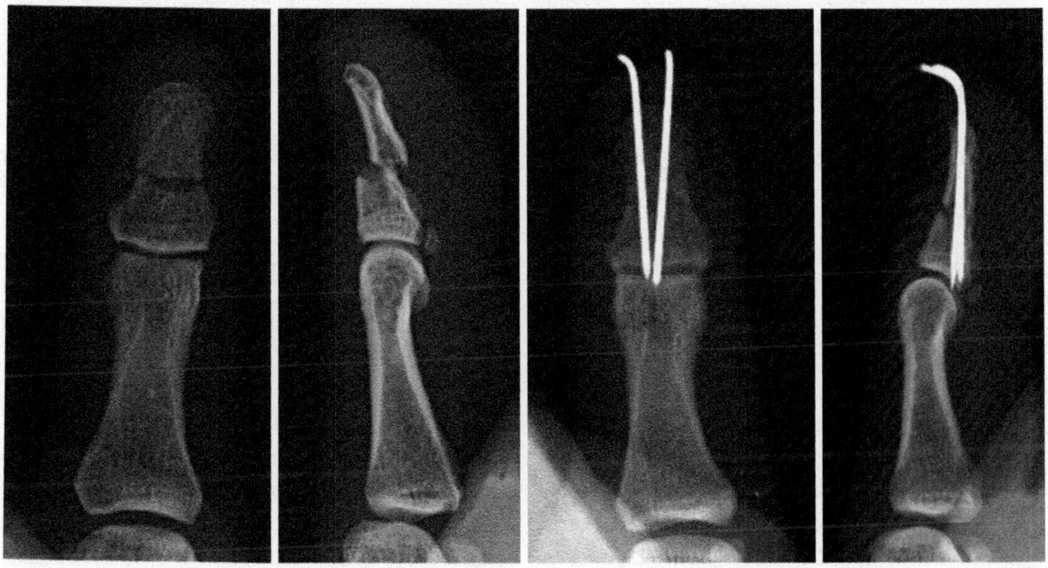

**Fig. 6.2** Transverse fracture of the distal phalanx of the thumb. Two longitudinal K-wires were driven to maintain reduction in a retrograde fashion from the distal hyponychium just under the nail plate across the fracture and into the head of the proximal phalanx

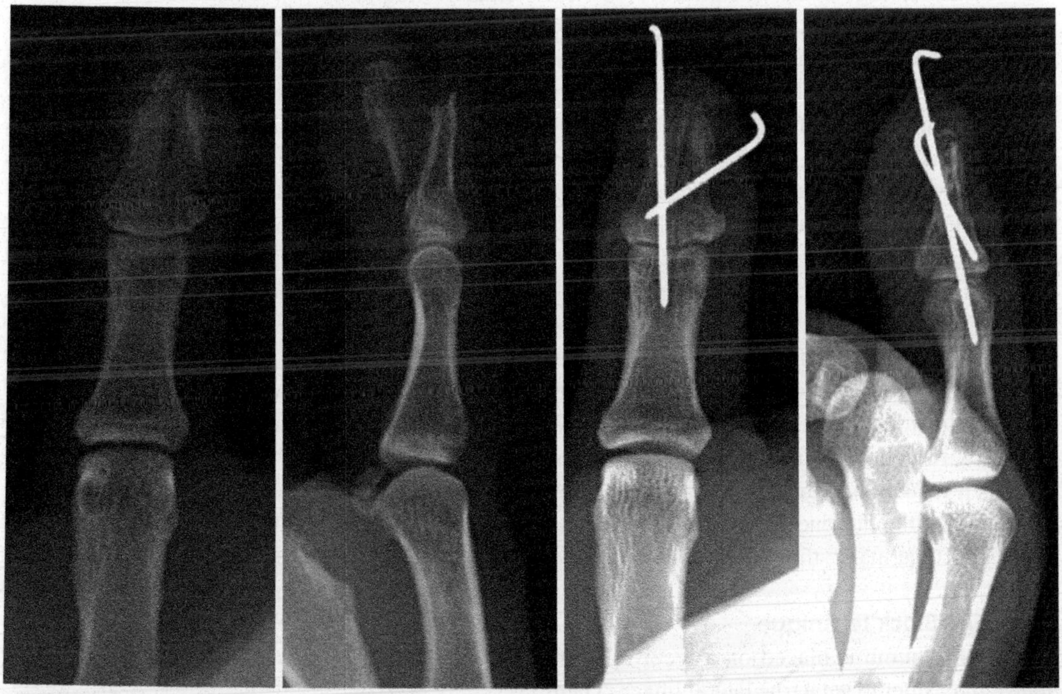

**Fig. 6.3** Open comminuted longitudinal fracture of the distal phalanx of the thumb. The fracture was reduced and pinned after repair of the nail matrix and reduction of the nail plate

Longitudinal extra-articular shaft fractures of the distal phalanx are not common, and these fractures are usually nondisplaced and stable. If displaced, the fracture can be reduced and pinned (Fig. 6.3). Seymour fractures are open fractures of the distal phalanx in children due to a fracture at the physis (Salter-Harris type I or II). Like other open fractures, Seymour fractures need operative irrigation and debridement. Then, the entrapped nail matrix should be pulled out to reduce the fractures.

## Intra-articular Fractures and Avulsions

### Mallet Thumb

Avulsion fractures of the dorsal base of the distal phalanx are designated a "mallet finger." Although mallet finger is a common fingertip injury, mallet thumb is relatively uncommon (only 2–3% of all mallet injuries). Like other mallet fingers, mallet thumb is caused by forced flexion of an extended fingertip. Less common hyperextension or hyperextension/axial loading tends to cause the larger fractures and volar subluxation of the distal phalanx. In children, mallet thumb causes Salter-Harris type III or IV fractures. The goal of treating mallet fractures is to establish a congruent joint and minimize the final extension lag. If the fracture involves less than 30% of the joint and without volar subluxation of the distal phalanx, it can be treated by continuous extension splinting of the IP joint for 6 weeks. However, the fractures associated with volar subluxation of the distal phalanx or joint incongruity and the fractures greater than 30% of the joint should be treated surgically to avoid consequences like traumatic osteoarthritis, swan neck deformity, and persistent IP joint stiffness. Various surgical techniques have been described to treat mallet fingers like extension block pinning, percutaneous direct fragment fixation, external fixator, tension band wire technique, pullout wire technique, internal suture, tenodesis, and open reduction with Kirschner wire fixation or fixation with plate and/or screws, and they can be used to treat mallet thumbs as well.

### Extension Block Technique

The mallet thumb is placed on a receiver of an image intensifier to get a true lateral image. Then, the IP joint of the thumb is in maximum flexion while checking the mallet fracture fragment to move distally and little bit volarly. A 0.9 mm K-wire is introduced just posterior to the fragment and driven into the proximal phalangeal head at an angle of 30–45° to its long axis. The fracture is reduced with the IP joint in traction and slight extension but still in 10° flexion. When the dorsal fragment is not reduced exactly, a second dorsal block wire can be needed to reduce it. The other 0.9 mm K-wire is then advanced from the volar or lateral side of the finger and across the IP joint to hold it in slight flexion [3]. The wires are cut short, and a volar aluminum splint is applied to protect. The wires are removed at 6 weeks, followed by intermittent volar splinting for 2 weeks.

### Open Reduction and Fixation

Occasionally an open reduction and fixation is required to reposition significantly displaced mallet fragments or chronic mallet fractures to remove the callus that prevents indirect reduction. There are several dorsal approaches using variants of extensile incision to the interphalangeal joint for the manipulation and fixation of the fracture fragments [4]. When indicated, a transverse crease incision is placed directly over the fracture site, which can be localized with the aid of fluoroscopy. Once the fracture site is exposed, the fracture fragment is intentionally displaced, and the hematoma, if present, is removed. Then, the fracture fragment is manipulated and reduced with the aid of a periosteal elevator or a similar instrument with blunt tip and fixed with 0.7 mm or smaller diameter K-wires or sometimes hypodermic needles to maintain its reduction. In this step, surgeons need to be careful not to break the small dorsal fragment with reduction forceps and not to damage the terminal tendon insertion. The wires are removed at 6 weeks, followed by intermittent volar splinting for 2 weeks. If the fragment is big enough, a specially designed plate like a hook plate can be applied to fix it (Fig. 6.4). The plate construct can be removed at 3 months when the fracture has healed completely.

## Avulsion Fractures of the Volar Lip

Avulsion fractures of the volar lip of the base of the distal phalanx usually represent impaction fractures after a dorsal IP dislocation or, rarely, avulsion of the flexor pollicis longus, called the

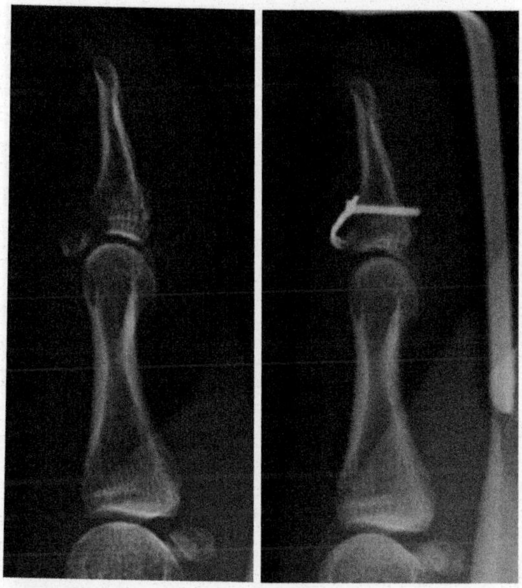

**Fig. 6.4** Mallet fracture of the distal phalanx of the thumb. A hook plate was applied to fix the displaced fragment with a dorsal approach

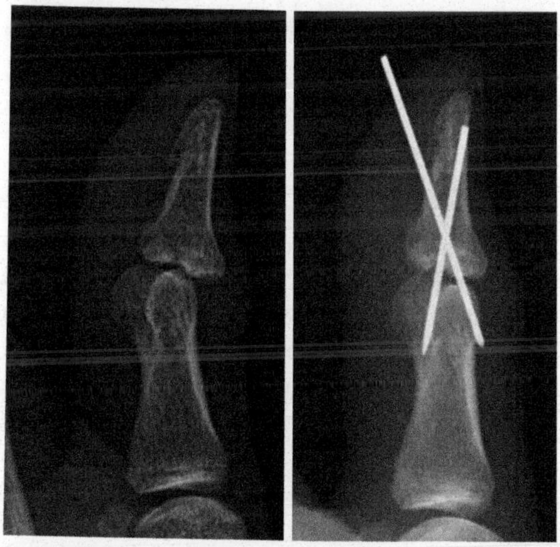

**Fig. 6.5** Volar lip fracture of the distal phalanx of the thumb with dorsal subluxation of the distal interphalangeal joint which was transfixed with two K-wires after reduction

bony jersey finger. If the avulsion fractures are associated with unstable IP joints, disruptions of the collateral ligaments and the volar plate will be present. In these cases, the IP joints can be transfixed with a K-wire to immobilize them for 4 weeks (Fig. 6.5). The bony jersey finger is uncommon but usually needs surgical fixation with suture anchor, pullout wire/button, or mini-screws depending on the size of bony fragments using a volar zigzag incision [5]. Open fixation is usually possible when that is diagnosed within 10 days of injury.

## Proximal Phalanx Fractures

Displaced spiral or oblique fractures of the proximal phalanx can be treated by percutaneous pinning or by open reduction using either Kirschner wires or interfragmentary screws. Transverse proximal phalanx fractures tend to angulate the apex volarly by the pull of the thenar intrinsics on the proximal fragment and the extensor pollicis longus on the distal fragment. If there is more than 20–30° of angulation in the lateral plane, it results in an extensor lag of the IP joint, so it should be reduced and maintained by percutaneous pinning or by open reduction with either Kirschner wires or interfragmentary screws (Fig. 6.6). If open reduction of a fracture of the proximal phalanx is indicated, a dorsal "Y"-shaped incision with sparing the extensor pollicis longus insertion is useful. Then, the fracture can be reduced indirectly or directly while moving the extensor pollicis longus side to side.

## Metacarpal Fractures

Fractures of the thumb metacarpal can occur in three locations: shaft and base fractures and intra-articular fractures of the trapeziometacarpal joint.

### Extra-articular Fractures

Extra-articular fractures through the base are common and are usually transverse or mildly oblique. Angulation up to 30° is acceptable for extra-articular thumb metacarpal fractures due to the motion at the TM joint. However, apex dorsal angulation of more than 30° will narrow the web space between the thumb and index finger and cause compensatory metacarpophalangeal joint hyperextension, which can result in unacceptable malunion. So, the extra-articular metacarpal frac-

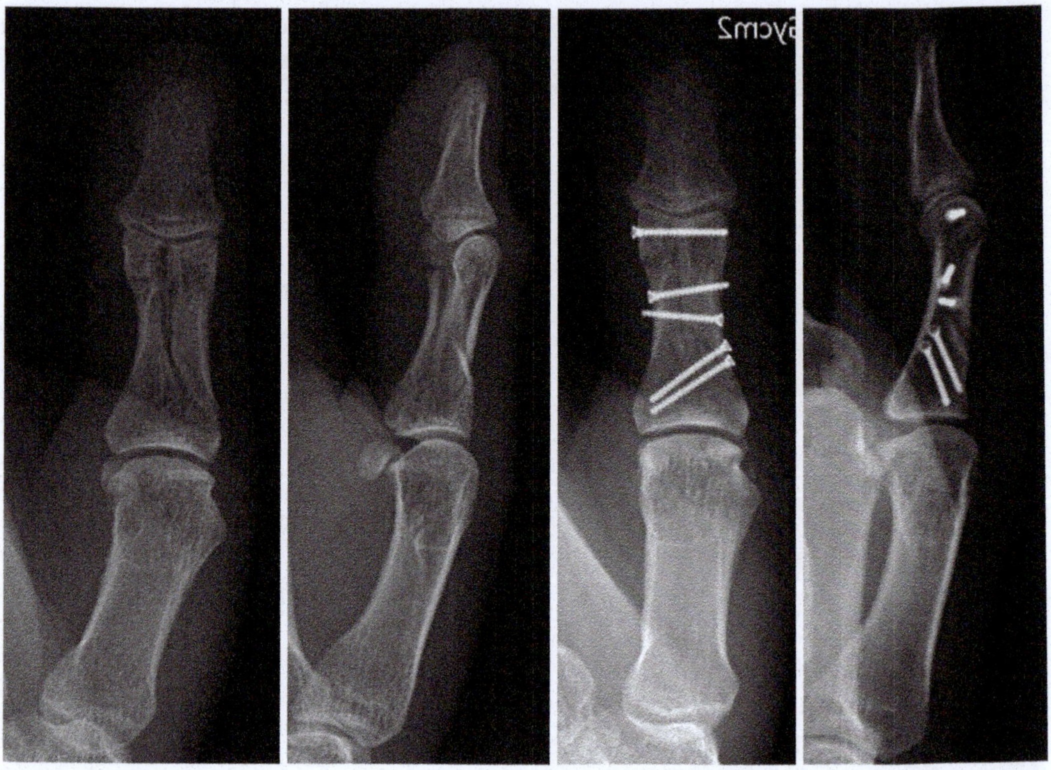


**Fig. 6.6** Bicondylar fracture of the proximal phalanx of the thumb. Multiple mini-screws were inserted after open reduction to fix the fragments of the proximal phalanx

tures which are angulated more than 30° are indicated for closed or open reduction to prevent unacceptable malunion. A true lateral radiograph, having superimposition of the thumb MP joint sesamoids, is necessary to evaluate the degree of angulation. The majority of extra-articular metacarpal fractures can be treated with immobilization in a thumb spica cast or splint that excludes the distal phalanx with or without reduction maneuver. The displaced thumb metacarpal fractures can be easily reduced by longitudinal traction, downward pressure on the apex of the fracture angulation with mild pronation of the distal fragment, and thumb extension. If an acceptable reduction cannot be maintained with immobilization alone, these fractures are needed to fix with crossed two Kirschner wires (Fig. 6.7). Some surgeons prefer open reduction and internal fixation with plate and screws because its construct provides a more stable fixation than K-wires that can permit earlier motion and return to daily activities. The fracture is approached by splitting the dorsal apparatus between the extensor pollicis longus and extensor pollicis brevis.

Comminuted thumb metacarpal shaft fractures are usually the result of direct trauma and are often associated with soft tissue injury. Fracture stabilization must be individualized. Open shaft fractures may require an external fixator to prevent metacarpal shortening and to allow soft tissue healing. Extension of the frame to the index metacarpal helps prevent a thumb/index finger web contracture.

## Intra-articular Metacarpal Fractures

### Metacarpal Head Fractures

Metacarpal head fractures are unusual because the longitudinally directed force that produces them is usually dissipated at the proximal metaphysis or trapeziometacarpal joint. Displaced intra-articular fractures require anatomic reduction. Fixation can be obtained with percutaneous Kirschner pins or by open reduction. The fracture is approached by splitting the dorsal apparatus

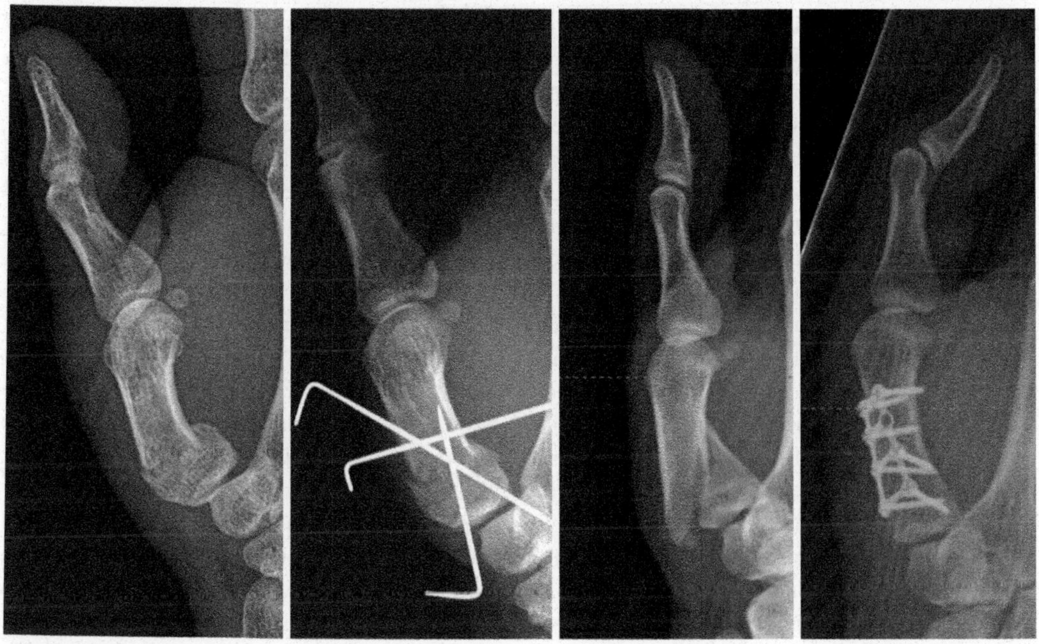

**Fig. 6.7** Extra-articular fracture of the metacarpal base of the thumb. Angulation could be reduced and fixed with closed or open method

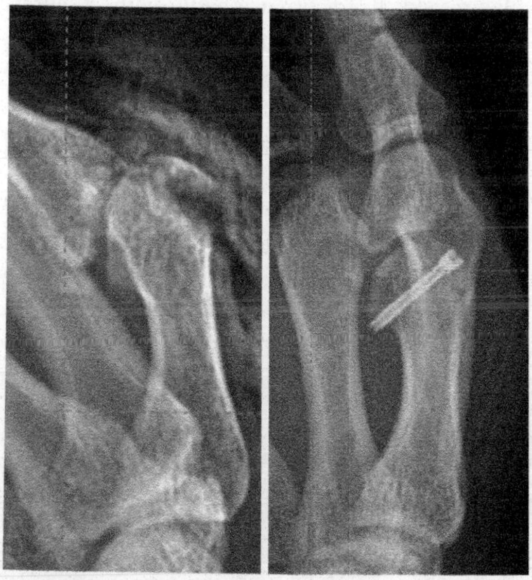

**Fig. 6.8** Fracture of the metacarpal head of the thumb. The fracture was approached by splitting the dorsal apparatus between the extensor pollicis longus and extensor pollicis brevis and fixed with a headless compression screw

between the extensor pollicis longus and extensor pollicis brevis (Fig. 6.8). With pin fixation, the thumb is immobilized for 2–3 weeks before initiating motion. With screw fixation, motion is initiated at 5–7 days postoperatively.

## Articular Fractures and Dislocations of Thumb Metacarpal Base

### Bennett's Fracture

Bennett's fracture refers to an intra-articular two-part fracture separating the volar-ulnar intra-articular fragment from the remaining thumb metacarpal. An indirect axial load on the partially flexed metacarpal can cause these fractures. The volar-ulnar fragment is held in place by the anterior oblique ligament (the beak ligament) to the trapezium, and the remaining metacarpal displaces dorsal, proximal, and radial direction by the pull of the abductor pollicis longus, extensor pollicis longus, extensor pollicis brevis, and the adductor pollicis longus [6–8]. These fractures are very unstable due to these tendons' pulls. Previously, Gedda classified the Bennett fractures into three types [8], with type 1 representing a fracture with a large single ulnar fragment and subluxation of the metacarpal base. A type 2 fracture represents an impaction fracture without subluxation of the thumb metacarpal. Lastly, a type 3 fracture represents a small ulnar avulsion fracture in association with metacarpal dislocation.

Axial traction, palmar abduction, and pronation of the metacarpal are applied to achieve proper reduction of the fracture while applying external pressure over the metacarpal base. Thumb extension (hitchhiker position) should be avoided to prevent the joint from displacement. The goal of reduction is less than 1 mm of articular step-off. Whereas Bennett advocated conservative treatment with a thumb spica cast, surgical fixation is needed because poor outcomes have been reported with casting alone [9–12]. So, while the reduction is held, we drill a Kirschner wire obliquely across the trapeziometacarpal joint or to the second metacarpal. An additional K-wire through the metacarpal to the volar-ulnar fragment may be added (Fig. 6.9) [13–15]. If the closed reduction fails, open reduction and internal fixation should follow, most commonly through a Wagner incision [14]. The longitudinal limb of this incision is over the subcutaneous border of the thumb metacarpal (between the abductor pollicis longus and the thenar muscles) and is extended proximally and ulnarly to the radial border of the flexor carpi radialis. The thenar muscles are reflected subperiosteally, the joint capsule is incised, and the fracture is visualized. When articular congruity has been restored, the Bennett fragment is held reduced with either reduction forceps or a small bone hook. Fixation of large fragments is secured with K-wires or a 1.5 mm or 2 mm small screw. An additional trans-articular pin fixation may be needed to protect the reduction. Postoperatively, if pins are used, the trans-articular pin is removed at 4 weeks, and the pins holding the fracture fragment are removed at 6 weeks.

## Rolando Fracture

The term *Rolando fracture* is applied to any comminuted intra-articular fracture of the base of the thumb but ideally should be reserved for Y- or T-pattern fractures that include the volar-ulnar Bennett fragment in addition to a dorsal radial fragment. When there are two large fragments, without considerable comminution, conduct open reduction and internal fixation through the Wagner incision as described earlier (Fig. 6.10). Longitudinal traction is applied first, and the two articular fragments are reduced with a reduction clamp and fixed provisionally with K-wires. Various methods of fixation have been described including K-wires, tension banding, and plate and screw fixation [16, 17].

For comminuted fractures, distraction and reliance on ligamentous reduction of the fragments may be used. Distraction can be achieved with oblique traction pinning. Alternatively, the fracture can be spanned and distracted using external fixation [18].

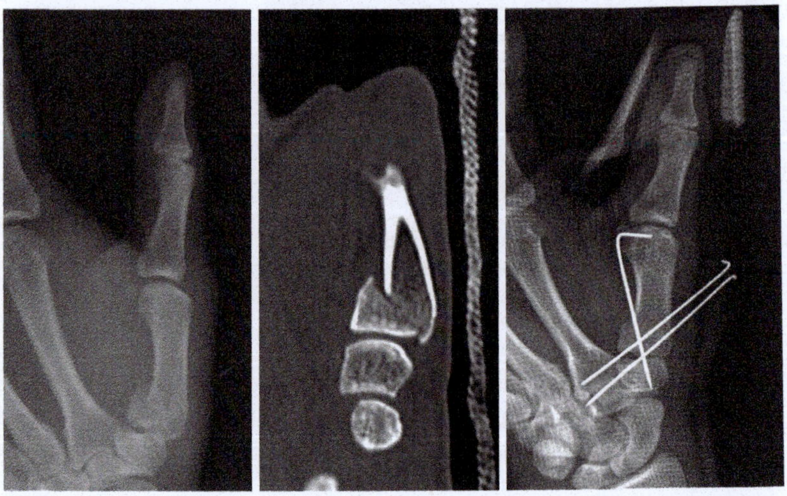

**Fig. 6.9** Bennett fracture of the thumb. Proper reduction was achieved with axial traction, palmar abduction, and pronation of the metacarpal while applying external pressure over the metacarpal base. Then, the fracture was stabilized using percutaneous pinning with two K-wires

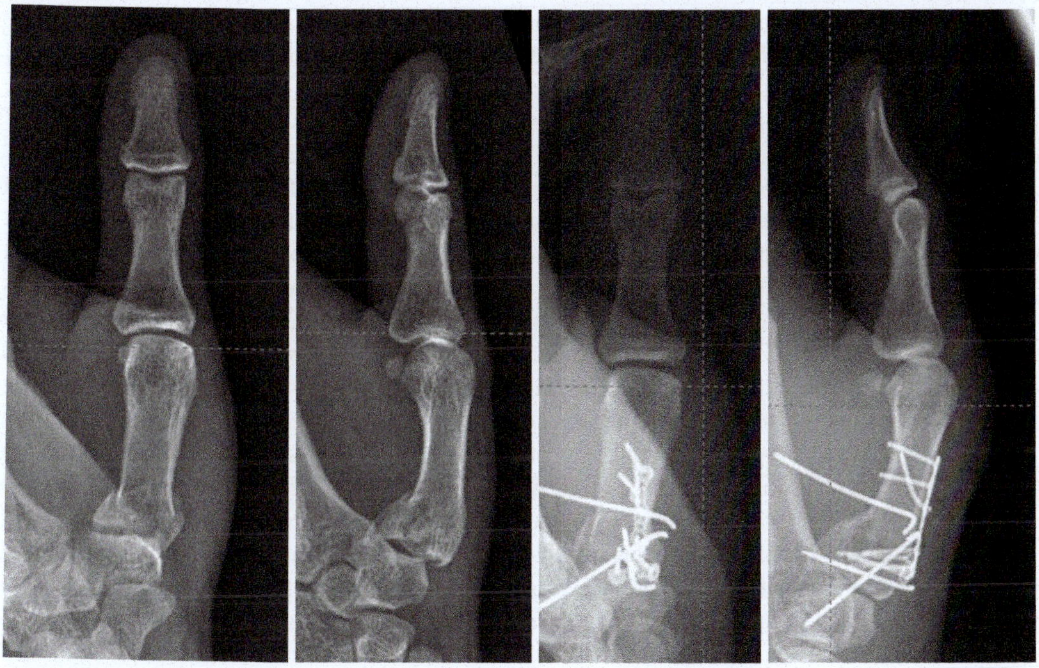

**Fig. 6.10** Rolando fracture of the thumb was reduced and fixed through the Wagner incision

## Dislocations

### Thumb IP Dislocations

Thumb IP joint dislocations are usually dorsal or lateral. Reduction can be easily accomplished with application of direct dorsal pressure on the distal phalanx while applying longitudinal traction under digital block anesthesia [19]. After reduction, stability of the joint should be assessed, and postreduction radiographs should be taken to evaluate for concentric reduction. Treatment consists of immobilization for 2–3 weeks in a finger splint. Instability after reduction is very uncommon.

Irreducible dislocations may be secondary to palmar plate interposition and require open reduction through a dorsal approach. The extensor pollicis longus terminal slip should be protected, and the interposed volar plate should be reduced over the proximal phalanx head. Sometimes partial excision or longitudinal split of the volar plate is required for accurate joint reduction [19]. Trans-articular pinning in full extension for 2–3 weeks is usually adequate if postreduction joint instability is noticed.

### Thumb MCP Dislocations

Thumb metacarpophalangeal dislocations are typically dorsal and occur secondary to a hyperextension injury with associated injuries to the collateral ligaments, volar plate, and capsule. Palmar MCP joint dislocations are relatively rare conditions. Dislocations are classified as simple or complex based on reducibility with closed maneuvers. The MCP dislocations present with a hyperextension deformity at the joint and metacarpal adduction. In complex dislocations, the proximally avulsed volar plate or the flexor pollicis longus tendon is often interposed [19, 20]. Before trying closed reduction, proper radiographic evaluation is necessary including standard posteroanterior and true lateral radiographs to evaluate for associated fractures. Closed reduction can be accomplished under local anesthesia with wrist flexion to relax the flexor tendons, gentle recreation of the hyperextension deformity at the MCP joint, and a palmar-directed force on the base of the proximal phalanx to reduce it onto the metacarpal head. Longitudinal traction should be avoided because the displaced flexor pollicis longus on the ulnar side of the metacarpal head and the displaced adductor pollicis muscle on the ulnar side of the metacarpal can strangle the metacarpal neck and can convert a reducible dislocation into an irreducible one.

If closed reduction fails, open reduction is required, most commonly via a dorsal or volar approach based on surgeon preference. The dorsal approach through the interval between the extensor pollicis brevis and longus has the advantage of minimal risk to the neurovascular bundles, whereas the volar approach with a Bruner incision has the advantage of allowing direct visualization of structures that may be impeding reduction like volar plate, sesamoids, and flexor pollicis longus. After reduction, the thumb is immobilized in a dorsal block splint with the metacarpophalangeal joint in 10° more flexion than the point of instability. Each week thereafter it is extended 10° until terminal extension is obtained. If, after reduction, the joint remains unstable and the collateral ligament is completely torn, operative repair is indicated.

## Thumb TM Joint Dislocations

Injuries to the thumb carpometacarpal or trapeziometacarpal joint may be complete or partial. Partial injuries are far more common and result in varying degrees of joint subluxation. Complete injuries with dislocation of the thumb carpometacarpal joint are relatively rare and occur when a flexed metacarpal is loaded axially. Dislocations are invariably dorsoradial and result in tearing of the dorsoradial ligament and volar oblique ligament [1]. These dislocations typically reveal adducted thumbs that reduce with a palmar-directed force or thumb extension. Radiologic evaluation must be performed to rule out associated fractures at the joints.

The dislocated joints need to be reduced immediately and assessed for joint stability. If the joint is well reduced and stable after reduction, immobilization in a thumb spica cast for 4–6 weeks may be sufficient to maintain reduction and achieve long-term stability. However, the joint frequently remains unstable, and if so, open reduction and repair of the dorsal radial ligament with trans-articular Kirschner wire fixation are indicated. If dislocations present more than 3 weeks after trauma or there is persistent instability after proper initial treatment, ligament reconstruction with a radial half of the distally is advised based on flexor carpi radialis tendon as described by Eaton and colleagues with a Wagner incision [21], a dorsoradial incision made along the proximal half of the first metacarpal curving ulnarward proximally around the base of the thenar eminence parallel with the distal flexor crease of the wrist. The carpometacarpal joint of the thumb is exposed subperiosteally, and the distal part of the flexor carpi radialis is isolated. A 6 cm distally based strip of the flexor carpi radialis is harvested from the radial side of the tendon and freed proximally. The thumb metacarpal is then reduced on the trapezium and secured with a Kirschner wire ensuring that its path will not interfere with the site through which the tendon transfer will eventually pass. A hole is drilled transversely through the base of the thumb metacarpal ulnar to the extensor pollicis brevis tendon exiting near the volar beak. The harvested tendon strip is passed through this tunnel deep to the abductor pollicis longus tendon and sutured to the periosteum near its exit. It is then looped around the flexor carpi radialis near its insertion and sutured to the base of the thumb metacarpal. Postoperatively, the thumb is immobilized for 4 weeks in extension and abduction.

## Summary

Fractures and dislocations of the thumb are relatively common. The thumb's unique orientation gives the hand great capability and predisposes the thumb to certain injuries, particularly of the metacarpal base. Given the greater movement of the thumb, some residual deformities from extra-articular thumb fractures are more acceptable than that of the other fingers. Rotational deformity rarely induces a disability. However, intra-articular fractures should be critically treated with the goal of anatomic joint reduction to avoid stiffness and pain with post-traumatic arthritis. Most traumatic dislocations of the thumb can be treated nonoperatively via closed reduction and immobilization. However, surgical treatment is necessary if the joint is not concentrically reduced or unstable after reduction.

## References

1. Strauch RJ, Behrman MJ, Rosenwasser MP. Acute dislocation of the carpometacarpal joint of the thumb: an anatomic and cadaver study. J Hand Surg Am. 1994;19(1):93–8.
2. Meals C, Meals R. Hand fractures: a review of current treatment strategies. J Hand Surg Am. 2013;38(5):1021–31; quiz 1031.
3. Lee SK, et al. Modified extension-block K-wire fixation technique for the treatment of bony mallet finger. Orthopedics. 2010;33(10):728.
4. Lee SK, et al. Modified pull-out wire suture technique for the treatment of chronic bony mallet finger. Ann Plast Surg. 2010;65(5):466–70.
5. Tuttle HG, Olvey SP, Stern PJ. Tendon avulsion injuries of the distal phalanx. Clin Orthop Relat Res. 2006;445:157–68.
6. Carlsen BT, Moran SL. Thumb trauma: Bennett fractures, Rolando fractures, and ulnar collateral ligament injuries. J Hand Surg Am. 2009;34(5):945–52.
7. Bettinger PC, Berger RA. Functional ligamentous anatomy of the trapezium and trapeziometacarpal joint (gross and arthroscopic). Hand Clin. 2001;17(2):151–68. vii
8. Gedda KO. Studies on Bennett's fracture; anatomy, roentgenology, and therapy. Acta Chir Scand Suppl. 1954;193:1–114.
9. Livesley PJ. The conservative management of Bennett's fracture-dislocation: a 26-year follow-up. J Hand Surg Br. 1990;15(3):291–4.
10. Foster RJ, Hastings H II. Treatment of Bennett, Rolando, and vertical intraarticular trapezial fractures. Clin Orthop Relat Res. 1987;(214):121–9.
11. Oosterbos CJ, de Boer HH. Nonoperative treatment of Bennett's fracture: a 13-year follow-up. J Orthop Trauma. 1995;9(1):23–7.
12. Thurston AJ, Dempsey SM. Bennett's fracture: a medium to long-term review. Aust N Z J Surg. 1993;63(2):120–3.
13. Gelberman RH, Vance RM, Zakaib GS. Fractures at the base of the thumb: treatment with oblique traction. J Bone Joint Surg Am. 1979;61(2):260–2.
14. Lutz M, et al. Closed reduction transarticular Kirschner wire fixation versus open reduction internal fixation in the treatment of Bennett's fracture dislocation. J Hand Surg Br. 2003;28(2):142–7.
15. Timmenga EJ, et al. Long-term evaluation of Bennett's fracture. A comparison between open and closed reduction. J Hand Surg Br. 1994;19(3):373–7.
16. Kahler DM. Fractures and dislocations of the base of the thumb. J South Orthop Assoc. 1995;4(1):69–76.
17. Soyer AD. Fractures of the base of the first metacarpal: current treatment options. J Am Acad Orthop Surg. 1999;7(6):403–12.
18. Marsland D, Sanghrajka AP, Goldie B. Static monolateral external fixation for the Rolando fracture: a simple solution for a complex fracture. Ann R Coll Surg Engl. 2012;94(2):112–5.
19. Owings FP, Calandruccio JH, Mauck BM. Thumb ligament injuries in the athlete. Orthop Clin North Am. 2016;47(4):799–807.
20. Kaplan EB. Dorsal dislocation of the metacarpophalangeal joint of the index finger. J Bone Joint Surg Am. 1957;39-A(5):1081–6.
21. Eaton RG, et al. Ligament reconstruction for the painful thumb carpometacarpal joint: a long-term assessment. J Hand Surg Am. 1984;9(5):692–9.

# Collateral Ligament Injuries

# 7

Ji Hun Park and Jong Woong Park

## Collateral Ligament Injuries of the Metacarpophalangeal Joint of the Thumb

The thumb collateral ligament ruptures at the metacarpophalangeal (MCP) joint are one of the most common injuries to the hand. Such injuries may result in joint instability, leading long-term pain and functional disability. In 1955, Campbell [1] described the "gamekeeper's thumb," referring to chronic attritional attenuation of the ulnar collateral ligament (UCL) in Scottish gamekeepers who repetitively received valgus stress while killing a wounded rabbit using the first web space between the thumb and index finger. On the other hand, it is possible that the injuries occurred acutely with sudden forced radial deviation of thumb. This acute injury to the UCL is termed "skier's thumb," because it is a common skiing-related injury [2]. In one study, UCL ligament injuries of the thumb accounted for 33% of all upper extremity injuries and 7% of all skiing injuries [3]. Radial collateral ligament (RCL) injury of the thumb occurs less frequently than UCL injury and approximately 10–40% of collateral ligament injuries of the thumb [4–6]. However, if they are not recognized and neglected, they lead to the similar complications and functional disability. Physical examination and management of UCL and RCL injuries appear similar, but there are anatomic differences between the two sides of MCP joint. They may dictate different approaches to injuries of these ligaments, and each requires special attention.

The clinical examination of collateral ligament injuries is crucial for distinguishing between partial and complete ruptures. Although acute and partial collateral ligament injury of the finger is usually managed conservatively, complete rupture combined with unacceptable instability should be repaired primarily, particularly in athletes or manual workers [7]. Effective management of both acute and chronic injuries requires an anatomically based examination, appropriate use of imaging studies, and proper decision for treatment. Attention must be directed toward repairing the collateral ligament to its anatomic insertion or origin. Chronic collateral ligament reconstructions with tendon graft, although less successful than acute repair, can restore stability of the thumb MCP joint. The purpose of this chapter is to describe the treatment algorithms and surgical techniques for collateral ligament injuries of the MCP joint.

## Anatomy

The MCP joint of the thumb is a diarthrodial condyloid joint. Primary movement is flexion–extension and secondarily allows motion planes

J. H. Park · J. W. Park (✉)
Department of Orthopedic Surgery, Korea University College of Medicine, Seoul, South Korea
e-mail: ziphun@korea.ac.kr; ospark@korea.ac.kr


S. H. Woo (ed.), *The Thumb*, https://doi.org/10.1007/978-981-10-4400-7_7

for abduction–adduction and pronation–supination. Joint motion varies from one individual to another widely according to the shape of the metacarpal head. In one study, rounder thumb metacarpal head showed greater MCP joint range of motion (ROM) than a flatter thumb metacarpal head [8].

Static stabilizers of the MCP joint include the articular surface congruity, the volar plate, the proper collateral ligaments, and accessory ligaments. Proper ligament arises from the lateral condyles of the metacarpal head and pass obliquely to insert on the volar third of the proximal phalanx. This structure becomes tight in flexion and loose in extension, serving as the primary restraint to valgus stress with the thumb MCP joint in flexion (Fig. 7.1a) [9]. The accessory collateral ligament originates more volar side on the metacarpal head and inserts onto the volar plate and sesamoid on either side of the joint. This structure becomes tight in extension and loose in flexion, serving as the primary restraint to valgus stress with the MCP joint in extension (Fig. 7.1b) [9]. Dynamic stabilizers of the thumb include the thumb intrinsic muscles (abductor pollicis brevis, flexor pollicis brevis, and adductor pollicis muscles) and extrinsic muscles (extensor pollicis longus, extensor pollicis brevis, and flexor pollicis longus muscles). The adductor pollicis muscle inserts onto the proximal phalanx and ulnar sesamoid and the adductor aponeurosis and serves as the primary dynamic stabilizer of the MCP joint and resists valgus stress (Fig. 7.2a). The similar mechanism exists on the radial side with the abductor pollicis brevis and flexor pollicis brevis muscles, which actively resist varus stress (Fig. 7.2b).

Anatomical origins of UCL and RCL are not mirror images of each other. Their origin and insertion sites are important concerns in anatomical repair. In one cadaveric study, UCL center of the metacarpal origin was reported 38% from the dorsal edge of the metacarpal head. The center of

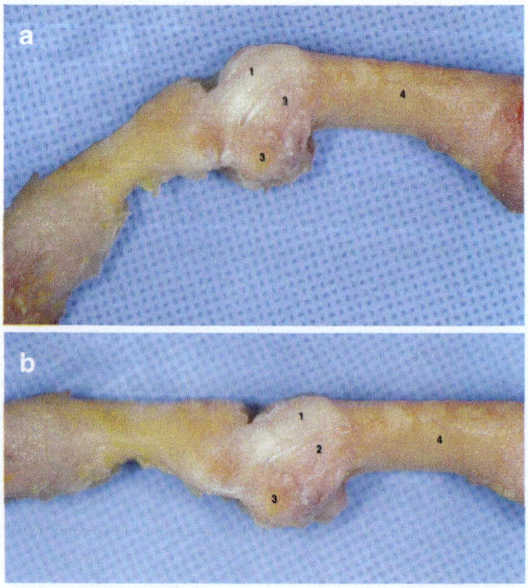

**Fig. 7.1** The collateral ligaments of the thumb metacarpophalangeal joint. (**a**) The proper ligament (*1*) becomes tight and accessory ligament (2) becomes loose in flexion. (**b**) The proper ligament becomes loose and accessory ligament becomes tight in extension (*3*, sesamoid; *4*, proximal phalanx)

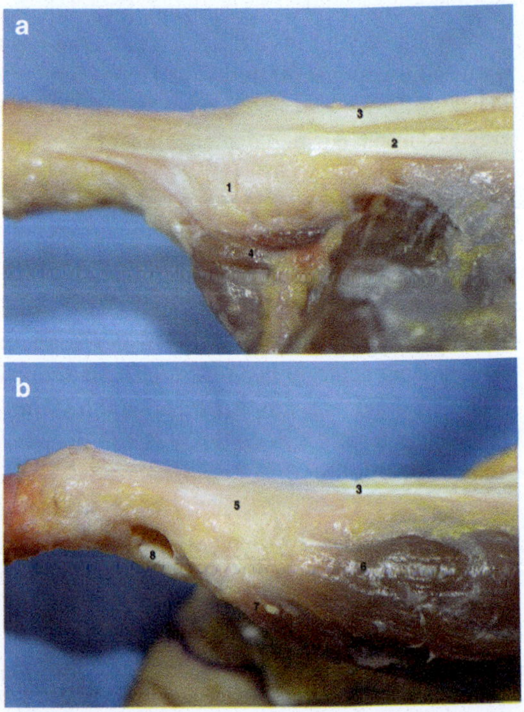

**Fig. 7.2** Dynamic stabilizers of the thumb metacarpophalangeal joint. (**a**) Ulnar side of the thumb. (**b**) Radial side of the thumb (*1*, adductor aponeurosis; *2*, extensor pollicis longus tendon; *3*, extensor pollicis brevis tendon; *4*, adductor pollicis; *5*, abductor aponeurosis; *6*, abductor pollicis brevis; *7*, flexor pollicis brevis; *8*, flexor pollicis longus tendon)

the phalangeal insertion was 24% from the volar edge of the proximal phalanx. Meanwhile, the RCL center of the metacarpal origin was reported 31% from the dorsal edge of the metacarpal head. The center of the phalangeal insertion was 29% from the volar edge of the proximal phalanx [10].

### Pathologic Anatomy

In 1962, Stener [9] observed interposition of the adductor aponeurosis between the torn UCL and the MCP joint in complete avulsion of the distal insertion of the UCL. He predicted that the adductor aponeurosis prevents apposition of the ligament back to its anatomic insertion and interferes spontaneous healing of UCL. The occurrence of a Stener lesion has been reported about 64% and 88% of complete ruptures of the UCL [9, 11]. This lesion is usually regarded as an indication for operative treatment, but this was not substantiated.

The lesion of UCL injury has higher incidence of distal avulsion compared with RCL injury. Mostly UCL avulse at its distal insertion, and less frequently, it also could be torn at midsubstance or at the metacarpal origin [9, 12]. The site of the tear of the RCL is more variable than is the site of UCL tears. The RCL may tear midsubstance or the metacarpal origin or proximal phalanx insertion. Coyle [13] demonstrated proximal tears in 55%, distal tears in 29%, and midsubstance tears in 16%. One possible explanation for greater incidence of proximal tears with RCL injury compared with UCL injury is the greater distal insertion size of the RCL [14].

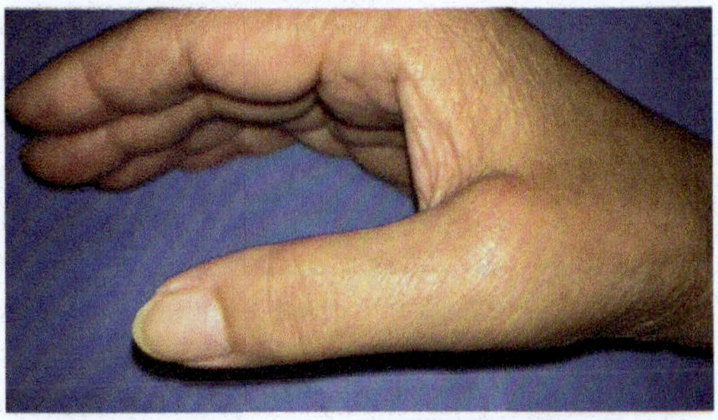

**Fig. 7.3** A bump can be palpated on the ulnar side of thumb metacarpophalangeal joint in cases of ulnar collateral ligament injury

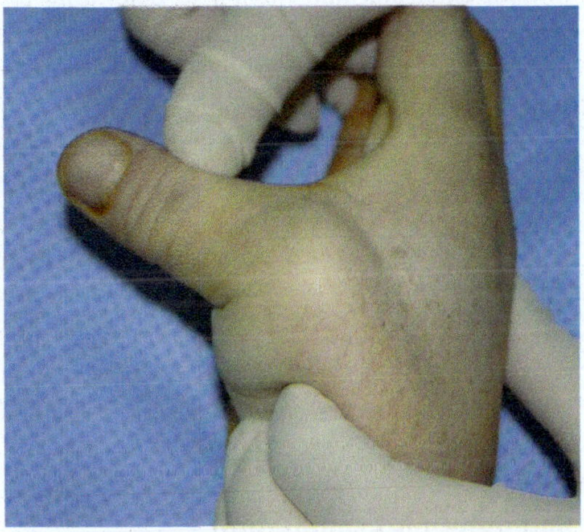

**Fig. 7.4** Valgus stress test of the thumb metacarpophalangeal joint. Absence of firm endpoint indicates rupture of ulnar collateral ligament

## Diagnosis

### Physical Examination

Patients with acute injuries usually have edema, ecchymosis, and tenderness on the ulnar or radial aspect of the MCP joint. The presence of a palpable bump on the ulnar aspect of the MCP joint may be indicative of a Stener lesion (Fig. 7.3). However, this finding is commonly absent or not prominent in chronic UCL injuries [11, 15].

Varus–valgus stress testing in UCL and RCL injuries has great diagnostic value (Fig. 7.4). Three-grade classification system is generally used description, but there was no formal validation. Grade 1 injury (sprain) is tenderness along the each collateral ligaments with symmetric laxity compared with that of the contralateral thumb. Grade 2 injury is a partial rupture with increased joint laxity compared with contralateral thumb. Grade 3 injury involves a complete rupture with definite MCP joint instability. If the MCP joint pain is too much to be examined stress test, local nerve block with lidocaine can be used to obtain adequate assessment.

The widely used criteria for determining UCL instability is 30° of laxity of the ulnar side of the joint when stressed radially in MCP extension and 40° of flexion [16]. Another criterion for instability is a relative opening of 15° compared with the contralateral side. In clinical situation, it is expected that manual testing and measuring angle are not precise enough to distinguish between 30° and 35°. Furthermore, in a study of 100 normal individuals, a variation of more than 10° was found between their uninjured thumbs [17]. According to these uncertainties of determining angle differences, we prefer to access partial or complete ruptures by identifying presence or absence of firm endpoint to each stress test.

Varus–valgus stress test should be performed in both extension and flexion to determine the status of the accessory and proper collateral ligaments, respectively. Heyman et al. [11] demonstrated specified tests examining the integrity of the UCL. At 30° of MCP joint flexion, greater than 35° of valgus laxity indicates rupture of the proper collateral ligament. At 0° of extension, the accessory collateral ligament is taut. In their study, valgus laxity greater than 35° when the joint was positioned in extension and then stressed consistently indicated the presence of tears of the proper and accessory collateral ligaments.

## Radiographic Examination

Plain radiographs including posteroanterior (PA), lateral, and oblique views of the thumb MCP joint should be taken before any maneuver or investigation of joint instability to rule out accompanying avulsion fracture. The use of stress radiographs has been described for diagnosing a UCL injury with >35° of valgus laxity or 10–15° of increased laxity compared with the contralateral thumb [18]. They are useful in the evaluation of patients with equivocal laxity, but not routinely performed when the physical examination is clear.

The making of stress radiographs can be limited by patient guarding and has demonstrated a high rate of false-negative results [19]. Dislocations of previously nondisplaced ligaments caused by taking stress radiographs have been reported [20]. Plain radiographs can also reveal small avulsion fractures at the base of the proximal phalanx combine with collateral ligament injury. However, the radiographic location of the fragment does not necessarily indicate location of the collateral ligament [21]. Hintermann et al. [22] noted that fracture fragments of UCL injury showed two types: a fragment was attached to the UCL and a fragment that was not attached to the UCL. The latter might represent shearing fracture without ligamentous attachment, and it does not imply joint stability even when they are nondisplaced [23].

Other diagnostic tests that have been reported in recent studies include ultrasound, magnetic resonance imaging (MRI), and magnetic resonance arthrography [24]. Ultrasound is a quick, noninvasive, and cost-effective imaging. Its usefulness has been reported throughout several studies [25–27]. As in other surgical fields, however, the results of ultrasound tend to be dependent on the examiner experience. A recent review of level 1 studies investigating ultrasound diagnosis of UCL rupture demonstrated a sensitivity of 76%, specificity of 81%, accuracy of 81%, positive predictive value of 74%, and negative predictive value of 87% [28].

Recent evolution of MRI with increased resolution allows precise evaluation of integrity of collateral ligaments. Previously reported cadaveric study of MRI for UCL injuries showed 100% sensitivity and 94% specificity for detecting Stener lesions [29]. Hergan et al. [30] directly compared ultrasound with MRI and demonstrated superior results with MRI: 100% specificity and sensitivity. One study reported MRA to be the most sensitive of tests for collateral ligament tears of the thumb MCP joint [31].

Despite their great success to diagnose UCL injuries, the cost-effectiveness of each techniques remains under question. Accurate clinical examination should precede, but when the test is unclear, further imaging investigation such as MRI or ultrasound is generally recommended.

## Treatment

### Acute Injuries

The preferred treatment for acute grade 1 and 2 UCL injuries is immobilization using a cast or splint. Immobilization of MCP joint in a thumb spica cast or splint with the interphalangeal (IP) joint free is usually maintained for 4 weeks. Active and passive ROM exercises are initiated immediately after immobilization, with avoidance of abduction or adduction forces at the MCP joint. Grip and pinch strengthening is started 6 weeks after the initiation of treatment. Surgical intervention is generally recommended for complete rupture of UCL. Although a Stener lesion is regarded as an indication for operative treatment, its clinical diagnosis is difficult. When its clinical finding is uncertain, advanced imaging techniques such as MRI of ultrasound help to rule out this lesion (Fig. 7.5). In cases of RCL, acute grade 1 and 2 injuries can be treated the same as the UCL. For grade 3 RCL injuries, recent literature favors surgical fixation to achieve a more predictable good results. Rationale for surgical fixation for grade 3 injuries is based on the fact that the ulnar pull of the extensor pollicis longus tendon maintains ulnar deviation of the MCP joint [5]. It may allow the ligament to heal in an elongated position. Untreated acute grade 3 injuries of the thumb collateral ligaments may progress to late symptomatic instability and degenerative arthritis of the MCP joint.

## Operative Approaches

Many techniques have been described for repair of the thumb collateral ligament. Both open and arthroscopic-assisted approaches have been reported [32, 33]. Torn ligament can be fixed with variable techniques including transosseous sutures [12, 34, 35], periosteal suture [9, 36], and suture anchors [7, 37–39]. Surgical repairs of acute UCL rupture have been demonstrated consistently satisfactory functional outcomes. In cases of distal avulsion, repair to the anatomical footprint is necessary to restore normal MCP joint motion [40]. Authors prefer open repair technique using a suture anchor.

## Surgical Technique of Open Repair of the Collateral Ligament Using a Suture Anchor

The ulnar or radial side of the involved joint was exposed through a lazy S-shaped incision centered at the joint line (Fig. 7.6). Branches of superficial radial nerve should be marked and protected throughout the operation (Fig. 7.7). In case of UCL repair, the adductor aponeurosis was cut and tagged. The adductor aponeurosis is cut 1 or 2 mm apart from the ulnar border of the extensor pollicis longus to facilitate later repair. In case of RCL repair, the abductor aponeurosis is incised at the radial border of the extensor pollicis brevis. After a transverse capsular incision, palmar and dorsal capsular flaps were gently elevated and tagged. Although midsubstance rupture can be repaired with nonabsorbable or slowly absorbable sutures, mostly they are avulsed distally. Distal avulsion at the base of the proximal phalanx is repaired using a small suture anchor

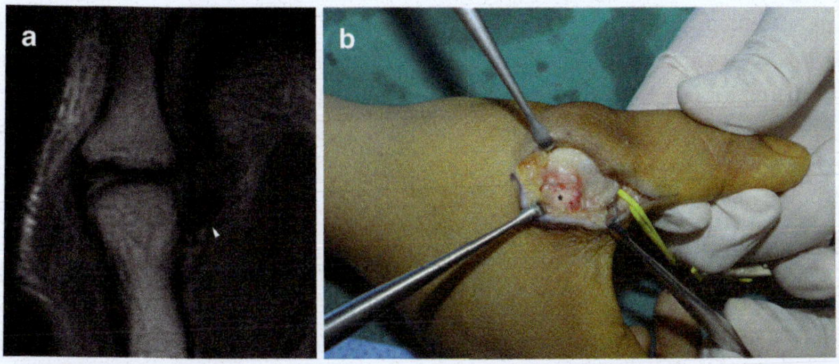


**Fig. 7.5** Magnetic resonance imaging (MRI) and intraoperative finding of acute ruptured ulnar collateral ligament (UCL) with Stener lesion. (**a**) Coronal MRI showed distal UCL avulsion with proximal retraction (arrowhead). (**b**) Intraoperatively, adductor aponeurosis was interposed between the thumb metacarpophalangeal joint and torn UCL fiber (asterisk) which was superficial to the adductor aponeurosis

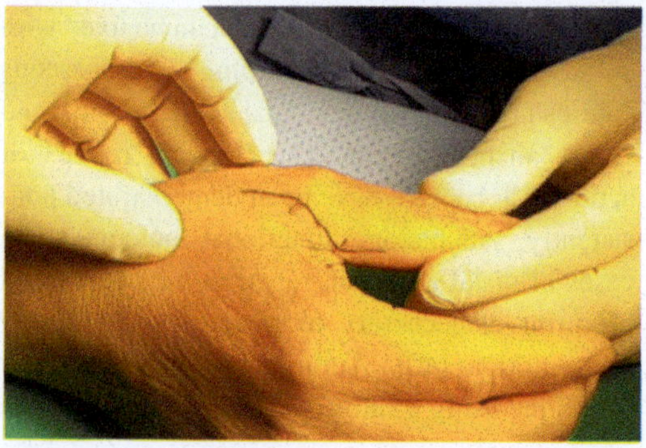

**Fig. 7.6** The ulnar side lazy S-shaped incision for the thumb ulnar collateral ligament repair

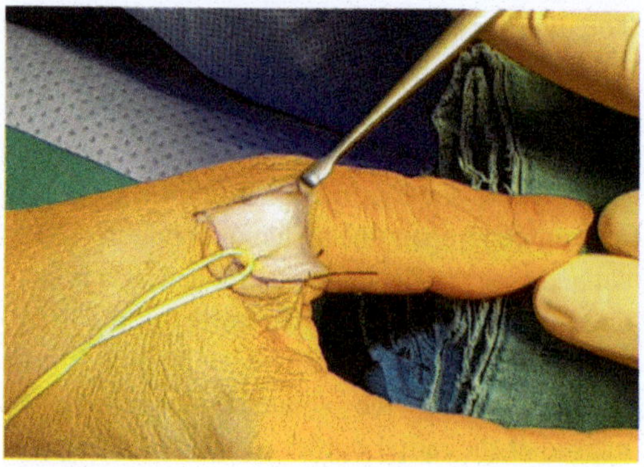

**Fig. 7.7** A branch of superficial radial nerve should be identified and protected during the dissection

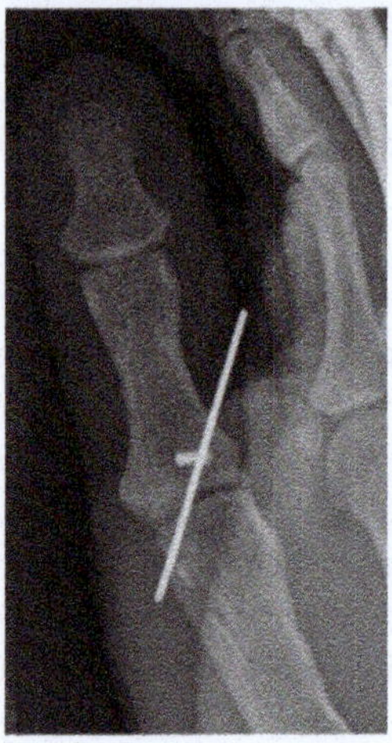

**Fig. 7.8** Repair of distal ulnar collateral ligament avulsion using a small intraosseous suture anchor and insertion of transfixing K-wire

(Fig. 7.8). Distal footprint of the ligament is carefully explored and prepared to reattachment by clearing adjacent soft tissues. We drill anchor hole at the distal footprint of the ligament which is placed slightly more volar than the lateral midline, accordingly to the reported anatomic attachment site of the ligament proper. The center of phalangeal insertion of UCL is 24% from the volar edge of the proximal phalanx. The center of phalangeal insertion of RCL is 29% from the volar edge of the proximal phalanx [10]. Drill tips are directed distally to the phalanx. After insertion of the suture anchor, we verify the stability of anchor by traction on two suture ends. Both needles are passed into the distal end of the avulsed ligament and knotted together. Some absorbable sutures can be additionally placed between the reattached ligament and surrounding structures.

Capsular flaps and the adductor (or abductor) aponeurosis are then repaired with an absorbable suture in layer by layer. After skin suturing, a short-arm thumb spica splint is applied in the operating room. Immobilization is maintained for 3–4 postoperative weeks, at which time active and gentle passive range of motion is started. We prefer transfixing the joint with the ligament repair, especially in patients with large capsular tear or with low compliance. The thumb MCP joint is held reduced in 10–15° of flexion and a 0.9-mm K-wire is placed. The K-wire is removed after 3 weeks in UCL repair and 4 weeks in RCL repair cases.

In the case of a bone avulsion, small fragment which involves MCP joint articular surface less than 10% can be removed. Then, the avulsed ligament is reattached into the bone defect using a small anchor. When there is larger bone fragment, it is reduced to an anatomical position into the defect site. It may be fixed with small K-wire, mini screws, or hook plate (Fig. 7.9).

## Chronic Injuries

Chronic instability leads to functional impairment including pain, weakness of thumb-to-digit pincer grasp, and progressive osteoarthritis. Acute and chronic injuries are generally distinguished using 6 weeks criterion. In the acute phase of injuries,

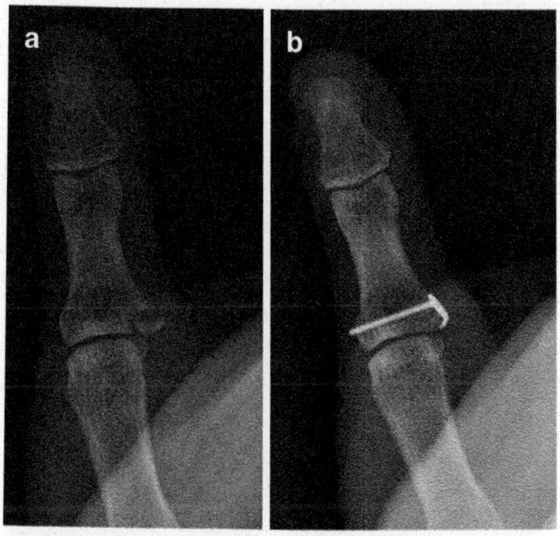


**Fig. 7.9** Refixation of ulnar collateral ligament avulsion fracture using a small hook plate. (**a**) Avulsion fracture at the base of the proximal phalanx with displacement. (**b**) Postoperative radiograph taken after reduction and hook plate fixation

the torn collateral ligament can be easily repaired because its remnant is usually preserved and easily identified, but in many chronic cases, direct repair is difficult, because remaining ligament tissues are frequently attenuated and absorbed not robust enough to repair. For chronic instability without arthritic changes, surgical repair or reconstruction is necessary. For chronic instability with arthritic changes, arthrodesis is preferable treatment considering patient symptoms and demands.

## Operative Approaches

Many surgical techniques for the reconstruction of chronic unstable collateral ligament injuries of the thumb and fingers have been described. Of the various available reconstruction techniques, a free tendon graft using palmaris longus tendon is the most reliable. However, the optimal graft configuration and adequacy of fixation methods remain subjects of debate. The commonly used surgical techniques are a tendon graft with a figure of eight configuration through bone tunnels [41, 42], a tendon graft with one drill hole at the base of the proximal phalanx [34], or a tendon graft through drill holes in the metacarpal and proximal phalanx [43]. In all cases, reconstructed tendon ends are passed through the bone tunnel, pulled out, and fixed with a button on the skin or attached to bone with a staple. These bone tunnel techniques are also commonly used for the reconstruction of PIP joint instability [44, 45]. An interference screw fixation technique for fixation of grafted tendon has recently been described [46]. The techniques for UCL reconstruction can be applied to RCL reconstruction [21], and most RCL reconstruction techniques use a free tendon graft with bone tunnels [6, 47]. Although these traditional fixation methods have produced favorable clinical results, making bone tunnels is technically demanding. Passing tendons through bone tunnels is sometimes difficult, and during passage of the tendon, there is a risk of breaking the bone bridge. Recently, intraosseous suture anchors have been widely used for ligament repair in the shoulder, elbow, and knee and offer the advantages of technical simplicity and mechanical stability. The successful application of intraosseous suture anchors for the treatment of MCP collateral ligament has been used in acute injury [7, 39, 48] and also in chronic injury [49].

## Surgical Technique of Anatomical Collateral Ligament Reconstruction Using Suture Anchors and a Free Tendon Graft

Author's preferred technique for reconstruction of the UCL ligament is using suture anchors and a free tendon graft (Fig. 7.10) [49]. The configurations of grafted tendons affect the stability and natural articulation of joints. When the traditional bone tunnel technique is used, it is difficult to reconstruct grafted tendons that approximate to original collateral ligaments due to the technical difficulty associated with safely making bone tunnels in narrow phalangeal bones. The collateral ligament reconstruction using suture anchors can minimize the risk of bone bridge breakage and feasible to provide a straightforward means of configuring grafts to approximate to the anatomical shapes of ligaments.

The exposure is the same as that described earlier for repair of acute ligament repairs. If remnants of collateral ligament do not exist, three suture anchors are used to hold the grafted tendon (Fig. 7.11). Two anchors are placed at the base of the proximal phalanx approximately 5 mm from

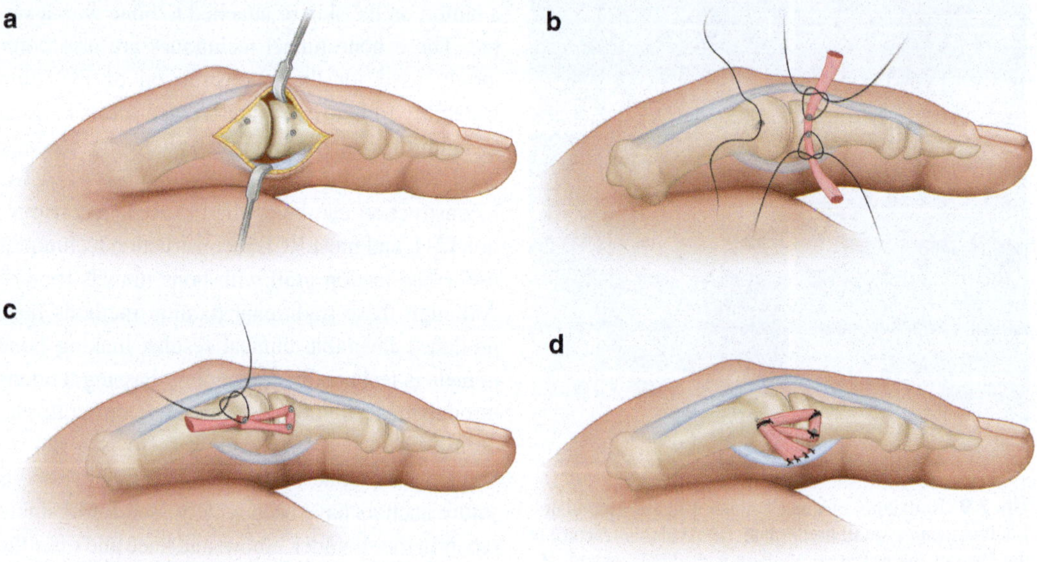


**Fig. 7.10** The reconstruction technique of the ulnar collateral ligament using three suture anchors and palmaris longus tendon graft. (**a**) Distal two and proximal one hole drilling for the placement of three anchors. (**b**) The tendon graft is sutured at the two distal anchors first. (**c**) Two limbs of the tendon graft are tied at the anchor of the metacarpal head. (**d**) The longer arm of the remaining graft is sutured to the volar plate

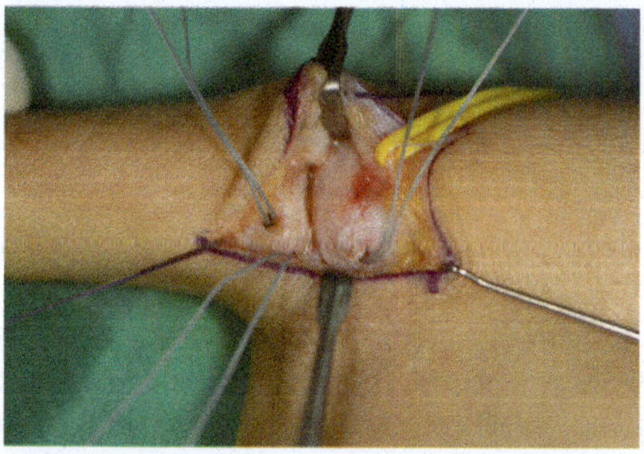

**Fig. 7.11** Three suture anchors are used to hold the grafted tendon. One of the distal suture anchors is fixed at the lateral center of the base of the proximal phalanx and the other at the lateral volar side of the bone. The proximal suture anchor is placed at the lateral center of the metacarpal head

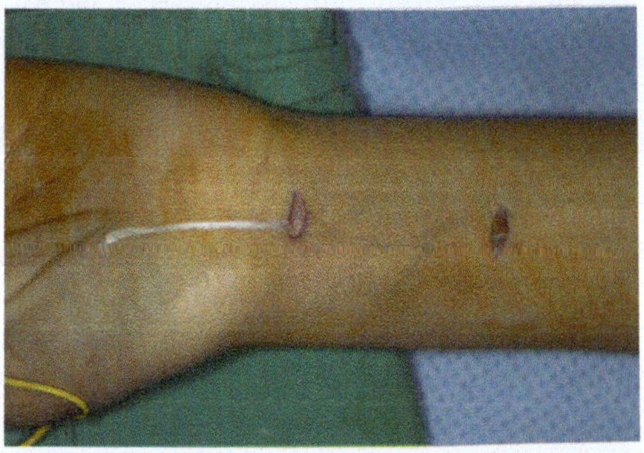

**Fig. 7.12** Two short transverse incisions are made at the distal wrist crease and 5 cm proximal to the first incision to harvest the half strip of the palmaris longus tendon

the joint line; one is fixed at the lateral center of the base of the proximal phalanx and the other at the lateral volar side of the bone. The proximal suture anchor is placed at the lateral center of the metacarpal head. If the remnants of collateral ligament tissue exist, only redundant end is trimmed and some ligament preserved at the metacarpal insertion site for the augmented suture with the grafted tendon after anchor suture.

After anchor fixation, a free tendon graft is harvested; the ipsilateral palmaris longus tendon is preferred. However, when the palmaris is not present, a one-third strip of flexor carpi radialis tendon can be used. To harvest the palmaris longus tendon, two short transverse incisions are made at the distal wrist crease and 5 cm proximal to the first incision (Fig. 7.12). Only a half strip of palmaris longus tendon is harvested using 2-0 nylon as a tendon stripper.

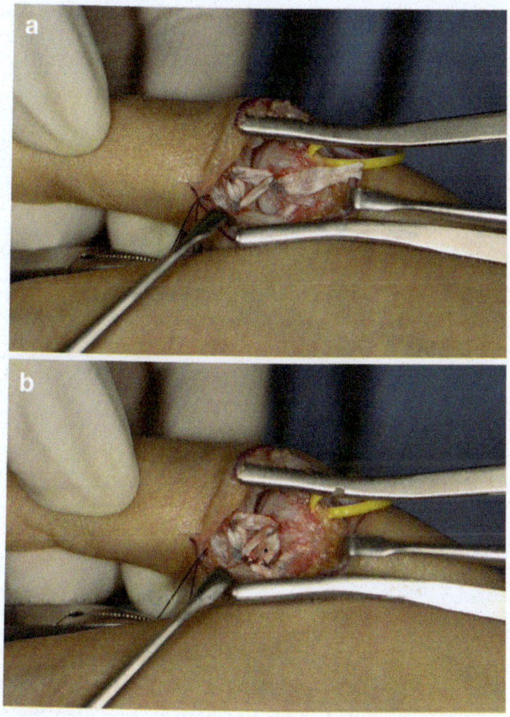

Fig. 7.13 Tying the tendon graft at the three suture anchors. (a) The tendon graft is sutured at the two distal anchors first. Then, two limbs of the tendon graft are tied at the anchor of the metacarpal head in reduced metacarpophalangeal joint. (b) The longer arm of the remaining graft (asterisk) is turned down and sutured at the volar plate to reconstruct the accessory collateral ligament

For anatomical reconstruction of the collateral ligament, a proper collateral ligament portion is first reconstructed by tying the tendon graft at the two suture anchors previously fixed at the base of proximal phalanx. While holding the graft under adequate tension, two limbs of the tendon graft are tied at the anchor of the metacarpal head. The longer arm of the remaining tendon is turned down to the palmar side and sutured to the volar plate for the reconstruction of the accessory collateral ligament (Fig. 7.13). The reconstructed graft is then gently tested by applying lateral stress to ensure adequate tensioning, and passive range of motion is checked to confirm that the reconstruction is not too tight. The joint is then transfixed with a 0.9-mm K wire, and each side of the incised capsule is repaired (Fig. 7.14). At anchor sites, the grafted tendon is sutured together with the capsule to promote healing of the graft. The adductor (or abductor) aponeurosis is then repaired with a 5-0 absorbable suture. After skin suturing, a short-arm thumb spica splint or simple finger splint is applied in the operating room.

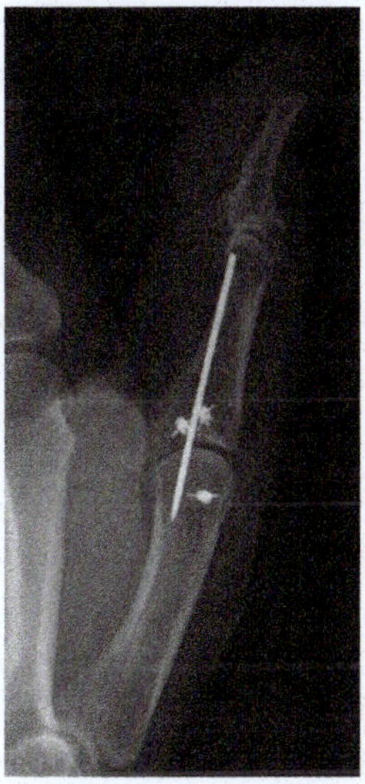

Fig. 7.14 Postoperative radiograph after ligament reconstruction shows the placement of three intraosseous suture anchors. Grafted tendon is protected by a temporary transfixing K-wire

Patients are splinted for 3–4 postoperative weeks, at which time the K-wire is removed and active and gentle passive range of motion is started. We tend to have longer period of immobilization of RCL injury than UCL because adductor muscle sometimes leads recurrent radial laxity. During the immobilization period, IP joint should be left free to move. Patient should be taught to avoid radial or ulnar deviation stress for 3 months. Full activity is allowed after 3 months postoperatively.

### Technical Tip

- Always identify and protect the branches of superficial radial nerve before incise the aponeurosis.
- Preserve 1–2 mm adductor (or abductor) aponeurosis from the ulnar (or radial) of the extensor pollicis tendon to facilitate later repair.
- Placed two anchors at the base of the proximal phalanx approximately 5 mm from the joint line; one is fixed at the lateral center and the

other at the lateral volar side of the bone to mimic anatomic insertion of the ligament.

- Place all three anchors before transfixing K-wire; later insertion of anchor can be failed due to crowding with K-wire.
- If it is difficult to maintain adequately reduced MCP joint while suturing graft tendon, transfixing K-wire can be inserted first to prevent ligament reconstruction in unexpected varus or valgus position.
- Suturing the graft tendon ends considering the reconstruction of the accessory ligament. The longer arm of the remaining tendon can be turned down to the volar side and sutured to the volar plate for the reconstruction of the accessory collateral ligament.

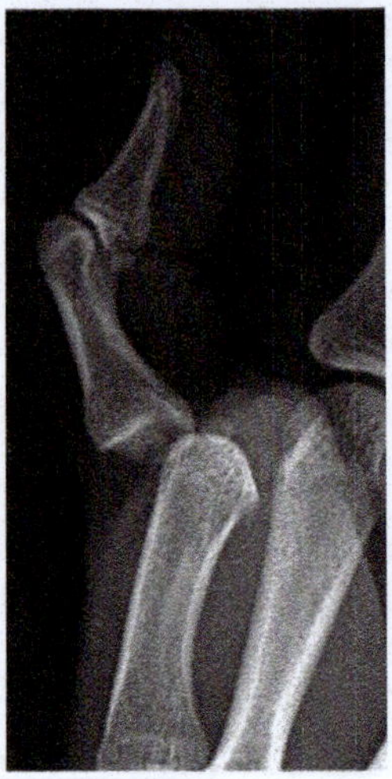

**Fig. 7.15** Radiographic appearance of dorsal dislocation of the thumb metacarpophalangeal joint

## Dislocation of the Metacarpophalangeal Joint of the Thumb

Most common dislocations of the thumb MCP joint are dorsal and occur from a forceful hyperextension injury. Patients with acute dislocation usually have edema, ecchymosis, and tenderness around the MCP joint. In dorsal dislocation, proximal phalanx is displaced dorsally and proximally, and bayonet-like deformity of the thumb can be observed due to the protrusion of the metacarpal head through the ruptured volar plate and intrinsic muscle (Fig. 7.15). Rupture of the volar plate usually ruptured proximally with the nondisplaced sesamoid. If volar plate is ruptured at the distal part, sesamoid is displaced proximally [50]. Dorsal dislocations are mostly reducible; however, some can be presented with irreducible dislocations. As first described by Kaplan [51], refer to instances in which the volar plate is avulsed from its attachment to the metacarpal and becomes interposed between the proximal phalanx and the metacarpus. Various interposing structures have been found to be responsible for the failure of closed reduction, typically the volar plate, the flexor and adductor tendon, the capsule interposition, and sesamoid bone incarceration.

Volar dislocations rarely occur as a result of hyperflexion of the MP joint or a blow to the dorsum of the proximal phalanx in flexion. They are mostly irreducible, and open reduction is usually required for the cases presenting with interposition of the extensor tendons [52–54]. In some cases, successful closed reduction has also been reported [53, 55].

### Treatment

The preferred reduction technique for dorsal dislocation is hyperextension of the dorsally angulated proximal phalanx with a gentle push over the base of the phalanx and the metacarpal head. Simple longitudinal traction can induce difficult reduction secondary to the strain of the adductor pollicis and flexor pollicis brevis [56, 57]. McLaughlin [58] demonstrated that if thumb dislocation is not reduced through a proper technique, simple complete dislocation could be converted to complex irreducible dislocation and may require operation.

After satisfactory reduction is achieved, stability should be assessed, and immobilization of the MCP joint is maintained for about 4 weeks. If significant instability of collateral ligament is observed after the reduction, it should be treated according to the acute UCL or RCL rupture. Occasionally, closed reduction is not possible, and open reduction is required. These cases may occur when the metacarpal head is entrapped into the rupture of the volar capsules and thenar muscle. In some cases, excessive contralateral traction may cause the buttonhole effect in the metacarpal head, resulting in over-tensioning of the surrounding soft tissue structures. Radial condyle of first metacarpal is anatomically larger and more protruded than ulnar condyle [59, 60]. Therefore, when this radial condyle is entrapped through the tear of radial part of volar plate during hyperextension injury, closed reduction may not be possible.

There has been no consensus which is the best surgical approach to treat these problems. Dorsal, volar, or lateral surgical approach can be determined by surgeon preference. The advantage of the volar approach is that it allows better visualization and protection of the digital nerves, which are not visible through a dorsal approach [61–63]. More recent evidence demonstrated that a dorsal approach more often results in successful reduction than does a volar approach. Because the volar plate has been displaced onto the dorsum of the metacarpal head, a dorsal approach provides ready access to this key structure [64]. Several authors describe how the volar plate can easily be identified and divided through the dorsal approach, allowing reduction of the joint with minimal soft tissue injury [65–67].

During surgical reduction, the soft tissue caught in the joints should be removed, and the ruptured volar plate, collateral ligaments, or sesamoid should be anatomically restored (Fig. 7.16). Postoperative care and rehabilitation protocol are

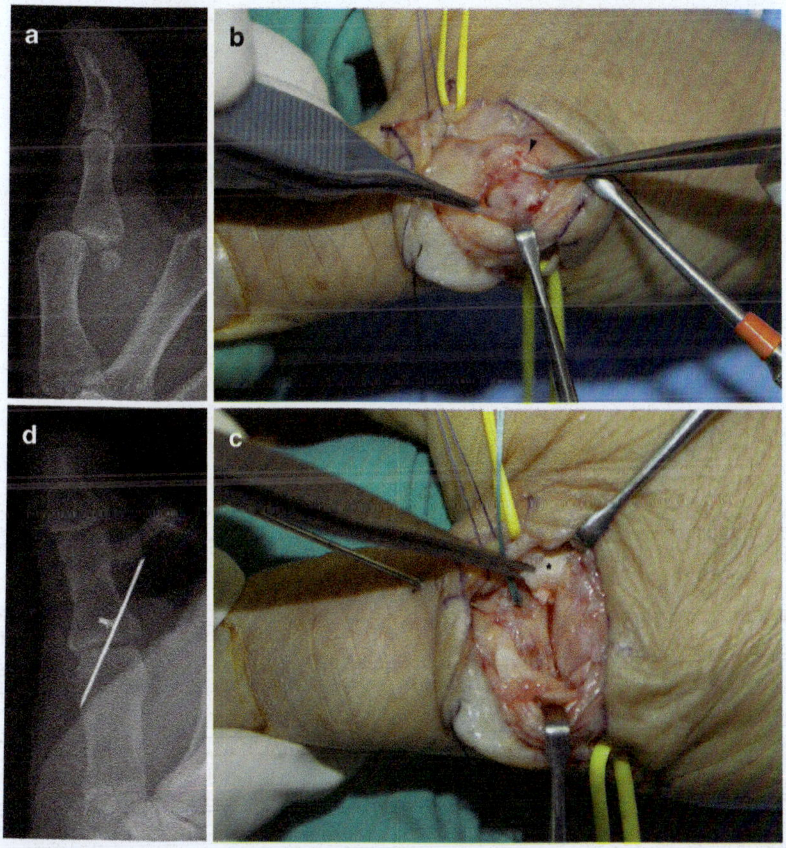


**Fig. 7.16** Volar dislocation of the thumb metacarpophalangeal (MCP) joint. (**a**) Plain radiograph lateral view shows volar dislocation of the right thumb MCP joint. (**b**) The intraoperative photograph demonstrates the metacarpal head protruded through a tear in the dorsal capsule (arrowhead). (**c**) After reduction, valgus instability and the proximal stump of the torn ulnar collateral ligament (UCL, asterisk) are observed. (**d**) Postoperative radiograph after suture anchor refixation of the torn UCL and capsular repair. Joint pinning is maintained for 4 weeks. (**e**) Thumb motion at 6 months follow-up

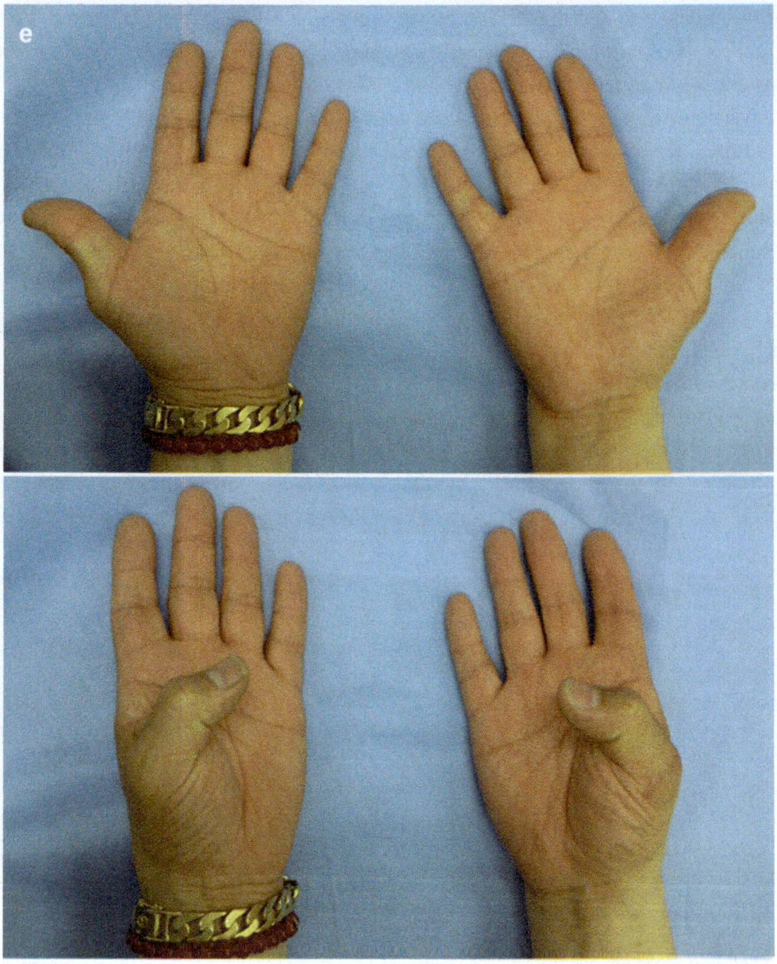


**Fig. 7.16** (continued)

similar with acute collateral ligament repair. Although favorable functional outcome is expected, stiffness is more common complication than instability. Patient should be counseled that they might have some loss of the thumb motion and strength. Frequently either ulnar or radial side of MCP joint can be prominent because of scar tissue formation at the area of injury and surgical repair.

## References


1. Campbell CS. Gamekeeper's thumb. J Bone Joint Surg Br. 1955;37-B:148–9.
2. Gerber C, Senn E, Matter P. Skier's thumb. Surgical treatment of recent injuries to the ulnar collateral ligament of the thumb's metacarpophalangeal joint. Am J Sports Med. 1981;9:171–7.
3. Warme WJ, Feagin JA Jr, King P, et al. Ski injury statistics, 1982 to 1993, Jackson Hole Ski Resort. Am J Sports Med. 1995;23:597–600.
4. Moberg E, Stener B. Injuries to the ligaments of the thumb and fingers; diagnosis, treatment and prognosis. Acta Chir Scand. 1953;106:166–86.
5. Edelstein DM, Kardashian G, Lee SK. Radial collateral ligament injuries of the thumb. J Hand Surg Am. 2008;33:760–70.
6. Melone CP Jr, Beldner S, Basuk RS. Thumb collateral ligament injuries. An anatomic basis for treatment. Hand Clin. 2000;16:345–57.
7. Kato H, Minami A, Takahara M, et al. Surgical repair of acute collateral ligament injuries in digits with the Mitek bone suture anchor. J Hand Surg Br. 1999;24:70–5.
8. Yoshida R, House HO, Patterson RM, et al. Motion and morphology of the thumb metacarpophalangeal joint. J Hand Surg Am. 2003;28:753–7.
9. Stener B. Displacement of the ruptured ulnar collateral ligament of the metacarpo-phalangeal joint of the

thumb—a clinical and anatomical study. J Bone Joint Surg Br. 1962;44:869–79.
10. Carlson MG, Warner KK, Meyers KN, et al. Anatomy of the thumb metacarpophalangeal ulnar and radial collateral ligaments. J Hand Surg Am. 2012;37:2021–6.
11. Heyman P, Gelberman RH, Duncan K, et al. Injuries of the ulnar collateral ligament of the thumb metacarpophalangeal joint. Biomechanical and prospective clinical studies on the usefulness of valgus stress testing. Clin Orthop Relat Res. 1993;292: 165–71.
12. Derkash RS, Matyas JR, Weaver JK, et al. Acute surgical repair of the skier's thumb. Clin Orthop Relat Res. 1987;216:29–33.
13. Coyle MP Jr. Grade III radial collateral ligament injuries of the thumb metacarpophalangeal joint: treatment by soft tissue advancement and bony reattachment. J Hand Surg Am. 2003;28:14–20.
14. Lyons RP, Kozin SH, Failla JM. The anatomy of the radial side of the thumb: static restraints in preventing subluxation and rotation after injury. Am J Orthop (Belle Mead NJ). 1998;27:759–63.
15. Stener B. Skeletal injuries associated with rupture of the ulnar collateral ligament of the metacarpophalangeal joint of the thumb. A clinical and anatomical study. Acta Chir Scand. 1963;125:583–6.
16. Harley BJ, Werner FW, Green JK. A biomechanical modeling of injury, repair, and rehabilitation of ulnar collateral ligament injuries of the thumb. J Hand Surg Am. 2004;29:915–20.
17. Malik AK, Morris T, Chou D, et al. Clinical testing of ulnar collateral ligament injuries of the thumb. J Hand Surg Eur Vol. 2009;34:363–6.
18. Bowers WH, Hurst LC. Gamekeeper's thumb. Evaluation by arthrography and stress roentgenography. J Bone Joint Surg Am. 1977;59:519–24.
19. Harper MT, Chandnani VP, Spaeth J, et al. Gamekeeper thumb: diagnosis of ulnar collateral ligament injury using magnetic resonance imaging, magnetic resonance arthrography and stress radiography. J Magn Reson Imaging. 1996;6:322–8.
20. Noszian IM, Dinkhauser LM, Straub GM, et al. Ulnar collateral ligament injuries of the thumb. Dislocation caused by stress radiography in 2 cases. Acta Orthop Scand. 1995;66:156–7.
21. Tang P. Collateral ligament injuries of the thumb metacarpophalangeal joint. J Am Acad Orthop Surg. 2011;19:287–96.
22. Hintermann B, Holzach PJ, Schutz M, et al. Skier's thumb—the significance of bony injuries. Am J Sports Med. 1993;21:800–4.
23. Giele H, Martin J. The two-level ulnar collateral ligament injury of the metacarpophalangeal joint of the thumb. J Hand Surg Br. 2003;28:92–3.
24. Lumens D, Lamraski G. [Treatment of a posttraumatic hyperextension instability of the metacarpophalangeal joint of the thumb using a free tendon graft and bone suture anchors]. Chir Main. 2007;26: 143–5.
25. Hergan K, Mittler C. Sonography of the injured ulnar collateral ligament of the thumb. J Bone Joint Surg Br. 1995;77:77–83.
26. Shinohara T, Horii E, Majima M, et al. Sonographic diagnosis of acute injuries of the ulnar collateral ligament of the metacarpophalangeal joint of the thumb. J Clin Ultrasound. 2007;35:73–7.
27. Jones MH, England SJ, Muwanga CL, et al. The use of ultrasound in the diagnosis of injuries of the ulnar collateral ligament of the thumb. J Hand Surg Br. 2000;25:29–32.
28. Papandrea RF, Fowler T. Injury at the thumb UCL: is there a stener lesion? J Hand Surg Am. 2008;33:1882–4.
29. Spaeth HJ, Abrams RA, Bock GW, et al. Gamekeeper thumb: differentiation of nondisplaced and displaced tears of the ulnar collateral ligament with MR imaging. Radiology. 1993;188:553–6.
30. Hergan K, Mittler C, Oser W. Ulnar collateral ligament: differentiation of displaced and nondisplaced tears with US and MR imaging. Radiology. 1995;194:65–71.
31. Ahn JM, Sartoris DJ, Kang HS, et al. Gamekeeper thumb: comparison of MR arthrography with conventional arthrography and MR imaging in cadavers. Radiology. 1998;206:737–44.
32. Ryu J, Fagan R. Arthroscopic treatment of acute complete thumb metacarpophalangeal ulnar collateral ligament tears. J Hand Surg Am. 1995;20:1037–42.
33. Slade JF 3rd, Gutow AP. Arthroscopy of the metacarpophalangeal joint. Hand Clin. 1999;15:501–27.
34. Smith RJ. Post-traumatic instability of the metacarpophalangeal joint of the thumb. J Bone Joint Surg Am. 1977;59:14–21.
35. Wilppula E, Nummi J. Surgical treatment of ruptured ulnar collateral ligament of the metacarpophalangeal joint of the thumb. Injury. 1970;2:69–72.
36. Downey DJ, Moneim MS, Omer GE Jr. Acute gamekeeper's thumb. Quantitative outcome of surgical repair. Am J Sports Med. 1995;23:222–6.
37. Zeman C, Hunter RE, Freeman JR, et al. Acute skier's thumb repaired with a proximal phalanx suture anchor. Am J Sports Med. 1998;26:644–50.
38. Kozin SH. Treatment of thumb ulnar collateral ligament ruptures with the Mitek bone anchor. Ann Plast Surg. 1995;35:1–5.
39. Weiland AJ, Berner SH, Hotchkiss RN, et al. Repair of acute ulnar collateral ligament injuries of the thumb metacarpophalangeal joint with an intraosseous suture anchor. J Hand Surg Am. 1997;22:585–91.
40. Bean CH, Tencer AF, Trumble TE. The effect of thumb metacarpophalangeal ulnar collateral ligament attachment site on joint range of motion: an in vitro study. J Hand Surg Am. 1999;24:283–7.
41. Alldred AJ. Rupture of the collateral ligament of the metacarpo-phalangeal joint of the thumb. J Bone Joint Surg Br. 1955;37-B:443–5.
42. Osterman AL, Hayken GD, Bora FW Jr. A quantitative evaluation of thumb function after ulnar collateral repair and reconstruction. J Trauma. 1981;21:854–61.

43. Glickel SZ, Malerich M, Pearce SM, et al. Ligament replacement for chronic instability of the ulnar collateral ligament of the metacarpophalangeal joint of the thumb. J Hand Surg Am. 1993;18:930–41.
44. Mantovani G, Pavan A, Aita MA, et al. Surgical reconstruction of PIP joint collateral ligament in chronic instability in a high performance athlete: case report and description of technique. Tech Hand Up Extrem Surg. 2011;15:87–91.
45. Morris SF, Yang D, Milne AD, et al. Reconstruction of the proximal interphalangeal joint collateral ligaments using the Mitek Micro Arc Anchor: an in vitro biomechanical assessment. Ann Plast Surg. 1999;42:124–8.
46. Rettig A, Rettig L, Welsch M. Anatomic reconstruction of thumb metacarpophalangeal joint ulnar collateral ligament using an interference screw docking technique. Tech Hand Up Extrem Surg. 2009;13:7–10.
47. Catalano LW 3rd, Cardon L, Patenaude N, et al. Results of surgical treatment of acute and chronic grade III [corrected] tears of the radial collateral ligament of the thumb metacarpophalangeal joint. J Hand Surg Am. 2006;31:68–75.
48. Rehak DC, Sotereanos DG, Bowman MW, et al. The Mitek bone anchor: application to the hand, wrist and elbow. J Hand Surg Am. 1994;19:853–60.
49. Lee JI, Jeon WJ, Suh DH, et al. Anatomical collateral ligament reconstruction in the hand using intraosseous suture anchors and a free tendon graft. J Hand Surg Eur Vol. 2012;37:832–8.
50. Miller RJ. Dislocations and fracture dislocations of the metacarpophalangeal joint of the thumb. Hand Clin. 1988;4:45–65.
51. Kaplan EB. Dorsal dislocation of the metacarpophalangeal joint of the index finger. J Bone Joint Surg Am. 1957;39-A:1081–6.
52. Alioto RJ, Pellegrini VD Jr. Complex palmar dislocation of the thumb metacarpophalangeal joint. A case report demonstrating paradoxical function of the extensor pollicis longus. Clin Orthop Relat Res. 1993;11:118–21.
53. Beck JD, Klena JC. Closed reduction and treatment of 2 volar thumb metacarpophalangeal dislocations: report of 2 cases. J Hand Surg Am. 2011;36:665–9.
54. Miyamoto M, Hirayama T, Uchida M. Volar dislocation of the metacarpophalangeal joint of the thumb—a case report. J Hand Surg Br. 1986;11:51–4.
55. Garcia Mata S, Hidalgo Ovejero A, Martinez Grande M. Volar dislocation of the first metacarpophalangeal joint. A case report and review of the literature. Acta Orthop Belg. 1991;57:323–8.
56. Green DP, Terry GC. Complex dislocation of the metacarpophalangeal joint. Correlative pathological anatomy. J Bone Joint Surg Am. 1973;55:1480–6.
57. Dutton RO, Meals RA. Complex dorsal dislocation of the thumb metacarpophalangeal joint. Clin Orthop Relat Res. 1982;4:160–4.
58. McLaughlin HL. Complex "locked" dislocation of the metacarpophalangeal joints. J Trauma. 1965;5:683–8.
59. Ishizuki M, Nakagawa T, Ito S. Hyperextension injuries of the MP joint of the thumb. J Hand Surg Br. 1994;19:361–7.
60. Hirata H, Tsujii M, Nakao E. Locking of the metacarpophalangeal joint of the thumb caused by a fracture fragment of the radial condyle of the metacarpal head after dorsal dislocation. J Hand Surg Br. 2006;31:635–6.
61. Dinh P, Franklin A, Hutchinson B, et al. Metacarpophalangeal joint dislocation. J Am Acad Orthop Surg. 2009;17:318–24.
62. Mudgal CS, Mudgal S. Volar open reduction of complex metacarpophalangeal dislocation of the index finger: a pictorial essay. Tech Hand Up Extrem Surg. 2006;10:31–6.
63. Hughes LA, Freiberg A. Irreducible MP joint dislocation due to entrapment of FPL. J Hand Surg Br. 1993;18:708–9.
64. Afifi AM, Medoro A, Salas C, et al. A cadaver model that investigates irreducible metacarpophalangeal joint dislocation. J Hand Surg Am. 2009;34:1506–11.
65. Patterson RW, Maschke SD, Evans PJ, et al. Dorsal approach for open reduction of complex metacarpophalangeal joint dislocations. Orthopedics. 2008;31:1099.
66. Bohart PG, Gelberman RH, Vandell RF, et al. Complex dislocations of the metacarpophalangeal joint. Clin Orthop Relat Res. 1982;4:208–10.
67. Vadala CJ, Ward CM. Dorsal approach decreases operative time for complex metacarpophalangeal dislocations. J Hand Surg Am. 2016;41:e259–62.

# Arthritis of the Interphalangeal Joint and Metacarpophalangeal Joint

8

Jae Hoon Lee

## Rheumatoid Arthritis

Rheumatoid arthritis is a systemic condition that affects synovial tissue. Rheumatoid arthritis is caused by hypertrophic synovitis, which eventually destroys the articular cartilage, causing erodes and ruptures of the tendons, compression of the surrounding nerves, and dislocation of the joints. The involvement of the thumb of rheumatoid arthritis causes a variety of deformities as synovitis begins in the joints. When synovitis begins at the thumb metacarpophalangeal joint, it results in boutonniere deformity (flexion of the metacarpophalangeal joint, palmar subluxation of the proximal phalanx, and hyperextension of the interphalangeal joint). Surgery is recommended when there is pain, deformity, and disability and includes synovectomy, tenodesis, tendon transfer, arthrodesis, and arthroplasty.

Thumb deformity due to rheumatoid arthritis was classified into five types by Nalebuff. This is based on initial deformity and secondary compensatory position of the metacarpal and phalanx.

Type 1 is the most common, followed by type 3. Types 2, 4, and 5 are rare.

J. H. Lee (✉)
Department of Orthopedic Surgery, Kyung Hee University Hospital at Gangdong, Seoul, South Korea

### Type 1 (Boutonniere Deformity)

It is most common and starts with proliferative synovitis that occurs in MPJ. MPJ synovitis stretches the joints and extensor hood, attenuates the insertion site of extensor pollicis brevis (EPB), and translates extensor pollicis longus (EPL) into ulnar and palmar. This change in force invokes MPJ hyperflexion, palmar subluxation of the proximal phalanx, and IPJ hyperextension. In the early stages, MPJ and IPJ deformities can be passively corrected. However, over time, fixed MPJ deformity occurs and then occurs in IPJ. In the early stages, splinting, medical treatment, and intermittent steroid injection may be used as conservative treatment to slow the pain relief and disease progression. Surgical treatment is determined by the severity of joint destruction, the possibility of passive correction of deformity, and the patient's expectation. In the early stages of the proliferative phase where pain is not controlled for conservative treatment and MPJ flexion and IPJ hyperextension can be passively corrected, surgical treatment includes MPJ synovectomy and extension tendon reconstruction. Extension tendon reconstruction is to reroute the EPL to the proximal phalanx base to provide additional power. For severely arthritic joints that can't be passively corrected and unstable or dislocated joints with articular defects, MPJ arthrodesis are recommended. It has been known that it allows rapid return with functional activity, low complication rate, and


S. H. Woo (ed.), *The Thumb*, https://doi.org/10.1007/978-981-10-4400-7_8

high fusion rate. In case of fixed MPJ and passively correctable IPJ, MPJ arthrodesis is recommended. When arthritis develops in MPJ and trapeziometacarpal joint (TMCJ), TMCJ arthroplasty and MPJ arthrodesis are recommended. If both MPJ and IPJ have a fixed deformity, MPJ arthrodesis and dorsal capsulotomy of IPJ can be performed. IPJ arthrodesis is recommended for severe IPJ deformities.

### Type 2

It is a rare and combination of type 1 and type 3. MPJ flexion, IPJ hyperextension, and TMCJ subluxation or dislocation are developed. Treatment is similar to treatment of type 1 and type 3.

### Type 3 (Swan Neck Deformity)

It is second most common and is characterized by MP joint hyperextension, IP joint flexion, and metacarpal adduction. Synovitis starts at TMCJ leading to dorsal and radial subluxation of TMCJ, adduction of the metacarpal bone, tightening of the extensor tendon, and eventually MPJ extension and IPJ flexion. If conservative treatment such as medication, splinting, and intermittent steroid injection fails and pain persists, resection arthroplasty with ligament reconstruction and tendon interposition may be performed. If MPJ deformity and joint destruction are advanced, MPJ arthrodesis and trapeziometacarpal resection arthroplasty are recommended.

### Type 4 (Gamekeeper Thumb)

It unusually occurs. As a result of MPJ synovitis, the ulnar collateral ligament is affected, resulting in laxity of ligament and deformity of the proximal phalanx with metacarpal adduction. In the early stages, MP synovectomy and collateral ligament reconstruction are performed. For more advanced, MPJ arthroplasty or arthrodesis is recommended.

### Type 5

MPJ hyperextension due to laxity of volar plate of MPJ occurs, and IPJ flexion due to tension of FPL occurs. This requires the differentiation with type 3 deformity. Treatment is to stabilize joints by MPJ capsulodesis or arthrodesis.

## Degenerative Arthritis

Degenerative arthritis is the most common joint disease of the hands and is characterized by articular cartilage deterioration. Cartilage changes appear as enlargement of joint, pain, swelling, stiffness, contracture, and angular deformity. Conservative treatment is the cornerstone of treatment. If conservative treatment is not effective, surgical treatment is required. This is for pain control and joint stability.

The osteophyte in the distal interphalangeal joint is called the Heberden node, and the mucoid cyst may occur at the joint boundary. The osteophyte arising from the proximal interphalangeal joint is called Bouchard node. Spur formation, cartilage fragmentation, and limited motion without dislocation are common. In the active phase, the pain is severe, and the joints and adjacent skin are inflamed. Direct trauma to the inflamed joints is particularly painful. TMCJ is the most common, followed by MPJ and IPJ. TMCJ is the most common site of primary osteoarthritis or post-traumatic arthritis. Trapeziometacarpal osteoarthritis is the result of gradual volar trapezial articular surface eburnation. MPJ is problematic by ligament instability, especially by the ulnar collateral ligament. Surgical treatment methods include synovectomy, soft tissue reconstruction, arthroplasty, and arthrodesis.

## Arthrodesis of Thumb Joints

Arthrodesis of the IPJ and MPJ of the thumb can be used in the treatment of rheumatoid arthritis, primary osteoarthritis, and traumatic arthritis. Traumatic arthritis can be caused by malunion and nonunion after intra-articular fractures of IPJ and MPJ and may lead to traumatic arthritis after instability due to injury of the ulnar collateral ligament of the MCJ. Arthrodesis can be applied in intractable pain, instability, and joint deformity. In rheumatoid arthritis, there are limitations in the selection of implant fixation during arthrodesis due to insufficient soft tissue and bone. In some cases, bone grafting may be required. The thumb should be fused so that the end of the fused thumb is in contact with the tips of all other fingers. The carpometacarpal joints of the thumb is abducted by about 40° and must be fixed at the 20° extension position to enable precise grasping operation using the tip of the thumb. The MPJ is recommended to be bent at 5–15°. IPJ is recommended to be in 0–10° flexion. For successful arthrodesis, a good cancellous-to-cancellous bone contact and firm fixation should be done with proper surface preparation. The most commonly used method for joint surface preparation is the flat cut technique. There is a problem of bone loss or shortening, but it is the most commonly used method. Finger joint fixation methods vary, ranging from K-wire to plate fixation techniques.

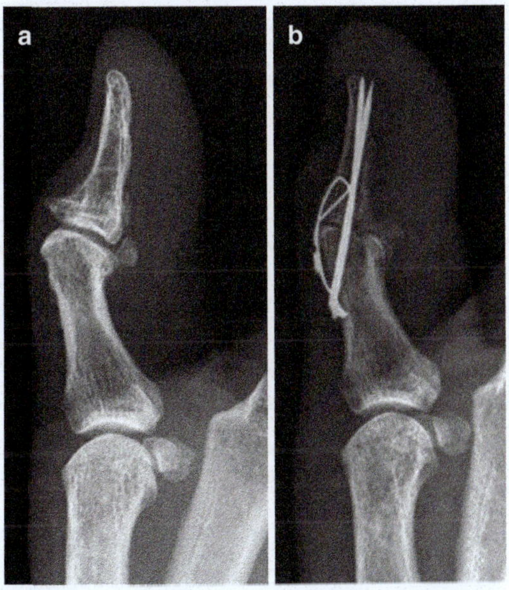


**Fig. 8.1** Radiographs showing arthrodesis (**b**) with tension band wiring in a patient with degenerative arthritis of interphalangeal joint of the thumb (**a**)

## IPJ Arthrodesis

The angle of the IPJ fusion of the thumb is fixed with neutral or slight bending. Longitudinal or crossed K-wires or tension band wiring (Fig. 8.1) for internal fixation using 0.045 or 0.062-in. K-wire is used. At present, intramedullary retrograde screw fixation using headless screws is most commonly used (Fig. 8.2).

Y-incision is made on the dorsal side of IPJ. After the skin flap is elevated, the extensor tendon is cut at the insertion site of the terminal tendon. Incise transversely the dorsal capsule and collateral ligaments. Remove the osteophyte around the joint. After exposing the joint surface by flexing the joints, the joint surface is cut to flat using small size saw, allowing the surface to bend about 5° when coapted. A guide wire is inserted through the intramedullary canal to the tip of distal phalanx tip. After reducing the joint, advance the guide wire through the fusion site to the middle phalanx. Fluoroscopy confirms the position of the wire and the extent of joint reduction. Measure the appropriate length, make an incision on the tip of the finger and drill to the proper length. Insert the headless screw.

## MPJ Arthrodesis

Arthrodesis is done at 5–15° flexion. Plate fixation, tension band wiring (Fig. 8.3), crossed K-wire fixation, and interosseous wiring with two orthogonal loops can be used. Currently, plate fixation is preferred (Fig. 8.4).

A 4 cm long longitudinal skin incision is made in the dorsal side of the MPJ of the thumb. The dorsal cutaneous nerve is well preserved, and the gap between the EPL and the EPB is exposed, and the joint capsule is exposed. The capsule is incised longitudinally, and then both collateral ligaments are cut. After flexing the joints, use a saw to cut the joint cartilage at an angle of 90°. After the joints are coapted, temporary K-wire fixation is performed, and fluoroscopy is performed to confirm the state of the cut and the angle of fixation. When the appropriate articular

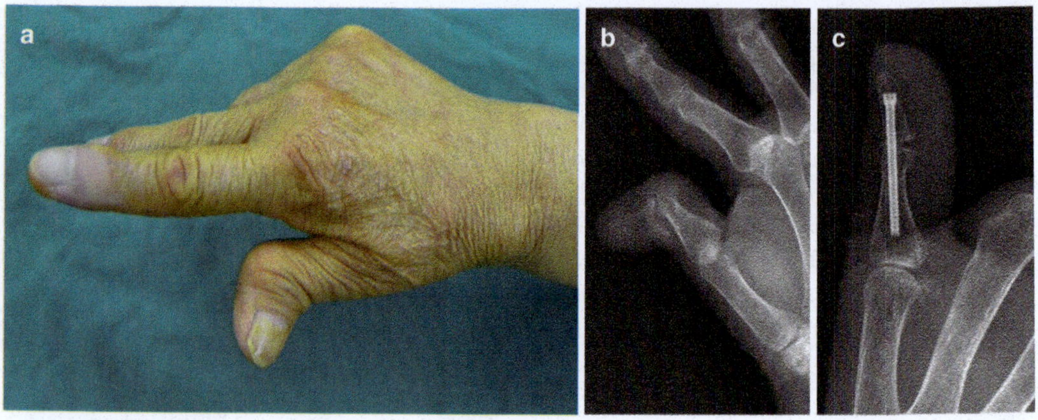


**Fig. 8.2** A 68-year-old female patient with joint deformity due to rheumatoid arthritis (**a**). Preoperative (**b**) and postoperative radiographs (**c**) after arthrodesis using headless screws

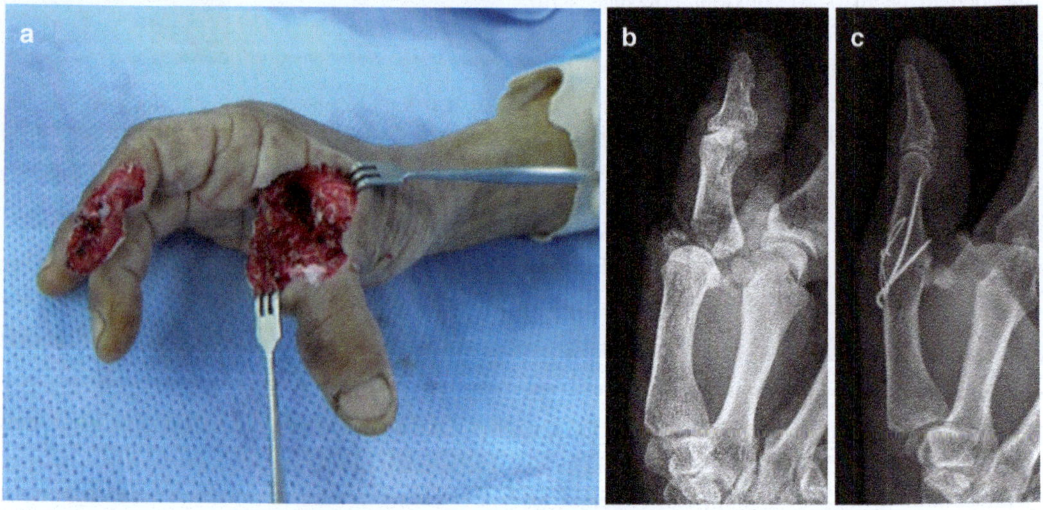


**Fig. 8.3** A 79-year-old male patient had saw injury and soft tissue defect at the metacarpophalangeal joint of the thumb (**a**). Preoperative radiography (**b**) and arthrodesis using tension band wiring (**c**)

**Fig. 8.4** A 56-year-old female patient with instability and arthritis due to bilateral collateral ligament injuries of the metacarpophalangeal joint the thumb (**a**) and radiography after plate fixation (**b**)

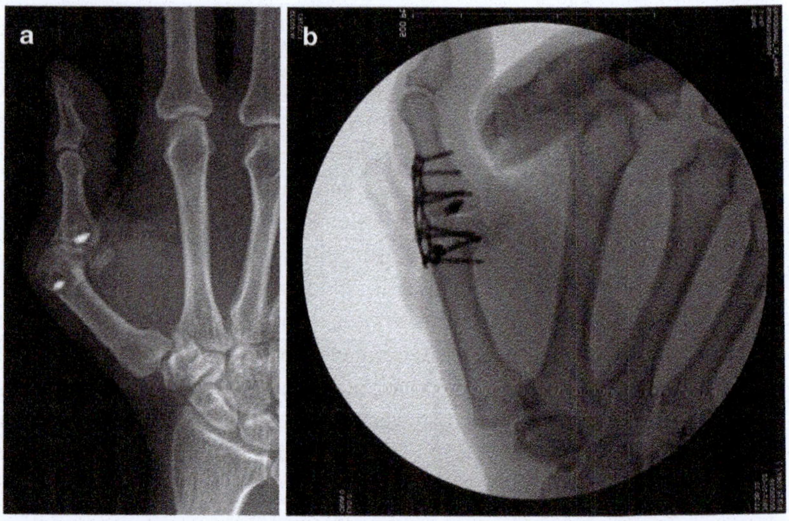

surface was gained, fuse the MPJ using a miniplate of 1.5–2.7 mm in size. After fixation, cover the plate with the joint capsule to prevent friction between plate and extensor tendon. Suture the skin using 4/0 nylon and immobilize with thumb spica short arm splint.

## Bibliography

Chung KC, Kotsis SV. Outcomes of hand surgery in the patient with rheumatoid arthritis. Curr Opin Rheumatol. 2010;22:336.

Day CS, Ramirez MA. Thumb metacarpophalangeal arthritis: arthroplasty or fusion? Hand Clin. 2006;22:211.

Feldon PG, Terrono AL, Nalebuff EA, et al. Rheumatoid arthritis. In: Green DP, Hotchkiss RN, Pederson WC, et al., editors. Operative hand surgery. 5th ed. Philadelphia: Churchill Livingstone; 2005.

Kahlenberg JM, Fox DA. Advances in the medical treatment of rheumatoid arthritis. Hand Clin. 2011;27:11.

King JA, Tomaino MT. Surgical treatment of the rheumatoid thumb. Hand Clin. 2001;17:275.

Nalebuff EA. Diagnosis, classification and management of rheumatoid thumb deformities. Bull Hosp Joint dis. 1968;29:119–37.

Rozental TD. Reconstruction of the rheumatoid thumb. J Am Acad Orthop Surg. 2007;15:118.

Sebastin SJ, Chung KC. Reconstruction of digital deformities in rheumatoid arthritis. Hand Clin. 2011;27:87.

Stanley JK, Smith EJ, Muirhead AG. Arthrodesis of the metacarpal-phalaneal joint of the thumb: a review of 42 cases. J Hand Surg. 1989;14:291–3.

# Arthritis of the Carpometacarpal Joint

9

Seok-Whan Song and Joo-Yup Lee

## Introduction

Osteoarthritis of the carpometacarpal (CMC) joint of the thumb is one of the most common symptomatic conditions of the hand. The prevalence of thumb CMC arthritis has been reported up to 15% of women and 7% of men in the middle years of life [1]. The wide range of motion contributes to the high prevalence of thumb CMC arthritis [2]. The condition may be acquired due to various underlying medical conditions, chronic trauma, advancing age, hormonal factors, and genetic influences [3]. Occupational factors are also believed to have a role in the development of thumb CMC arthritis [4].

This review will briefly introduce the pathophysiology and clinical features of the CMC arthritis and will discuss the possible surgical options including ligament reconstruction, extension osteotomy, simple trapeziectomy, interposition arthroplasty, trapezium excision and ligament reconstruction procedures, arthrodesis, and prosthetic arthroplasty. Clinical outcomes after different surgical procedures are also presented.

S.-W. Song
Department of Orthopedic Surgery,
Yeouido St. Mary's Hospital, The Catholic University of Korea, Seoul, South Korea
e-mail: sw.song@catholic.ac.kr

J.-Y. Lee (✉)
Department of Orthopedic Surgery,
St. Paul's Hospital, The Catholic University of Korea, Seoul, South Korea

## Pathophysiology

The CMC joint of the thumb is a biconcave-convex or reciprocal saddle joint with inherent instability. Because of the lack of bony stability, the stability of the joint is dependent on ligamentous structures. Although there is an association between CMC joint instability and the subsequent development of arthritic changes, there is no consensus on which ligament is primarily responsible for the joint stability. There are four primary ligamentous stabilizers in the CMC joint of the thumb: the anterior oblique ligament, the dorsoradial ligament, the intermetacarpal ligament, and the posterior oblique ligament. The primary stabilizer of the thumb CMC joint is the deep anterior oblique ligament. Eaton reported that the anterior oblique or volar beak ligament, which originated from the palmar tubercle of the trapezium and inserting to the volar aspect of the first metacarpal, is the primary restraint to dorsoradial subluxation [5]. This theory is supported by anatomic studies showing a direct correlation between the degeneration of the carpometacarpal articular surface and the integrity of the beak ligament.

Dorsoradial ligament is another important structure to contribute the thumb CMC joint stability. Strauch and colleagues performed serial sectioning of the ligaments of the CMC joint and showed that the primary restraint to dorsal dislocation was the dorsoradial ligament that connects the dorsal and radial aspect of the trapezium to


S. H. Woo (ed.), *The Thumb*, https://doi.org/10.1007/978-981-10-4400-7_9

the dorsum of the metacarpal base [6]. The intermetacarpal ligament, which originated from the dorsoradial aspect of the index metacarpal and inserting to the ulnar aspect of the first metacarpal, was determined to be the primary stabilizer to dorsal and radial subluxation according to Pagalidis and colleagues [7]. The posterior oblique ligament, which originated from the dorso-ulnar aspect of the trapezium and inserting on the palmar-ulnar aspect of the first metacarpal base, was the primary stabilizer according to Harvey and Bye [8].

Osteoarthritis of the thumb CMC joint occurs in a predictable pattern. High compressive and shear forces occur across the thumb CMC joint during pinch motion. Eaton and Littler observed that the dorsoradial facet of the CMC joint was the first site of articular wear. Subsequent study by Pellegrini et al. showed that arthritic changes usually occurred in the palmar compartment, and the area of cartilage eburnation corresponds to the primary loading area during lateral pinch [9]. Pellegrini concluded that the degeneration of the anterior oblique ligament results in dorsal translation of the metacarpal during lateral pinch motion. The beak ligament is the focus of many procedures designed to stabilize the thumb especially in the pronated position.

## Clinical and Radiologic Findings

Clinical symptoms and signs of the arthritis of thumb CMC joint are variable according to the stages of the disease. From the vague pain and discomfort to the frank swelling and instability, the level of derangements of the anatomical structures and biomechanics of thumb CMC joint determines the clinical and radiologic findings. Usually the symptoms start with vague discomfort at the CMC joint and often aggravated with powerful pinch and grasp. It is possible to identify the maximum tender point on the radial side of thumb basal joint. However, sometimes the patient cannot locate the tender point at the joint and describes as the pain of whole or part of the thumb. With the advancement of the arthritis, physical examination reveals swelling around the joint, tenderness at the joint, sometimes pain radiating to the radial aspect of the forearm, and decreased pinch power. Crepitus over the joint can be felt, and the grind test is positive when it causes pain and/or crepitus at the joint [10].

Finally, if the stabilizing ligaments, especially anterior oblique and/or dorsoradial ligaments, were attenuated, instability of the joint is established with dorsoradial protrusion of the base of the first metacarpal bone. The subluxation can be described as dynamic or fixed. In dynamic subluxation stage, i.e., an active instability stage, the CMC joint subluxes and reduces during active pinch and release. However, when the arthritis progresses, narrowing of the joint space and development of osteophytes decrease and prevent the subluxation of joint and result to fixed deformity as adducted position of the CMC joint and/or hyperextended metacarpophalangeal joint of the thumb [11].

Radiographic examination includes anterior-posterior (AP), lateral, semi (45°)-pronated, and semi-supinated oblique views. Hyperpronated Robert view and oblique stress view (Fig. 9.1) are also helpful to view the joint space clearly [12]. In general MRI or CT examinations are not needed in preparation of an operation. However if there is a severe deformity of the joint, CT

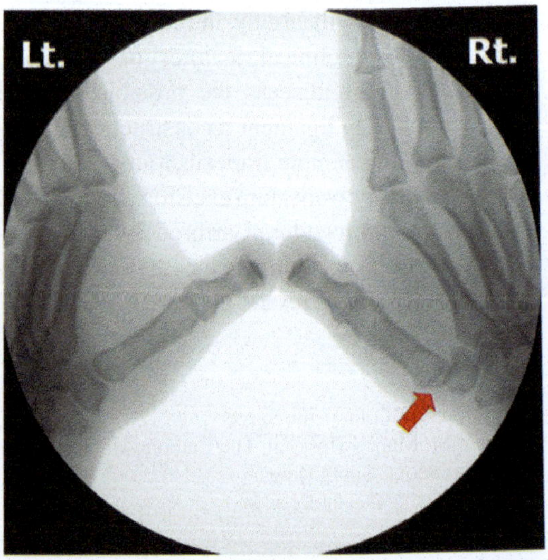


**Fig. 9.1** Posteroanterior oblique stress view of the thumb showing subluxation of the right thumb carpometacarpal joint (arrow)

examination can be used to plan a more detailed operative preparation [13] and MRI examination for the detection of soft tissue pathology [14].

Burton classified the carpometacarpal joint arthritis into a four-stage system, based on clinical signs, symptoms, and radiographic findings (Table 9.1). Stage I involves early degeneration of the joint characterized by pain, ligamentous laxity, and a dorsoradial subluxation. Stage II demonstrates increased instability, chronic subluxation, and degenerative changes in radiographs. Stage III is a further progression of the degeneration to involve the scaphotrapezial joint or trapeziotrapezoid or carpometacarpal joint of the index finger. Stage IV is either stage II or III with metacarpophalangeal joint changes [15].

Eaton and Littler introduced a classification system for staging the severity of CMC joint arthritis in 1973, and Eaton and Glickel adapted this to include degenerative changes to the scaphotrapezial joint in 1987 (Table 9.2) [16, 17]. The Eaton classification remains the most common system employed to determine the stage of the disease. Although this is the most useful staging system clinically, it relies on radiographic changes only without the patient's subjective and objective findings.

**Table 9.1** Burton classification for thumb carpometacarpal arthritis

| Staging | Description |
|---|---|
| I | Pain, ligamentous laxity, slight subluxation |
| II | Instability, chronic subluxation, radiographic degenerative changes |
| III | Involvement of the scaphotrapezial joint |
| IV | Stage II or III with the metacarpophalangeal joint arthritis |

**Table 9.2** Eaton classification system for thumb carpometacarpal arthritis

| Staging | Description |
|---|---|
| I | Normal joint or slight widening as a result of coexisting synovitis |
| II | Joint narrowing due to cartilage wear and osteophytes < 2 mm |
| III | Joint narrowing and osteophytes > 2 mm, sclerosis, and cystic changes |
| IV | Scaphotrapezial involvement with advanced carpometacarpal arthritis |

**Table 9.3** Arthroscopic classification system suggested by Badia

| Staging | Description |
|---|---|
| I | Intact articular cartilage, disruption of the dorsoradial ligament and diffuse synovial hypertrophy, inconsistent attenuation of the anterior oblique ligament |
| II | Frank eburnation of the articular cartilage on the ulnar third of the base of first metacarpal and central third of the distal surface of the trapezium |
| III | Widespread, full-thickness cartilage loss with or without a peripheral rim on both articular surfaces |

Badia recently introduced a classification with carpometacarpal arthroscopy (Table 9.3) and recommended this arthroscopic staging to ensure better judgment of this condition in order to provide the most adequate treatment option to patients who have this disabling condition [18].

## Treatment for Early Arthritis

In early CMC arthritis, nonoperative treatment is always recommended before surgical intervention. Nonsteroidal anti-inflammatory drugs and thumb spica splint/brace may be helpful to relieve pain and to return to an adequate level of function [19]. Intra-articular steroid injections can offer short-term pain relief in patients with early arthritis [20]. Hypertonic dextrose injection may be effective in reducing pain [21].

Because volar ligamentous laxity contributes to carpometacarpal instability and arthritis progression, it has been suggested to reconstruct the weak volar ligaments to treat early carpometacarpal joint arthritis. Eaton and Littler described a procedure to reconstruct the volar ligaments by using the half-slip of flexor carpi radialis tendon through the base of the first metacarpal [16]. It has been reported to slow the radiologic progression of arthritis in more than 90% of patients. Although the patients have mild pain, they are generally satisfied with the procedure. Another procedure that can be done in early disease is dorsal wedge extension osteotomy. This osteotomy can extend and abduct the metacarpal and unload the joint. It has the added benefit of correcting adduction contracture that may be present. Tomaino reported good to excellent long-term pain relief in more than 90% of patients [22]. This procedure is contraindicated in patients with global joint laxity and irreducible subluxation.

## Treatment for Advanced Arthritis

### Simple Trapeziectomy

Simple trapezial excision without soft tissue interposition was first described by Gervis [23]. Based on the simplicity and low morbidity of the procedure, trapeziectomy with hematoma arthroplasty has been increasingly used in clinical practice. Many authors agree that significant pain relief can be achieved with trapeziectomy alone. Although grip and pinch strength are often decreased after surgery, the absence of pain results in improved overall function. Multiple studies have demonstrated the clinical success of simple trapezial excision. Dhar and colleagues reported that excellent pain relief and reasonable strength and motion were obtained at the last follow-up [24]. Hollevoet and colleagues found no significant difference in motion, strength, and trapezial height between simple trapeziectomy and tendon interposition arthroplasty [25].

A prospective study comparing trapeziectomy alone, trapeziectomy with palmaris longus tendon interposition, or trapeziectomy with ligament reconstruction and tendon interposition was performed by Dowing et al. [26]. They showed that no statistically significant decrease was seen in the trapezial space ratio in the three treatment groups. In contrast, De Smet et al. reported trapezial height was much better preserved in the ligament reconstruction group, and the remaining trapezial space did significantly correlate with key pinch force [27].

Trapeziectomy with K-wire fixation has continued to gain support as a reliable technique for treating painful CMC arthritis. The results have improved with modification to develop of a fibrous pseudarthrosis from maturation of the postoperative hematoma in the arthroplasty space. Slightly overdistracting the first metacarpal also enhances the ability of the thumb to heal with adequate stability [28]. This procedure is especially useful in patients with low demand and high morbidity.

### Ligament Reconstruction

In Eaton stage I or II of the thumb CMC joint arthritis, a ligament reconstruction may be enough to prevent the further progression of the disease [16]. If there is a chronic long-standing instability with the weakness of ligaments, it may lead to a potential osteoarthritis of the joint [29]. Ligament reconstruction has been proved to improve the stability of the joint in a biomechanical study [30]. It stabilizes the joint and reduces those shear forces on the CMC joint [31]. It has generally been felt that ligament reconstruction be reserved for patients with very mild articular changes and that it is contraindicated in patients with stage III and IV disease.

Gervis described one of the oldest surgical procedures, the concept of trapeziectomy without suspension arthroplasty or tendon interposition [23]. Based on the work by Gervis [23] on trapeziectomy and by Eaton and Littler [16] on volar ligament reconstruction using the flexor carpi radialis tendon, Burton et al. [32] described the ligament reconstruction and tendon interposition (LRTI) arthroplasty and used the flexor carpi radialis tendon and a bone tunnel at the base of the thumb metacarpal to maintain the trapezial height after resection of the trapezium and thus, theoretically, preserve thumb strength [33]. Although there is a debate between anterior oblique ligament and dorsoradial ligament as a principal stabilizer of the thumb CMC joint, the technique of ligament reconstruction with flexor carpi radialis (FCR) tendon slip is routed functionally and reconstructs both the anterior oblique and dorsoradial ligaments [31].

## Operative Technique of Ligament Reconstruction (Fig. 9.2)

The basal joint is opened through Wagner's approach. After the skin incision, along the radial border of the first metacarpal bone and trapezium, thenar muscles are sharply dissected subperiosteally, and the dissection is extended to the CMC and scaphotrapeziotrapezoidal (STT) joints. The deeper dissections include "T"-shaped incision over the ligament-capsule of the CMC joint, the transverse fascial fibers overlying the FCR tendon, and the dorsal and volar soft tissues of first to second metacarpal bases.

The inflammatory synovium is cleaned. After the debridement of any osteophytes, manually reduce the CMC joint. To avoid injury, the terminal branch of the superficial radial nerve and extensor pollicis brevis (EPB) tendon is retracted in either direction. Between the insertions of the EPB and abductor pollicis longus (APL) tendons, the periosteum is sharply incised longitudinally, about 1 cm distal to the CMC joint, and dissected subperiosteally.

About 1 cm distal to the CMC joint, a 0.062 in. K-wire is inserted at the base of the metacarpal, parallel to the joint and perpendicular to the metacarpal long axis. On the fluoroscopic examination, the correct position of the

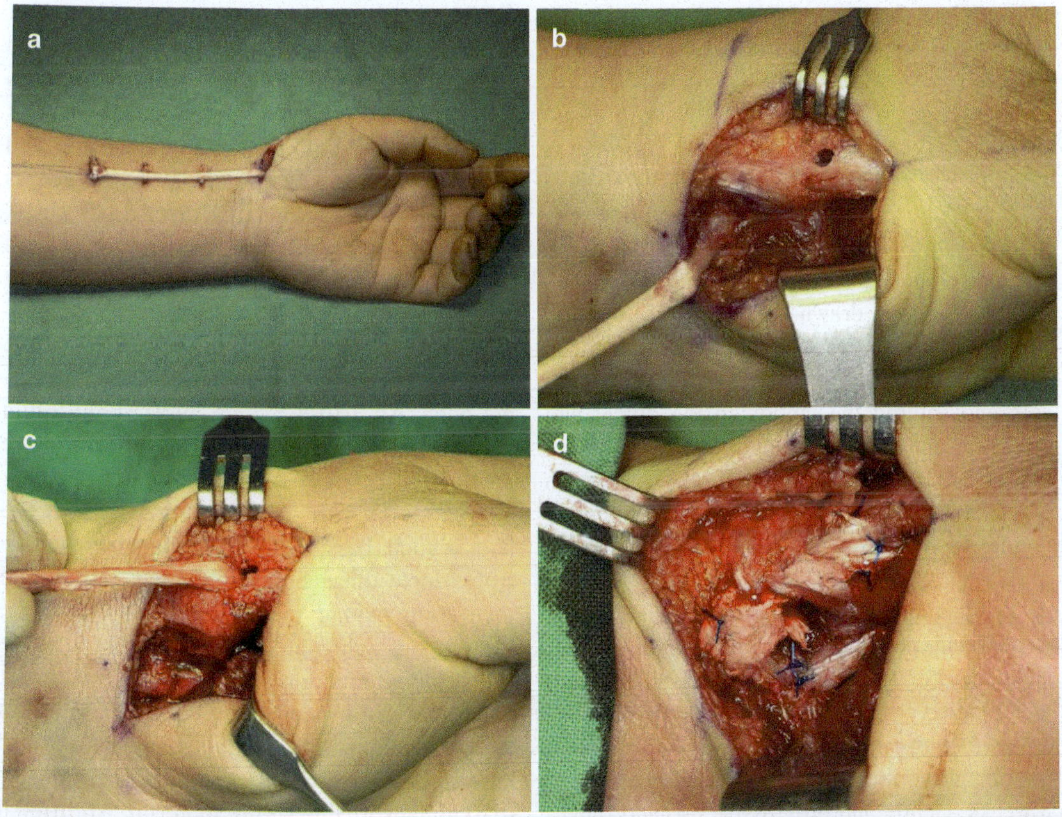


**Fig. 9.2** (**a**) The FCR tendon slip is harvested in half, while the distal portion is attached to the insertion. (**b**) The drill hole is placed through the thumb metacarpal base and above the abductor pollicis longus tendon. (**c**) The FCR tendon slip is passed through the hole and is directed volarly along the radial side of the carpometacarpal joint. (**d**) The reconstruction is completed by passing the FCR tendon slip beneath the intact part of the FCR volarly and then back dorsally beneath the APL tendon to which it is sutured (*FCR* flexor carpi radialis, *APL* abductor pollicis longus)

K-wire is confirmed, and then 2.5 or 3.2 mm drill bit is used to create a hole at the base of the metacarpal. The size of the hole depends on the size of the metacarpal and thickness of the half of FCR tendon.

Half of distal FCR tendon is harvested as follows. The distal insertion of FCR is identified, passing medial to the scaphoid tubercle. About 10–12 cm proximal to the wrist crease, usually at the musculotendinous area, proximal FCR tendon is identified, and 2 cm longitudinal skin incision is made over the tendon. Using #2-0 nylon suture material, without needle, pass through the distal half of FCR tendon, and pass the both ends of nylon subcutaneously and preferably intra-FCR fascial proximally. The nylon material is pulled proximally in seesaw motion until the desired length of FCR is separated in half. Cut the radial half of FCR tendon proximally and retrieve through the distal incision. The proximal incision is closed.

A folded end of #28 wire is passed dorsal to volar through the drill hole. The 2–4 mm free end of FCR tendon is inserted between the folded ends of wire and drawn volar to dorsal through the hole. The free graft end is passed under the APL tendon insertion and across the volar capsule and sutured the tendon to the dorsal and volar capsules and the metacarpal periosteum using #3-0 nonabsorbable suture. If FCR tendon length is enough, the tendon graft is looped around the sutured FCR tendon and sutured to itself.

The tendon is kept in a moist sponge, and it is important not to overtighten the graft. If possible the "T" incised capsule and soft tissues are repaired, and the thenar muscles also are repaired with absorbable suture. A short arm thumb spica splint is applied and is removed at 3 weeks. Gentle and progressive use and range-of-motion exercises are begun. Unlimited activities, including sports, are permitted at 6 weeks postoperatively.

The author used to use the radial half of extensor carpi radialis longus (ECRL) tendon instead of FCR, to make a simple first to second intermetacarpal ligament reconstruction, as in the following technique (Fig. 9.3).

Through the modified Wagner incision, the CMC joint of the thumb is opened dorsoradially. A second incision on the mid-forearm, about the musculotendinous area of the ECRL muscle, is made about 2 cm in length. ECRL tendon insertion on the dorsal second metacarpal base is identified and longitudinally separated in half. #2-0 nylon suture is passed through the mid-ECRL tendon, and both ends of nylon are passed to the proximal incision through intra-tendon sheath space. Using see-sawing movement, the nylon, without needle, is pulled proximally until the desired length of ECRL is separated in half. Cut the radial half of ECRL tendon proximally and retrieve through the distal incision. The proximal incision is closed.

T-incision on the dorsoradial capsule and first to second intermetacarpal base area is made and exposes the two metacarpal bases. From dorso-ulnar base of the first metacarpal base, 2.5 mm drilling is made to the palmar radially, and then another drilling, from dorso-ulnar base of second metacarpal base, is made to the palmar radial base of the second metacarpal bone. All drill holes are made about 5 mm distal from the proximal articular surface of the metacarpals.

Using #28 wire loop, the prepared ECRL half tendon passed the first metacarpal base from dorso-ulnar hole to palmar radial and then from palmar radial hole to dorso-ulnar. Pulling and tightening the tendon should make the proper reduction of the first CMC joint under the vision, and the ECRL tendon from the dorso-ulnar hole of the second metacarpal base sutured to the ECRL tendon insertion with #2-0 nonabsorbable suture material. Additional suture of the ECRL end can be done to the capsule. Avoid too much tightening, because it may make a limitation of motion or pain on motion. We do not use K-wire to fix the joint and apply short arm thumb spica splint for 3 weeks. After

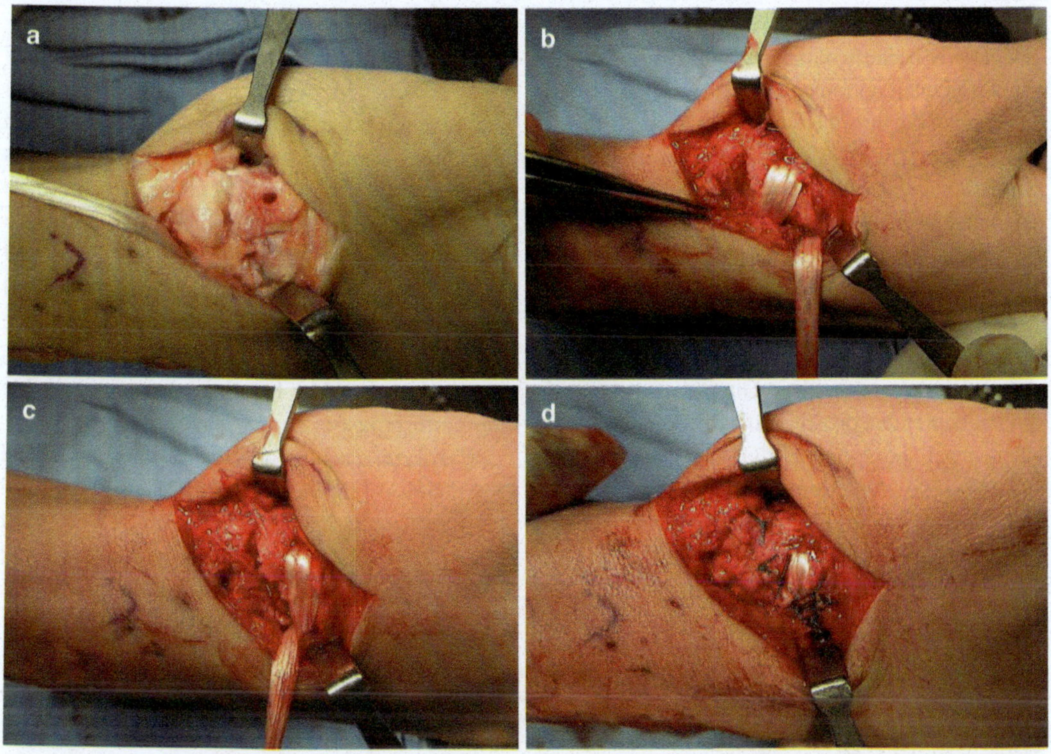


**Fig. 9.3** (**a**) The ECRL tendon slip is harvested in half, while the distal portion is attached to the insertion. (**b**) The drill hole is placed through the thumb and second metacarpal base. (**c**) The ECRL tendon slip is passed through the holes and is tightened to reduce the first carpometacarpal joint under the vision. (**d**) The reconstruction is completed by passing the ECRL tendon slip beneath the intact part of the ECRL tendon and sutured itself (*ECRL* extensor carpi radialis longus)

6 weeks the thumb is allowed to use activities of daily living and 3 months later for normal activities.

## Prosthetic Arthroplasty

Once an arthritic change is established, the joint cannot be made asymptomatic only with ligament reconstruction. Prosthetic arthroplasty can provide some benefits compared to trapeziectomy only and trapeziectomy with ligament reconstruction. The potential advantages include preservation of joint biomechanics, avoidance of metacarpal subsidence, and prevention of possible later adjacent joint problems [34]. Vitale et al. provided a summary of the trapezium prosthetic options that have emerged over the past five decades [34]. First-generation implants were primarily Swanson silicone prostheses, which have been reported as preserving good range of motion and grip strength and minimizing pain [35]. Several other studies have reported the outcomes of silicone implants with varying results. Frequently identified problems include the development of silicone synovitis, breakage, subluxation/dislocation, bony erosion, loosening, and long-term implant failure. Therefore, these implants are no longer available [36]. Interestingly, Umarji and colleagues have recently reported their experience with ten patients who had revision surgery with a silastic finger joint implant spacer following failure of simple trapeziectomy [37]. At an average follow-up of 53 months, 9 of the 10 patients reported improvement in pain and were generally satisfied with their function. Silicone arthroplasty has fallen out of favor because of the availability of numerous other treatment options.

Implant arthroplasty of the thumb CMC joint has met with varied, if not unpredictable, results. Several other devices have been developed and used. These include the de la Caffinière prosthesis which is a semiconstrained ball-and-socket design with both components cemented. The metacarpal component is made of cobalt chromium, and the trapezium component is a polyethylene cup. The Guepar prosthesis is also a cemented prosthesis with cobalt-chrome metacarpal component that snap-fits into a polyethylene trapezium component and functions in a constrained fashion. The Elektra prosthesis is a modular design made of cobalt-chrome and threads into the trapezium. The Braun prosthesis is a cemented design that consists of a metallic metacarpal and a polyethylene socket. The Avanta CMC prosthesis is a cemented total joint surface replacement with matching sloped, saddle-shaped components approximating the natural contours of the base of the first metacarpal and the articular surface of the trapezium, with the trapezium component made of cobalt-chrome and the first metacarpal component made of polyethylene [38]. More recent implant designs have focused on resurfacing devices with the hope of producing a stable hemiarthroplasty.

Pyrolytic carbon prosthesis has been used to develop replacement arthroplasties and hemiarthroplasties of the thumb CMC joint (Figs. 9.4 and 9.5), including the pyrolytic carbon anatomic interposition arthroplasty,

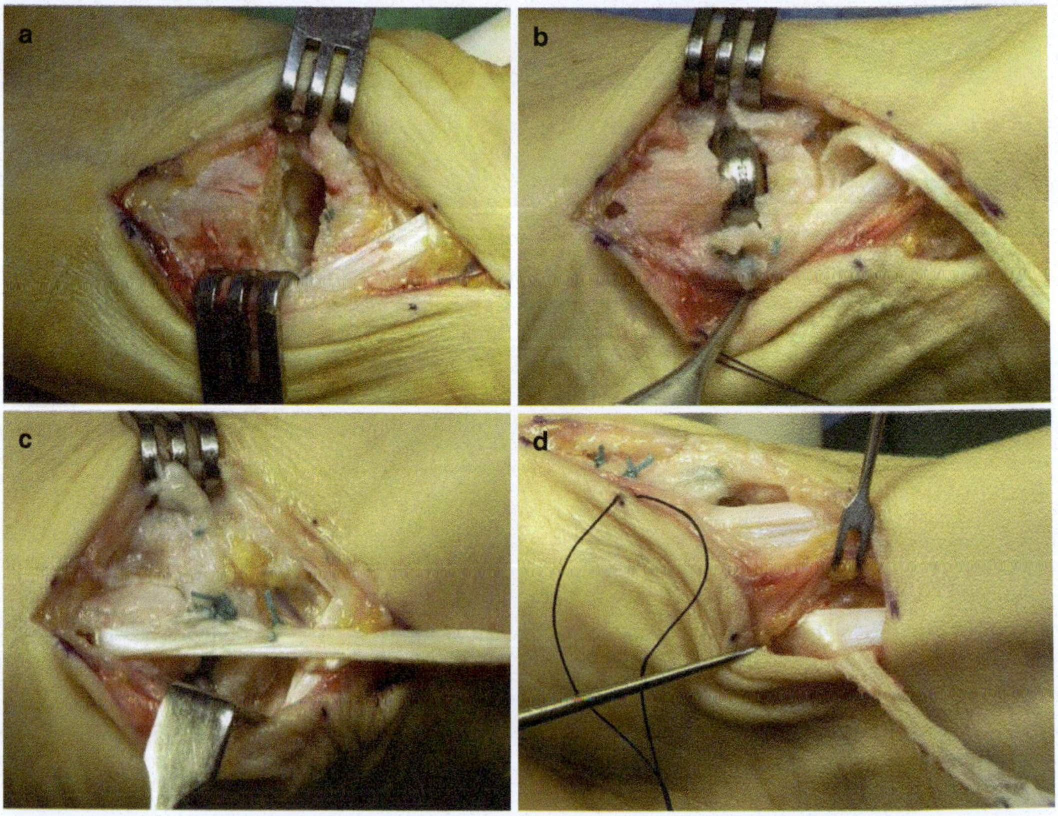


**Fig. 9.4** (**a**) Part of the trapezium and the first metacarpal is resected to make a space for pyrocarbon implant. (**b**) The drill hole is placed through the trapezium and the first metacarpal with trial implant. (**c**) Once the implant is placed, APL tendon slip is passed through the holes and is tightened. (**d**) Remaining tendon is passed under the FCR tendon to stabilize the carpometacarpal joint

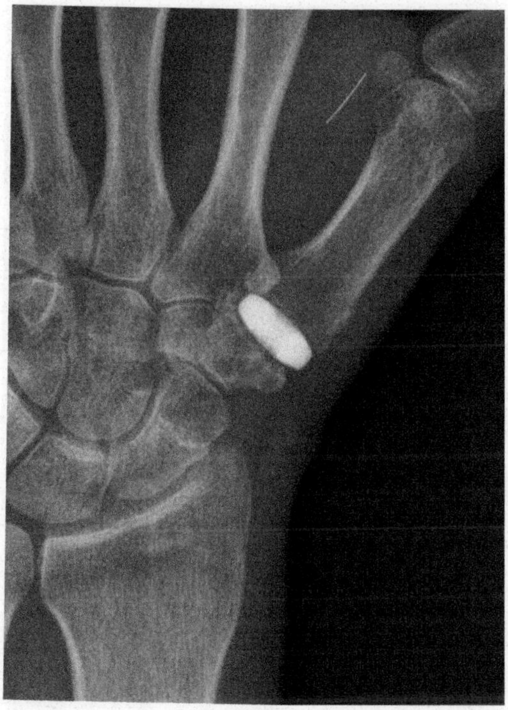

**Fig. 9.5** Postoperative radiograph showing pyrocarbon implant placed in the carpometacarpal joint

the pyrocarbon implant (BioProfile/Tornier, Montbonnot-Saint-Martin, France), and the pyrocarbon interposition implant (Pyrodisk, Integra Life Sciences, Plainsboro, NJ). This prosthesis has been used in patients with stage II or III disease. A recent prospective study of trapeziectomy alone versus trapeziectomy and pyrocarbon hemiarthroplasty assessed outcomes in 38 patients [39]. There was no significant difference in functional scores and pain and grip strength between two groups, although there was a higher complication rate in the pyrocarbon group.

Confidence in many of these devices is hampered by its relatively recent use and high loosening rates. Metallic implant arthroplasty has improved to address shortcomings and failures of previous implant design. Subsidence, instability, and implant loosening have all been reported with metallic implant and have decreased their popularity. Newer synthetic materials are also available on the market. However, care should be taken to use these implants as no long-term studies are available at the moment.

## Carpometacarpal Arthrodesis

Arthrodesis of the carpometacarpal joint of the thumb has proven to be a reliable option for advanced arthritis. It has been reported to provide satisfactory pain relief and obtain a strong, stable, and functional hand at the expense of mobility. Patient selection for this procedure is important for a successful outcome. This procedure is usually reserved for young high-demand patients under 50 as older patients were thought to be prone to progression of pantrapezial arthritis [40]. However, recent report proved that this procedure can be used successfully for the older patients [41]. To be indicated for carpometacarpal joint arthrodesis, the patient should not have degenerative changes in scaphotrapezial and metacarpophalangeal joints. Arthrodesis is also indicated for patients with soft tissue laxity as there will be a high probability of dislocation or mechanical failure of the implant arthroplasty. Arthrodesis is contraindicated in patients with scaphotrapezial and metacarpophalangeal joint arthritis or in patients requiring a mobile carpometacarpal joint.

Although there are several techniques for thumb carpometacarpal arthrodesis, the position of fusion is constant. The thumb is placed in the "position of a clenched fist" in which the distal phalanx of the thumb comfortably rests on the middle phalanx of the index finger with a fully clenched fist [42]. The optimal position for carpometacarpal arthrodesis is 35° of palmar abduction and 10° of radial deviation with 15° of pronation. Excellent results have been reported from arthrodesis of thumb CMC joint (Fig. 9.6). Leach and Bolton found that 89% of patients had excellent results with no pain after fusion. Although there was reduced motion, it did not hinder their function [43]. Stark and colleagues reported all patients had pain relief and felt that the gain in stability and strength compensated for the slight loss in motion [44].

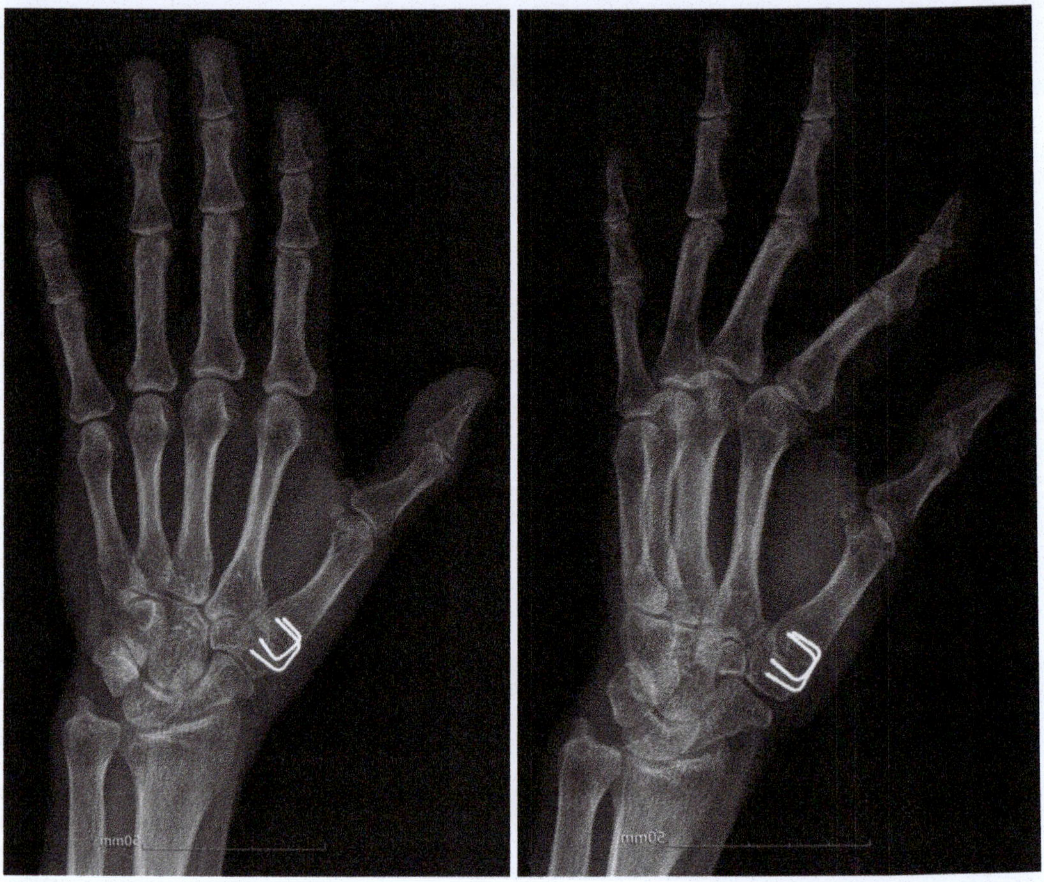

**Fig. 9.6** Postoperative radiograph showing carpometacarpal joint arthrodesis using two staples

Bamberger and colleagues reported that functional outcome after arthrodesis revealed a 72% decrease in the adduction/abduction arc of motion and a 61% decrease in flexion/extension arc of motion. Despite this loss of motion, there were minimal subjective functional complaints (Fig. 9.7). Complications of carpometacarpal arthrodesis include progression to pantrapezial arthritis and nonunion [45].

Arthrodesis of the carpometacarpal joint of the thumb may be useful for advanced arthritis in the high-demand patient. This procedure creates a pain-free, strong, stable thumb at the expense of full range of motion. Arthrodesis remains an excellent option for patients who need a strong pain-free thumb.

## Comparison of Clinical Results

There have been many prospective, randomized, clinical trials comparing different surgical procedures. De Smet et al. compared trapeziectomy alone and trapeziectomy with ligament reconstruction and tendon interposition procedure [27]. They found the results showed no differences in pain relief and functional outcome although trapezial height was better maintained after ligament reconstruction. Davis et al. conducted prospective randomized trials comparing trapeziectomy alone and trapeziectomy with ligament reconstruction tendon interposition [46]. They found that there was no difference in pain relief, hand function, and thumb strength between groups. This group

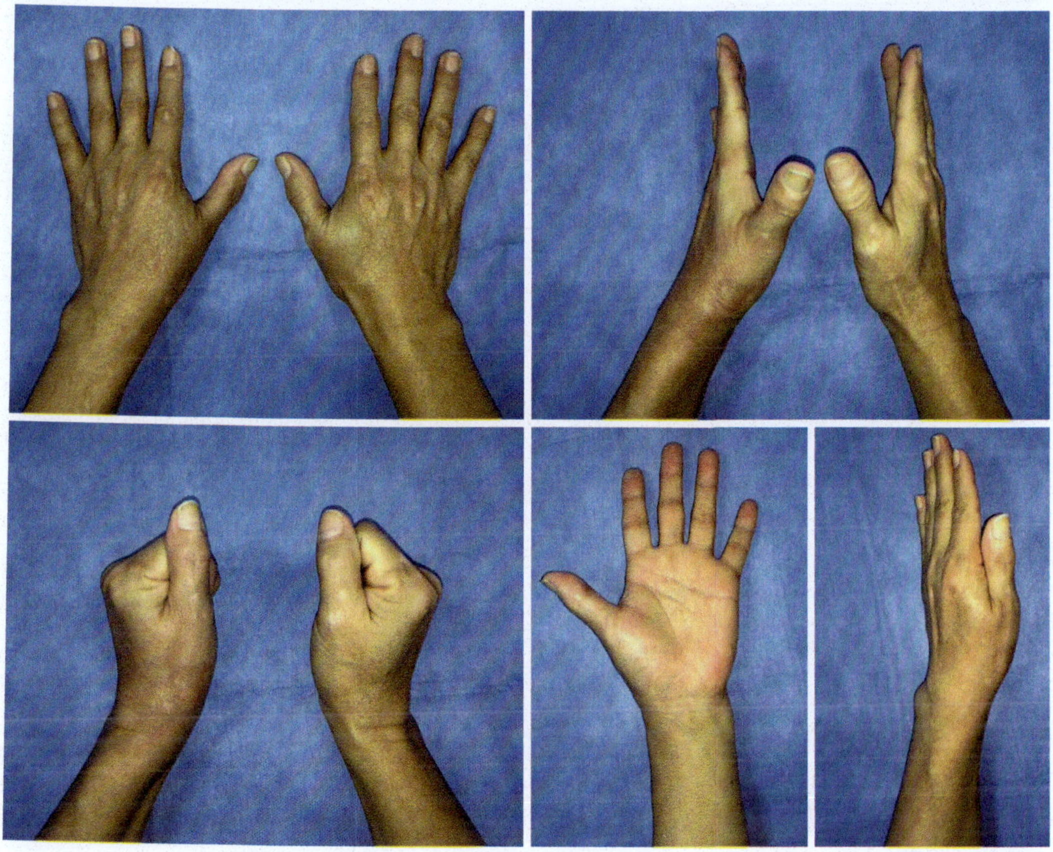

**Fig. 9.7** Range of motion after thumb carpometacarpal arthrodesis. Compensatory motions occur in scaphotrapezial and metacarpophalangeal joint

subsequently compared simple trapeziectomy and trapeziectomy with ligament reconstruction and tendon interposition and additional Kirschner wire stabilization [47]. There were no significant differences between the two treatment groups in any subjective or objective outcome measures.

At present, there is no evidence to suggest that any one surgical procedure is superior to another. Based on the Cochrane Database Systematic Review, they recommended trapeziectomy alone for the treatment of carpometacarpal arthritis [48]. However, a recent survey showed that trapeziectomy with ligament reconstruction and tendon interposition is the most popular procedure among members of the American Society for Surgery of the Hand [49].

## Conclusions

Thumb carpometacarpal arthritis is one of the most common causes of pain in the hand. There are several surgical options for this condition; however, to date, no single method has emerged superior, although each method has specific advantages and disadvantages for the surgeon to consider. Until the ideal prosthetic implant is developed by innovations, trapeziectomy with ligament reconstruction and/or tendon interposition remains the most commonly performed procedure for patients who want mobile thumb. Arthrodesis can still be a valid option for patients who want strong stable thumb at the expense of mobility.

## References


1. Haara MM, Heliovaara M, Kroger H, Arokoski JP, Manninen P, Karkkainen A, et al. Osteoarthritis in the carpometacarpal joint of the thumb. Prevalence and associations with disability and mortality. J Bone Joint Surg Am. 2004;86-A:1452–7.
2. Barron OA, Glickel SZ, Eaton RG. Basal joint arthritis of the thumb. J Am Acad Orthop Surg. 2000;8:314–23.
3. Cicuttini FM, Spector TD. The epidemiology of osteoarthritis of the hand. Rev Rhum Engl Ed. 1995;62:3S–8S.
4. Fontana L, Neel S, Claise JM, Ughetto S, Catilina P. Osteoarthritis of the thumb carpometacarpal joint in women and occupational risk factors: a case-control study. J Hand Surg Am. 2007;32:459–65.
5. Eaton RG, Lane LB, Littler JW, Keyser JJ. Ligament reconstruction for the painful thumb carpometacarpal joint: a long-term assessment. J Hand Surg Am. 1984;9:692–9.
6. Strauch RJ, Behrman MJ, Rosenwasser MP. Acute dislocation of the carpometacarpal joint of the thumb: an anatomic and cadaver study. J Hand Surg Am. 1994;19:93–8.
7. Pagalidis T, Kuczynski K, Lamb DW. Ligamentous stability of the base of the thumb. Hand. 1981;13:29–36.
8. Harvey FJ, Bye WD. Bennett's fracture. Hand. 1976;8:48–53.
9. Pellegrini VD Jr. Osteoarthritis of the trapeziometacarpal joint: the pathophysiology of articular cartilage degeneration. I. Anatomy and pathology of the aging joint. J Hand Surg Am. 1991;16:967–74.
10. Matullo KS, Ilyas A, Thoder JJ. CMC arthroplasty of the thumb: a review. Hand (N Y). 2007;2:232–9.
11. Klinefelter R. Metacarpophalangeal hyperextension deformity associated with trapezial-metacarpal arthritis. J Hand Surg Am. 2011;36:2041–2; quiz 2043.
12. Oheb J, Lansinger Y, Jansen JA, Nguyen JQ, Porembski MA, Rayan GM. Radiographic assessment of the robert and lateral views in trapeziometacarpal osteoarthrosis. Hand Surg. 2015;20:251–9.
13. Saltzherr MS, van Neck JW, Muradin GS, Ouwendijk R, Luime JJ, Coert JH, et al. Computed tomography for the detection of thumb base osteoarthritis: comparison with digital radiography. Skeletal Radiol. 2013;42:715–21.
14. Dumont C, Lerzer S, Vafa MA, Tezval M, Dechent P, Sturmer KM, et al. Osteoarthritis of the carpometacarpal joint of the thumb: a new MR imaging technique for the standardized detection of relevant ligamental lesions. Skeletal Radiol. 2014;43:1411–20.
15. Burton RI. Basal joint arthrosis of the thumb. Orthop Clin North Am. 1973;4:331–8.
16. Eaton RG, Littler JW. Ligament reconstruction for the painful thumb carpometacarpal joint. J Bone Joint Surg Am. 1973;55:1655–66.
17. Eaton RG, Glickel SZ. Trapeziometacarpal osteoarthritis. Staging as a rationale for treatment. Hand Clin. 1987;3:455–71.
18. Badia A. Trapeziometacarpal arthroscopy: a classification and treatment algorithm. Hand Clin. 2006;22:153–63.
19. Weiss S, LaStayo P, Mills A, Bramlet D. Prospective analysis of splinting the first carpometacarpal joint: an objective, subjective, and radiographic assessment. J Hand Ther. 2000;13:218–26.
20. Joshi R. Intraarticular corticosteroid injection for first carpometacarpal osteoarthritis. J Rheumatol. 2005;32:1305–6.
21. Jahangiri A, Moghaddam FR, Najafi S. Hypertonic dextrose versus corticosteroid local injection for the treatment of osteoarthritis in the first carpometacarpal joint: a double-blind randomized clinical trial. J Orthop Sci. 2014;19:737–43.
22. Tomaino MM. Treatment of Eaton stage I trapeziometacarpal disease with thumb metacarpal extension osteotomy. J Hand Surg Am. 2000;25:1100–6.
23. Gervis WH. Excision of the trapezium for osteoarthritis of the trapezio-metacarpal joint. J Bone Joint Surg Br. 1949;31B:537–9, illust.
24. Dhar S, Gray IC, Jones WA, Beddow FH. Simple excision of the trapezium for osteoarthritis of the carpometacarpal joint of the thumb. J Hand Surg Br. 1994;19:485–8.
25. Hollevoet N, Kinnen L, Moermans JP, Ledoux P. Excision of the trapezium for osteoarthritis of the trapeziometacarpal joint of the thumb. J Hand Surg Br. 1996;21:458–62.
26. Downing ND, Davis TR. Trapezial space height after trapeziectomy: mechanism of formation and benefits. J Hand Surg Am. 2001;26:862–8.
27. De Smet L, Sioen W, Spaepen D, van Ransbeeck H. Treatment of basal joint arthritis of the thumb: trapeziectomy with or without tendon interposition/ligament reconstruction. Hand Surg. 2004;9:5–9.
28. Gray KV, Meals RA. Hematoma and distraction arthroplasty for thumb basal joint osteoarthritis: minimum 6.5-year follow-up evaluation. J Hand Surg Am. 2007;32:23–9.
29. Freedman DM, Eaton RG, Glickel SZ. Long-term results of volar ligament reconstruction for symptomatic basal joint laxity. J Hand Surg Am. 2000;25:297–304.
30. Koff MF, Shrivastava N, Gardner TR, Rosenwasser MP, Mow VC, Strauch RJ. An in vitro analysis of ligament reconstruction or extension osteotomy on trapeziometacarpal joint stability and contact area. J Hand Surg Am. 2006;31:429–39.
31. Glickel SZ, Gupta S. Ligament reconstruction. Hand Clin. 2006;22:143–51.
32. Burton RI, Pellegrini VD Jr. Surgical management of basal joint arthritis of the thumb. Part II. Ligament reconstruction with tendon interposition arthroplasty. J Hand Surg Am. 1986;11:324–32.
33. Vermeulen GM, Slijper H, Feitz R, Hovius SE, Moojen TM, Selles RW. Surgical management of pri-

mary thumb carpometacarpal osteoarthritis: a systematic review. J Hand Surg Am. 2011;36:157–69.
34. Vitale MA, Taylor F, Ross M, Moran SL. Trapezium prosthetic arthroplasty (silicone, Artelon, metal, and pyrocarbon). Hand Clin. 2013;29:37–55.
35. Zschock-Holle A, Reik M, Wolfle O, Sauerbier M. [Treatment of basal joint osteoarthritis by Swanson's trapezium implant arthroplasty]. Handchir Mikrochir Plast Chir. 2015;47:7–16.
36. Lanzetta M, Foucher G. A comparison of different surgical techniques in treating degenerative arthrosis of the carpometacarpal joint of the thumb. A retrospective study of 98 cases. J Hand Surg Br. 1995;20:105–10.
37. Umarji SI, Arnander MW, Evans DM. The use of Swanson silastic interposition arthroplasty in revision thumb-base surgery for failed trapeziectomy; a case series of 10 patients. J Hand Surg Eur Vol. 2012;37:632–6.
38. Pendse A, Nisar A, Shah SZ, Bhosale A, Freeman JV, Chakrabarti I. Surface replacement trapeziometacarpal joint arthroplasty—early results. J Hand Surg Eur Vol. 2009;34:748–57.
39. Colegate-Stone TJ, Garg S, Subramanian A, Mani GV. Outcome analysis of trapezectomy with and without pyrocarbon interposition to treat primary arthrosis of the trapeziometacarpal joint. Hand Surg. 2011;16:49–54.
40. Carroll RE. Arthrodesis of the carpometacarpal joint of the thumb. A review of patients with a long postoperative period. Clin Orthop Relat Res. 1987;220:106–10.
41. Fulton DB, Stern PJ. Trapeziometacarpal arthrodesis in primary osteoarthritis: a minimum two-year follow-up study. J Hand Surg Am. 2001;26:109–14.
42. Eaton RG, Littler JW. A study of the basal joint of the thumb. Treatment of its disabilities by fusion. J Bone Joint Surg Am. 1969;51:661–8.
43. Leach RE, Bolton PE. Arthritis of the carpometacarpal joint of the thumb. Results of arthrodesis. J Bone Joint Surg Am. 1968;50:1171–7.
44. Stark HH, Moore JF, Ashworth CR, Boyes JH. Fusion of the first metacarpotrapezial joint for degenerative arthritis. J Bone Joint Surg Am. 1977;59:22–6.
45. Kenniston JA, Bozentka DJ. Treatment of advanced carpometacarpal joint disease: arthrodesis. Hand Clin. 2008;24:285–94, vi–vii.
46. Davis TR, Brady O, Dias JJ. Excision of the trapezium for osteoarthritis of the trapeziometacarpal joint: a study of the benefit of ligament reconstruction or tendon interposition. J Hand Surg Am. 2004;29:1069–77.
47. Davis TR, Pace A. Trapeziectomy for trapeziometacarpal joint osteoarthritis: is ligament reconstruction and temporary stabilisation of the pseudarthrosis with a Kirschner wire important? J Hand Surg Eur Vol. 2009;34:312–21.
48. Wajon A, Carr E, Edmunds I, Ada L. Surgery for thumb (trapeziometacarpal joint) osteoarthritis. Cochrane Database Syst Rev. 2009;(2):CD004631.
49. Wolf JM, Delaronde S. Current trends in nonoperative and operative treatment of trapeziometacarpal osteoarthritis: a survey of US hand surgeons. J Hand Surg Am. 2012;37:77–82.

# Part IV

# Tendon Problems

# Flexor Tendon

# 10

SuRak Eo

## Introduction

The thumb has only one extrinsic flexor tendon, which is the flexor pollicis longus (FPL) that flexes the interphalangeal (IP) joint of the thumb. The FPL originates from two heads: the radial head originates from the proximal radius and interosseous membrane, and an accessory head originates from the coronoid process of the ulna and from the medial epicondyle of the humerus. It inserts into the proximal base of the thumb distal phalanx and is innervated by the anterior interosseous branch of the median nerve. It is involved in bending both the interphalangeal and metacarpophalangeal joints of the thumb.

The FPL is structurally and functionally quite different from the flexor tendons of the other fingers. The thumb flexor is simpler, in that it lacks the lumbrical muscle and superficialis tendon. Anatomically, the FPL lies within the radial bursa, and soft tissues, such as the abductor pollicis brevis (AbPB), flexor pollicis brevis (FPB), and superficial palmar branch, and the recurrent motor branch of the median nerve overlie the FPL. This makes surgical exposure of the FPL difficult, and surgeons should be particularly careful in their approach.

S. Eo (✉)
Department of Plastic and Reconstructive Surgery, DongGuk University Hospital, University of DongGuk School of Medicine, Goyang-si, Gyeonggi-do, South Korea

The FPL is an individual unit covered by its own sheath and moves two phalanges beneath three pulleys: two annular and one oblique (Fig. 10.1). The FPL has the blood supply from the osseous insertion, vinculum brevis, mesotenon, and musculotendinous junction, which makes it important for hand surgeons to avoid the avascular zone in FPL repair (Fig. 10.2) [1–3]. Lundborg suggested that the FPL blood supply was superior to that in the other fingers and showed better results in FPL tenorrhaphies [4].

Reconstruction of the FPL function is desired to restore the IP joint flexion and pinch in particular. Because full IP joint mobility is not necessary for proper thumb function, FPL repairs provide better results compared to that of the other digits [5]. Even an arthrodesis of the IP joint of the thumb permits acceptable results [6]. However, FPL dysfunction might cause serious impairment in thumb movement, especially in precise pinch with gripping, which requires strength, stability, and dexterity. The thicker FPL tendon is known to be related to these actions in healthy individuals and causes resting tremor in Parkinson's disease [7].

Through a biomechanical analysis, Cooney and Chao evaluated the tension load on the thumb tendons and noted that during pinch and grasp, the FPL generated greater force than all the other thumb tendons [8]. Therefore, lacerations or avulsions of the FPL should be properly repaired with greater skill and perfection of technique. In addition to the FPL, the thenar intrinsic muscles,



S. H. Woo (ed.), *The Thumb*, https://doi.org/10.1007/978-981-10-4400-7_10

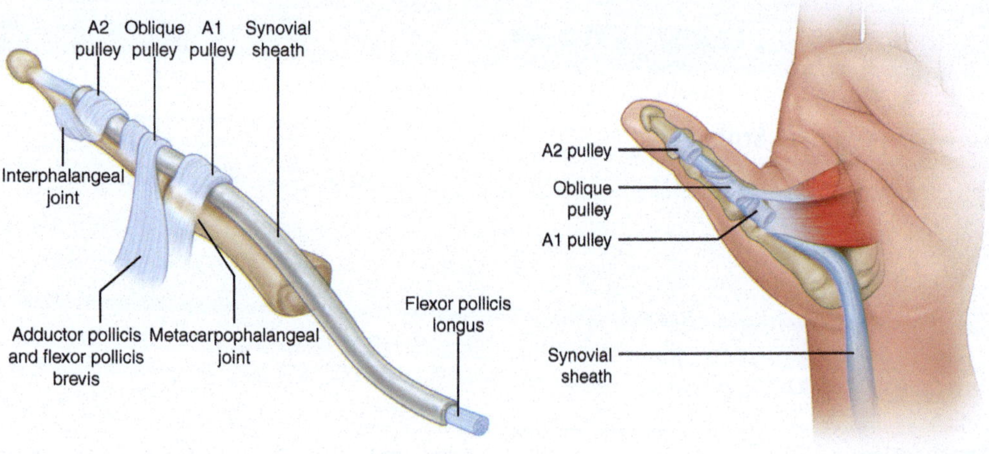


**Fig. 10.1** Flexor pollicis longus (FPL) tendon and its pulleys; annular pulleys A1 and A2 and oblique pulley (O)

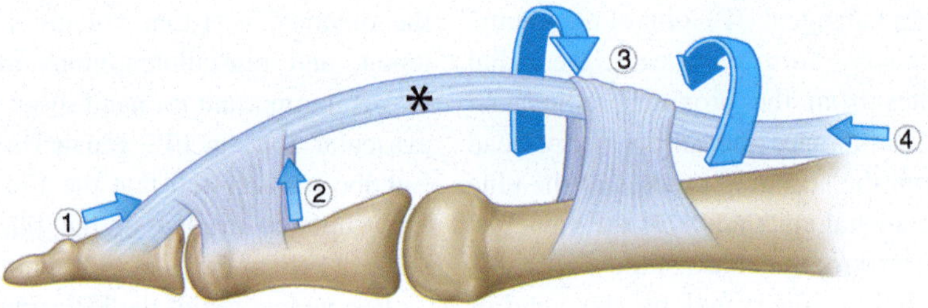


**Fig. 10.2** Vascularity of FPL. Asterisk depicts the avascular zones between the vinculum brevis and the mesotenon. (1) osscous insertion; (2) vinculum brevis; (3) mesotenon, attached to tendon volarly; and (4) musculotendinous junction. (redrawn from Hergenroeder et al., Clin Orthop Relat Res. 1982;162:298–303)

including the FPB and AbPB, also contribute to the stability of the MCP joint and the range of motion of the trapeziometacarpal joint. This is important in the pinch grip between the thumb and index finger. When the FPB is paralyzed, transfer of the flexor superficialis tendon of the third or the ring finger is used, as described by Bunnel [9].

In addition to the FPL rupture, IP joint flexion of the thumb is impossible in numerous clinical settings, such as congenital absence of the FPL, anomalous insertion of the FPL, tenovaginitis of the FPL tendon sheath, and anterior interosseous nerve palsy.

The absence of the FPL associated with or without aplasia of the thenar muscles has been described [10], and it should be differentiated from the FPL rupture. Uchida proposed a classification of the absence of the FPL with associated anomalies [10]. Anomalous insertion of the FPL to the proximal phalanx or transverse carpal ligament causes the inability to flex the IP joint of the thumb [11]. The rarest variation of the Linburg-Comstock anomaly, which represents simultaneous flexion of the thumb and fingers, has been also reported [12]. Because of the anomalous interconnecting tendinous bands between the FPL and FDP of the index finger, this may jeopardize the healing process after FPL repair, especially when the range of motion of index finger is not monitored.

In this chapter, the flexor tendon problems in the thumb, including trigger thumb, acute injury, and secondary reconstruction of the FPL, are described.

## Trigger Thumb

Since its initial description by Jahss in 1936, trigger thumb afflicts both children and adults, due to the pathology of the FPL tendon or A1 pulley. Clicking or locking of the IP joint on thumb movement can cause pain, swelling, and the loss of thumb function. Although the mechanism and pathology of triggering is the same in both age groups, the etiology is known to be different.

In addition to the A1 pulley, the variable annular (Av) pulley is also known to be a normal anatomical structure, which might provide an additional site of stenosis (Fig. 10.3) [13, 14]. Therefore, care must be taken not to cause bowstringing during surgical procedures while severing both A1 and Av pulleys.

### In Children

Trigger thumb occurs due to pathology of the FPL or A1 pulley with an incidence in infants and children of 0.05–0.3% [15]. It is characterized by the formation of a nodule within the tendon at the volar side of the metacarpophalangeal (MCP) joint level, which is called Notta's nodule, and thickening of the tendon sheath where it passes through the pulleys of the thumb [16]. Trigger thumb is usually not present at birth but rather develops with postnatal growth. Although rarer bilateral involvement is sometimes associated with genetic disorders, controversy has existed regarding the etiology of this condition, and it is still debatable whether it is truly congenital or acquired. As some studies revealed that it is an acquired, rather than a congenital problem [15–17], the term "pediatric trigger thumb" is currently preferred.

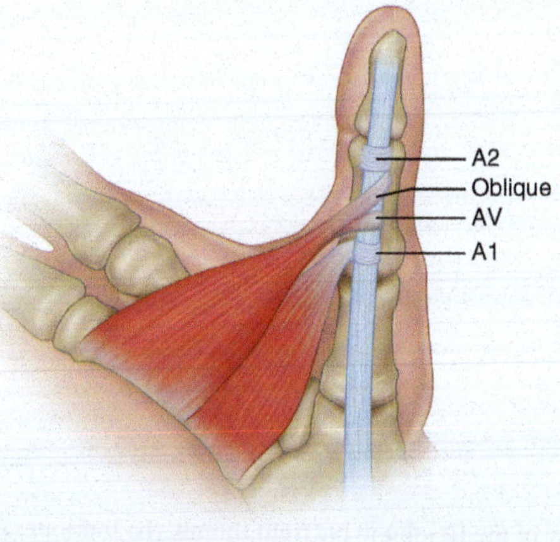


**Fig. 10.3** Variable annular (Av) pulley is commonly noted between the A1 and oblique pulleys. (redrawn from Schubert MF et al., J Hand Surg [Am]. 2012;37:2278–85).

Usually, children show the locked thumb in flexion deformity of the IP joint, rather than triggering (Fig. 10.4). The pathology reveals an enlarged FPL tendon and thickening of the annular pulley, as in the case of acquired stenosing tenosynovitis in adults. However, it is unclear whether the primary pathology involves the pulley system [18] or the FPL tendon itself [19].

Watanabe classified pediatric trigger thumb into four stages according to the symptoms: stage 0, only palpable mass on the MCP joint without restriction of motion; stage 1, the thumb IP joint can be actively flexed and extended without snapping; stage 2, the locked IP joint can be passively flexed or extended with snapping; and stage 3, the locked IP joint cannot be passively flexed or extended [20].

Pediatric trigger thumb is usually passively correctable and non-painful. Nonsurgical options have been proposed, such as watchful waiting, extension stretching exercises, splinting, and steroid injections. Many studies show that surgical intervention is not urgent, and delaying the surgery even beyond the age of 3–5 years does not interfere with the result [21]. Therefore, attempting conservative treatment is the preferable option before elective surgery. However, because leaving the trigger unreleased may lead to contracture of the thumb at the IP joint, release sooner, rather than later, is generally recommended after 3 years [22]. Surgical treatment involving release of the A1 pulley on the FPL is only indicated when there is painful triggering or the thumb is not passively correctable (Fig. 10.4). Pediatric trigger thumb responds

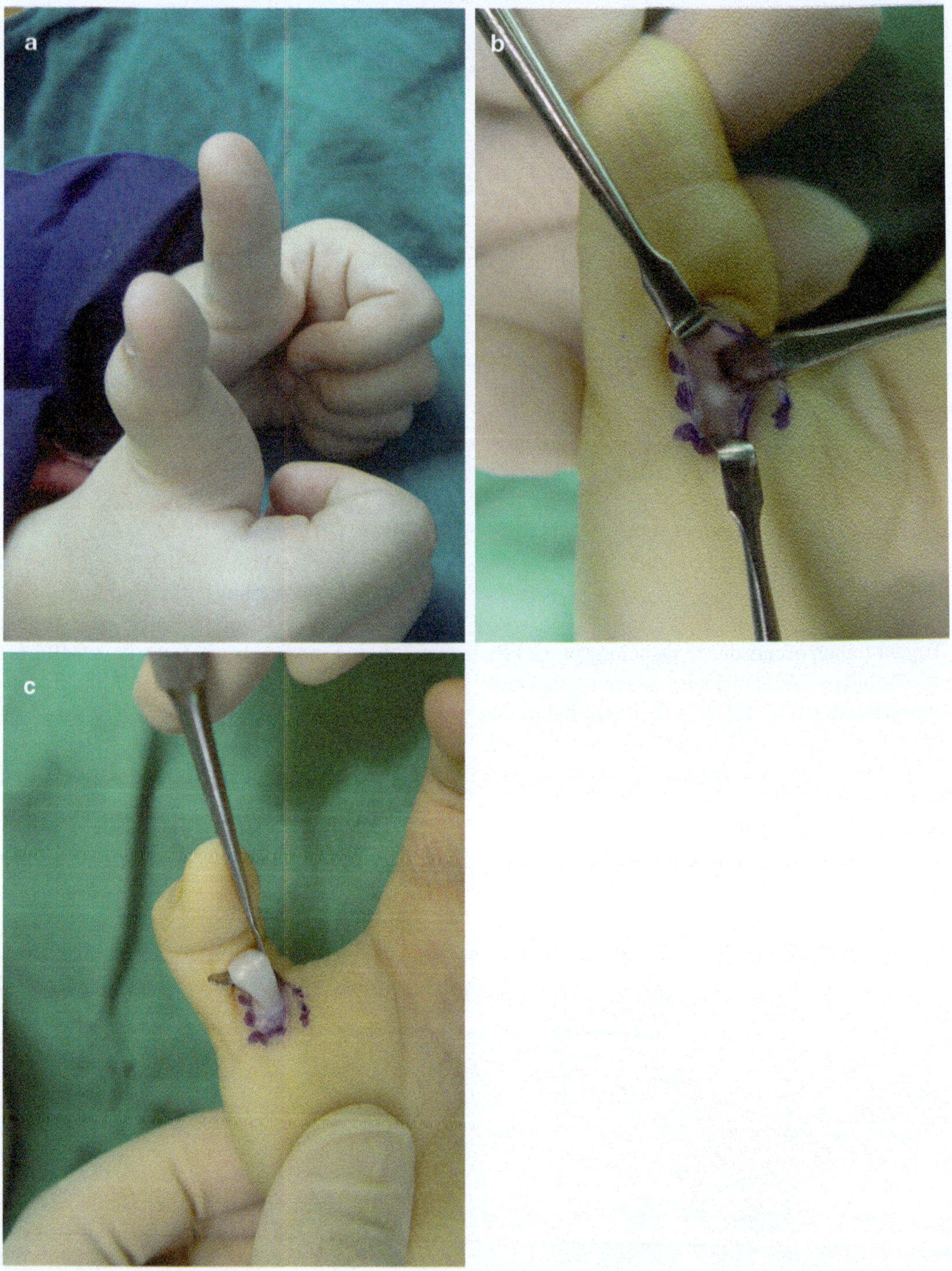


**Fig. 10.4** (**a**) This 4-year-old boy revealed the flexion deformity of the IP joint in his right thumb. (**b**) Intraoperatively, thickened A1 pulley was noted. (**c**) After release of the A1 pulley, FPL was retracted using Ragnell retractor

predictably to A1 pulley release, preferably before age 4 years, although milder cases may resolve spontaneously.

### In Adults

Painful snapping of the thumb may be caused by [1] stenosing tenosynovitis of the FPL at the level of the A1 pulley; [2] connective tissue disorders from systemic diseases, such as rheumatoid arthritis, gout, and diabetes; or [3] tumors of the tendon sheath, loose body, and osteophyte on the MCP joint level. Seybold et al. reported trigger thumb due to the impingement of the FPL tendon by an enlarged radial sesamoid [23]. As a stenosing tenosynovitis, trigger thumb is more common in diabetic patients than in nondiabetic patients, and when multiple digits are involved, the possibility of diabetes should be considered.

Conservative treatment includes activity modification, splinting, nonsteroidal anti-inflammatory drugs, and corticosteroid injection. Surgical release of the thickened A1 pulley is advocated in patients who are not responsive to those conservative approaches. Complications, such as radial digital nerve injury, persistent triggering, residual flexion contracture, and bowstringing, should be prevented with careful surgical procedures.

## Injury

Jaeger and Mackin described the FPL zones, in comparison to the other digit flexor zones, and Verdan divided the FPL into five zones (Fig. 10.5) [24]: zone I, IP joint–thumb tip; zone II, IP joint–midportion of the proximal phalanx; zone III, midportion of the proximal phalanx–metacarpophalangeal joint; zone IV, thenar area; and zone V, wrist area. The ideal repair is direct suture of the lacerated FPL, and as much as 3 months should be allowed for direct repair [25]. Because the FPL has no lumbrical muscle that causes intrinsic tightness, some proximal retraction is permitted in the FPL repair. Furthermore, a slightly flexed IP joint of the thumb is not problematic for thumb function.

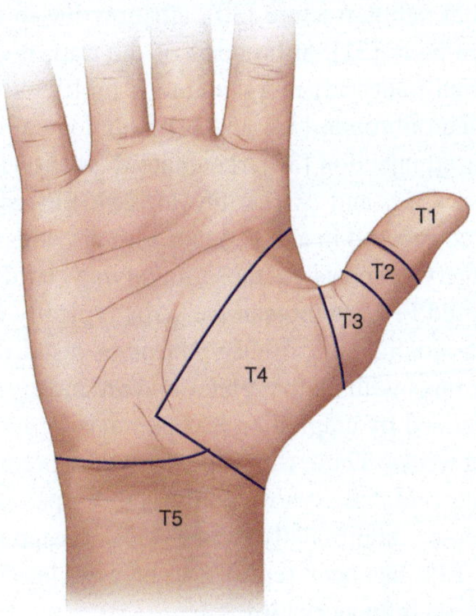

**Fig. 10.5** Five zones of flexor system of the thumb

### Acute Injury

FPL ruptures have been reported to occur less frequently than other flexor tendons, because the FPL is much stronger, and is an individual unit, compared to the other digits. The lack of interconnections to other fingers results in the FPL leading to more proximal tendon retractions.

In children, FPL injury is quite rare, and many authors preferred primary repair and early rehabilitation in the same way as that of adults [26]. Unawareness of thumb dysfunction in young children and overlooking the FPL rupture might delay proper FPL repair. However, better blood supply to the flexor tendons and more pliable adhesions in children explain the absence of requirement for tenolysis after tendon repair [27].

FPL rupture may occur not only by a trauma but also spontaneously without an event [28]. It has been documented secondary to various contributing factors, such as [1] mechanical, non-united scaphoid fracture [29], volar plating of the distal radius fracture [30], attrition due to a foreign body [31], arthrodesis of the trapeziometacarpal joint [32], intratendinous proliferation of a neurofibroma, [33] and [2] pathological, local steroid injection [34], rheumatoid arthritis infections [35], and osteoarthrosis [28]. FPL should be considered in any patients with previous wrist surgery, especially those involving hardware. Closed FPL ruptures at the wrist typically occur 3–6 months after osteosynthesis of distal radius fractures with palmar plates and are mostly characterized by crepitation and pain lasting for several weeks. These can be prevented by premature plate removal, synovectomy, and carpal tunnel release. Additionally, some closed rupture of the FPL has been reported to be associated with genetic influences [36].

When there is no history of trauma to the thumb, it is also necessary to differentiate it from the anterior interosseous nerve (AIN) palsy, because peripheral nerve injury and spinal cord injury can cause FPL dysfunction. This is important, because surgical exploration should be avoided for an intact FPL tendon. Pressing the musculocutaneous junction of the FPL firmly with the examiner's thumb and noting the thumb IP joint flexion demonstrate if the FPL unit is intact [37]. A tendon irritation test provides a way to elicit a sign of FPL tendon irritation after the volar plate fixation [38]. In addition to the physical exams using the tenodesis effect [37], MRI scanning, sonography, and electroneurophysiological studies are helpful to make differential diagnosis of FPL ruptures from AIN palsy or congenitally absent FPL [39]. Succinylcholine is also used to distinguish FPL rupture from FPL dysfunction due to nerve injury [40]. When disruption of the FPL tendon is detected, it should be repaired to restore the thumb function.

Even when the FPL is completely severed, it may be possible to actively flex the thumb interphalangeal joint, in the case where the vinculum brevis remains attached to the volar plate [2]. Because this might cause a misdiagnosis of an intact FPL, hand surgeons should in all cases always keep in mind any possibility of FPL injury.

Most lacerations of FPL occur at the metacarpophalangeal joint level. The excursion of FPL at the thumb interphalangeal (IP) joint is 10–12 mm, while that of the other profundus tendons is only 5 mm so avulsion at the FPL insertion site is relatively rare [41]. If injury happens while the fingers are flexed, distal cut ends of the FPL tendon shift distally. When the FPL lacerations occur distal to the MCP joint, the FPL usually retracts to the thenar area or wrist, and this makes surgical exploration difficult. Kasashima et al. compared the results in zone II injury with those in zones I and III and found that the results were less satisfactory due to the presence of a pulley system and an avascular region of the tendon (Fig. 10.6) [42].

Surgical repair of the FPL is well established as the optimum treatment for FPL lacerations, and it reveals better results than that of the other fingers, because the anatomy of the FPL is simpler as it includes just one tendon and one IP joint. Furthermore, IP motion is not critical for satisfactory thumb function [26, 43].

The repair technique is dependent on the time and zone of injury and the state of the tendon bed and muscle. Direct tendon repair is the procedure of choice in the acute stages of less than 2 months after injury [25]. If the delay is more than 2–3 months, the proximal tendon stump retracts more proximally, and the tendon sheath is scarred, which impedes the advancement and lengthening of the injured FPL. In those situations, secondary FPL reconstruction is needed.

General theories of flexor tendon repair are also applied to FPL repair. The strength of flexor tendon repair is known to be directly proportional to the number of sutures crossing the repair site [44]. The knots-outside technique initially reveals greater strength than the knots-inside technique, although there is no significant difference at 6 weeks postoperation [45]. Considering that tendon nutrition after tendon injury is mainly from the imbibition of synovial fluid, dorsal placement of core sutures represents the best mechanical location for tendon repair [46]. The epitenon repair not only improves the contour of tendon repair but also increases the strength of the tendon repair.

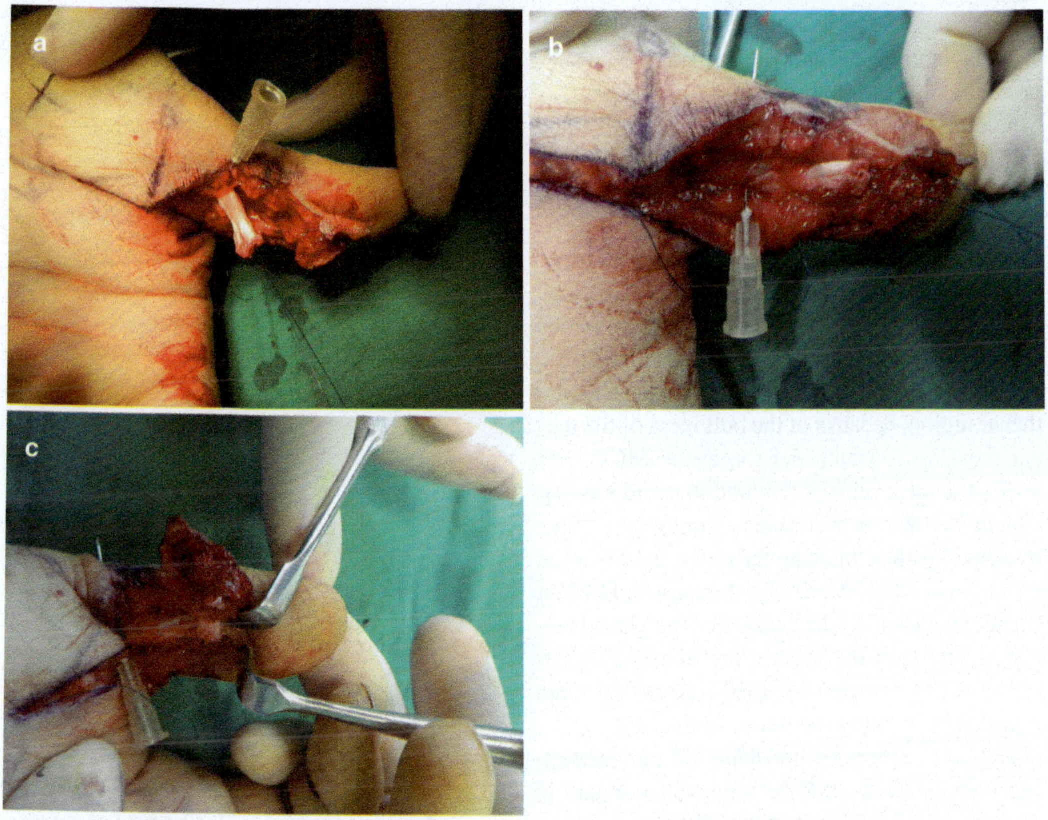

**Fig. 10.6** This 45-year-old man sustained a glass injury on his left thumb. (**a**) Proximal stump of the FPL was retrieved and fixed temporarily using 32-gauge needle. (**b**) It was passed through the A1 and oblique pulley to prevent the bowstring of the FPL tendon. (**c**) Proper tenorrhaphy of the FPL was performed using four-stranded modified Kessler technique

Deeper epitenon sutures provide more increased strength than superficial epitenon sutures [47]. It is recommended that tendon lacerations of less than 60% of the cross-sectional area of the tendon be treated without tenorrhaphy and with early mobilization. Comparison of the tendon sheath repair, tendon sheath excision, and tendon sheath grafting revealed no significant difference in the final results [48]. Because the epitenon seems to be the most active portion of the early phase of tendon repair, epitenon suture results in an increase in repair strength and a significant reduction in the tendency for gapping at the repair site.

Generally, primary FPL repair with early mobilization is the treatment of choice for FPL injuries. The FPL heals through both extrinsic and intrinsic mechanisms. Extrinsic tendon healing relates to the peripheral adhesions via cells brought to the site of injury by the ingrowth of capillaries and fibroblasts. Intrinsic healing occurs from epitenocytes and endotenocytes that migrate into the tendon gaps. The goal of FPL repair is to encourage both intrinsic and extrinsic tendon healing without the formation of thick adhesions, which would limit tendon excursion, and ultimately results in restricted motion of the finger.

## Surgical Technique for FPL Tenorrhaphy

Under tourniquet control, local anesthesia is preferred for the primary repair of the FPL. Some surgeons nowadays prefer wide-awake hand surgery for FPL repair. The proper timing for the primary repair is not settled, and even 4 weeks after the injury is acceptable. Urbaniak even suggested a direct repair of the FPL as late as 3 months after the laceration, if tendon damage and muscle retraction are minimal [25]. Bruner incision on the palmar surface is favored over the midlateral incision on the thumb (Fig. 10.7). Because of the fewer pulleys and absence of superficialis tendon, the retracted FPL can be retrieved more easily through the fibro-osseous tunnel. To retrieve the FPL, an incision at the wrist level is recommended, rather than in the thenar region, because of the bulkiness of the thenar muscles. A small incision at the MCP joint level or wrist level is performed to avoid passing a blunt tendon retriever blindly through the fibro-osseous sheath or incising the entire thumb at the thenar area. After identifying the retracted FPL, a small catheter or feeding tube may be placed retrograde through the sheath, and the end of the retracted FPL is sutured to the catheter [49]. This is pulled back out of the injured site of the thumb to prepare the proper tenorrhaphy. A transversely oriented needle secures the tendons for repair. If surgical incision for the total FPL exposure is needed, three basic incisions may be applied (Fig. 10.7) [25]. The proximal end of the ruptured FPL is usually adhered to the clotted blood in the synovium, which is the clue to detect the retracted FPL tendon. The severed tendons are held in approximation by small needles, and the tendon ends are minimally trimmed and arranged. It is beneficial that partial excursion of the FPL provides excellent thumb function contrary to the other finger flexor tendons.

The preferred suture technique consists of atraumatic handling of the tendon ends with placement of proper core sutures. The type and technique of suture placement are controversial. The ideal suture material should be nonreactive, strong enough, easy to handle, of small size, pliable, and capable of maintaining a stable knot. Nonabsorbable sutures are widely used, due to the advantages of easy handling, good biocompatibility, and minimal loss of tensile strength after knotting. Various techniques of the tenorrhaphy of ruptured FPL have been performed according to the site and condition of the tendon injury (Fig. 10.8).

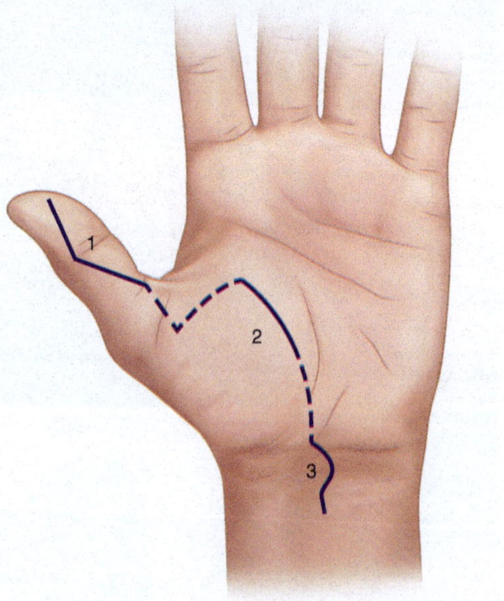


**Fig. 10.7** Three basic incisions may be needed for retrieving the retracted FPL tendon (redrawn from Urbaniak, Hand Clin 1985;1:69–76)

When the FPL tendon was avulsed at its insertion site on the distal phalanx, a Becker type of suture is widely used, using anchor suture ends (Fig. 10.8). If the distal phalanx is too weak to bear the anchor, the traditional pullout suture using plastic buttonhole can be replaced. Keith needles are drilled through the base of the distal phalanx, and thread ends are tied over a button placed on the nail plate beyond the lunula to avoid nail deformity (Fig. 10.9).

Although two-strand suture methods, i.e., the Kessler and modified Kessler and the Tajima techniques, are still being widely used, newer multistrand suture methods, such as the Strickland, cruciate, Becker, Savage, Winters, and Mantero techniques [50], have been suggested with increasing frequency because of the stronger tension and increased resistance to repair site gapping (Fig. 10.10).

Direct tenorrhaphy of FPL is mostly difficult in the thenar area, due to the bulkiness of the surrounding structures. Tendon divisions in zones II and III can be repaired by a modified Kessler suture using either 4–0 Prolene or 4–0 Ethibond and a circumferential running suture of 6–0 Prolene (Fig. 10.11). A Kessler core suture and a reinforced

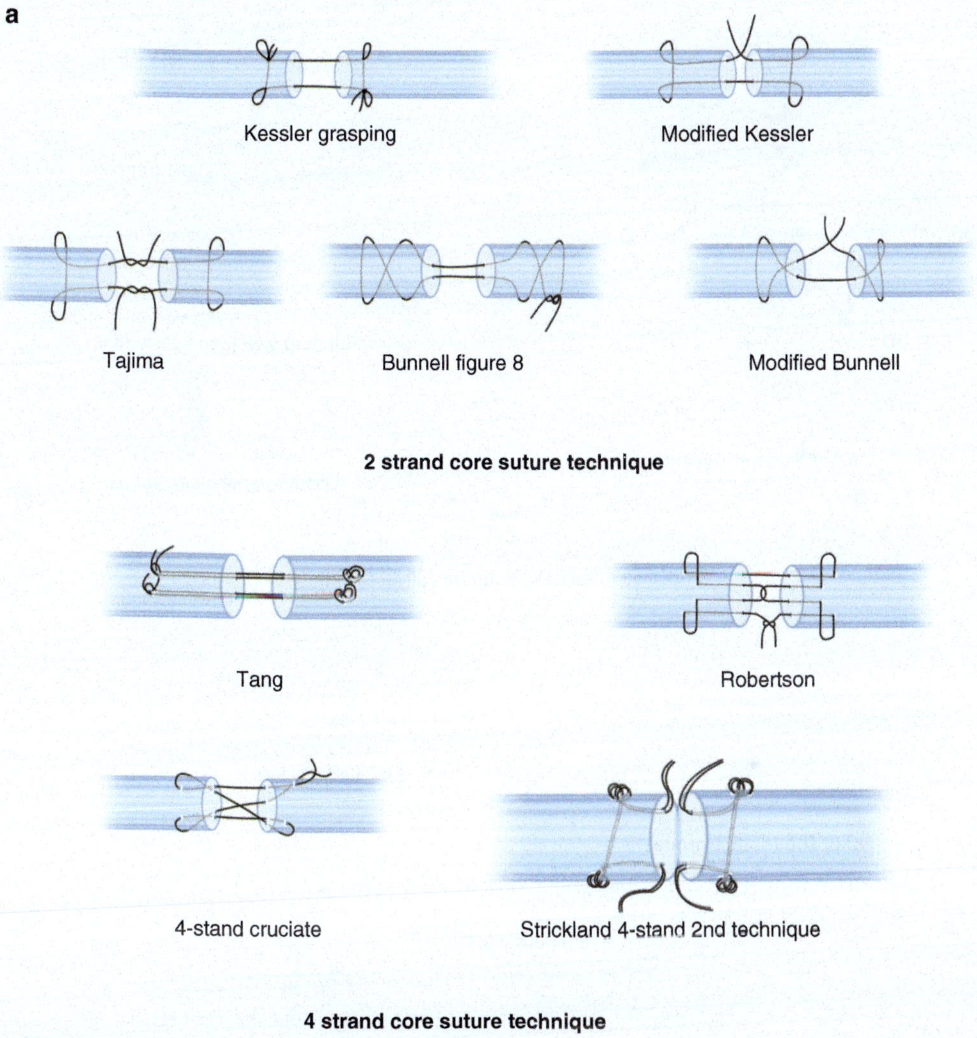


**Fig. 10.8** Various techniques for tenorrhaphy of FPL

epitendinous suture, two-Kessler two-strand core sutures and a strengthened circumferential suture [51], have also been proposed (Fig. 10.11). In zones III, IV, and V injuries, Stark used an interposition graft (Fig. 10.8) [52]. It is generally recommended to escape zone III, to avoid injury to the recurrent motor branch of the median nerve.

Many authors have indicated that epitendinous sutures reinforce the main tendon suture, including the modified Kessler and Becker methods [25, 53], although Noonan et al. found no statistical importance of the epitenon suture [54]. 6–0 nylon sutures are placed circumferentially through the epitendon. We have used a needle with a looped suture 4–0 in diameter for the tenorrhaphy of FPL using the Tsuge technique or Tajima repair using 4–0 Ethibond® loop suture (Fig. 10.12). In infants or very young children, Zolotov restored the FPL by a modified Tsuge suture technique using a looped suture 5–0 [55]. Tang described the technique of inserting three Tsuge sutures arranged in a three-dimensional configuration [56]. The Tsuge sutures were carried out using a 4–0 Ticron

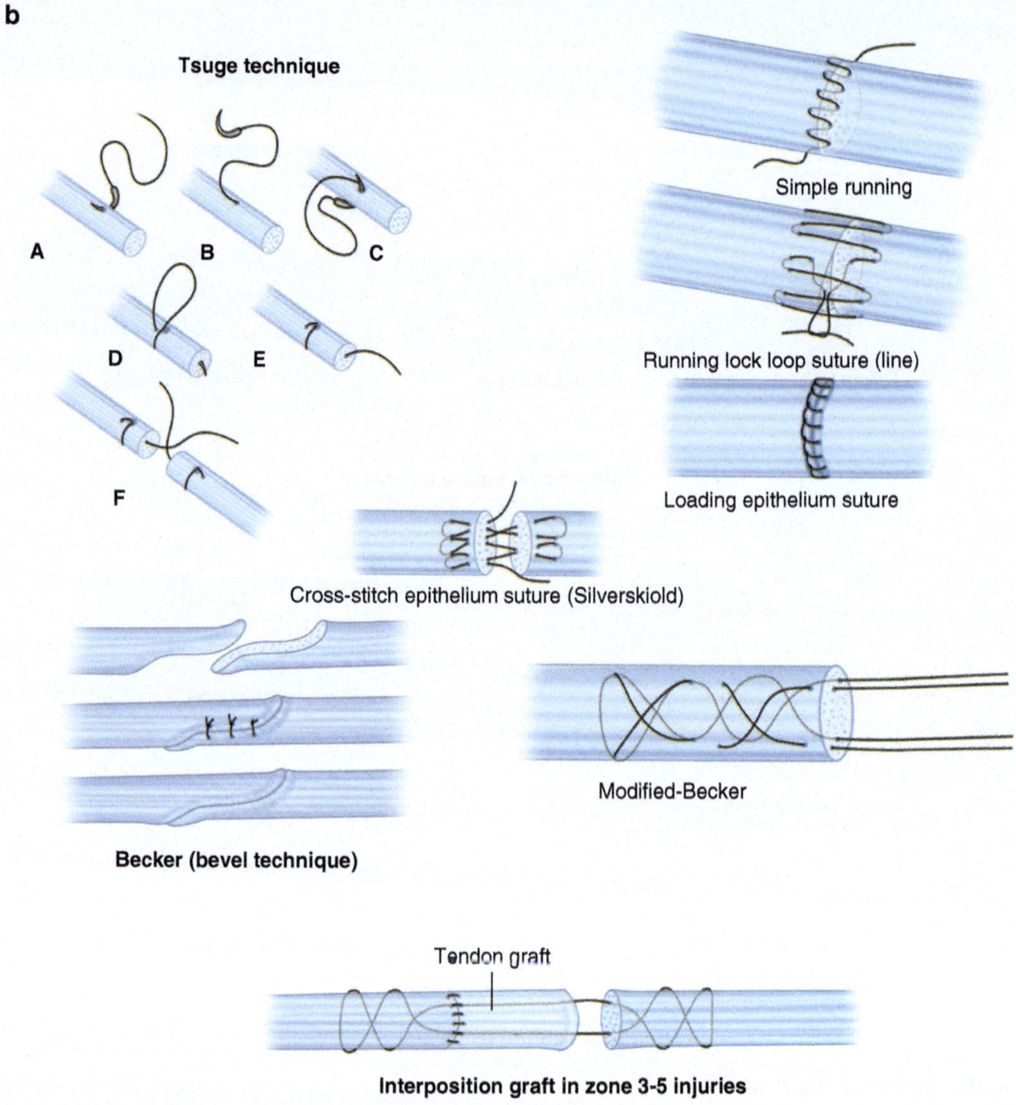


**Fig. 10.8** (continued)

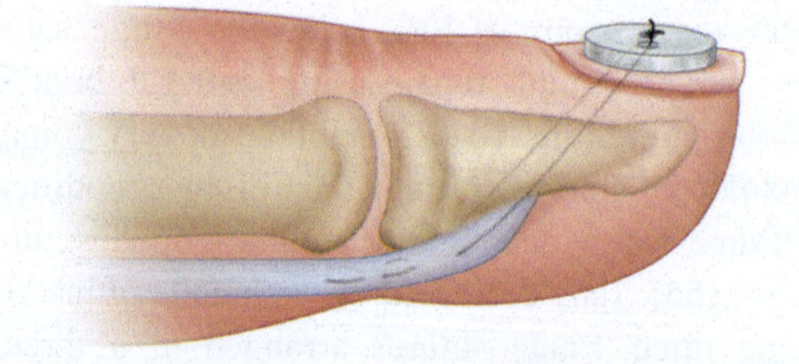

**Fig. 10.9** Pullout suture using buttonhole is commonly used when the FPL tendon was avulsed at its insertion site on distal phalanx of the thumb

suture core suture on a round needle with a loop thread (Tendi-Loop, Aesculap AG and Co. KG, Tuttlingen, Germany).

Although pulley reconstruction is usually not required in the thumb, the oblique pulley, which is the most important of the three pulleys in the thumb [57], should be repaired, to prevent bowstring by the tendon grafts using the palmaris longus [58] or triple-loop plantaris tendon [59]. Closed rupture of the thumb flexor tendon pulleys is extremely rare. Fazilleau

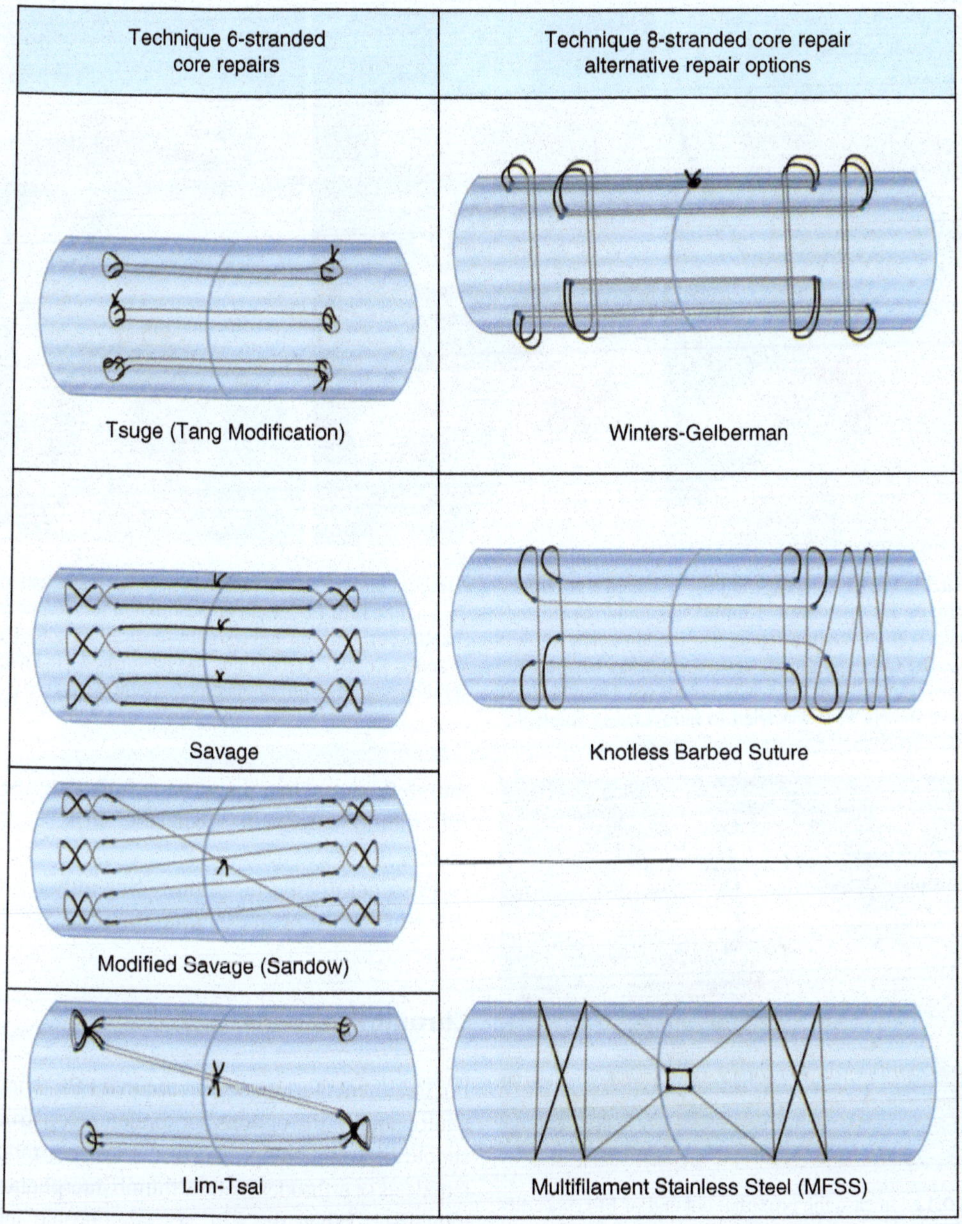


**Fig. 10.10** Multistrand suture methods for FPL tenorrhaphy

described a single, free palmaris longus (PL) autograft for thumb pulley reconstruction [58]. Kutsumi et al. recommended that after the FPL tenorrhaphy, the oblique pulley should if possible be left intact, because when the partial excision of the distal end of the pulley of the thumb was performed, the gliding resistance was increased [60].

If it is needed to lengthen the FPL by more than 1 cm, Z-plasty lengthening technique can be applied at the musculocutaneous junction (Fig. 10.13) [25]. Stepwise lengthening is the useful option, especially in the FPL avulsion at its insertion site. Advancement and lengthening is sometimes easier and less complicated than the tendon graft. When more than 3 or 4 cm of length

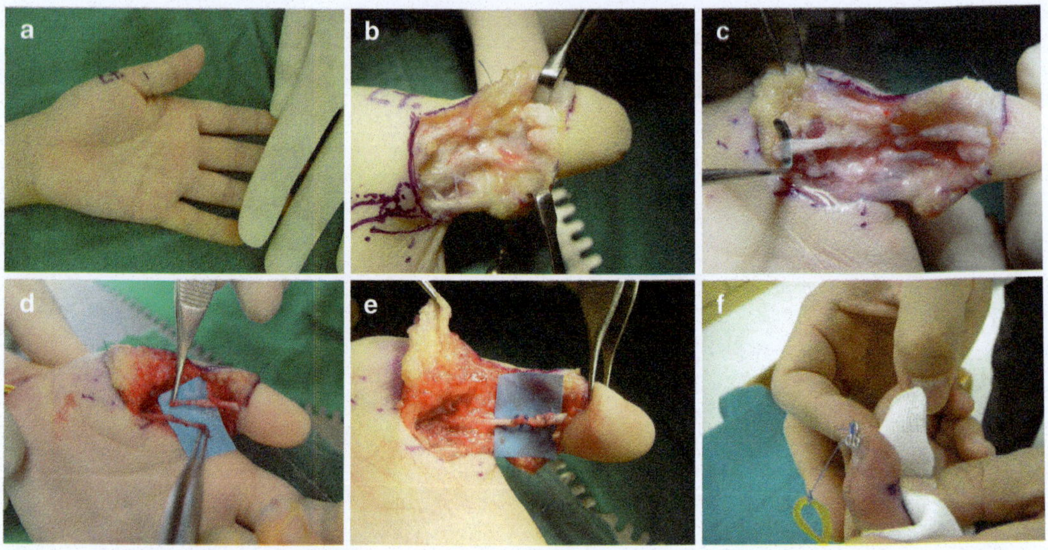


**Fig. 10.11** (**a**) This 7-year-old boy sustained a cut injury by knife on his left thumb 3 months ago and healed secondarily without tendon repair. He couldn't flex his left thumb. (**b**) On exploration, severe adhesion of the FPL and surrounding structures was noted. (**c**) The proximal stump of the cut FPL was tried to retract using Ragnell® retractor, and the distally cut end of FPL was revealed. (**d**) Two cut ends of FPL were approximated for proper tenorrhaphy. (**e**) With an appropriate tension, modified four-stranded Kessler's technique was performed. (**f**) Dynamic splint was applied immediate postoperatively

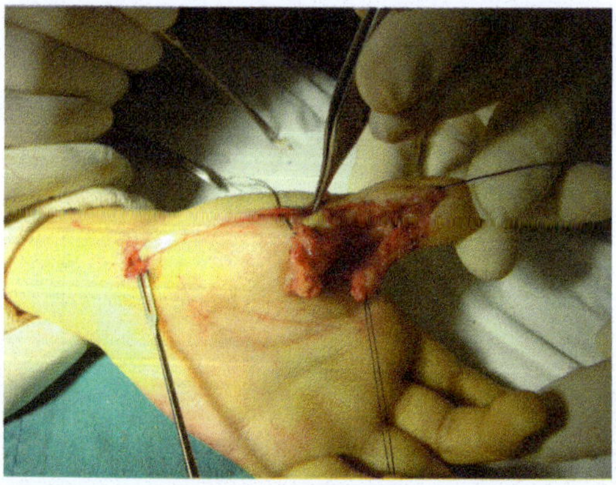

**Fig. 10.12** In case the proximal cut end of FPL was difficult to locate intraoperatively, the wrist incision is helpful to retrieve the injured FPL tendon

is needed, a tendon graft would be the choice. The donor site would be the palmaris longus or one of the extensor digitorum communis tendons of the toes. The Pulvertaft, end-weave method is preferred for stronger repair (Fig. 10.14). The appropriate length of the tendon graft is determined with the proper tension by either complete thumb flexion when the wrist is fully extended or full thumb extension when the wrist is completely flexed.

Postoperatively, the thumb was either placed in a plaster cast or in dynamic traction.

## Chronic Problems

For treatment of a neglected, ruptured FPL tendon in adult patients, the options for tendon reconstruction should be weighed up against the less complicated tenodesis or arthrodesis of the thumb interphalangeal joint [61]. When the FPL reveals chronic tendon injuries with primarily the inability to repair, or the musculotendinous complex of FPL does not show proper function, surgical options include tendon transfer, tendon graft, and IP joint arthrodesis. Many factors must also be assessed, such as age, etiology, and the experience of the surgeon.

Another infrequent FPL tendon problem is the Linburg-Comstock syndrome, which may cause unexplained chronic pain in the distal forearm, resulting from post-traumatic inflammation of the intertendinous connections. This

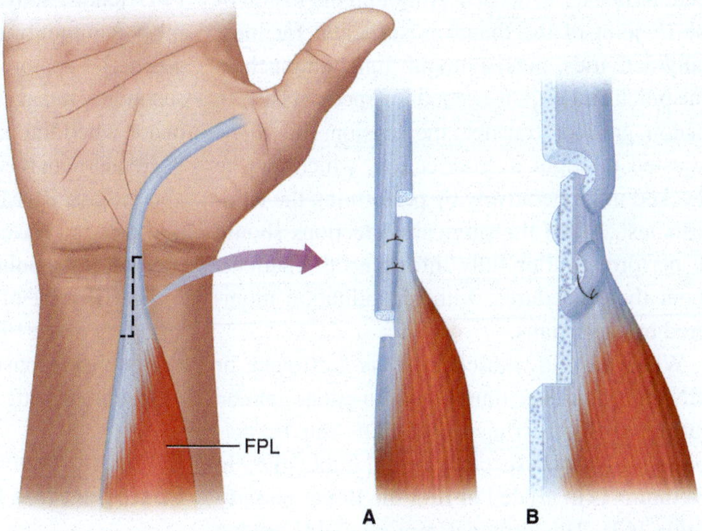


**Fig. 10.13** Distal advancement and lengthening of the FPL at the wrist level (redrawn from Urbaniak, Hand Clin 1985;1:69–76)

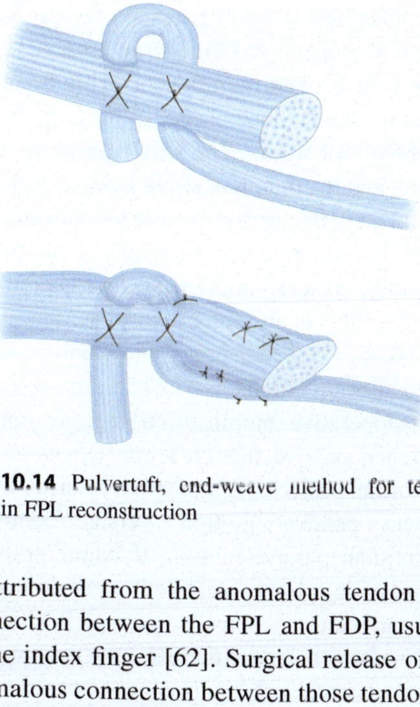

**Fig. 10.14** Pulvertaft, end-weave method for tendon graft in FPL reconstruction

is attributed from the anomalous tendon slip connection between the FPL and FDP, usually of the index finger [62]. Surgical release of the anomalous connection between those tendons is an effective treatment.

## Secondary Reconstruction of FPL

FPL reconstruction could be performed as one-stage [5, 63] or two-stage [64, 65]. Two-stage tendon reconstructions are usually required in patients with more than 4 weeks after an initial cut injury or extensive trauma accompanying infection that is not feasible for immediate repair. The Hunter two-stage silicone rod technique is infrequently applied for FPL reconstruction, especially in severe scarring or contracture [66]. Passing through the original FPL path should always be tried. After at least 2 months, the silicone rod is replaced with a tendon graft.

Contrary to the flexor tendons in the other fingers, the FPL runs at 90° to the line of pull of the muscle when the thumb is in full abduction. Therefore, FPL reconstruction is more difficult than that of the other fingers. Interestingly, Urbaniak emphasized that adequate FPL muscle excursion is present more than 15 years after FPL laceration, because the severed proximal tendon moves with its adjacent tendons in the forearm [57].

Reconstruction after acute or chronic loss of FPL function should be considered when restoration of pinch and grip strength is needed. For treatment of a ruptured FPL tendon in adult patients, the options for tendon reconstruction should be weighed up against the less complicated tenodesis or arthrodesis of the thumb. When the FPL ruptures over a long period of time, primary repair is hindered by hypertrophied tenosynovium, tendon defect with fibrous tissue, and tendon retraction. Therefore, IP joint arthrodesis or tendon reconstruction using tendon graft or tendon transfer is needed. Although the fusion of the IP joint of the thumb is sufficient for most daily activities, precise thumb function, such as fine pinch and grip, is needed for special tasks. In tendon graft or transfer, the tension should be adjusted to slight overcorrection, which can be checked intraoperatively by performing the tenodesis test. All of the surgical corrections should be performed after fully informing the patients about the procedures, with rehabilitation monitored by physicians.

When the FPL muscle belly is destroyed, or AIN palsy causes thumb malfunction, tendon transfer from the ring finger FDS can be performed [67]. It is especially useful if the injury to the thumb is in grade I or II of the Boyes classification [63]. This provides a more viable tendon and motor, if there is direct damage to the FPL muscle belly or to its nerve supply.

In FPL deficiency, commonly used tendon transfers that can augment the thumb opposition strength are the Huber abductor digiti minimi muscle transfer and the FDS opposition transfer. The former increases thenar bulk, but does not provide additional tissue for metacarpophalangeal stability.

In a severely paralyzed hand, the thumb grip can be restored by split FPL tenodesis. Considering that the key grip includes a flexion force applied from the tip of the thumb to the radial aspect of the middle phalanx, Mohamed et al. positioned the thumb optimally and provided limited active flexion of the IP joint for tetraplegic hands [68]. The positive Froment's sign due to intrinsic paralysis of the thumb could also be corrected with splint distal FPL tenodesis [69, 70] which uses a radial half of the FPL tendon rerouted dorsally and inserted into the extensor pollicis longus tendon. Compared to the IP joint arthrodesis, the patient can re-establish pulp pinch positioning, while the thumb maintains its IP joint mobility.

## Complications of Primary and Delayed FPL Tenorrhaphy

Complications, such as tendon re-ruptures, adhesions, and joint contractures-stiffness, can be minimized with proper postoperative care after FPL tenorrhaphy. Tendon rupture after repair most commonly occurs in zone II repairs; and when the rupture is immediately diagnosed, a secondary repair should be performed. Adhesions occur when the passive range of motion (ROM) is greater than the active ROM. When both active and passive ROM are limited, joint contractures develop and have to be properly treated. If the oblique or A2 pulley is severed, attempted flexion of the IP joint of the thumb might cause bowstringing of the FPL. Therefore, oblique pulley is sometimes reconstructed by tendon graft or wrist retinaculum graft.

## Postoperative Care

There has been no fixed policy for the postoperative management of FPL tendon repairs in the thumb. Postoperative FPL is to be managed in the same way as other digit flexors. With the proper dressing, dorsal block plaster splint is applied on the thumb for weeks. The wrist is held in 30° of flexion and the thumb in slight flexion. Although controlled active or passive flexion movement is urged by some surgeons, there is no proven advantage for early motion of the repaired FPL [25, 71]. This is attributed to the fact that whole excursion is not mandatory in thumb function, unlike the other digits.

Postoperative mobilization regimes include shortened passive flexion/active extension versus normal passive flexion/active extension, continuous passive motion versus controlled intermittent passive motion, dynamic splintage versus static splintage, active flexion versus rubber band traction, controlled passive flexion with active extension (modified Kleinert) versus controlled passive mobilization (modified Duran), and grasping suture and early controlled active mobilization versus modified Kessler technique with early controlled passive mobilization [6, 48, 72]. Some authors have reported no differences between patients with static or dynamic splinting [54], and Urbaniac stated that there is no advantage to early mobilization of a repaired FPL [25]. However, by performing a cadaveric study, Rappaport et al. provided a biomechanical basis for early passive and active exercise to an isolated thumb IP joint [73].

According to the author's regimen, protected active flexion is begun after 3 weeks of FPL repair, and full active extension is started at 6 weeks. Percival noted that the postoperative dynamic controlled mobilization improves the repair results, particularly in zone II, which is where most FPL divisions occur [6]. Forceful stretching is recommended for at least 8 weeks postoperation.

## Outcomes After FPL Reconstruction

Unlike the other digits, better functional recovery is expected in FPL repair, because of its simpler anatomy and less permitted excursion in thumb function. However, the re-rupture rate after FPL repair is relatively high compared to that in flexor tendons of the other fingers. This is attributed to the comparative difficulty of FPL tendon repair, due to the surrounding soft tissues, the relative avascularity of the FPL tendon in zone II, and the increased mobility of the thumb [1, 51, 54]. According to Kasashima, age, accompanying neurovascular damage, and timing of repair did not affect the results of FPL tenorrhaphy [42].

The functional evaluation after FPL repair is also different from that of FDP and FDS. In addition to the range of motion, pinch grip and the ability to perform the activities of daily living should be assessed. When evaluating the reconstruction after acute or chronic loss of FPL function, restoration of proper pinch strength is an important criterion. To get optimal results, a properly planned hand therapy program is critical. The best indicator of thumb function is tip-to-tip pinch grip and a fully functional hand.

Children display tremendous healing potential after FPL tendon repair, because they have a better blood supply on the tendon surface with shorter vincula than adults and the ability to remodel scars is greater [27]. In very young children, the zone of injury in the thumb seems to have little effect on the postoperative range of motion, and many authors recommend strict immobilization by above-elbow cast [74].

## Other Problems

In systemic disease, such as rheumatoid arthritis, the FPL is severely involved as marked tendon sheath widening, synovial proliferation, loss of the normal homogeneous fibrillary echotexture, and a large intratendinous tear [75]. These conditions with FPL tenosynovitis might cause carpal tunnel syndrome [76]. Additionally, calcific tendinitis of the FPL should be differentiated from trauma, septic arthritis, tenosynovitis, or even a soft tissue mass, because in most cases, the symptoms mimic each other [77].

When the IP joint was dislocated while the FPL was wrapped around the radial condyle of the proximal phalanx, the displaced FPL hinders the closed reduction of the displaced IP joint [78].

## References


1. Hergenroeder PT, Gelberman RH, Akeson WH. The vascularity of the flexor pollicis longus tendon. Clin Orthop Relat Res. 1982;(162):298–303.
2. Armenta E, Fisher J. Anatomy of flexor pollicis longus vinculum system. J Hand Surg [Am]. 1984;9:210–2.
3. Azar CA, Culver JE, Fleegler EJ. Blood supply of the flexor pollicis longus tendon. J Hand Surg [Am]. 1983;8:471–5.
4. Lundborg G. The vascularization of the human flexor pollicis longus tendon. Hand. 1979;11:28–33.
5. Pulvertaft RG. Tendon grafts for flexor tendon injuries in the fingers and thumb; a study of technique and results. J Bone Joint Surg Br. 1956;38-B:175–94.
6. Percival NJ, Sykes PJ. Flexor pollicis longus tendon repair: a comparison between dynamic and static splintage. J Hand Surg Br. 1989;14:412–5.
7. Toktas H, Dundar U, Kusbeci OY, et al. FPL tendon thickness, tremor and hand functions in Parkinson's disease. Open Med (Wars). 2016;11:16–20.
8. Cooney WP, 3rd, Chao EY. Biomechanical analysis of static forces in the thumb during hand function. J Bone Joint Surg Am. 1977;59:27–36.
9. Riordan DC. Tendon transfers in hand surgery. J Hand Surg [Am]. 1983;8:748–53.
10. Uchida M, Kojima T, Sakurai N. Congenital absence of flexor pollicis longus without hypoplasia of thenar muscles. Plast Reconstr Surg. 1985;75:413–6.
11. Nakamura J, Kubo E. Bilateral anomalous insertion of flexor pollicis longus. J Hand Surg Br. 1993;18:312–5.

12. Linburg RM, Comstock BE. Anomalous tendon slips from the flexor pollicis longus to the flexor digitorum profundus. J Hand Surg [Am]. 1979;4:79–83.
13. van Loveren M, van der Biezen JJ. The congenital trigger thumb: is release of the first annular pulley alone sufficient to resolve the triggering? Ann Plast Surg. 2007;58:335–7.
14. Schubert MF, Shah VS, Craig CL, Zeller JL. Varied anatomy of the thumb pulley system: implications for successful trigger thumb release. J Hand Surg [Am]. 2012;37:2278–85.
15. Slakey JB, Hennrikus WL. Acquired thumb flexion contracture in children: congenital trigger thumb. J Bone Joint Surg Br. 1996;78:481–3.
16. Ty JM, James MA. Failure of differentiation: Part II (arthrogryposis, camptodactyly, clinodactyly, madelung deformity, trigger finger, and trigger thumb). Hand Clin. 2009;25:195–213.
17. Vyas BK, Sarwahi V. Bilateral congenital trigger thumb: role of heredity. Indian J Pediatr. 1999;66:949–51.
18. Hueston JT, Wilson WF. The aetiology of trigger finger explained on the basis of intratendinous architecture. Hand. 1972;4:257–60.
19. Fahey JJ, Bollinger JA. Trigger-finger in adults and children. J Bone Joint Surg Am. 1954;36-A:1200–18.
20. Watanabe H, Hamada Y, Toshima T. Conservative management of infantile trigger thumb: indications and limitations. Tech Hand Up Extrem Surg. 2003;7:37–42.
21. Chalise PK, Mishra AK, Shah SB, Adhikari V, Singh RP. The treatment of trigger thumb in children: conservative or surgical? Nepal Med Coll J. 2013;15:122–4.
22. Edwards DS, Richards RH. Risk stratification for the recurrence of trigger thumb after surgical release in the paediatric patient. Eur J Orthop Surg Traumatol. 2016;26:587–90.
23. Seybold EA, Warhold LG. Impingement of the flexor pollicis longus tendon by an enlarged radial sesamoid causing trigger thumb: a case report. J Hand Surg [Am]. 1996;21:619–20.
24. Verdan CE. Half a century of flexor-tendon surgery. Current status and changing philosophies. J Bone Joint Surg Am. 1972;54:472–91.
25. Urbaniak JR. Repair of the flexor pollicis longus. Hand Clin. 1985;1:69–76.
26. Grobbelaar AO, Hudson DA. Flexor pollicis longus tendon injuries in children. Ann R Coll Surg Engl. 1995;77:135–7.
27. Arons MS. Purposeful delay of the primary repair of cut flexor tendons in "some-man's-land" in children. Plast Reconstr Surg. 1974;53:638–42.
28. Webb JB, Elliot D. Spontaneous rupture of the flexor pollicis longus tendon on a sesamoid bone. J Hand Surg Br. 1997;22:381–2.
29. Saitoh S, Hata Y, Murakami N, et al. Scaphoid nonunion and flexor pollicis longus tendon rupture. J Hand Surg [Am]. 1999;24:1211–9.
30. Chilelli BJ, Patel RM, Kalainov DM, Peng J, Zhang LQ. Flexor pollicis longus dysfunction after volar plate fixation of distal radius fractures. J Hand Surg [Am]. 2013;38:1691–7.
31. Yang SS, Bear BJ, Weiland AJ. Rupture of the flexor pollicis longus tendon after 30 years due to migration of a retained foreign body. J Hand Surg Br. 1995;20:803–5.
32. Kanaya K, Kanaya K, Iba K, Yamashita T. Attrition rupture of the flexor pollicis longus tendon after arthrodesis of the trapeziometacarpal joint: a case report. Hand Surg. 2015;20:474–6.
33. Kawabata H, Masada K, Kawai H, Masatomi T. Rupture of the flexor pollicis longus in von Recklinghausen's disease. J Hand Surg [Am]. 1991;16:666–9.
34. Taras JS, Iiams GJ, Gibbons M, Culp RW. Flexor pollicis longus rupture in a trigger thumb: a case report. J Hand Surg [Am]. 1995;20:276–7.
35. Mannerfelt L, Norman O. Attrition ruptures of flexor tendons in rheumatoid arthritis caused by bony spurs in the carpal tunnel. A clinical and radiological study. J Bone Joint Surg Br. 1969;51:270–7.
36. Qureshi A, Wong KY, Cormack G, Gillespie P. Bilateral closed flexor pollicis longus musculotendinous junction ruptures. BMJ Case Rep. 2015;2015
37. Melton JT, Murray JR, Lowdon IM. A simple clinical test of flexor pollicis longus rupture. J Hand Surg Br. 2005;30:624–5.
38. Suganuma S, Tada K, Tsuchiya H. Reducing the risk of flexor pollicis longus tendon rupture after volar plate fixation for distal radius fractures: validation of the tendon irritation test. Eur J Orthop Surg Traumatol. 2014;24:1425–9.
39. Shamsian N, Exton R, Shibu M. Reconstruction of a congenitally absent flexor pollicis longus in an adult. Can J Plast Surg. 2010;18:143–4.
40. Doyle JR, Semenza J, Gilling B. The effect of succinylcholine on denervated skeletal muscle. J Hand Surg [Am]. 1981;6:40–2.
41. Urbaniak JR, Goldner JL. Laceration of the flexor pollicis longus tendon: delayed repair by advancement, free graft or direct suture. A clinical and experimental study. J Bone Joint Surg Am. 1973;55:1123–48.
42. Kasashima T, Kato H, Minami A. Factors influencing prognosis after direct repair of the flexor pollicis longus tendon: multivariate regression model analysis. Hand Surg. 2002;7:171–6.
43. Nunley JA, Levin LS, Devito D, Goldner RD, Urbaniak JR. Direct end-to-end repair of flexor pollicis longus tendon lacerations. J Hand Surg [Am]. 1992;17:118–21.
44. Thurman RT, Trumble TE, Hanel DP, Tencer AF, Kiser PK. Two-, four-, and six-strand zone II flexor tendon repairs: an in situ biomechanical comparison using a cadaver model. J Hand Surg [Am]. 1998;23:261–5.
45. Papandrea R, Seitz WH Jr, Shapiro P, Borden B. Biomechanical and clinical evaluation of the epitenon-first technique of flexor tendon repair. J Hand Surg [Am]. 1995;20:261–6.
46. Soejima O, Diao E, Lotz JC, Hariharan JS. Comparative mechanical analysis of dorsal ver-

sus palmar placement of core suture for flexor tendon repairs. J Hand Surg [Am]. 1995;20:801–7.
47. Diao E, Hariharan JS, Soejima O, Lotz JC. Effect of peripheral suture depth on strength of tendon repairs. J Hand Surg [Am]. 1996;21:234–9.
48. Gelberman RH, Woo SL, Amiel D, Horibe S, Lee D. Influences of flexor sheath continuity and early motion on tendon healing in dogs. J Hand Surg [Am]. 1990;15:69–77.
49. Sourmelis SG, McGrouther DA. Retrieval of the retracted flexor tendon. J Hand Surg Br. 1987;12:109–11.
50. Schaller P. Repair of the flexor pollicis longus tendon with the motion-stable Mantero technique. Scand J Plast Reconstr Surg Hand Surg. 2010;44:163–6.
51. Sirotakova M, Elliot D. Early active mobilization of primary repairs of the flexor pollicis longus tendon with two Kessler two-strand core sutures and a strengthened circumferential suture. J Hand Surg Br. 2004;29:531–5.
52. Stark HH, Anderson DR, Zemel NP, et al. Bridge flexor tendon grafts. Clin Orthop Relat Res. 1989;(242):51–9.
53. Ozturk K, Orhun E, Polatkan O, Polatkan S. Long-term results of early primary repair of flexor pollicis longus tendon injuries. Acta Orthop Traumatol Turc. 2004;38:50–3.
54. Noonan KJ, Blair WF. Long-term follow-up of primary flexor pollicis longus tenorrhaphies. J Hand Surg [Am]. 1991;16:653–62.
55. Zolotov AS. Repair of the flexor pollicis longus tendon in an infant. Hand Surg. 2008;13:31–5.
56. Tang JB, Shi D, Gu YQ, Chen JC, Zhou B. Double and multiple looped suture tendon repair. J Hand Surg Br. 1994;19:699–703.
57. Doyle JR. Anatomy of the flexor tendon sheath and pulley system: a current review. J Hand Surg [Am]. 1989;14:349–51.
58. Fazilleau F, Cheval D, Richou J, Le Nen D. Reconstruction of closed rupture of thumb flexor tendon pulleys with a single free palmaris longus tendon graft: a case report and review of literature. Chir Main. 2014;33:51–4.
59. Kosiyatrakul A, Jitprapaikulsarn S, Durand S, Oberlin C. Closed flexor pulley rupture of the thumb: case report and review of literature. Hand Surg. 2009;14:139–42.
60. Kutsumi K, Amadio PC, Zhao C, Zobitz ME, An KN. Gliding resistance of the flexor pollicis longus tendon after repair: does partial excision of the oblique pulley affect gliding resistance? Plast Reconstr Surg. 2006;118:1423–8; discussion 1429–1430
61. Uekubo K, Itoh S, Yoshioka T. Closed traumatic rupture of the flexor pollicis longus tendon in zone T I: a case report. Hand Surg. 2015;20:145–7.
62. Badhe S, Lynch J, Thorpe SK, Bainbridge LC. Operative treatment of Linburg-Comstock syndrome. J Bone Joint Surg Br. 2010;92:1278–81.
63. Boyes JH. Flexor-tendon grafts in the fingers and thumb; an evaluation of end results. J Bone Joint Surg Am. 1950;32-A:489–99; passim
64. Unglaub F, Bultmann C, Reiter A, Hahn P. Two-staged reconstruction of the flexor pollicis longus tendon. J Hand Surg Br. 2006;31:432–5.
65. Frakking TG, Depuydt KP, Kon M, Werker PM. Retrospective outcome analysis of staged flexor tendon reconstruction. J Hand Surg Br. 2000;25:168–74.
66. Hunter JM, Salisbury RE. Flexor-tendon reconstruction in severely damaged hands. A two-stage procedure using a silicone-dacron reinforced gliding prosthesis prior to tendon grafting. J Bone Joint Surg Am. 1971;53:829–58.
67. Schneider LH, Wiltshire D. Restoration of flexor pollicis longus function by flexor digitorum superficialis transfer. J Hand Surg [Am]. 1983;8:98–101.
68. Mohammed KD, Rothwell AG, Sinclair SW, Willems SM, Bean AR. Upper-limb surgery for tetraplegia. J Bone Joint Surg Br. 1992;74:873–9.
69. Ejeskar A, Dahlgren A, Friden J. Split distal flexor pollicis longus tenodesis: long-term results. Scand J Plast Reconstr Surg Hand Surg. 2002;36:96–9.
70. Van Heest A, Hanson D, Lee J, Wentdorf F, House J. Split flexor pollicus longus tendon transfer for stabilization of the thumb interphalangeal joint: a cadaveric and clinical study. J Hand Surg [Am]. 1999;24:1303–10.
71. Orhun E, Polatkan S, Polatkan O, Nuzumlali E, Kantarci U. Repair of zone 2 flexor pollicis longus lacerations in children. J Hand Surg Br. 1999;24:54–5.
72. Strickland JW, Glogovac SV. Digital function following flexor tendon repair in Zone II: a comparison of immobilization and controlled passive motion techniques. J Hand Surg [Am]. 1980;5:537–43.
73. Rappaport PO, Thoreson AR, Yang TH, et al. Effect of wrist and interphalangeal thumb movement on zone T2 flexor pollicis longus tendon tension in a human cadaver model. J Hand Ther. 2015;28:347–354; quiz 355.
74. Fitoussi F, Mazda K, Frajman JM, Jehanno P, Pennecot GF. Repair of the flexor pollicis longus tendon in children. J Bone Joint Surg Br. 2000;82:1177–80.
75. Filippucci E, Garofalo G, Grassi W. Thumb troubles in rheumatoid arthritisReumatismo. 2004;56:211–4.
76. Manfield L, Thomas M, Lee SW. Flexor pollicis longus tenosynovitis in patients with carpal tunnel syndrome. Am J Phys Med Rehabil. 2014;93:524–7.
77. Kheterpal A, Zoga A, McClure K. Acute calcific tendinitis of the flexor pollicis longus in an 8-year-old boy. Skelet Radiol. 2014;43:1471–5.
78. Naito K, Sugiyama Y, Igeta Y, Kaneko K, Obayashi O. Irreducible dislocation of the thumb interphalangeal joint due to displaced flexor pollicis longus tendon: case report and new reduction technique. Arch Orthop Trauma Surg. 2014;134:1175–8.

# 11 Extensor Tendon

Young Ho Lee

## Extensor Tendon

Injuries to the extensor tendon more frequently occur than flexor tendon injuries. With regard to thumb tendon injuries, extensor tendon is more significantly involved than the flexor tendon [1]. Among open extensor tendon injuries, injuries to the thumb are the most frequent, followed by those to the index finger [2]. The following components may contribute to this data. Open extensor tendon injuries lack overlying subcutaneous tissue. Open extensor tendon injuries are superficially located and more associated with sports injury. But the management of extensor tendon injury is frequently underemphasized. The composite system of extensor mechanism with extensor retinacula structures and both extrinsic and intrinsic tendon may contribute to the difficult management. Moreover, the extensor tendon apparatus are superficially located with thin soft tissue structures that are very close to the bones, which make them prone to soft tissue or tendon loss and underlying fracture dislocation. In a given situation, a thorough understanding of the anatomy and extensor mechanism is necessary to provide appropriate treatment (see Chap. 2).

The extensor muscle bellies become an extensor tendon at the lower third of the forearm and transmit muscle forces. At the level of the wrist, the extensor tendon passes the six compartments beneath the extensor retinaculum. The extensor retinaculum forms fibro-osseous tunnel and acts to prevent bowstrings. The thumb extensors lie within the first (APL, abductor pollicis longus, and EPB, extensor pollicis brevis) and third (EPL, extensor pollicis longus) dorsal extensor compartments. After passing through the extensor retinaculum, the extensor tendons become more thin and flat. According to Doyle's measurement, the thickness of the extensor mechanism in the fingers is within a range of 1.75 mm in zone 6 to 0.65 mm at zone 1, and similar range applies to the thumb [3]. Therefore, standard core sutures become technically impossible when dealing with extensor tendon apparatus at this level.

## Extensor Mechanism of the Thumb

The thumb has two extrinsic extensor tendons (extensor pollicis brevis on the radial side and extensor pollicis longus on the ulnar side) and three short muscles (flexor pollicis brevis and abductor pollicis brevis muscles on the radial side and the adductor pollicis muscle on the ulnar side) that contribute to the extensor apparatus. The EPB inserts into the base of the proximal phalanx or the extensor tendon apparatus of the thumb at varying levels and extends the MP joint of the thumbs and may be able to extend the IP joint of the thumb.

Y. H. Lee (✉)
Department of Orthopedic Surgery, Seoul National University Hospital, Seoul, South Korea
e-mail: orthoyhl@snu.ac.kr


S. H. Woo (ed.), *The Thumb*, https://doi.org/10.1007/978-981-10-4400-7_11

The EPL tendon inserts into the base of the distal phalanx of the thumb and extends the joint of the thumb and contributes to abduction and extension of the wrist. When checking the EPL tendon of the thumb, the examiner must hold the metacarpophalangeal joint and must test carefully for active extension of the interphalangeal joint and active retropulsion of the thumb toward the dorsum of the hand. Because an intact EPB can actively extend the thumb as a unit, although the EPB cannot extend the interphalangeal joint alone, the thumb intrinsic muscles assist with interphalangeal extension in some patients. The diagnosis of extensor tendon injuries is often evident. However, physical examination is less reliable in children, and finger motion can be limited by the pain. Also, partial lesions can be missed if the remaining tendon is strong enough to create some extension force. As a general rule, open lesions should therefore be surgically explored to identify the extent of the injury and prevent secondary ruptures. A detailed neurovascular examination is essential.

## Diagnostic Imaging

Plain radiographs are usually obtained at the time of the initial assessment to evaluate the accompanying bone injury or retained foreign body. Diagnostic ultrasound and MRI may be useful to evaluate the continuity of tendon, but they are not always needed. When a definite diagnosis of tendon injury cannot be made, surgical exploration is usually indicated.

## Classification of Extensor Tendon Injuries of the Thumb

Treatment strategies vary according to the zone of injury, the chronicity of the injury, and accompanying injuries of the adjacent structures (bone and soft tissue). The thumb is described with its own alternative classification system (Kleinert and Verdan system) [4] because it has one less phalanx than the other digits. Zone T1 includes the thumb interphalangeal joint, and zone T2 includes the proximal phalanx. Zone T3 is at the metacarpophalangeal joint, and zone T4 is over the thumb metacarpal. Finally, zone T5 includes the third extensor compartment and the area of the first dorsal compartment. The extensor pollicis longus, extensor pollicis brevis, and abductor pollicis longus tendons may be injured in this zone.

"Acute" injury is within 4–8 weeks after original injury. With an acute presentation, treatment depends on whether the injury is open or closed. Usually, a primary tendon repair is done within the first 12 h of injury. A so-called delayed primary repair is one that is done within 24 h to approximately 10 days. After 10–14 days, the repair is considered to be secondary; and after about 4 weeks, the secondary repair is a "late" secondary repair. "Chronic or old injury" is considered when more than 8 weeks has passed from original injury. In chronic injury, tendon reconstruction should be considered, because tendon is widely separated and fibrosis of muscle is progressed.

## General Principles

### Exposures

For wound exploration and tendon manipulation, appropriate local or general anesthesia is required. A wide-awake approach is recommended in select patients with extensor tendon injuries (see Chap. 12). Various types of incisions can be used for open repair based on surgeon's preference and the shape of the previous laceration. The skin incision should be planned so that it can be extended proximally or distally and enough for the exploration of the injured tendon. The IP joint is opened through an "H" incision or a reverse "Y" incision or a 90° Z-plasty or lazy S-shaped incision (Fig. 11.1). On the dorsal side of the thumb, where a relative abundance of skin is present, lazy S-shape or Z-plasty can also be used according to the surgeon's preference (Fig. 11.2).

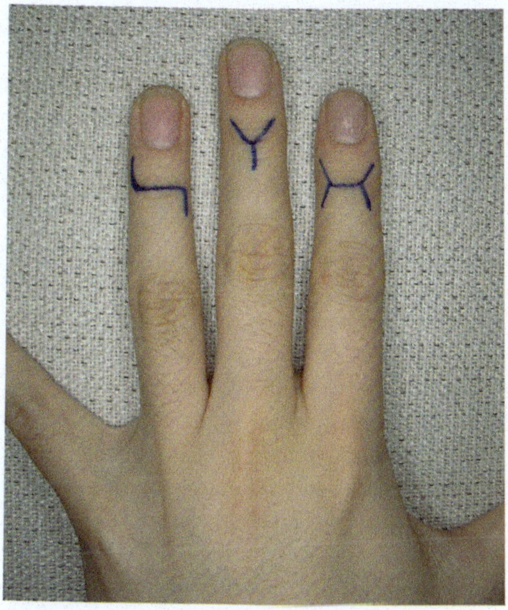

**Fig. 11.1** The incision of IP joint of the thumb

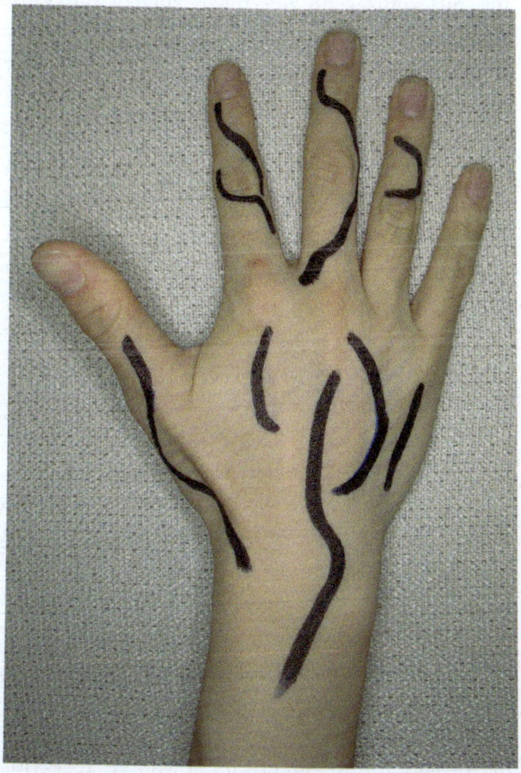

**Fig. 11.2** The incision of the thumb

## Sutures

The strength of tendon suture is affected by the number of suture strands passing through the repair site, the suture diameter, the suture material properties, and the suture method. Currently used suture materials are nylon, Prolene (polypropylene), PDS (polydioxanone), and Mersilene. Including Mersilene, Ethibond, Tircon, and FiberWire, the braided polyester sutures provide sufficient resistance, easy handling, and secure knot characteristics. In the past, monofilament stainless steel was used due to the highest tensile strength. However, it tends to pull through the tendon, makes a large knot, and provides handling difficulties. Including catgut and the polyglycolic acid group (Dexon, Vicryl), most absorbable sutures become weak too early after the repair. Consequently, these materials are not suitable for tendon surgery. A variety of different suture techniques have been described in the treatment of tendon injuries.

Generally, the suture method and suture caliber depend on the tendon thickness at the level of injury. Four or more sufficient number of strands passing through the repair site, appropriate suture calibers of the suture that are equal to or greater than 4-0, the suture purchase no less than 7–10 mm, and the size of the lock or grasp equal to or greater than 2 mm are essential. However, the extensor tendons become thin and flat distally, and extensor tendons cannot accommodate core sutures. Traditionally, a four-strand core suture and a supplemental epitendinous suture have been used for extensor tendon repairs [5–12]. Clinically, repairs with 4-0 sutures are commonly used in extensor tendon repair. Larger 3-0 suture can be used in the more proximal portions of the tendon such as zone T5. The extensor tendons are thicker and rounder in proximal portion and are capable of holding core sutures like flexor tendons.

There are few studies on biomechanics of suture techniques for extensor tendon injuries compared with flexor tendon injuries. Newport reported that the Kleinert-modified Bunnell technique and the modified Kessler techniques were the strongest methods in zones 4 and 6 [8, 9]. Howard and colleagues show the augmented Becker (MGH) technique to be biomechanically superior to the modified Bunnell technique and the Krackow-Thomas technique for extensor tendon repairs in zone 6 [10]. In a 2005 study, Woo and colleagues found the modified Becker technique to be the biomechanically strongest repair than the double figure-of-eight, a double-modified Kessler, and six-strand double-loop for extensor tendon zone 6 injuries [11]. More recently, Lee and colleagues compared the modified Bunnell and the augmented Becker techniques with a new, running interlocking horizontal mattress technique [12]. They found the running interlocking horizontal mattress technique was significantly stronger and led to less shortening of tendon. Furthermore, the technique was faster to perform than the other two techniques.

Doyle proposed the suture techniques for extensor tendon repair according to the anatomical site of lesion [3]. For T1 injuries, 5-0 running suture incorporating the skin and tendon or 5-0 dorsal cross-stitch is recommended. For T2 and T3 injuries, modified Kessler suture of 4-0 synthetic material in the thickest area and 5-0 dorsal cross-stitch are recommended. For T4 and T5 injuries, the same as for T2 and T3 is indicated.

## Surgical Management

### Zones T1 and T2

#### Mallet Thumb

Closed mallet injuries are uncommon in the thumb, because the terminal extensor tendon is thicker on the thumb [13]. The EPL injuries in these zones can be treated successfully with prolonged splinting for 8–12 weeks. According to Doyle's classification of mallet finger [3], open tendon injuries (types 2 and 3) are indications for surgical repair. If the EPL tendon is cleanly cut at these zones, the proximal segment does not retract appreciably, because the adductor pollicis, abductor pollicis brevis, and extensor pollicis brevis insert into the extensor expansion; consequently, it can be repaired primarily or secondarily without grafting or tendon. The tendon is broad and flat in this region and can be treated by a fine running mattress 4-0 or 5-0 nonabsorbable suture that approximates the tendon ends without shortening of the tendon. Additionally, the IP joint is stabilized in the extension using one or two transarticular Kirschner wires. For T1 and T2 injuries, I frequently use several mattress sutures of 5-0 Prolene to reapproximate the tendon anatomically. If the tendon laceration is irregular, mattress suture is more useful for regular margin approximation. Furthermore, in running suture method, there is only one knot present, and if the knot is loosened or ruptured, the hold suture fails. With several mattress sutures, there is less chance of failure of the whole of the knot. Secure fixation is achieved with several mattress sutures, but irritation of the skin due to the increased knot is possible. But the frequency is not high, because the 5-0 sutures do not make such a big knot (Figs. 11.3 and 11.4).

If the distal stump of the tendon is too short to repair, the bone anchor is used. Approximately 2–3 mm of the scar tissue at the distal end of the tendon is resected, and the tendon is advanced into the bone via a pullout suture or suture anchor. At the base of the distal phalanx, the periosteum was peeled off to insert the anchor. To use a suture anchor for an avulsion injury, insert the bone suture anchor before K-wire fixation. After the bone anchor is seated into the bone, check the stability by pulling the accompanying thread. A 0.045-in. Kirschner wire was placed across the IP joint in full extension. The accompanying suture, which passed through the hub of the anchor, was then sutured to the terminal extensor tendon in a half-horizontal mattress fashion (Fig. 11.5).

#### Tenodermodesis

For chronic resistant mallet thumb, preferred operative procedure is tenodermodesis.

The combined suture of the tendon and skin is performed following elliptical wedge resection of the skin and scarred tendon. The IP joint is pinned with transarticular Kirschner wire in full extension for 4–6 weeks.

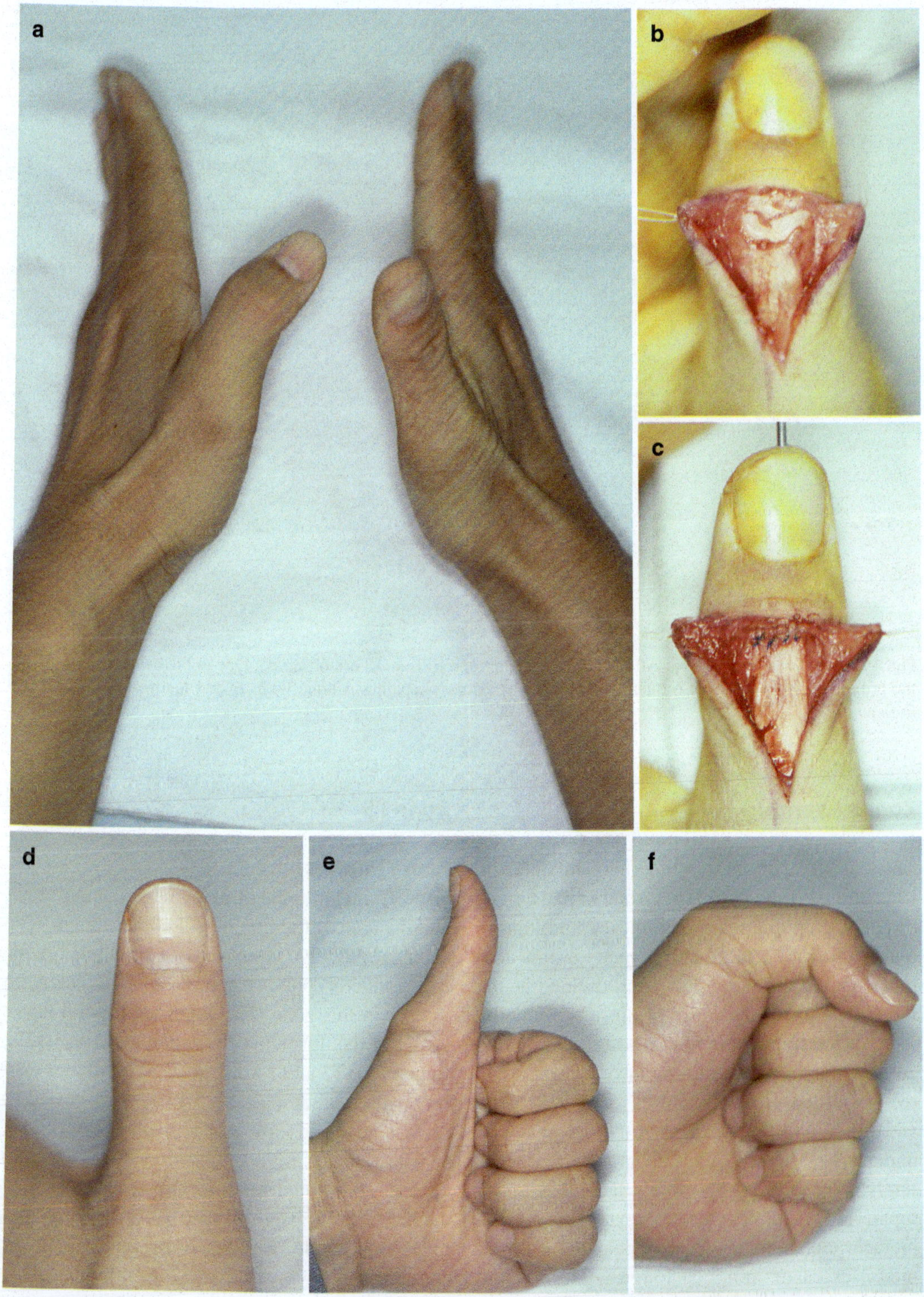


**Fig. 11.3** (**a**) The closed tendinous mallet thumb. Preoperative photograph is showing inability to extend the left thumb. (**b**) After exploration, ruptured EPL at T1 are observed. (**c**) The IP joint is stabilized in the extension using one transarticular Kirschner wire. Several mattress sutures of 5-0 Prolene were done to reapproximate the tendon anatomically. (**d–f**) One year after operation, the scar is minimal and obtained full range of motion

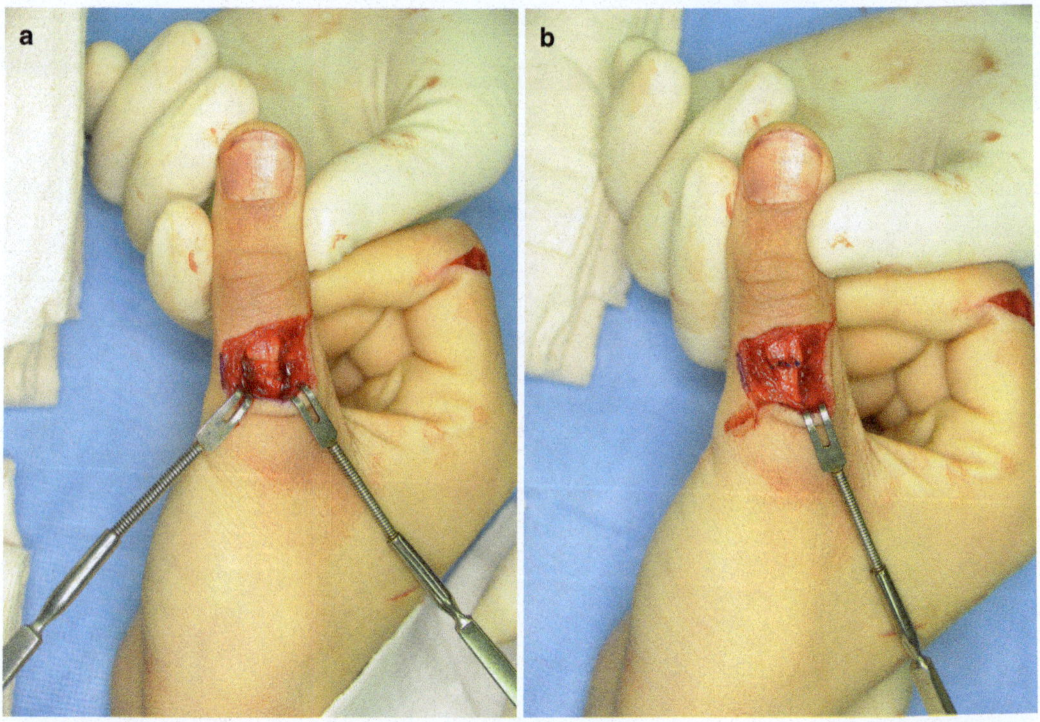


**Fig. 11.4** (**a**) Laceration on T2. After exploration, ruptured EPL at T2 are observed. Due to the extensor expansion, the proximal stump does not retract appreciably. (**b**) Primary repair was done with several mattress sutures of 5-0 Prolene

## Zones T3 and T4

Lacerations over these zones may involve the EPL and EPB, or both. The broad expansion of the metacarpophalangeal joint of the thumb makes laceration of all components in this area rare. When the tendon has been divided at the metacarpophalangeal joint or more proximally, its proximal segment retracts rapidly. In this zone, a standard core suture may be used. I use two modified Kessler sutures of 4-0 Prolene and finish with a 5-0 cross-stitch sutures. The underlying MP joint capsule is repaired separately. EPB is rare to be solely lacerated, so its repair is debatable, because extension of the metacarpophalangeal joint is possible with an intact extensor pollicis longus. During the wound exploration, if injuries to the EPB in these zones are noted, repairing the EPB is recommended to avoid potential MP joint subluxation (Figs. 11.6 and 11.7).

## Zone T5

### Acute Injuries

Zone T5 includes the third extensor compartment and the area of the first dorsal compartment. The extensor pollicis longus, extensor pollicis brevis, and abductor pollicis longus tendons may be injured in this zone. The superficial radial nerve also is at risk for injury. Repair at this zone is the same as for T3 and T4. Large nerve branches may be repaired when possible or the ends buried to prevent neuroma formation (Figs. 11.8 and 11.9).

The extensor retinaculum may be released to expose the injured tendon. However, repairs to the retinaculum itself may be too bulky or sometimes impossible. But the retinaculum of these compartments typically does not require subsequent repair. The retinaculum may be step-cut or Z-lengthened so that wound closure is possible and the repaired tendons are allowed to glide smoothly under it.

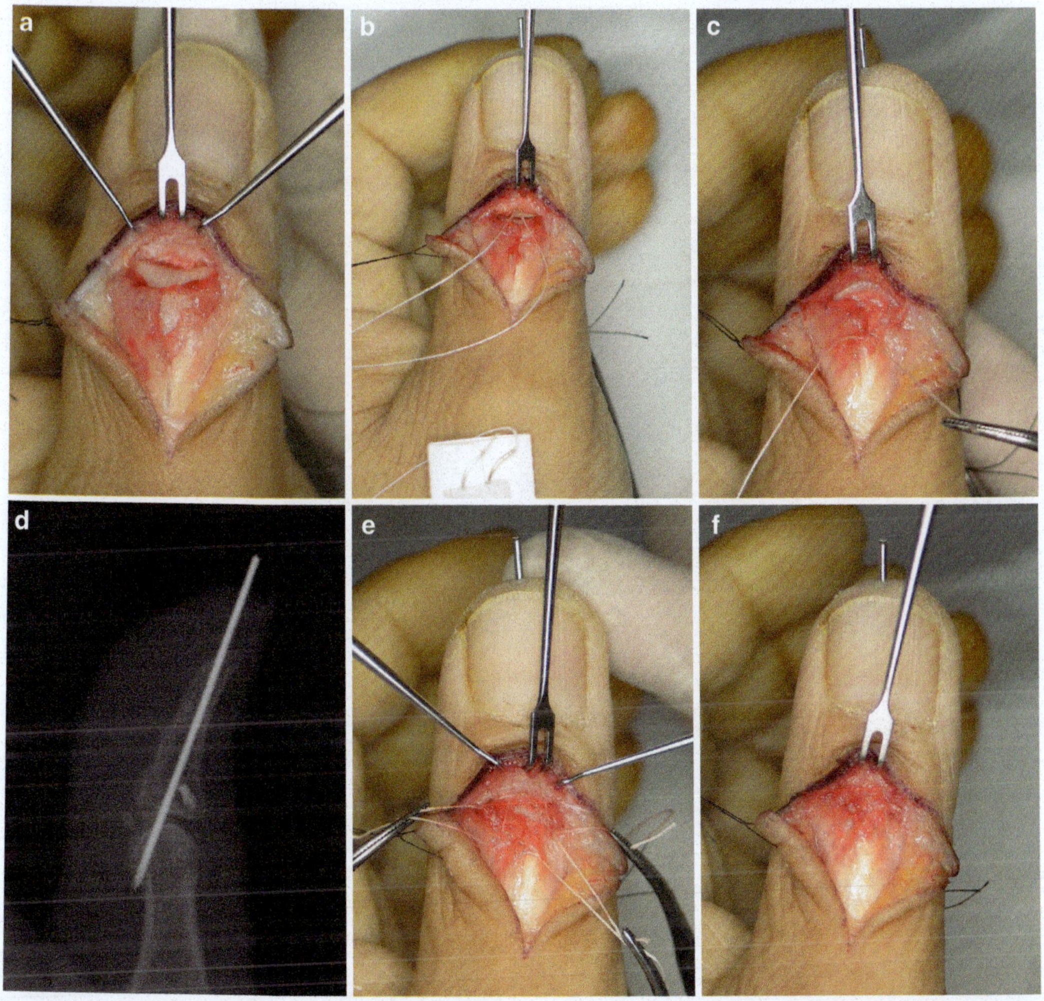


**Fig. 11.5** (a) The closed tendinous mallet thumb. Distal stump of the tendon is too short to repair. (b) At the base of the distal phalanx, the anchor was inserted. And a 0.045-in. Kirschner wire across the IP joint was placed in full extension. (c, d) Checking the position of anchor and Kirschner wire. (e, f) The terminal extensor tendon was sutured in a half-horizontal mattress fashion

## Chronic Injuries or Segmental Tendon Loss of EPL Tendon

If the tendon has segmental degeneration, it will not support a direct repair without undue tension and must be reconstructed. The transfer of extensor indicis proprius (EIP) or tendon graft using the palmaris longus tendon is most widely used for reconstructing the EPL. Good clinical results have been reported for both techniques [14, 15].

### EIP Transfer

This procedure is simple and fast and can easily be used even for additional shortening of the proximal end which may occur through myostatic contracture, if the presentation is delayed.

Although functional loss or weakness of the donor index or an extensor lag is not reported frequently [16], the strength of index extension may be reduced as much as 49% [17, 18]. Other findings such as loss of dexterity and loss of independent extension of the index finger also have been reported [19]. It is preferable not to use the EIP as a donor tendon in patients who require great independence of motion of the index finger such as musicians, surgeons, and secretaries or in the

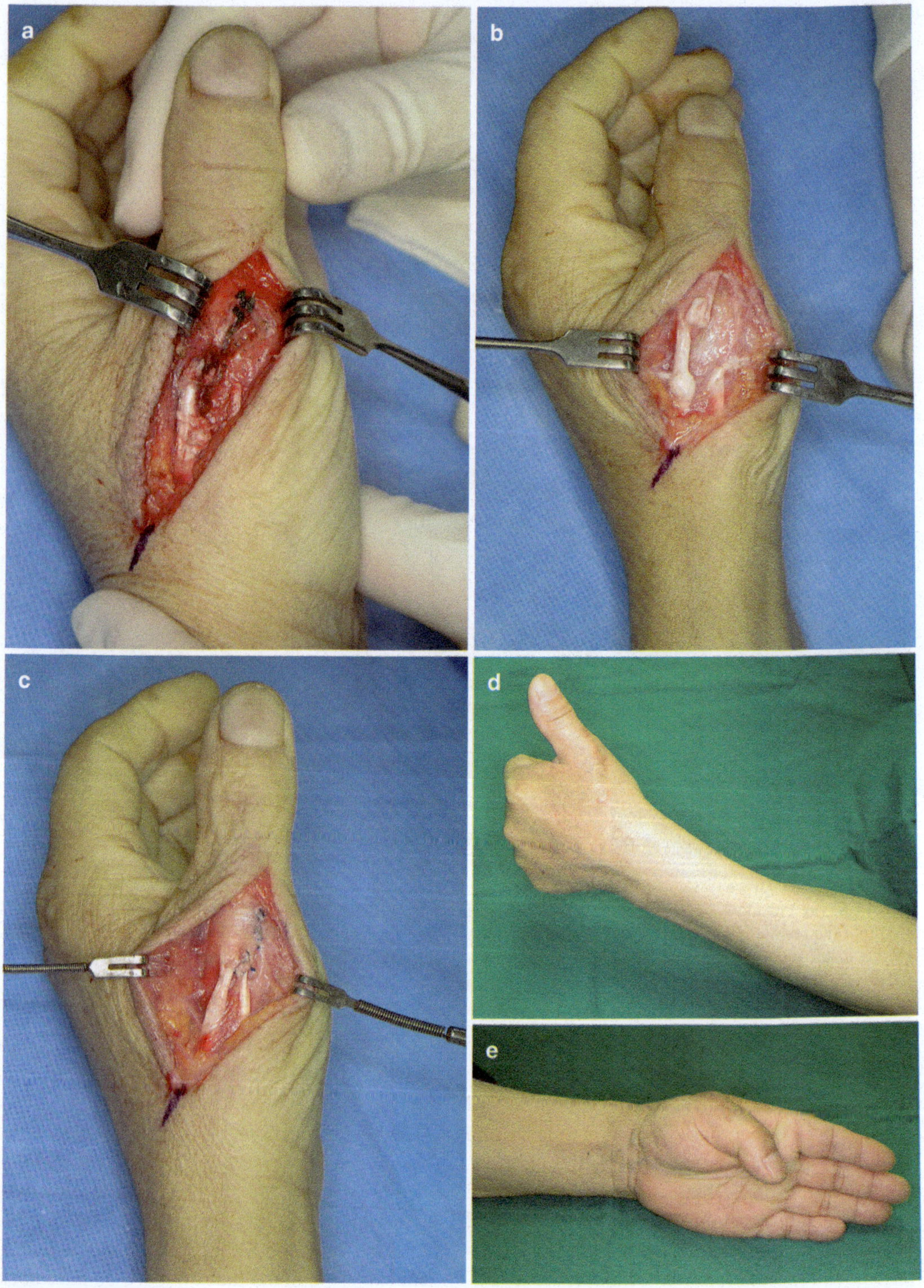

**Fig. 11.6** Oblique laceration from T3 to T4. (**a**) Highly contaminated wound due to sawing machine injury was observed. (**b**) Radical debridement of all foreign bodies and contaminated tissue was done. Partially ruptured EPL (more than 50%) and complete ruptured EPB were observed. (**c**) Both tendons were sutured and MP joint capsule is repaired separately. (**d**, **e**) Six months after the operation, achieved full range of motion and observed no MP joint subluxation

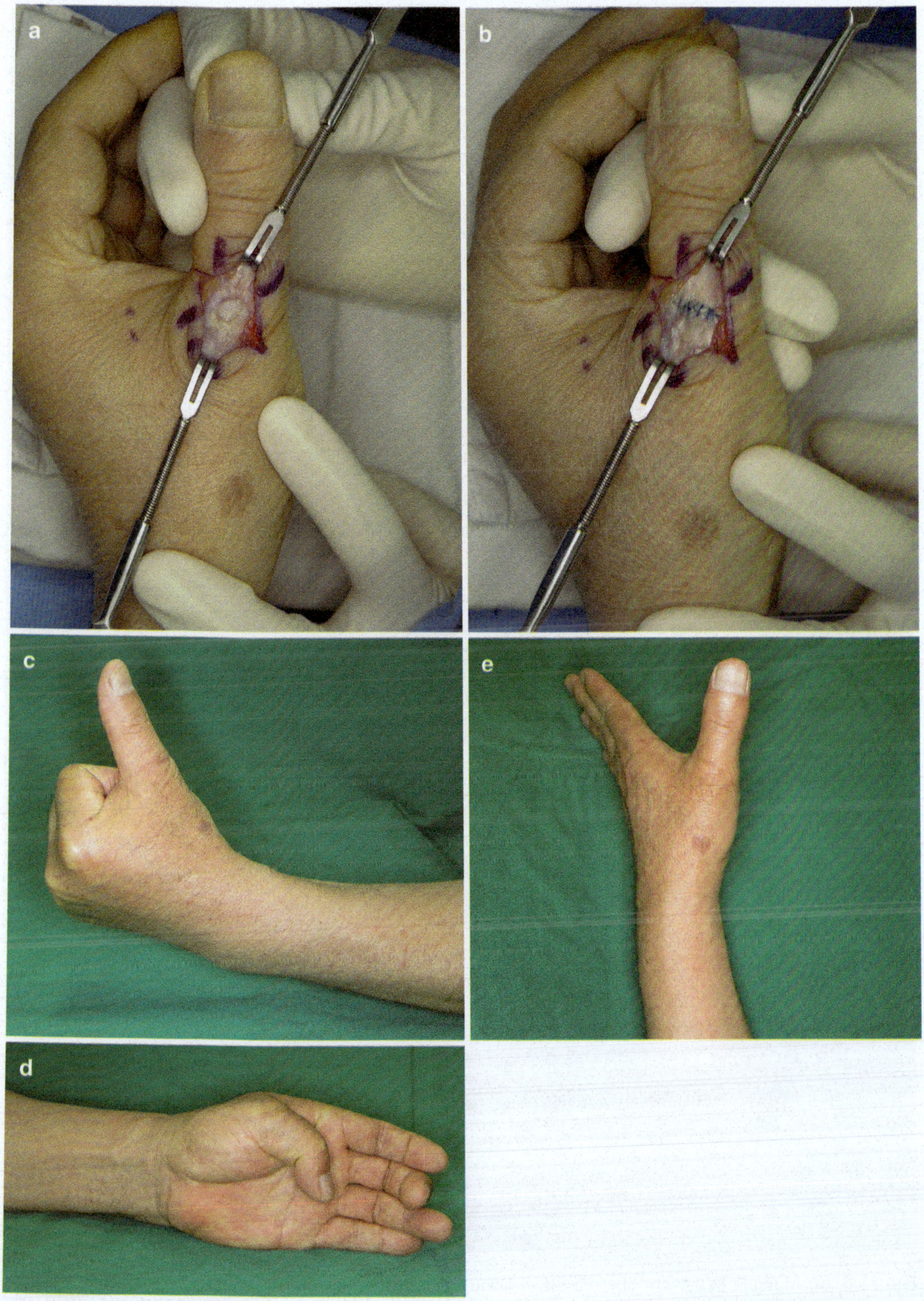


**Fig. 11.7** (**a**) EPL and EPB injuries on T4. (**b**) Two modified Kessler sutures were placed, and additional cross-stitch suture was done to augment the repair further. (**c**–**e**) One year after the operation, achieved full range of motion and observed no MP joint subluxation

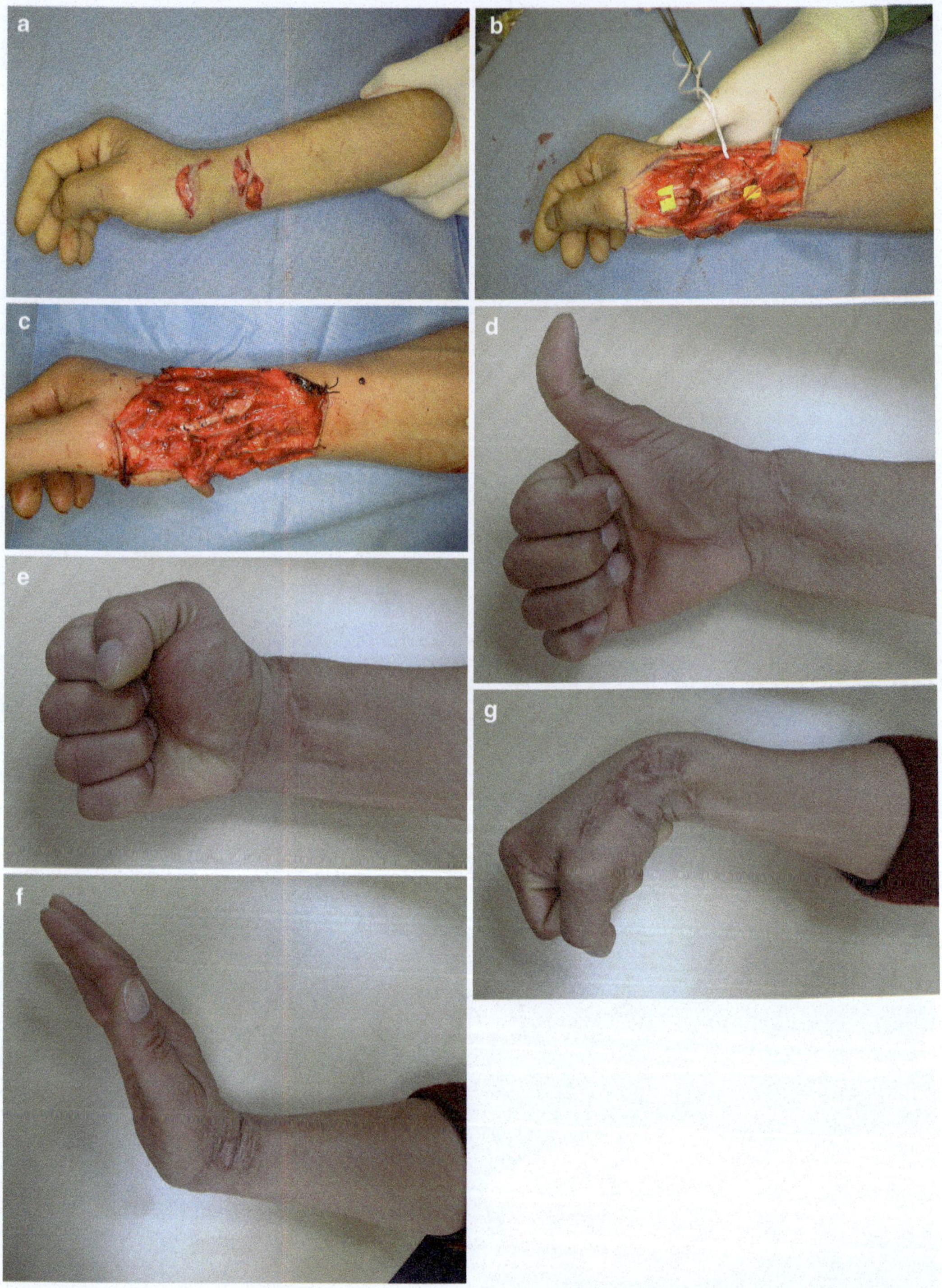


**Fig. 11.8** (**a**) Multiple lacerations after electrical lawn trimmer injury. (**b**) After wound exploration, demonstrates a segmental defect in the APL, EBP, and EPL. Additionally, ECRL, ECRB, and FCR tendon injuries, superficial radial nerve injury, and radial artery injury were observed. (**c**) The segmental defect of EPL, EPB, and APL was reconstructed with PL graft from the bilateral wrist. And tenorrhaphy of the ECRL and ERCB, arteriorrhaphy, and neurorrhaphy were also done. (**d**–**g**) Ten months after the surgery, he was very satisfied with the results

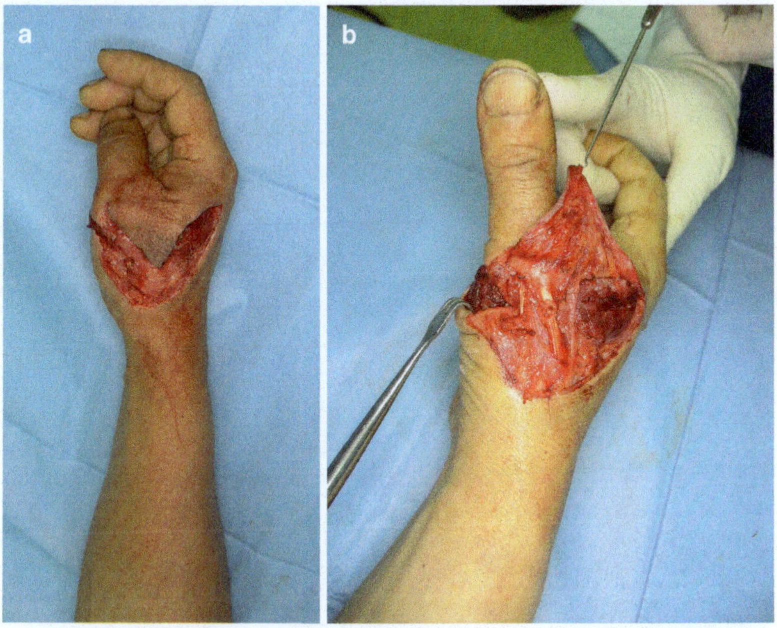

**Fig. 11.9** (**a**) Degloving injuries resulting flap-like wound and extensor tendon ruptures from T4 to T5. (**b**) After radical debridement, primary tenorrhaphy of EPL and EPB and neurorrhaphy of branch of superficial radial nerve were done

presence of multiple ruptured tendons secondary to rheumatoid disease.

A small transverse or longitudinal incision is made just proximal to the index MCP joint. The EIP is found ulnar and deep to the EDC tendon at the index finger MCP joint and is released subcutaneously to the level of the wrist retinaculum. It is transected proximal to the sagittal band. A second incision is made overlying the EIP tendon just distal to the retinaculum, and the tendon is then retrieved to this level. A third longitudinal incision is made overlying the EPL tendon at metacarpal level, close to the MP joint. The EIP is tunneled subcutaneously to the distal end of nonfunctioning EPL tendon. It is not necessary to dissect out the rupture site of EPL tendon. When tunneling is done, not ensnaring any EDC tendons in the passage is important. A Pulvertaft weave with 3-0 nonabsorbable sutures is performed. Setting tension during graft interposition is a critical issue to obtain balance between flexion and extension of thumb. Standard tension is obtained by full extension of the thumb with 30° flexion of wrist, whereas over-tension is obtainable with full extension of the thumb and wrist in neutral position. I recommend slight over-tensioning, because during the rehabilitation period, the transferred EIP muscle could be lengthened at the muscular portion. Postoperatively, a thumb spica cast is placed for 4 weeks and removable thumb spica splint for another 2 weeks with allowing active motion (Figs. 11.10 and 11.11).

## Interpositioning Tendon Graft

The most common donor tendons used in such conditions are the palmaris longus and the plantaris longus, but extensor indicis proprius and EDM have also been used as a valid graft option for tendon reconstruction. Interposition tendon grafting using PL tendon is rare in literature [20]. This procedure requires two tendon repair sites and has the difficulty of overcoming myostatic contracture for appropriate tensioning. And the risk in avascular necrosis of the autograft which increases the risk of ruptures may be a limiting factor. However, I recommend this procedure because

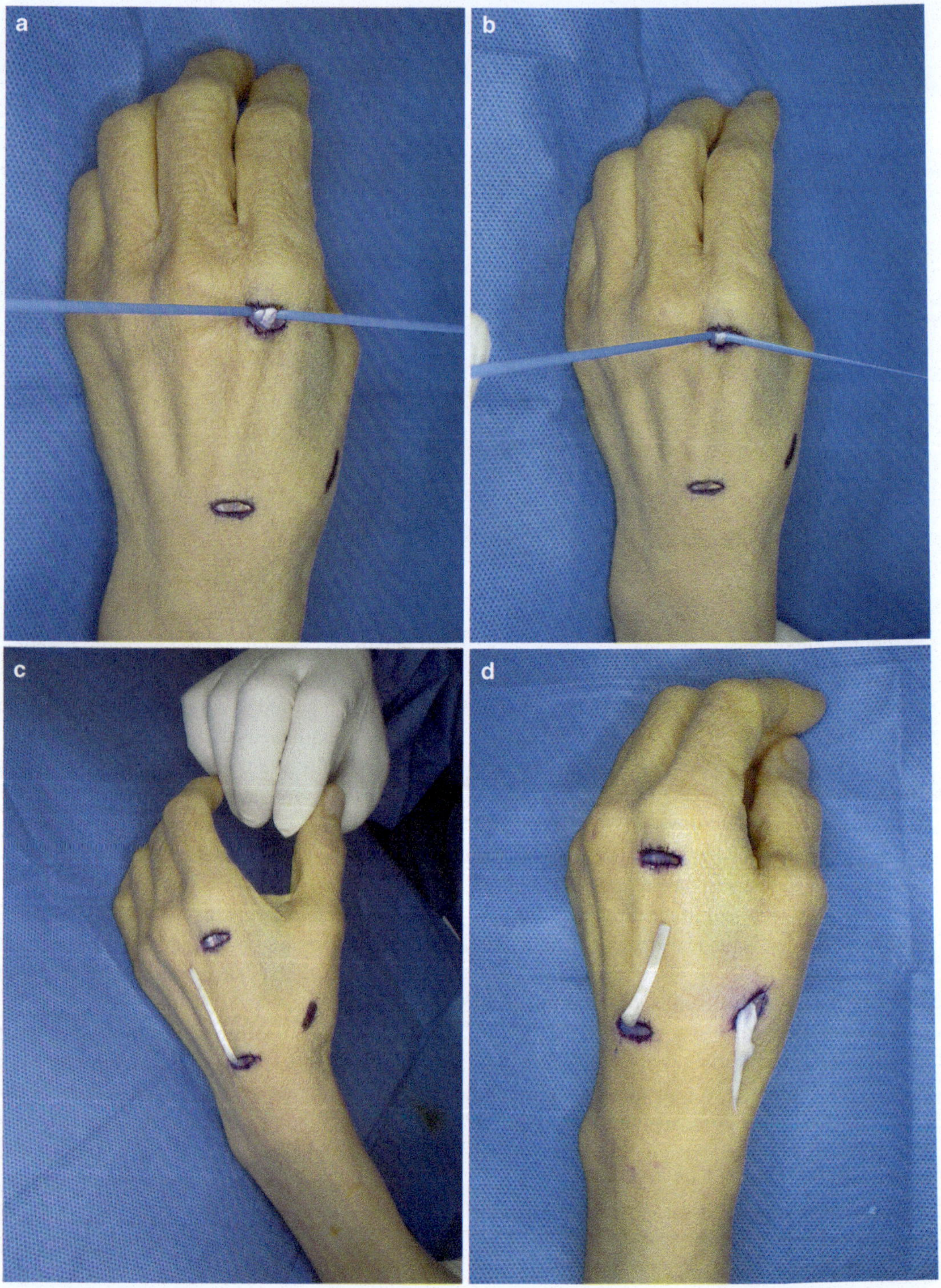


**Fig. 11.10** EIP to EPL transfer. (**a**) Incisions used for EIP to EPL transfer. Just proximal at the index MP joint, a first transverse incision is made. (**b**) The EIP tendon is located at the most ulnar side. (**c**) The EIP is transected proximal to the sagittal band and withdrawn through subcutaneously to distal margin of extensor retinaculum. A second transverse incision is made in this point, and the EIP is reflected to this location subcutaneously. (**d**) A third longitudinal incision is made overlying EPL tendon at metacarpal level. Here, the distal stump of EPL is observed. (**e**) The EIP tendon is passed subcutaneously and sutured with weaving method

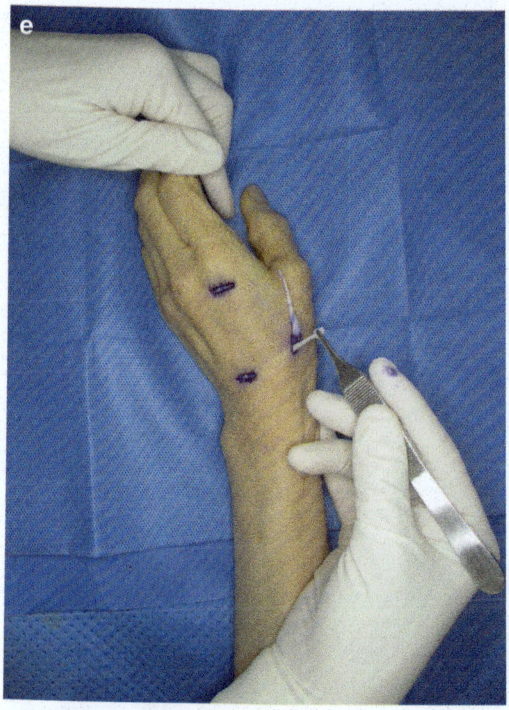


**Fig. 11.10** (continued)

the original EPL muscle can be used and proper tension and amplitude can be obtained. Additionally, no cortical rearrangement and adaption are needed. And donor site morbidity should be minimal with the use of a palmaris longus graft.

### Palmaris Longus Tendon Graft

The presence of this tendon should be determined before any grafting procedure; its presence can be exhibited by having the patient appose the tips of the thumb and little finger while flexing the wrist. A short transverse incision is made directly over the tendon just proximal to the flexion crease of the wrist. The distal end of the tendon is clamped with a hemostat and held taut, while the stripper is advanced proximally. A second transverse incision is made over the tendon at the junction of proximal third of the forearm. The tendon is identified and divided (Fig. 11.12).

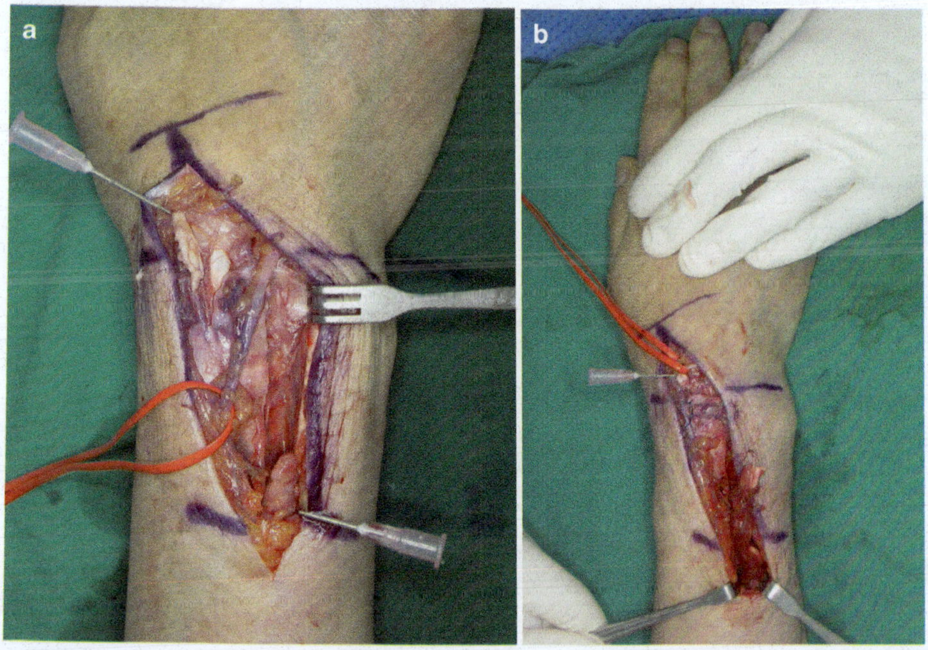


**Fig. 11.11** EIP transfer, clinical case. EPL rupture, 2 months after volar plating. No offending screws are observed. (**a**) Preoperative plan was EPL reconstruction by interpositioning PL graft. After exploration along the course of EPL, ruptured ends of the EPL were identified. (**b**) Ends of EPL tendon after resection of the degenerated part on either side. Ends of the EPL were identified; the degenerated parts were excised. (**c**) Due to severe myofibrosis, EPL was avulsed from its origin during excursion modulation. (**d**) EIP transfer to EPL was done with end-to-side interweave suture with 3-0 Prolene. Tension of the reconstruction was set by full extension of the thumb in neutral position of the wrist. (**e–g**) Six months after the surgery, nearly full range of motion of the thumb was obtained, and no extension lag on index finger was observed

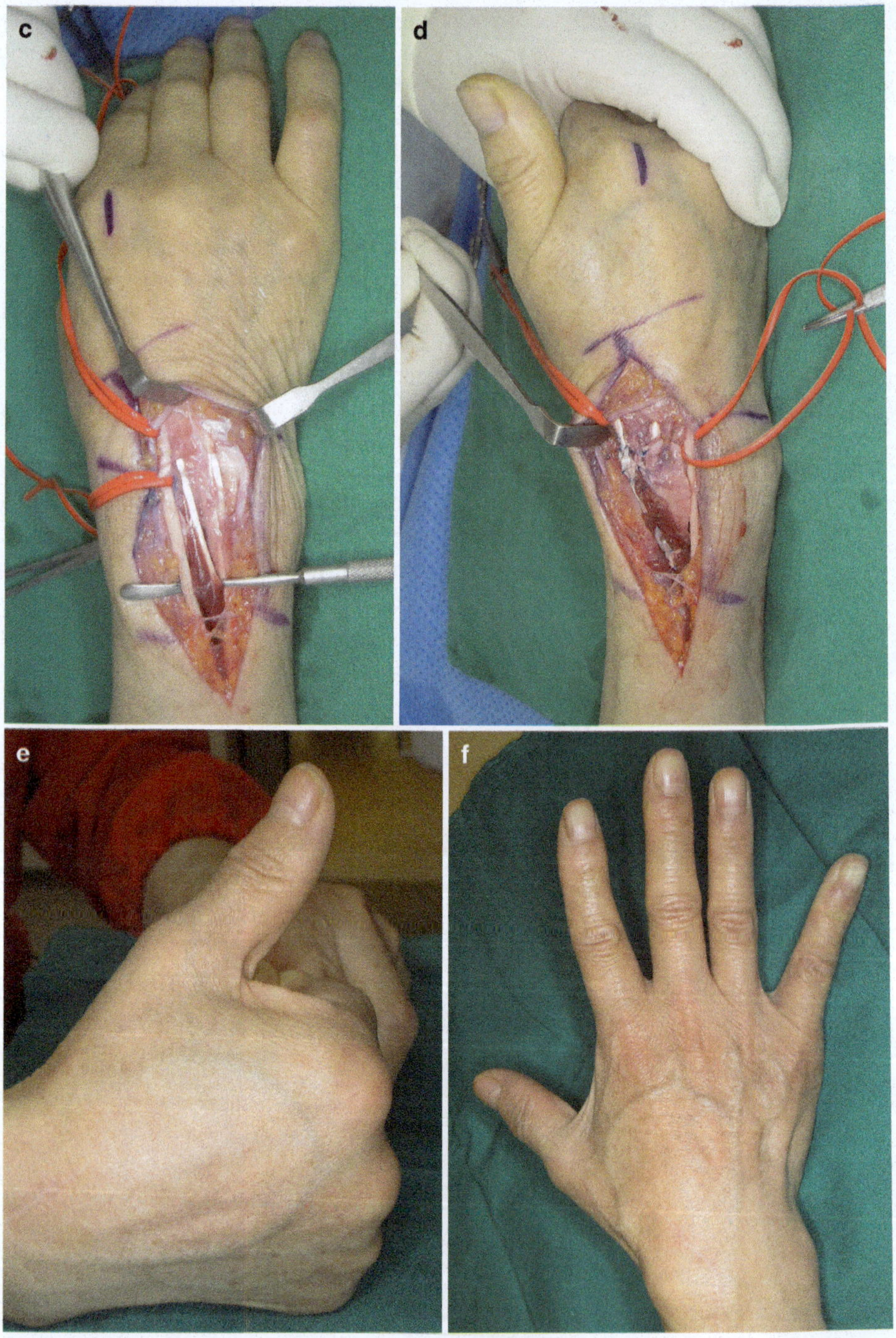


**Fig. 11.11** (continued)

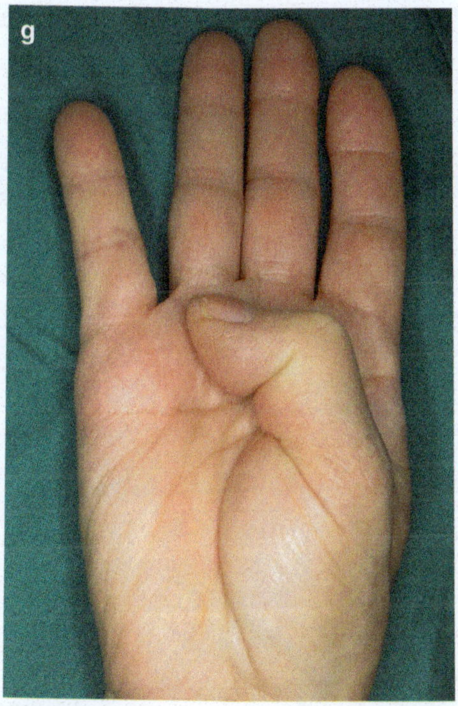

**Fig. 11.11** (continued)

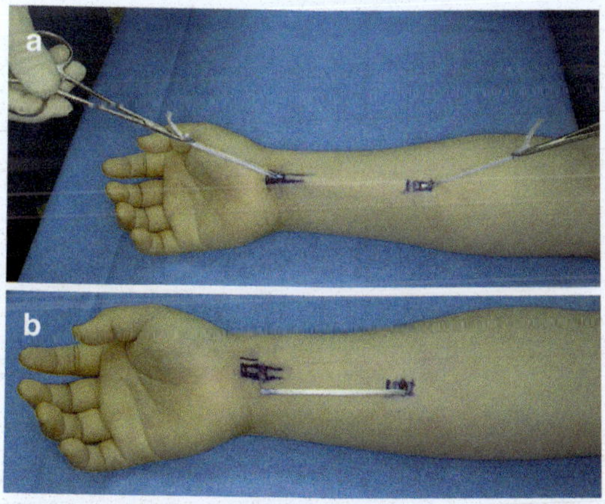

**Fig. 11.12** Palmaris longus tendon graft. (**a**) A short transverse incision is made directly over the tendon just proximal to the flexion crease of the wrist. And the distal end of the tendon is ligated with a sling and held taut. (**b**) A second transverse incision is made over the tendon at the junction of proximal third of the forearm

## Procedure

Along the course of EPL, ruptured ends of the EPL were identified, and the degenerated parts were excised. Appropriate length of ipsilateral palmaris longus was harvested and grafted between the ends of the EPL. Grafted tendons can be sutured using the Pulvertaft technique in proximal stump and modified Kessler technique at that of distal stump with 3-0 polydioxanone (PDS, Ethicon). But I prefer end-to-side interweave technique with 3-0 Prolene. I recommend slight over-tensioning like EIP transfer procedure, because during the rehabilitation period, the grafted PL could be loose and the adaptation process could occur. Third dorsal compartment retinaculum was sutured beneath the graft. The grafted tendon was left subcutaneously and not imbedded in the third dorsal extensor compartment. The grafted tendon should be rerouted from around the Lister tubercle to avoid adhesion and abrasion of the graft (Fig. 11.13).

Previous published series reported a 4.4–8.6% incidence of extensor tendon rupture following volar plating [21, 22]. If there is offending screws during EPL exploration, removal is needed, because it might cause damage subsequently. Plate removal should not be attempted as it may not be possible or might cause refracture of the radius. But, after confirmation of the fracture union, plate removal can be attempted. Wounds were then closed, and postoperative managements are the same with EIP transfer.

## Complicated Injury

Injuries of the extensor tendon of the thumb are frequently complicated by lesions of the bone and joint and soft tissue defect. These complicated injuries are difficult to treat for surgeon. Before repair or reconstruction of the extensor

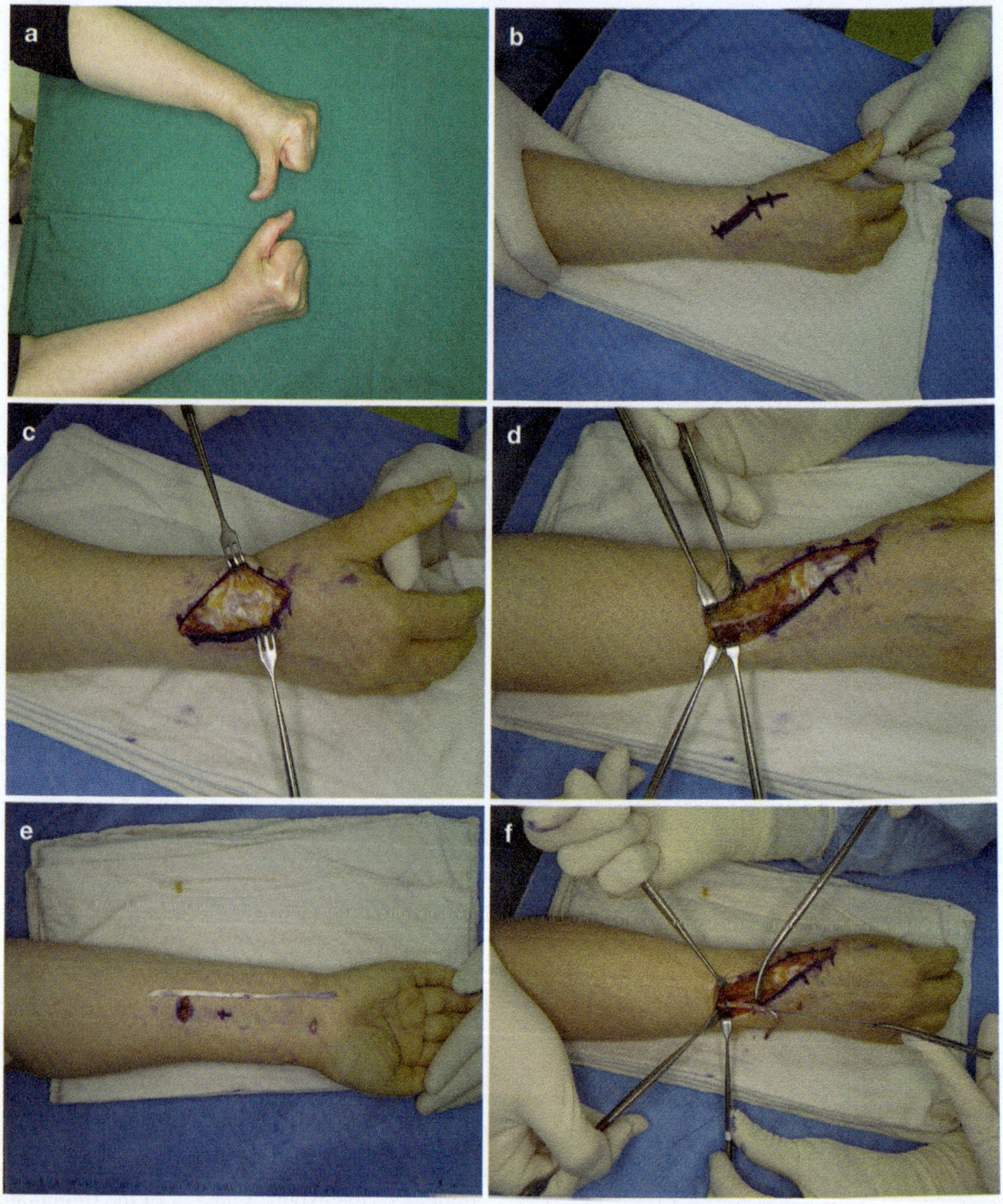


**Fig. 11.13** Reconstruction of a ruptured extensor pollicis longus (EPL) tendon with the use of a palmaris longus tendon graft. (**a**) Preoperatively, she cannot extend her right thumb actively. (**b–d**) After exploration along the course of EPL, ruptured ends of the EPL were identified. (**e**) Harvest of the ipsilateral palmaris longus tendon as a graft. (**f**) The proximal stump of the tendon was sutured with the graft end-to-side interweave suture with 3-0 Prolene. (**g**, **h**). Maintaining appropriate tension, distal stump was sutured with the same method. (**i**) The grafted tendon was left subcutaneously and not imbedded in the third dorsal extensor compartment. (**j**, **k**) Two years after the surgery, full range of motion was obtained

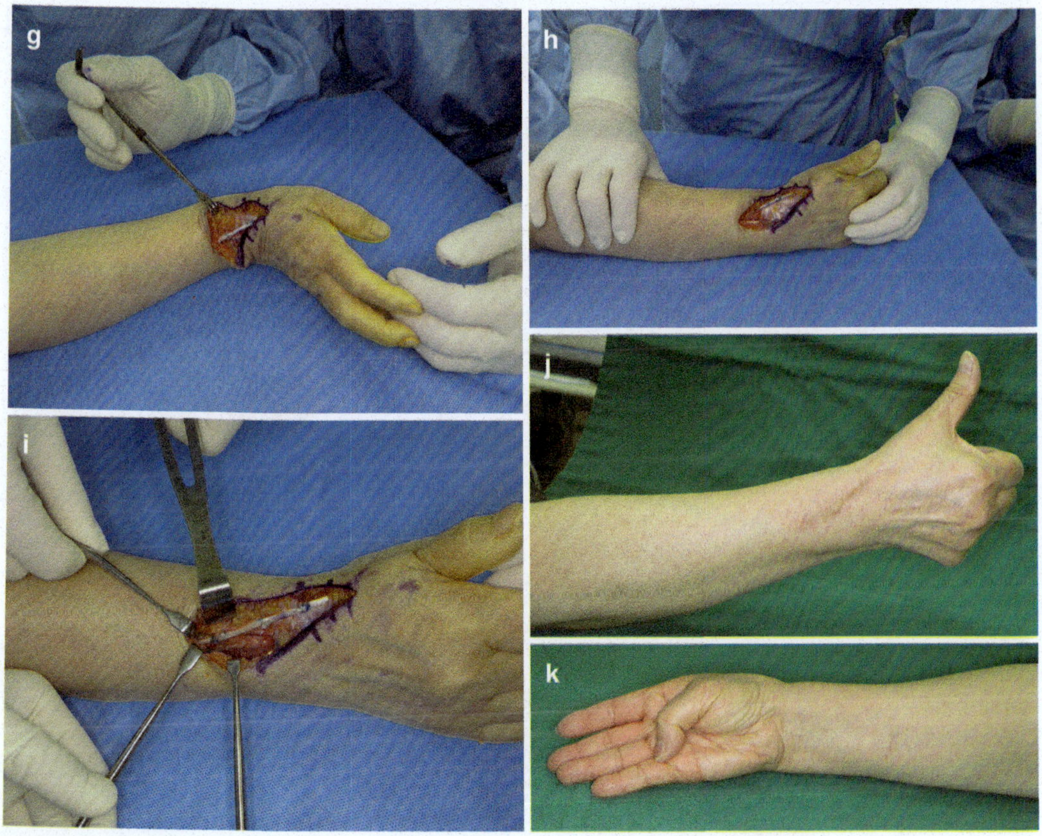


**Fig. 11.13** (continued)

tendons, the basic reconstructive principles are also applied as in other multiple complicated injuries. First of all, radical debridement of all contaminated and devitalized tissue in order to prevent infection is mandatory. Second, bone and joint stabilization must be obtained before soft tissue surgery. Third, osseous structures and tendons must be provided with durable and healthy soft tissue coverage. Therefore, primary or delay flap surgery is often necessary. Traditionally, staged procedures have been addressed, but more recently, one-stage procedures for defects involving the mutilating injuries have been reported with excellent results [23–25]. The primary tendon reconstruction or transfer can be performed at the time of soft tissue surgery. Staged reconstruction of extensor tendons using silicone rods is not necessary, because the creation of tendon sheath is not critical [26, 27] (Figs. 11.14 and 11.15).

## Partial Tendon Injury

For lacerations that are more than 50% of the tendon cross-sectional area, repairing the tendon is usually accepted. If the cross-sectional area lacerated is less than 50%, tendon is either repaired or debrided. There have been considerable debates; my preference is repairing the tendon using a core suture method and a circumferential suture (Fig. 11.16).

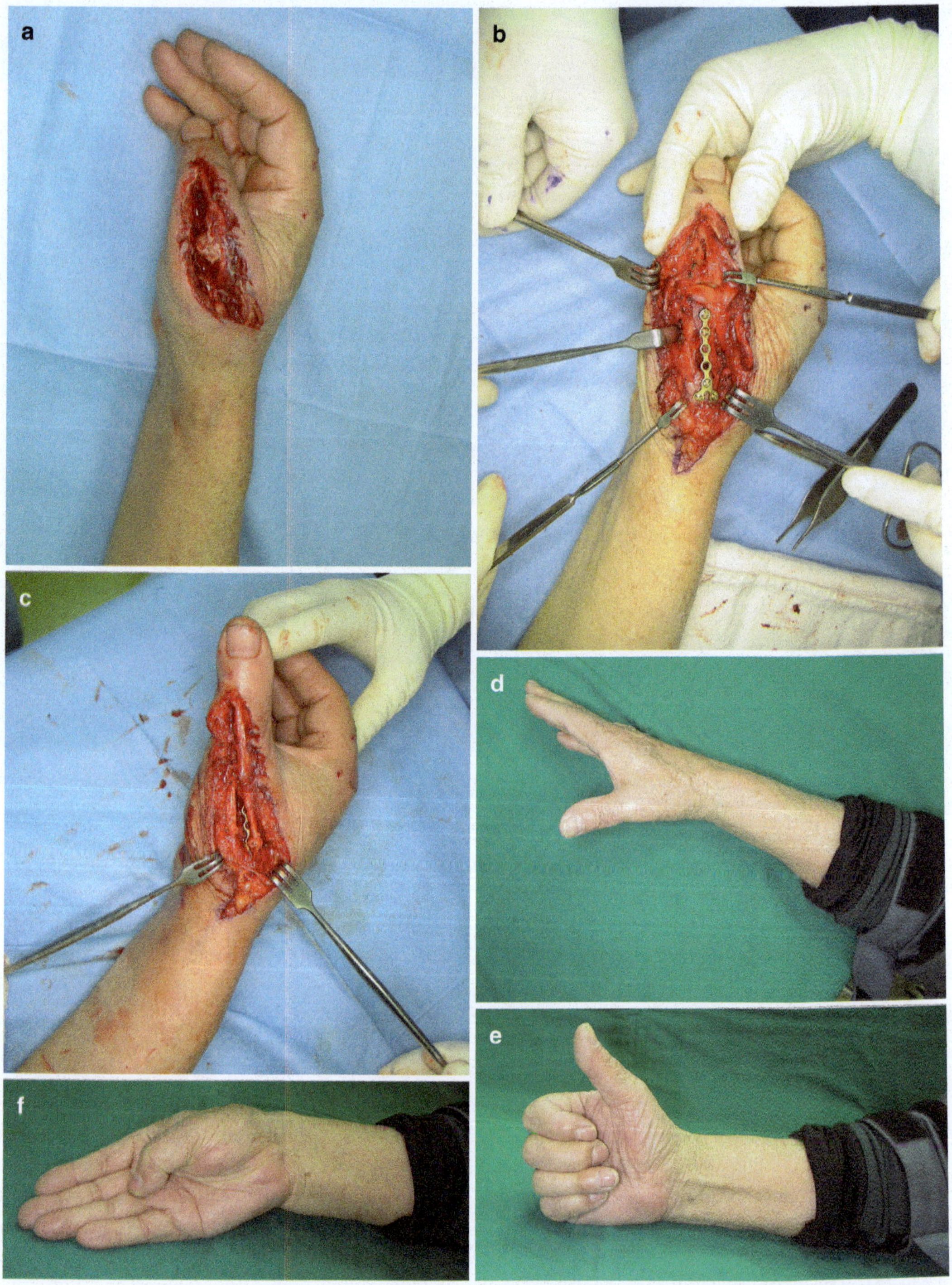


**Fig. 11.14** (**a**) Rollover motor vehicle crash resulting in open MP joints and exposed tendons from T2 to T5. (**b**) After radical debridement, fixation with screws and plate was done. It is important to stabilize the bone, smooth all rough surfaces, and close the periosteum to prevent re-rupture of the tendon. (**c**) EPL and EBP repair was done. (**d–f**) One year after surgery, achieved full range of motion, and bone union was confirmed on the X-rays

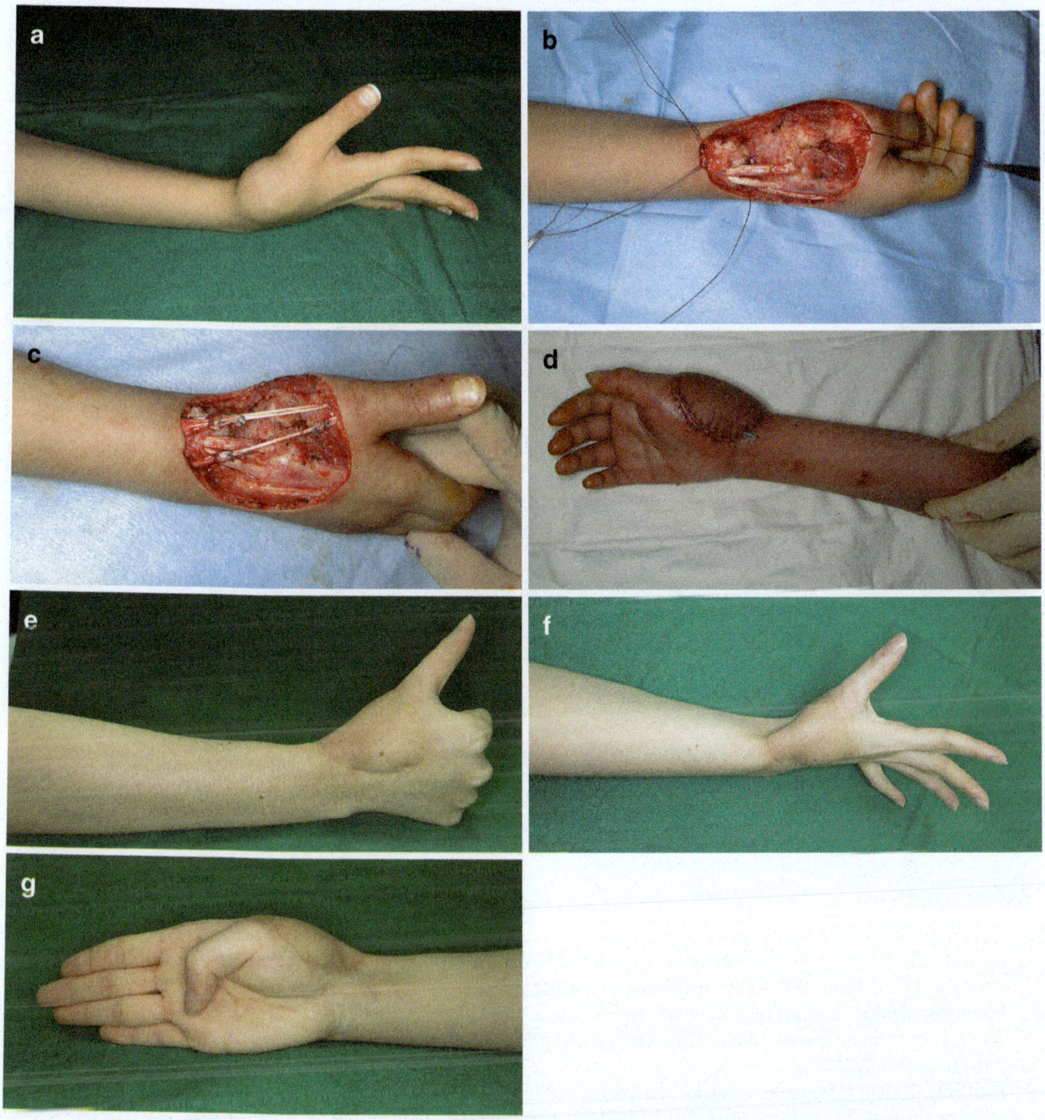


**Fig. 11.15** (**a**, **b**) An 8-year-old girl with small cell sarcoma on her right wrist; wide excision was done by tumor surgeon. (**c**, **d**) Harvest of the ipsilateral and contralateral palmaris longus tendon as a graft. Reconstruction of EPL and EPB was done. And the flap operation was done simultaneously. (**e**–**g**) Ten years after the operation, excellent results were obtained

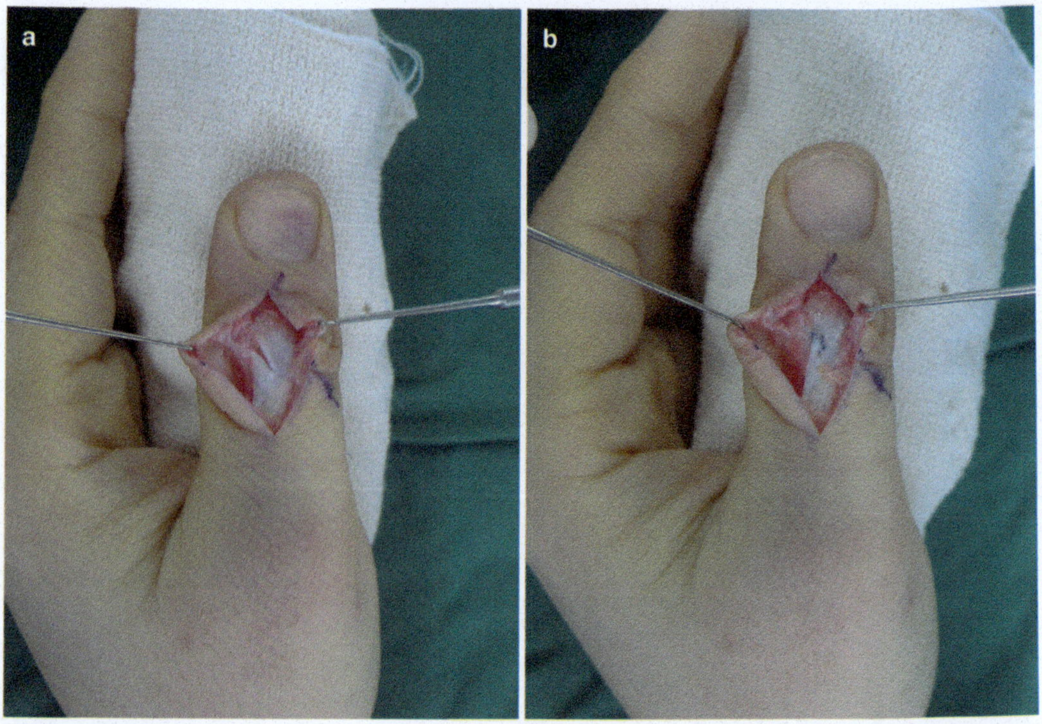

**Fig. 11.16** Partial laceration. (**a**) Less than 50% of the tendon is lacerated. (**b**) After debridement, the tendon was repaired with a circumferential suture

## References


1. de Jong JP, Nguyen JT, Sonnema AJ, Nguyen EC, Amadio PC, Moran SL. The incidence of acute traumatic tendon injuries in the hand and wrist: a 10-year population-based study. Clin Orthop Surg. 2014;6(2):196–202.
2. Patillo D, Rayan GM. Open extensor tendon injuries: an epidemiologic study. Hand Surg. 2012;17(1):37–42.
3. Doyle JR. Extensor tendons: acute injuries. In: Green DP, Hotchkiss RN, Pederson WC, et al., editors. Green's operative hand surgery. 5th ed. New York: Churchill Livingstone; 1999. p. 195–1987.
4. Kleinert HE, Verdan C. Report of the committee on tendon injuries (International Federation of Societies for Surgery of the Hand). J Hand Surg Am. 1983;8(5 Pt 2):794–8.
5. Strauch RJ. Extensor tendon injury. In: Wolfe SW, Hotchkiss RN, Pederson WC, Kozin SK, editors. Green's operative hand surgery. 6th ed. New York: Churchill Livingstone; 2011. p. 165–8.
6. Henderson J, Sutcliffe M, Gillespie P. Epitendinous suture techniques in extensor tendon repairs—an experimental evaluation. J Hand Surg Am. 2011;36(12):1968–73.
7. Henderson J, Sutcliffe M, Gillespie P. The tension band principle and angular testing of extensor tendon repairs. J Hand Surg Eur. 2001;36(4):297–302.
8. Newport ML, Williams CD. Biomechanical characteristics of extensor tendon suture techniques. J Hand Surg Am. 1992;17(6):1117–23.
9. Newport ML, Pollack GR, Williams CD. Biomechanical characteristics of suture techniques in extensor zone IV. J Hand Surg Am. 1995;20(3):650–6.
10. Howard RF, Ondrovic L, Greenwald DP. Biomechanical analysis of four-strand extensor tendon repair techniques. J Hand Surg Am. 1997;22(5):838–42.
11. Woo SH, Tsai TM, Kleinert HE, Chew WY, Voor MJ. A biomechanical comparison of four extensor tendon repair techniques in zone IV. Plast Reconstr Surg. 2005;115(6):1674–81.
12. Lee SK, Dubey A, Kim BH, et al. A biomechanical study of extensor tendon repair methods: introduction to the running-interlocking horizontal mattress extensor tendon repair technique. J Hand Surg Am. 2010;35:19–23.
13. Patel MR, Lipson L-B, Desai SS. Conservative treatment of mallet thumb. J Hand Surg Am. 1986; 11:45.

14. Schaller P, Baer W, Carl HD. Extensor indicis-transfer compared with palmaris longus transplantation in reconstruction of extensor pollicis longus tendon: a retrospective study. Scand J Plast Reconstr Surg Hand Surg. 2007;41(1):33–5.
15. Chung US, Kim JH, Seo WS, et al. Tendon transfer or tendon graft for ruptured finger extensor tendons in rheumatoid hands. J Hand Surg Eur. 2010;35:279–82.
16. Noorda RJ, Hage JJ, de Groot PJ, et al. Index finger extension and strength after extensor indicis proprius transfer. J Hand Surg Am. 1994;19:844–9.
17. Lemmen MHM, Schreuders TAR, Stam HJ, Hovius SER. Evaluation of the restoration of the extensor pollicis function by transfer of the extensor indicis. J Hand Surg Br. 1999;24:46–9.
18. Magnussen PA, Harvey FJ, Tonkin MA. Extensor indicis proprius transfer for rupture of the extensor pollicis longus tendon. J Bone Joint Surg Br. 1990;72:881–8.
19. Stahl S, Wolff TW. Delayed rupture of the extensor pollicis longus tendon after nonunion of a fracture of the dorsal radial tubercle. J Hand Surg Am. 1988;13:338–41.
20. Choi JC, Kim WS, Na HY, Lee YS, Song WS, Kim DH, Park TH. Spontaneous rupture of the extensor pollicis longus tendon in a tailor. ClinOrthop Surg. 2011;3(2):167–9.
21. Al-Rashid M, Theivendran K, Craigen MA. Delayed ruptures of the extensor tendon secondary to the use of volar locking compression plates for distal radial fractures. J Bone Joint Surg Br. 2006;88:1610–2.
22. Zwetkow AN, Schibli SI, Canova MA, Mark GI, Sommer CH. Rupture of the extensor tendons: a complication following volar locking compression plate osteosynthesis of the distal radius. Br J Surg. 2005;92:900–18.
23. Scheker LR, Langley SJ, Martin DL, et al. Primary extensor tendon reconstruction in dorsal hand defects requiring free flaps. J Hand Surg Br. 1993;18:568–75.
24. Sundine M, Scheker LR. A comparison of immediate and staged reconstruction of the dorsum of the hand. J Hand Surg Br. 1996;21:216–21.
25. Ulusal BG, Lin YT, Ulusal AE, et al. Free lateral arm flap for 1-stage reconstruction of soft tissue and composite defects of the hand: a retrospective analysis of 118 cases. Ann Plast Surg. 2007;58:173–8.
26. Bevin AG, Hothem AL. The use of silicone rods under split thickness skin grafts for reconstruction of extensor tendon injuries. Hand. 1978;10:254–8.
27. Cautilli D, Schneider LH. Extensor tendon grafting on the dorsum of the hand in massive tendon loss. Hand Clin. 1995;11:423–9.

# Wide-Awake Tendon Surgery

# 12

Myung Jae Yoo and Sang Hyun Woo

## Introduction

Wide-awake anesthesia without the use of a tourniquet or sedation is widely used in hand surgery. This procedure is well described by WALANT, the wide-awake local anesthesia no tourniquet technique [1, 2]. The only two medications required for treatment would then include lidocaine for anesthesia and epinephrine for hemostasis. In addition, the technique provides additional benefits such as eliminating the need for intravenous insertion, constant monitoring, routine preoperative testing, and fasting for the patient.

The advent of increasingly safe general anesthesia before 1950 generated the era of bloodless tourniquet hand surgery that dominated the field for the past 15 years. Although it was once taboo, the early 2000s brought solid evidence that epinephrine hemostasis in the finger and hand is safe [2–5] and that the use of the tourniquet and its requirement for sedation are no longer essential to perform hand surgery.

**Electronic Supplementary Material** The online version of this chapter (https://doi.org/10.1007/978-981-10-4400-7_12) contains supplementary material, which is available to authorized users.

M. J. Yoo (✉) · S. H. Woo
W Institute for Hand and Reconstructive Microsurgery, W Hospital, Daegu, South Korea

## Dosage of Local Anesthesia in Wide-Awake Surgery of the Thumb

The use of tumescent local anesthesia to a tourniquet-free extravascular Bier block in which subcutaneous injections of lidocaine with epinephrine are administered only when necessary. In this technique, the epinephrine substitutes the tourniquet to achieve hemostasis. Although some literature supports the safe use of 35 mg/kg of lidocaine with epinephrine [6], the generally accepted maximal dose is 7 mg/kg. Therefore the average 70 kg person can safely receive 50 cc 1% lidocaine with epinephrine. This mixture remains quite effective when diluted with up to 150 cc of saline to attain the frequently used 0.25% lidocaine with 1:400,000 epinephrine [7].

Special precaution must be taken with the volume so that "top-ups" are never required. If 50 cc or less is needed, the use of 1% of lidocaine with 1:100,000 epinephrine is recommended. If anywhere between the ranges of 50 and 100 cc is required, 0.5% lidocaine with 1:200,000 epinephrine will be satisfactory. For any necessary quantities between 100 and 200 cc, the use of 0.25% lidocaine with 1:400,000 epinephrine is ideal. Concentrations of bicarbonate are used to neutralize the acidic average pH of 4.7 of 1% lidocaine with 1:100,000 epinephrine, but the preferred ratio is 10 cc lidocaine to 1 cc 8.4% bicarbonate to decrease injection pain [8] (Fig. 12.1).



S. H. Woo (ed.), *The Thumb*, https://doi.org/10.1007/978-981-10-4400-7_12

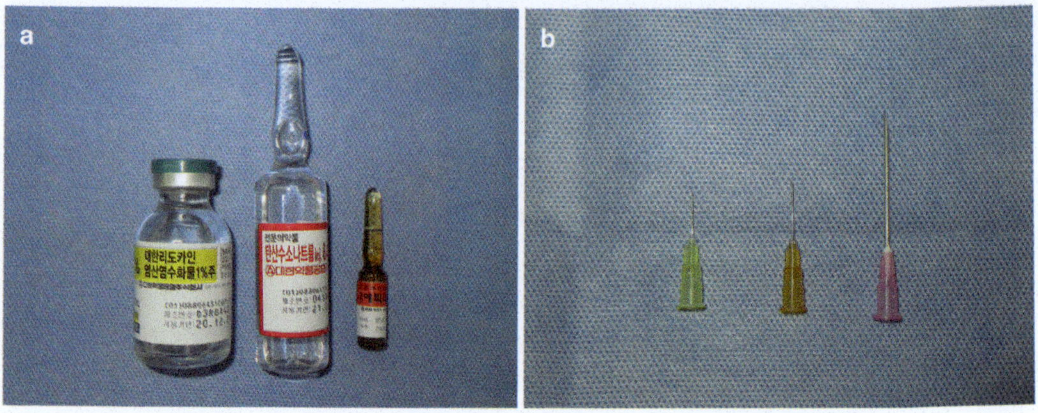


**Fig. 12.1** (**a**) The anesthetic solution used for injection (1% lidocaine, 1:100,000, 8.4% bicarbonate, epinephrine), (**b**) the injection needle (30-gauge needle, 25-gauge needle, and 18-gauge needle)

## Minimal Pain Injection Tumescent Local Anesthesia

A 27-gauge needle causes less pain going in the patient's skin than a 25-gauge needle, and it helps remind the injector to slow down. The injector should start by injecting 2 cc slowly, just below the skin. The use of 30-gauge needles for children or patients who are particularly sensitive is recommended. The pain can be alleviated by creating sensory noise in the area of injection which is icing the skin or vibrating.

Nerves in the dermis are akin to trees with sensitive leaves, and the fatter areas to sturdier branches and tree trunks. So administrating the injection in the dermis causes more pain than in subcutaneous fat. When the needle is inserted, an injection of 0.5 mL with a perpendicular needle just under the dermis and pausing until the patients say the needle pain is gone is advisable.

Also, precaution must be taken to never let the needle get ahead of the local anesthetic [9]. If this happens, the sharp needle tip will irritate nerve endings that have not been numbed. As a precautionary measure, the mental repetition of a phrase such "blow slow before you go" while injecting the area will assist in slowing down and exercising patience. If the injection is administered in an anterograde direction while advancing gradually and steadily under the skin, the sharp needle tip will only enter numbed territory.

## Technique for Injecting Local Anesthesia

The local anesthetic is injected in the digits of the patient in the waiting area, 30 min prior to applying anesthesia. The injection starts proximally with a fine needle (25- or 30-gauge). Between 10 and 15 mL of infiltration is injected in the most proximal part next to the area likely to be dissected to block the nerves distally. In this way, the large volume of the first injection will bathe all of the nerves leading to the area of later injections. In making the first injection, the needle is inserted perpendicularly to the skin into the subcutaneous fat to reduce the pain of injection [10]. The syringe is then stabilized by propping the fingers on the skin to avoid needle wobble. The first 0.5 mL is injected for a duration of 5 s and followed by a 15–45 s pause, until the patient reports that the sting is gone. The rest of infiltration is then injected very slowly, for a duration of more than 5 min, while keeping the needle still. About 10–15 min after the first injection, the whole distal area of dissection is almost or completely numb. As a result, the next injections will be pain-free. The next three injections are used mainly for the epinephrine vasoconstriction effect for digital nerves.

In the finger, the 1% lidocaine with 1:100,000 epinephrine is injected into the subcutaneous fat in the middle of the base of the phalanges,

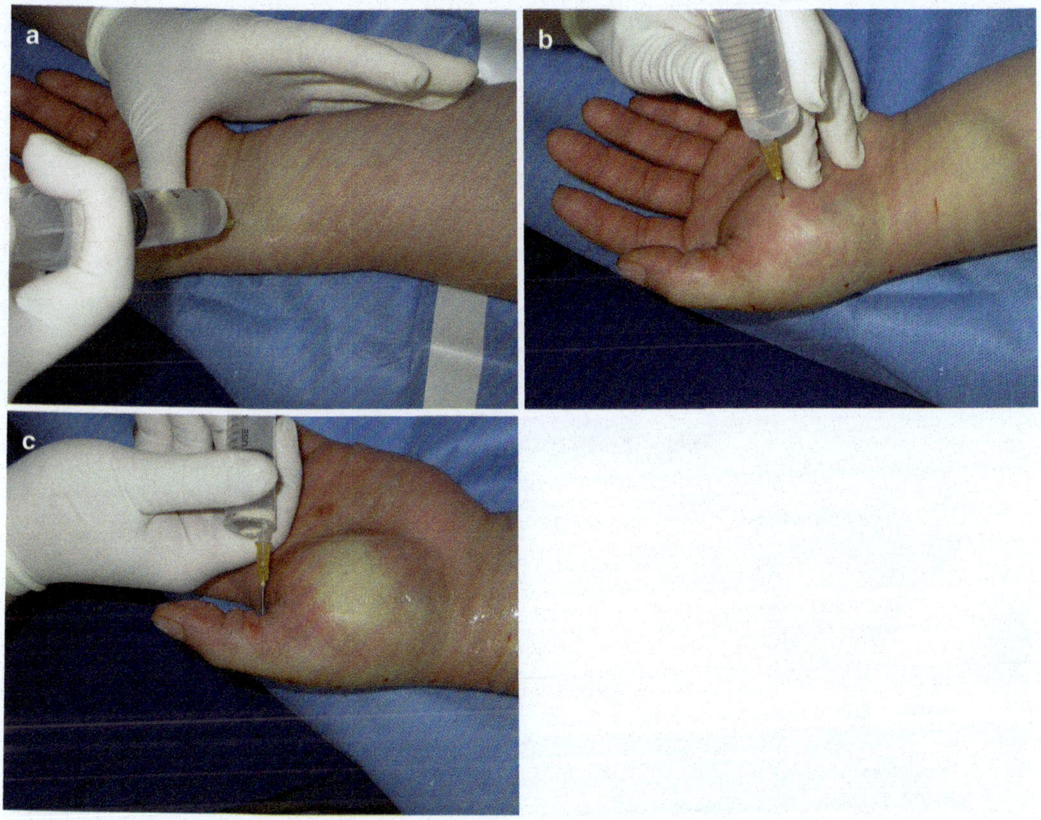

**Fig. 12.2** Wide-awake local anesthesia for flexor pollicis longus (FPL) in the thumb. (**a**) Between 10 and 15 mL of 1% lidocaine with 1:100,000 epinephrine buffered with 10:1 8.4% bicarbonate is injected with a 27-gauge needle in the palm more proximal than the most proximal incision possible. The local anesthesia is injected slowly just under the skin in the fat without moving the needle. (**b**) Fifteen minutes after the first injection, the second injection (10 mL) was performed subcutaneously at the more proximal palmar area between both digital nerves. (**c**) The final injection (2 mL) was performed immediately after the second injection under the skin at the palmar digital crease between both digital nerves

between both digital nerves. This ensures that the bevel of the needle does not lacerate the fascicles. In the proximal and middle palmar phalanges, 2 mL is injected. In the distal phalanx, 1 mL is injected. The routine injection of 10–15 mL in the palm follows wherever dissection will be performed (Figs. 12.2 and 12.3) (Video 12.1).

## Advantages of WALANT

There are several advantages of flexor tendon repair in wide-awake surgery. The most important advantage is intraoperative testing which can reveal the gapping of a weak repair and decrease rupture rates [11]. These repairs get less tenolysis because intraoperative testing of the repair guides the surgeon to vent pulleys that impede the full flexion or extension of the thumb [12]. Surgeons can educate the lucid patient during surgery, so they understand how to avoid rupture and getting stuck [13]. Intraoperative flexor tendon repair testing guides the surgeon in the decision to maintain a superficialis repair or resect a superficialis slip [14]. Seeing full active flexion and extension with no gap during the surgery empowers the surgeon to allow up to half a fist of true active postoperative flexion (not place and hold) 3–5 days after surgery [15].

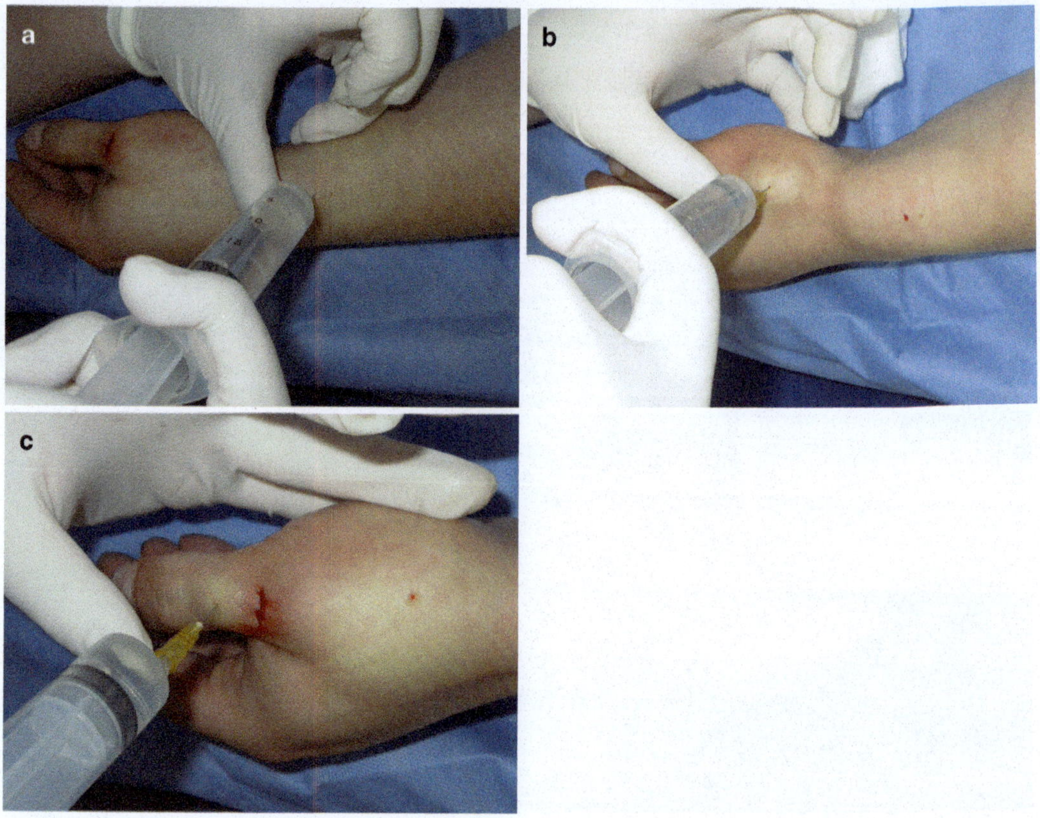


**Fig. 12.3** Wide-awake local anesthesia for extensor pollicis longus (EPL) tendon in the thumb. (**a**) Between 10 and 15 mL of 1% lidocaine with 1:100,000 epinephrine buffered with 10:1 8.4% bicarbonate is injected with a 27-gauge needle in the palm more proximal than the most proximal incision possible. The local anesthesia is injected slowly just under the skin in the fat without moving the needle. (**b**) Fifteen minutes after the first injection, the second injection (10 mL) was performed subcutaneously at the more proximal palmar area between both digital nerves. (**c**) The final injection (2 mL) was performed immediately after the second injection under the skin at the dorsal proximal phalanx of the thumb

## Flexor Pollicis Longus (FPL) Repair of the Thumb

When the proximal ends of the tendon are pulled out to length, patients will sometimes actively pull the flexor tendon away from the surgeon. This is usually easily dealt with by asking the patient to relax the finger. If that does not work, the patient is asked to actively extend the finger, which causes a reflex that relaxes the involved flexor tendon. The flexor tendon is then brought out to length and skewered into position with 22-gauge hypodermic needles [14]. The flexor pollicis longus (FPL) tendon is repaired with a six-strand core suture repair (Prolene 4–0 suture, M-Tang method using looped suture, or M-Becker's method). Repeatedly testing the patient's full active flexion and extension of the thumb after each core and epitenon suture is advised to make sure that there is no gap and that the repair fits through the pulleys. Before the skin closure, there are three tests that should be conducted: full active extension to verify that there is no gapping between the tendon ends; smooth active flexion to verify smooth gliding of the tendon and its repair site; and active flexion to almost fully flex the digit to verify that no pulley prevents tendon gliding. Surgeons can repair any gaps and vent pulleys as required to get a full range of motion [16]. In postoperative therapy, immobilize and elevate the hand until swelling, friction, and the work of flexion are

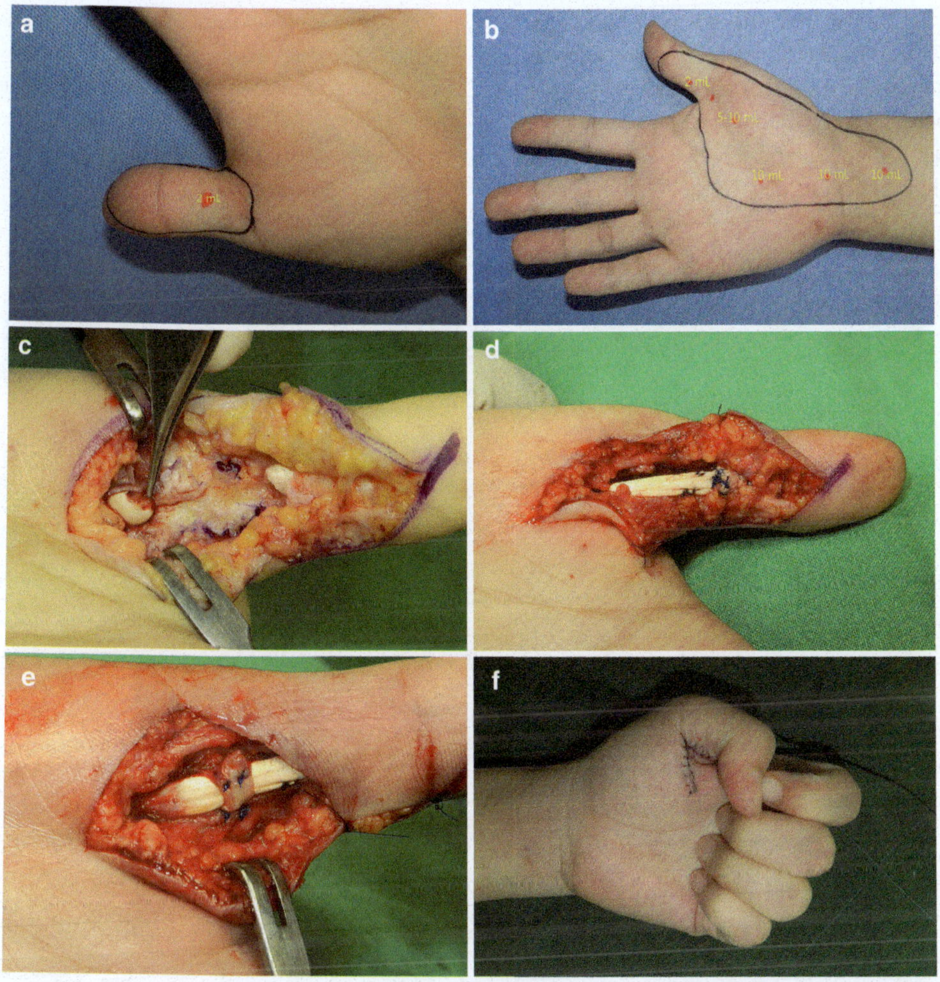


**Fig. 12.4** (**a**) Simple distal thumb block. When you inject 2 mL of 1% lidocaine with 1:100,000 epinephrine (buffered at a ratio 10 mL of 8.4 sodium bicarbonate) in subcutaneous fat in the red spot point. (**b**) The flexor pollicis longus (FPL) in carpal tunnel may benefit from a median nerve block of 10 mL of 1% lidocaine with 1:100,000 epinephrine and 1 mL of 8.4% sodium bicarbonate under the skin and under the distal forearm fascia in the proximal red spot. Up to 20 mL of the same solution wound go in the palm, starting with 10 mL over the carpal tunnel, then 10 mL over the thenar eminence, and 2 mL in the thumb proximal phalanx injection point just under the skin. (**c**) A 39-year-old patient hurt by a knife ruptured the flexor pollicis longus (FPL). Thirty minutes after the local anesthesia injection, the epinephrine takes effect. The wound was exposed through the A1 pulley stepladder and was opened. (**d**) This FPL shown was repaired with a 6-strand M-Tang technique. (**e**) After FPL repair, the patient actively extended and flexed the thumb to perform the extension-flexion test. A1 pulley was reconstructed with fourth FDS radial slip about bowing of FPL. (**f**) After skin suture, the patient actively flexed the thumb

gone (3–5 days). Initiate up to half a fist of true active movement (not place and hold) from day 4 or 5. In the initial first to second week, patients keep the active flexion within only one-third of the range of motion with dynamic splint. Patients should avoid full range of active flexion in the first 2 to 3 weeks. Full range of active motion starts at 4 weeks post-repair (Fig. 12.4) (Video 12.2).

## Extensor Pollicis Longus (EPL) Tendon Repair of the Thumb

Surgeons ask the patients to flex the thumb to get the extensor to relax. The extensor pollicis longus (EPL) tendon is repaired with a six-strand core suture repair (Prolene 4–0 or 5–0 suture, Silfverskiöld epitendinous suture, or M-Becker's method). Surgeons then test the following areas:

full fist flexion and full extension after repair to verify that there is no gapping between the ends of the tendons and smooth active flexion to verify the smooth gliding of the tendon. In postoperative therapy, immobilize and elevate the hand until swelling, friction, and work of flexion are gone (3–5 days). Patients then must comply with controlled active mobilization exercises which involve active joint extensions and limiting joint flexion with a palmar splint in the initial 1–2 weeks. Full range of active motion with dynamic splint starts at 3 weeks post-repair (Fig. 12.5).

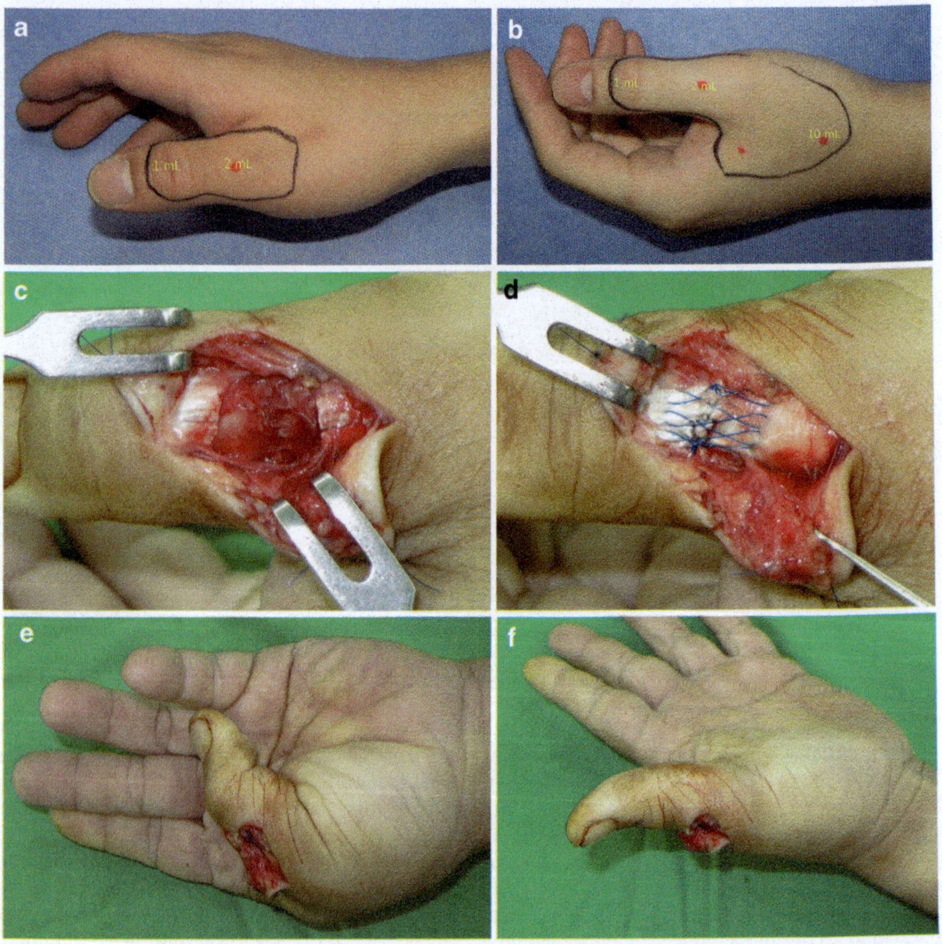


**Fig. 12.5** (**a**) Dorsal thumb proximal phalanx block. When you inject 2 mL of 1% lidocaine with 1:100,000 epinephrine (buffered at a ratio 10 mL of 8.4 sodium bicarbonate) in subcutaneous fat in the red spot point. (**b**) When extensor pollicis longus (EPL) tendon is ruptured at more proximal area, 10 mL of anesthetic mixture of 1% lidocaine with epinephrine (1: 100,000) buffered with 10:1 8.4% bicarbonate is injected with a 27-gauge needle in just dorsal distal wrist red spot point. Fifteen minutes after the first injection, the second injection (5–10 mL) was performed subcutaneously at the more proximal dorsal area between both superficial radial sensory nerves. The final injection (2 mL) was performed immediately after the second injection under the skin at the dorsal proximal phalanx of the thumb. (**c**) A 47-year-old patient hurt by a sickle ruptured the extensor pollicis longus (EPL) tendon. Thirty minutes after the local anesthesia injection, the epinephrine takes effect. Thumb flexed and extended on the table. After that, the wound was exposed. (**d**) This EPL shown was repaired with a Silfverskiöld epitendinous suture. (**e**, **f**) After EPL repair, the patient actively extended and flexed the thumb to perform the extension-flexion test before the skin closure. It could ensure to no gapping between the tendon ends and smooth active flexion to verify smooth gliding of the tendon

## Tenolysis of the Thumb

Tenolysis in the thumb after tendon surgery or trauma is effective in wide-awake surgery. The patient can actively move the thumb to ensure that tenolysis is adequate and that the tendon is strong enough to move the tendon. The surgeons can intraoperatively ask the patient to actively flex or extend the thumb to see the active gliding of the tendon. If the tenolysis is sufficient, the surgery is complete. If the tenolysis is insufficient, further release of scar around the tendon is necessary.

Tendons are sometimes found frayed during surgery. Active motions by the patient can help the surgeon test the strength of such tendons. If the tendon is remarkably elongated or is broken when the digits or the hand is in movement, tendon reconstruction using a tendon grafting should be considered. During active motion, the strength of the pulley can be tested as well, and whether the pulleys restrict tendon gliding can be assessed. If the pulleys are broken during active tendon motion, important annular pulleys may need reconstruction. Restriction of the tendon gliding from the pulleys may need further release of adhesions or a pulley plasty or pulley shortening procedure.

Patients can watch themselves move the thumb through a full range of motions before the skin is closed. They know that their thumb will function well once they overcome the postoperative discomfort and stiffness through putting effort in therapy. Early active motion is a key factor in the success of any tenolysis procedure and should be instituted as soon as possible. If hemostasis is not a concern and the pain is tolerable, rehabilitation in the operating room is preferable. Splinting is usually not necessary. Formal therapy continues until the patient has reached a plateau in recovery, with no improvement in active range of motion over 3 weeks [16] (Fig. 12.6) (Video 12.3).

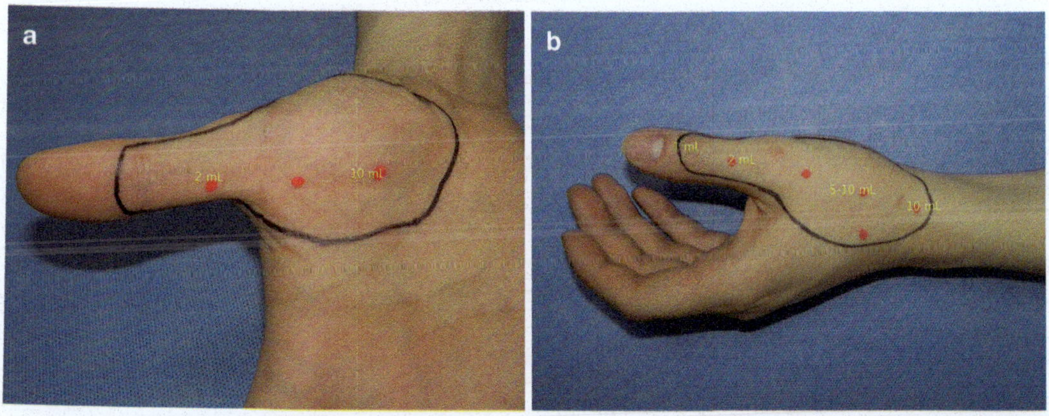


**Fig. 12.6** (**a**) The flexor pollicis longus (FPL) in hypothenar may benefit from a median nerve sensory branch block of 10 mL of 1% lidocaine with 1:100,000 epinephrine and 1 mL of 8.4% sodium bicarbonate under the skin in the proximal red spot. Starting with 10 mL over the thenar eminence and 2 mL in the thumb proximal phalanx injection point just under the skin. (**b**) 10 mL of anesthetic mixture of 1% lidocaine with epinephrine (1:100,000) buffered with 10:1 8.4% bicarbonate is injected in just dorsal distal wrist red spot point. The second injection (5–10 mL) was performed subcutaneously at the more proximal dorsal area between both superficial radial sensory nerves. The final injection (2 mL) was performed immediately after the second injection under the skin at the dorsal proximal phalanx of the thumb. (**c**) After a 27-year-old patient was repaired of flexor pollicis longus (FPL), the thumb was flexion contracture. Thirty minutes after the local anesthesia injection, the epinephrine takes effect. The thumb flexed and extended on the table. After that, the wound was exposed. (**d**) The tenolysis of FPL was done, and volar plate and joint capsule in interphalangeal joint of the thumb were released. (**e**, **f**) After that, the patient actively extended and flexed the thumb to perform the extension-flexion test. It could ensure to smooth active flexion to verify smooth gliding of the tendon

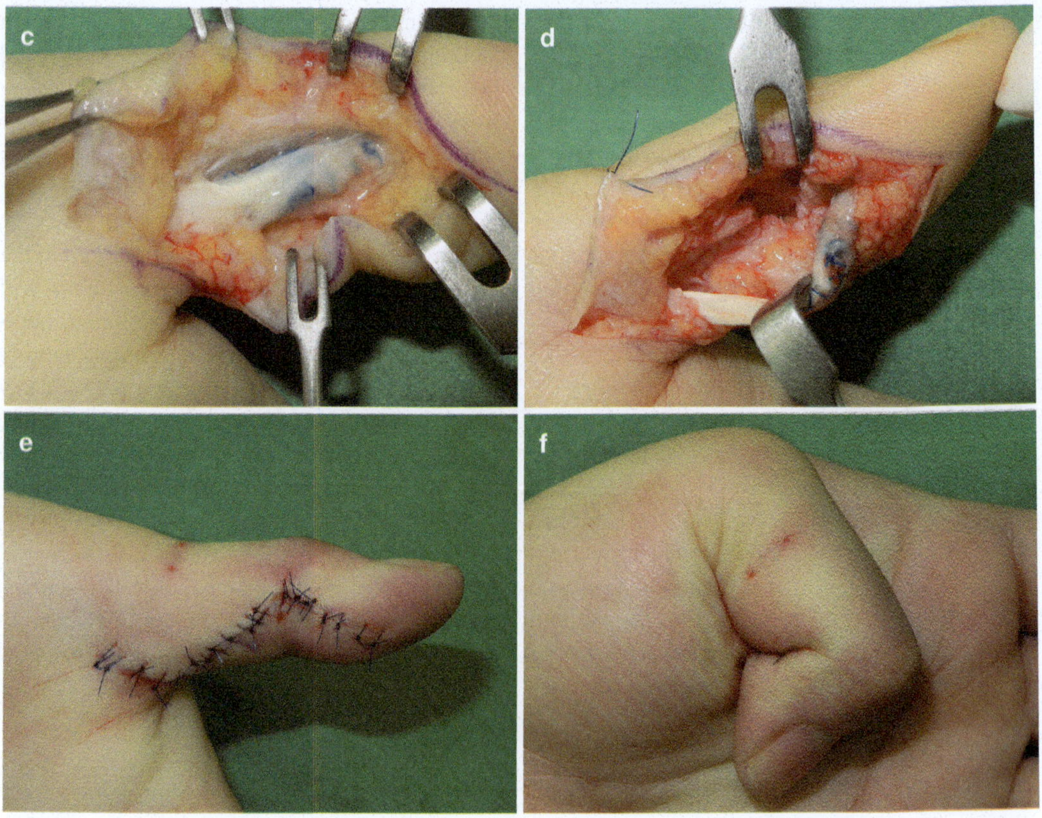


**Fig. 12.6** (continued)

## Extensor Indicis Proprius (EIP) to Extensor Pollicis Longus (EPL) Tendon Transfer

Rupture of the EPL is most frequently seen after a fracture of the radius. The transfer of the EIP is simple, synergistic, readily available, and anatomically close. Patients do not have to learn about this transfer and can cooperatively move the thumb immediately on the operating table while remaining wide awake.

Tendon transfer is best indicated during wide-awake surgery, while adjusting for the tension of the transfer has always been difficult during conventional surgery. With the patient being awake, they can move actively to determine the appropriate tension of the transfer. It is easy to make a tendon transfer too tight to too loose. Surgeons can see that tour tendon transfer tension is correct by watching the patient take the thumb through a full range of motion before closing the skin [17].

The EIP and EPL tendon stumps are overlapped so that the thumb position looks good with wrist flexion and wrist extension, as is done under motor block anesthesia. Two temporary mattress sutures are placed between the two tendons. One suture may not be enough to hold the tendons with active movement. The patient is then asked to extend the thumb as if hitchhiking, to test whether the tension is tight enough. The patient is then asked to touch their little finger with their thumb, to make sure the tension is not too tight. Tension is adjusted until it is just right, and then a Pulvertaft weave is carried out [18].

Rehabilitation in patients who have already seen themselves perform a full range of motions on the operating table is greatly facilitated compared with those who have been sedated and told that the procedure will be successful after surgery. Motion with dynamic splint begins 4 days after post-repair (Fig. 12.7) (Video 12.4).

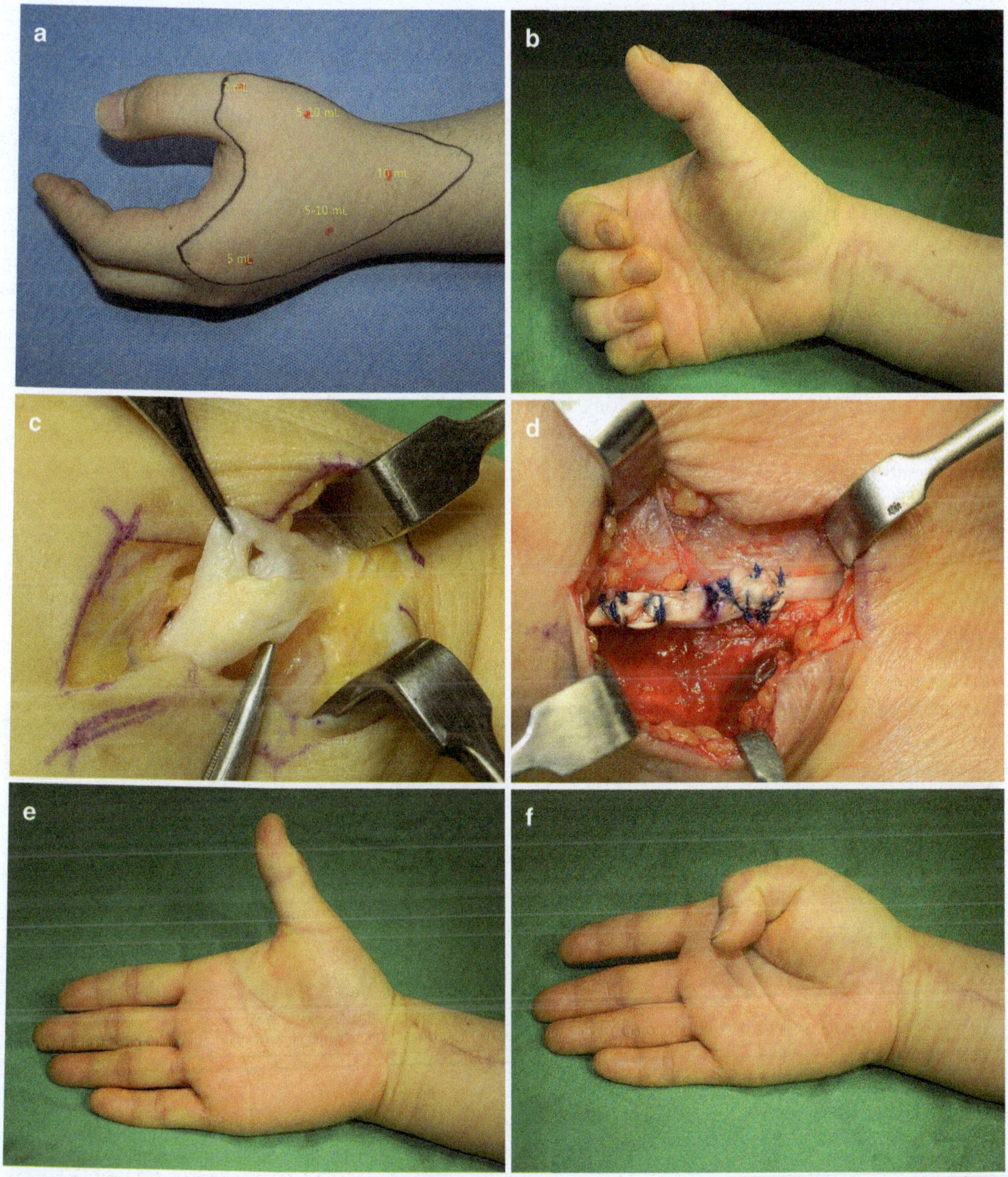


**Fig. 12.7** (**a**) 10 mL of anesthetic mixture of 1% lidocaine with epinephrine (1:100,000) buffered with 10:1 8.4% bicarbonate is injected in dorsal wrist red spot point. The second injection (5–10 mL) was performed subcutaneously at the more proximal dorsal area (the index and thumb) between both superficial radial sensory nerves. The final injection (2 mL) was performed immediately after the second injection under the skin at the dorsal proximal phalanx of the thumb and metacarpophalangeal joint of the index finger. (**b**) A 64-year-old patient ruptured the spontaneous extensor pollicis longus (EPL) tendon. Thirty minutes after the local anesthesia injection, the epinephrine takes effect. On table, the thumb actively extended and flexed in intraoperative field. (**c**) The wound was exposed with tourniquet help for bloodless surgical field. (**d**) This EIP to EPL shown was repaired with a Pulvertaft weave. (**e**, **f**) After tendon transfer, the patient actively extended and flexed the thumb to perform the extension flexion test

## Flexor Digitorum Superficialis (FDS) of the Long or Ring Finger to Flexor Pollicis Longus (FPL) Tendon Transfer

The flexor pollicis longus (FPL) flexes the interphalangeal (IP) joint of the thumb, and the loss of this motion impedes precision pinch activities. The flexor digitorum superficialis (FDS) tendon transfer of the ring or the long finger is a good option for FPL reconstruction under WALNAT. The harvest of the flexor digitorum superficialis (FDS) of the ring or the long finger is not difficult through small incisions, replacing the FPL entirely without supplement by a tendon graft. The procedure also requires little reeducation.

When the FPL is exposed, the normal retinacular pulley system is preserved. The FDS of the ring or the long finger is harvested after verified FDS movement. A third transverse incision is made at the base of the ring finger, and the FDS is cut, leaving the distal 1 cm and its insertion intact. The FDS is then withdrawn into the distal forearm wound and redirected into the thumb flexor tendon sheath. Two temporary mattress sutures are placed between the two tendons. The patient is then asked to extend the thumb as if hitchhiking, to test whether the tension is tight enough. Tension is adjusted until it is just right, and then a Pulvertaft weave is carried out.

Splinting and rehabilitation after FPL reconstructions are akin to primary repair like early active mobilization in a protective dorsal splint. It is necessary to include a dorsal splint behind the fingers as well as behind the thumb and prevent finger gripping activities, as these are followed by movement of the thumb into tight flexion over the dorsum of the index finger, which may rupture any suture of the FPL (Fig. 12.8) (Video 12.5).

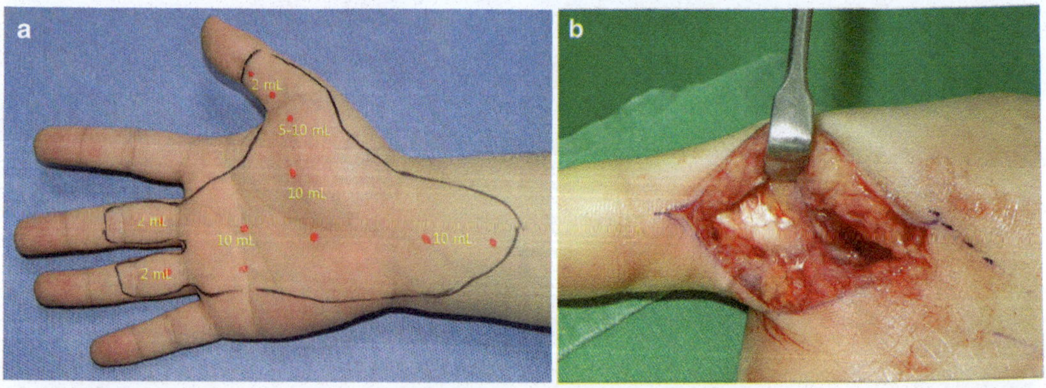


**Fig. 12.8** (**a**) The harvested flexor digitorum superficialis (FDS) of the ring or long finger in carpal tunnel may benefit from a median nerve block of 10 mL of 1% lidocaine with 1:100,000 epinephrine and 1 mL of 8.4% sodium bicarbonate under the skin and under the distal forearm fascia in the proximal red spot. Up to 20 mL of the same solution wound goes in the palm, starting with 10 mL over the carpal tunnel, then 10 ml over the thenar eminence, and 2 mL in the thumb proximal phalanx injection point just under the skin. Additional injection (2 mL) was performed immediately after the second injection under the skin at proximal phalanx of the ring or long finger. (**b**) A 45-year-old patient ruptured the spontaneous flexor pollicis longus (FPL). Thirty minutes after the local anesthesia injection, the epinephrine takes effect. On the table, the thumb actively extended and flexed in intraoperative field. The wound was exposed with tourniquet help for bloodless surgical field. (**c**) The FDS of the ring or the long finger is harvested after verified FDS movement. The FDS is then withdrawn into the distal forearm wound and redirected into the thumb flexor tendon sheath. (**d**) Two temporary mattress sutures are placed between the two tendons. The patient is then asked to extend the thumb as if hitchhiking, to test whether the tension is tight enough. (**e, f**) After tendon transfer, the patient actively extended and flexed the thumb to perform the extension-flexion test

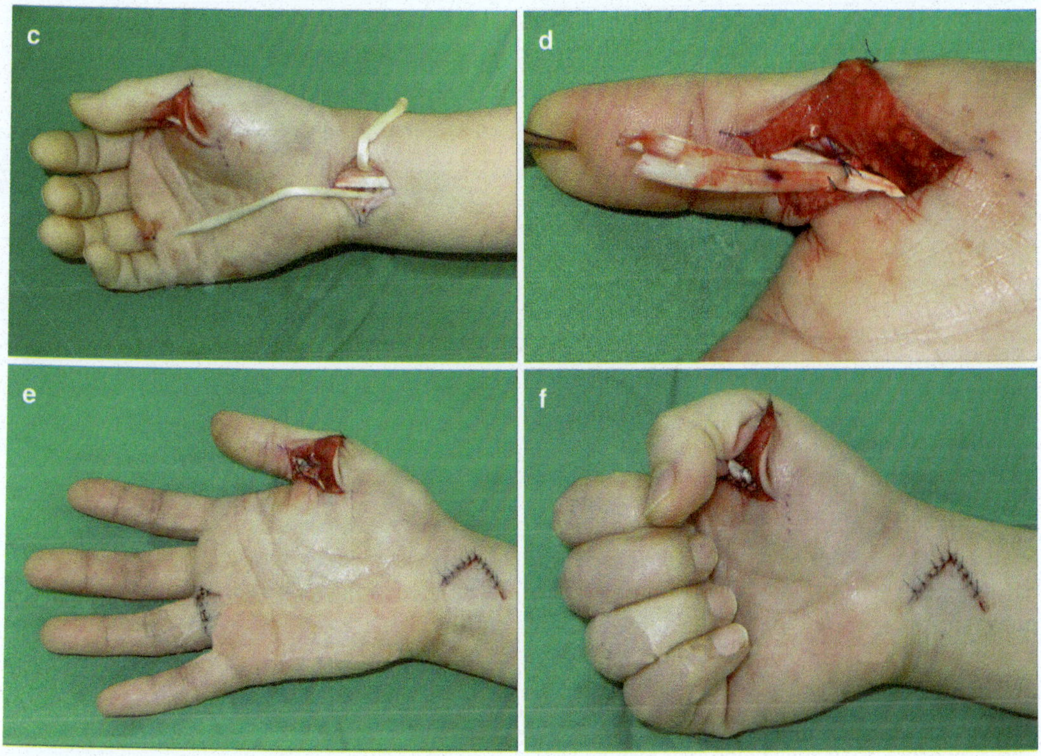


**Fig. 12.8** (continued)

## Complications and Limitations

The white thumb after injection with epinephrine was seen when performing this procedure. If it should occur and the surgeon is uncomfortable with it, 1 mg of phentolamine (an alpha-adrenergic blocking agent introduced in 1957 as antihypertensive agent in pheochromocytoma management) can be diluted into 5–10 mL of saline solution and injected wherever epinephrine has been introduced. This is done to reverse vasoconstriction. Generally, capillary refill returns within 1 h [3)] (Fig. 12.9).

Wide-awake anesthesia has its own limitations. There is a constraint on the time in which the surgery can be carried out and a risk of enlarging the dissection and surgery areas. In addition, there is a risk of bleeding at the initial stage of surgery. These limitations can be addressed and minimized. Lidocaine's effect lasts 2 h, providing enough time for the surgery to be carried out. In addition, the enlargement of the surgery area can be prevented by diluting the injection and carrying out the procedure. Lastly, utilizing a tourniquet at 200 mmHg during the first 20 min of the surgery can be used to combat any initial bleeding.

## Improved Results with Tendon Surgery

The ability to detect and repair gapping that can be seen during a WALANT flexor tendon repair has decreased the rupture rate [18]. In addition, full flexion and extension by a comfortable, cooperative, tourniquet-free patient allows the surgeon to vent pulleys and trim the repair so that the full range of flexion and extension of the finger can be obtained intraoperatively before the

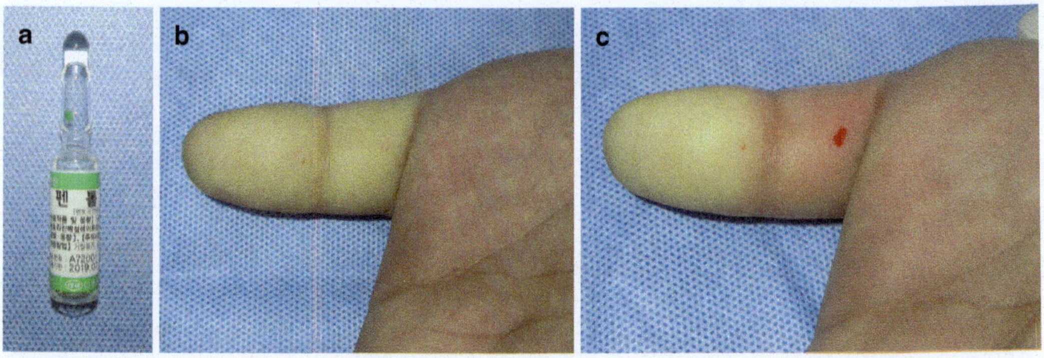


**Fig. 12.9** (**a**) Phentolamine is the rescue agent for epinephrine vasoconstriction in the thumb. (**b**) The white thumb after injection with epinephrine was seen. (**c**) 1 mg of phentolamine can be diluted into 5–10 mL of saline solution and injected wherever epinephrine has been introduced. This is done to reverse vasoconstriction. Generally, capillary refill returns within 1 h

skin is closed; this decreases the need for subsequent tenolysis [15, 16]. Obtaining an optimal tendon transfer is challenging because transfers can be either too tight or too loose. With this approach, the extensor indicis to extensor pollicis longus transfer can be adjusted during the procedure to achieve optimal results [12]. Incorporating intraoperative mobilization using "wide-awake" surgery could emerge to further improve tendon outcomes. However, good surgical approach, meticulous surgery, up-to-date physiotherapy regimens, and patient education remain the cornerstone of obtaining optimal outcomes.

## Conclusion

Patients who are wide awake are comfortable, cooperative, and educable and are able to assist the surgeon set the correct tension for the transfer. Surgeons flex and extend the finger before the skin is closed to make sure that the transfer is not too tight or too loose. In addition, remembering the fine movements of the finger during surgery assists patients when they are in postoperative hand therapy. Surgeons can also ensure the more accurate results of tendon surgery in both the intra- and postoperation stages.

In conclusion, wide-awake no tourniquet surgery, which allows tendons to actively move during surgery, greatly benefits surgeons by allowing them to test tendon function and ensure the tendon is properly repaired before leaving the operating table.

## References

1. Lalonde DH. Reconstruction of the hand with wide awake surgery. Clin Plast Surg. 2011;38:761–9.
2. Lalonde DH, Martin A. Epinephrine in local anesthesia in finger and hand surgery: the case for wide-awake anesthesia. J Am Acad Orthop Surg. 2013;21:443–7.
3. Nodwell T, Lalonde DH. How long does it take phentolamine to reverse adrenaline-induced vasoconstriction in the finger and hand? A prospective randomized blinded study: the Dalhousie project experimental phase. Can J Plast Surg. 2003;11(4):187–90.
4. Lalonde DH, Bell M, Benoit P, et al. A multicenter prospective study of 3,110 consecutive cases of elective epinephrine use in the fingers and hand: the Dalhousie project clinical phase. J Hand Surg Am. 2005;30(5):1061–7.
5. Thomson CJ, Lalonde DH, Denkler KA, et al. A critical look at the evidence for and against elective epinephrine use in the finger. Plast Reconstr Surg. 2007;119(1):260–6.
6. Burk RW III, Guzman-Stein G, Vasconez LO. Lidocaine and epinephrine levels in tumescent technique liposuction. Plast Reconstr Surg. 1996;97(7):1379–84.
7. Lalonde DH. Dosage of local anesthesia in wide awake hand surgery. J Hand Surg Am. 2013;38(10):2025–8.
8. Frank SG, Lalonde DH. How acidic is the lidocaine we are injecting, and how much bicarbonate should we add? Can J Plast Surg. 2012;20(2):71–3.
9. Strzar AR, Leynes PG, Lalonde DH. Minimizing the pain of local anesthesia injection. Plast Reconstr Surg. 2013;132:675.

10. Higgins A, Lalonde DH, Bell M, et al. Avoiding flexor tendon repair rupture with intraoperative total active movement examination. Plast Reconstr Surg. 2010;126:941–5.
11. Lalonde DH, Kozin S. Tendon disorders of the hand. Plast Reconstr Surg. 2011;128:1e–14e.
12. Lalonde DH. How the wide awake approach is changing hand surgery and hand therapy: inaugural AAHS sponsored lecture at the ASHT meeting, San Diego, 2012. J Hand Ther. 2013;26:175–8.
13. Lalonde DH. Finger flexor tendon repair. Wide awake hand surgery. Boca Raton, FL: CRC; 2016. ISBN 9781498714792.
14. Lalonde DH. Wide awake flexor tendon repair and early mobilization in zones 1 and 2. In: Bo Tang J, Lee SK, eds. Hand clinics tendon repair and reconstruction. Hand Clin. 2013;29(2):207–13.
15. Tang JB. Wide-awake primary flexor tendon repair, tenolysis, and tendon transfer. Clin Orthop Surg. 2015;7(3):275–81.
16. Alba CD, LaStayo P. Postoperative management of functionally restrictive muscular adherence, a corollary to surgical tenolysis: a case report. J Hand Ther. 2001;14:43–50.
17. Lalonde DH. Wide-awake extensor Indicis Proprius to extensor Pollicis longus tendon transfer. J Hand Surg Am. 2014;39(11):2297–9.
18. Bezuhly M, Sparkes GL, Higgins A, et al. Immediate thumb extension following extensor indicis proprius to extensor pollicis longus tendon transfer using the wide awake approach. Plast Reconstr Surg. 2007;119(5):1507–12.

# Part V

# Nerve Problems

# Sensory Loss

# 13

Jong Won Hong

## Introduction

Human evolution is characterized by parallel increases in brain size and hand development. Brain enlargement, along with the development of thought and intelligence, increased together with the area of cerebral cortex that is associated with the hand. "Cortex man or cortical homunculus" emphasizes how much area of the cerebral cortex is associated with the hand, particularly the thumb. This is also the reason that motor and/or sensory loss of the thumb causes considerable inconvenience and suffering for patients.

The skin of the palm and volar fingers is different from other types of skin. Fingertips are covered with glabrous skin, which is tough, durable, and resistant to pressure and tearing. Pulp supports glabrous skin and protects the underlying bone and tendon. Glabrous skin and its supporting pulp tissue contain a high concentration of specialized nerve endings that are critical to its function [1]. Swartz distinguishes sensory recovery as the critical sensibility of fingertips and the protective sensibility of the palm and dorsum [2]. This is important to consider during the reconstruction of sensory loss that is due to soft tissue defects.

The loss of sensation alone does not affect the motor area. However, movement control requires a continuous and reciprocal exchange of information between the motor and the task programs and the elaborating proprioceptive sensory system [3]. For example, a patient with nerve defects will not feel the proper pressure during a pinch or holding. These patients will flex a thumb more to prevent drop instead of using opposition. Additionally, these patients often use unnecessary movement to complete small tasks and compensate for sensory loss with eyesight.

First, the loss of sensation from the thumb feels uncomfortable to the patient, in addition to the secondary effects in the motor area due to loss of sensation. Patients express that the thumb feels numb and like the flesh of another person. The skin is easily damaged because it does not feel pain from trauma, and this can cause wounds and soft tissue infection. Occasionally, the patient may burn themselves while performing hyperthermia on the region that has experienced sensory loss. Therefore, loss of sensation of the thumb should not be considered simply as a loss of sensation but should also be treated for its role in affecting movement.

## Nerve Anatomy

### Sensory Nerve from the Median Nerve and Radial Nerve

The median nerve and the radial nerve are the sensory nerves in the thumb. The median nerve

J. W. Hong (✉)
Department of Plastic and Reconstructive Surgery, Yonsei University, Severance Hospital, Seoul, South Korea


S. H. Woo (ed.), *The Thumb*, https://doi.org/10.1007/978-981-10-4400-7_13

dominates the senses of the volar area of the thumb and the dorsal area below the interphalangeal (IP) joint. In contrast, the radial nerve controls the dorsal side of the thumb. As the median nerve progresses through the upper arm, there is no branching of the motor and sensory nerves. After the cubital fossa, the motor nerve first branches toward the pronator teres. Thereafter, it travels between the flexor digitorum superficialis (FDS) and the flexor digitorum profundus (FDP), and the motor nerve branches to the forearm. The median nerve continues and branches into the palmar cutaneous nerve at 5 cm above the wrist flexion crease, to allow sensing of the radial side palm. The remaining median nerve passes through the carpal tunnel. This passing median nerve branches into the recurrent median nerve for the thenar muscles. Finally, the proper digital nerves are then branched to fingers 1, 2, and 3 and the radial side of fourth finger [4].

The radial nerve is divided into a deep branch and a superficial branch at the elbow level. The superficial branch runs between the brachioradialis and extensor carpi radialis longus (ECRL), but clinically it lies under the brachioradialis and runs adjacent to the radial artery at the forearm. Proximal 9 cm from the radial styloid, the superficial radial nerve passes out between the brachioradialis and ECRL at the subcutaneous layer. After that, it travels in the direction of the radial styloid to the dorsal side of fingers 1, 2, and 3 and the radial side of finger 4. The cephalic vein runs through the forearm past the radius distal epicondyle. Superficial radial nerves can easily be seen traveling along with the cephalic vein (Fig. 13.1).

The proper digital nerve, which runs through the volar part of the thumb, is divided into three types. Type I consists of two proper digital nerves. One nerve runs on the radial side of the thumb, and the other runs into the first web space that is divided by the ulnar side of the thumb and the radial side of the index finger. Type II also consists of two proper digital nerves. One nerve runs on the radial and ulnar sides of the thumb, and the other runs into the first web space that is divided by both sides of the index finger. Type III branches into three proper digital nerves and travels to the radial side, the ulnar side of the thumb, and the radial side of the index finger (Fig. 13.2). The most common type is Type I. Although there is some debate, Type II is considered the second most common [5].

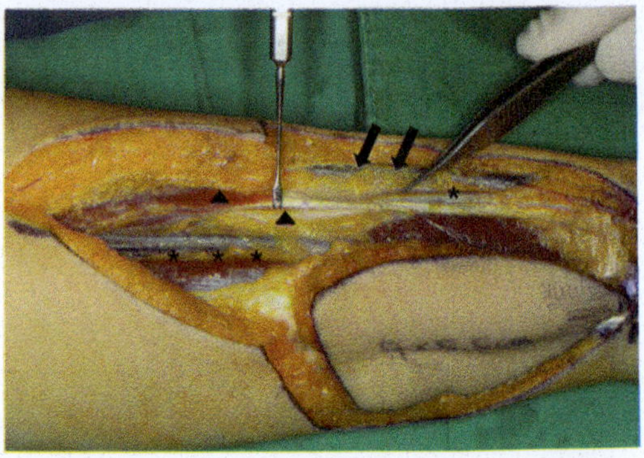

**Fig. 13.1** Superficial radial nerve in the forearm. The superficial radial nerve runs under the brachialis (★) and passes between brachialis and ECRL. Under the brachialis, the nerve runs near the radial artery (▲). After passing into the subcutaneous layer, the nerve runs parallel with the cephalic vein (*)

The nerves enter the IP joint of the thumb from both sides, on the dorsal and volar sides. The volar side nerve branches from the proper digital nerve at 20 mm proximal to the IP joint line, and the emergence angle is an average of 40°. The dorsal side nerve branches from the superficial radial nerve. The radial side nerve branches at an average of 20 mm proximal and the ulnar side branches at about 13 mm proximal. The emergence angle is also an average of 40° for these nerves [6] (Fig. 13.3). The sensory nerve distribution in the hand may differ between regions due to multiple displacements or communication branches [7].

## Sensory Receptor

The most prominent sensory receptors are the Meissner's corpuscles, which are easily seen

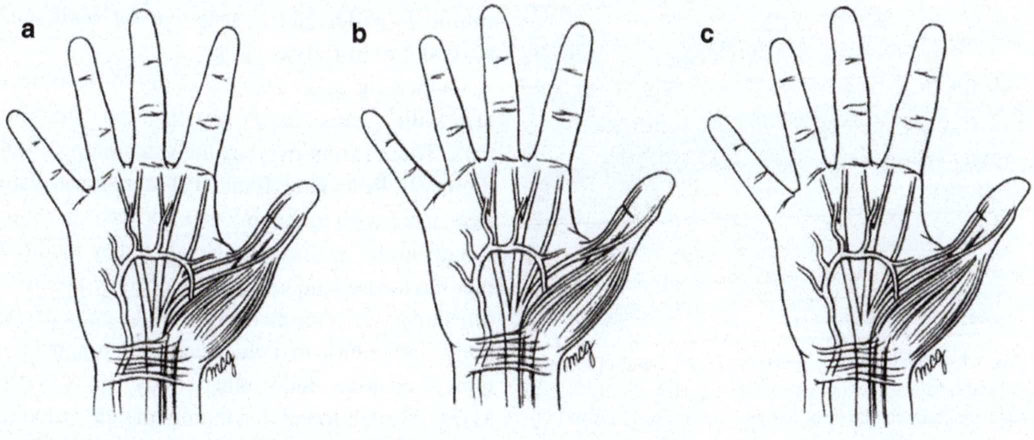


**Fig. 13.2** Patterns of the proper digital nerve in relation to the thumb. (**a**) Type I is two proper digital nerves divided by the radial side of the thumb and first web space between the index and ulnar side of the thumb. (**b**) Type II is also two proper digital nerves that are divided to both sides of the thumb and index finger. (**c**) Type III is three proper digital nerves for each side of the thumb and index finger (from Jolley et al. [5])

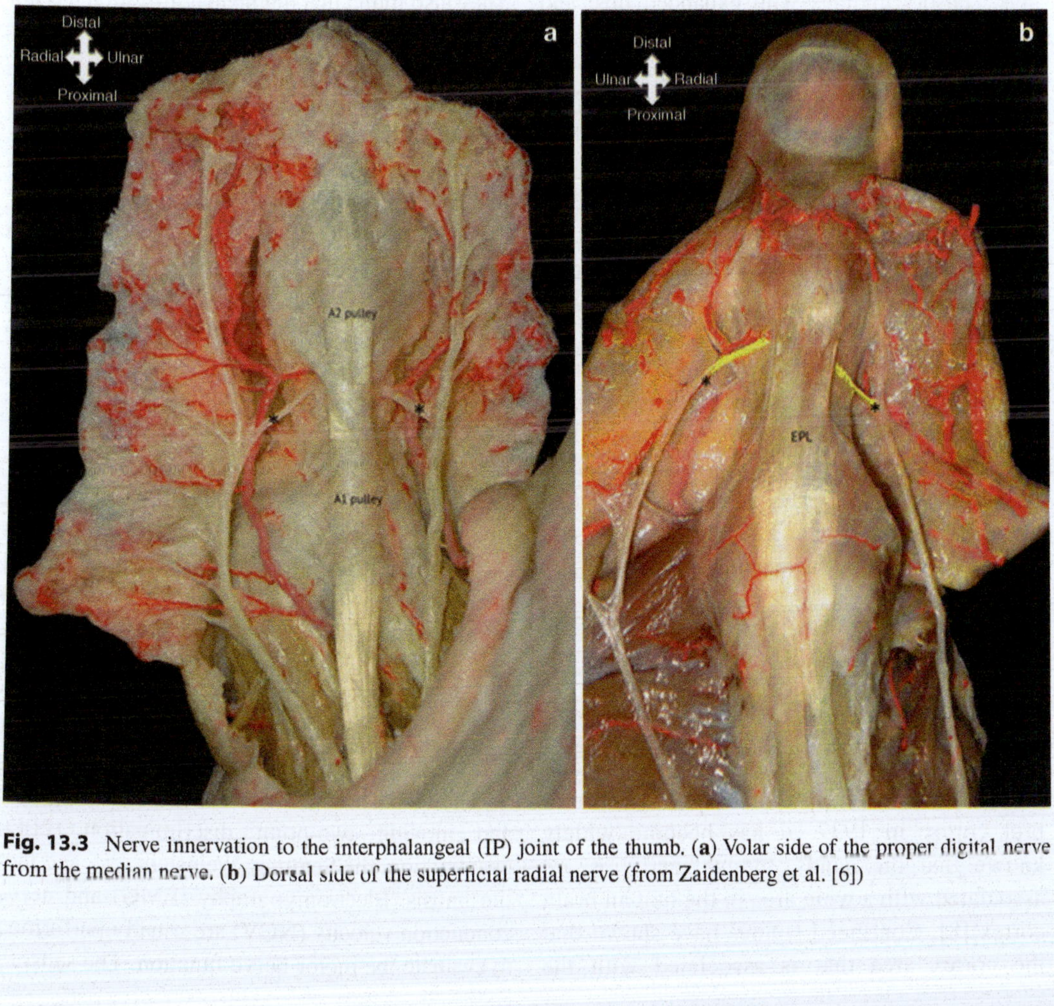


**Fig. 13.3** Nerve innervation to the interphalangeal (IP) joint of the thumb. (**a**) Volar side of the proper digital nerve from the median nerve. (**b**) Dorsal side of the superficial radial nerve (from Zaidenberg et al. [6])

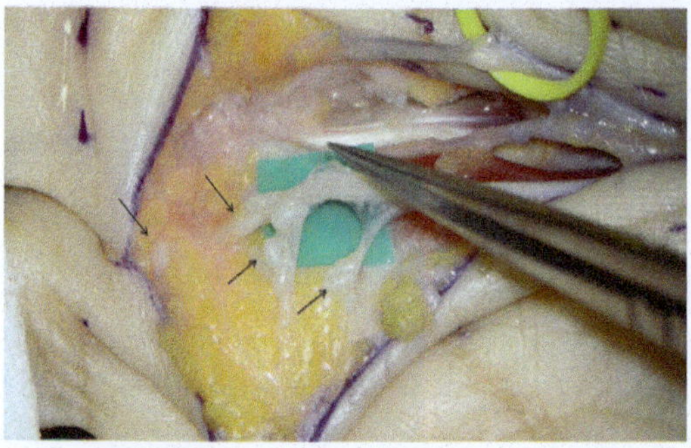

**Fig. 13.4** Meissner's corpuscles in the hand. The most common sensory receptor in the hand can be easily seen in the subcutaneous layer of the palm and finger (arrow)

during a hand operation. It is evident when observed by the naked eye and looks like rice under a microscope (Fig. 13.4). Sensory nerves are divided into three patterns: free sensory endings, sensory endings with expanded tips, and encapsulated sensory endings. Free sensory endings are unencapsulated and are responsible for sensing pain and temperature. Sensory endings with expanded tips are Merkel cells, which characterize glabrous skin. Ruffini complexes are sensors in hairy skin. Meissner's corpuscles and Pacinian corpuscles are considered encapsulated sensory endings. In particular, Meissner's corpuscles are responsible for tactile gnosis and discrimination [1].

Meissner's corpuscle and Pacinian corpuscles are composed of fast adapting myelinated nerve fibers. They provide touch, vibration, and tactile gnosis. If sensory receptors are considered part of the treatment of soft tissue defects of the thumb, we recommend a similar region of glabrous skin and receptors, such as a toe pulp or palm flap.

## Sensory Representation of the Human Thumb in Cortex

Since Penfield and Boldrey described somatic motor and sensory representations in the cerebral cortex in 1937, it has become widely known that the hands, tongue, and lips are associated with a wide area in the human brain cortex [8]. Continued studies have shown that the cortex area that is associated with the thumb is wider and is sensitive for both sensory and motor areas [9–11].

Sutherling et al. found that thumb is associated with a larger cortex area than the other fingers. There is non-overlapping somatotopy of all digits [9]. Roux et al. found that more areas were associated with the thumb than for the other four fingers in the hemisphere. Notably, they reported that the mean hand and tongue positive intensity thresholds were lower than for other parts of the body, indicating that the hand and tongue are more sensitive than other body parts [10]. Martuzzi et al. found that thumb magnification in the cortex is not due to a larger skin region of the thumb but more likely reflects a higher number of neurons and/or a larger associated cortex volume. This perspective is important when considering the human thumb's role in tactile perception. They also found that thumb magnification has not been observed in nonhuman primates [11].

Thus, the thumb and the hand are very significant in the context of the brain cortex. In modern society, traditional hand function remains important, but small motor function and hand sensitivity have become more meaningful as computer use increases. In recent years, the relationship between the hand and the brain cortex has been an important aspect of hand transplantation and the required neural remapping.

## Sensory Physical Examination

In general, sensory test evaluations should be distinguished according to the purpose of the sensory test, such as identifying any abnormality of the central nervous system (CNS) and evaluation of peripheral sensory nerve function after injury or recovery. The hand surgeon should be focused more on evaluating sensory loss and recovery using the range of sensory loss and the degree of sensation.

The sensory test for the hand includes the static and moving two-point discrimination (2PD) examination, the Semmes-Weinstein test, and tactile gnosis. Electromyography (EMG) and nerve conduction velocity (NCV) are usually performed to evaluate the motor nerve function. The sensory

NCV (sNCV) is used to evaluate the large diameter myelinated sensory nerve. Because small nerve fibers are not detectable by sNCV, this kind of test is not performed to evaluate hand peripheral nerves. Therefore, a thorough physical examination of the senses should be performed to confirm sensory loss and determine the cause of abnormal sensations. In addition to physical examination, a thorough medical history taking should aid in diagnosis and the choice of treatment plan options.

Sensory tests depend on patient cooperation and reliable reporting between the examiner and the patient. If normal communication is not possible, such as in cases of severe trauma, underlying CNS issues, or irritability, a complete sensory test cannot be performed. In addition, extra care should be taken in the sensory evaluation of children because their expression and understanding of various senses are immature.

Sensory transmission tracts are the spinothalamic tract and the dorsal column tract. Pain and temperature sensations are transmitted via the spinothalamic tract. Vibration, proprioception, and touch localization are transmitted via the dorsal column tract. Alcohol cotton is used regardless of the presence of pain, to test the anesthetic level in a brachial plexus block (BPB) or regional block. This test is based on the transmission of pain and temperature along the same nerve route. Pins and toothpicks are used for pain tests, and a tuning fork is used for vibration tests. However, these tests are not often used to assess the peripheral senses because they are gross testing methods that evaluate the subtle sensory states of each hand and the resin itself.

## Two-Point Discrimination (2PD)

This is the routine and basic method for sensory evaluation of hands. For this test, the patient closes his eyes, and the examiner touches two different points. The minimum distance at which the patient feels two points of contact is called the 2PD. Typically, this test uses a standardized device; however, if you do not have such a tool, to improve test accuracy, it is helpful to take repeated measurements.

The 2PD value is determined by the size of the receptive field. As the number of sensory receptors per unit area increases and the area of the same nerve decreases, the accuracy of the representation improves [12].

Sometimes, there is a poor correlation between the 2PD value and nerve recovery. The moving 2PD test compensates for this limitation because it is performed while moving the two-point measurement, in order to identify the fast adapting sensory system [13]. Moving 2PD correlates well with nerve recovery and has high interobserver reliability [14, 15]. Conventional 2PD is also called static 2PD to distinguish it from moving 2PD.

## Semmes-Weinstein Test

The Semmes-Weinstein test is usually used to compare sensory loss and sensory recovery. This test is for tactile and pressure sensations and is performed using a kit of monofilaments with varying thickness to fit the target force. The monofilament is pressed perpendicularly against the skin until it bends on the finger and palm. The examiner starts with a small filament.

## Tactile Gnosis

Tactile gnosis tests for the ability to recognize or identify different stimuli by touch. It can be performed using various objects of different sizes. Typically, various shapes of nuts, buttons, and other objects from daily life are used. For all objects, the patient must adjust his or her tactile senses without the use of sight.

# Symptoms and Cause

Although numbness and a tingling sensation are the typical symptoms for a sensory loss patient, the expression of this condition by the patient may be different. Patients express feelings such as "it does not feel like my own skin" or "it feels like bugs crawling." Some patients feel numb, an itch not resolved by scratching, or the sensation of wearing a rubber glove. Some patients do not complain much about numbness but require frequent massage.

Most causes of sensory loss in the thumb are the result of trauma. Trauma is characterized by direct nerve injury and soft tissue damage of the thumb. It is analogous to the concept of a landline phone and electrical wiring, where the electrical wiring is the nerve and the telephone is the sensory skin and soft tissue. In this context, treatment can be viewed as repairing the wiring and telephone or as using other home telephone wirings. As with all traumas, the mechanism of the trauma, any accompanying trauma, the patient's past history, vital signs, and general condition must be considered. The sensory loss of the thumb can be relevant to other diseases such as CNS disease, c-spine symptoms, or carpal tunnel syndrome, and any association must be confirmed.

Nerve injuries can be divided to high median nerve injuries, lower median nerve injuries, high radial nerve injuries, and lower radial nerve injuries. Damage to the area of the thumb itself can be distinguished into damage to the proper digital nerve itself and damage to the soft tissue unit. Nail is also important for the finger's sensory abilities. Nails enhance pulp sensitivity, increase pulp stability, and are necessary for fine prehension [16].

In severe paralysis such as poliomyelitis, the movement of the hands is poor, but the sensation is normal. Multiple difficult motions are required to perform a task, but there is no skin damage or infection of the thumb due to sensory loss. Digital nerve laceration has no direct effect on motor function. However, the patient's thumb behavior is clumsy, or use of their thumb requires the patient to look at the hand.

In lower median nerve injury, there is palsy and sensory loss in thenar muscles at fingers 1, 2, and 3 and the radial side of finger 4. Sensory recovery tends to be poor if the motor recovery is poor. High median nerve damage affects the motor function of the forearm and hands. In this case, it is more important to recover motor function than recover sensation in the hand. Cutaneous sensation should be restored before performing a tendon transfer to treat median nerve palsy, if possible.

## Treatment

If nerve damage is caused by direct laceration, the best choice of treatment is direct repair with meticulous and atraumatic methods without a gap or tension. If there is a nerve defect, a nerve graft or nerve conduit can be used. In the case of severe damage to the thumb itself or thumb amputation, the toe-to-thumb can be considered for whole tissue reconstruction, including nerve reconstruction. This is a good method to recover the thumb's function and aesthetic appearance [17, 18].

The degree of sensory loss due to a soft tissue defect of the thumb depends on the size and depth of the defect. A small range of damage can be solved by a skin graft, which can restore some of the sensation. However, if there is a large defect, a sensory flap is used. Many surgeons perform sensory flaps, and these have various names according to their preferred methods. But if we classified these flaps, they are divided into pedicled flaps and free flaps that include sensory nerves. In much of the literature, the pedicled flaps include two overlying methods. First, there is a cutaneous flap of the ulnar side of the third finger that uses the proper digital artery. This method includes sensory nerves based on the Littler flap. Second, there is a cutaneous flap of the dorsal side of the second finger that uses the interosseous artery. This method includes sensory nerves based on the kite flap. In the pedicled flap, the most important issue is the failure of sensory switching, in which the sensation of the flap is not accepted as a thumb. This phenomenon is characterized by double sensitivity, erroneous localization, or allachesthesia. To overcome allachesthesia, the nerve of island flap is cut and connected to the recipient nerve [19–22]. A free flap for sensory loss reconstruction is performed using a toe pulp free flap and a palmar free flap

[23, 24]. The sensory nerve of the toe pulp is a proper plantar digital nerve, and the sensory nerve of a palmar cutaneous flap is mainly the palmar cutaneous branch of the median nerve.

Pedicled flaps and free flaps all have advantages and disadvantages, none of which are absolute. The pedicled flap requires a wider dissection within the hand itself because the pedicle must be shifted to the thumb. However, there is an advantage in that anastomosis is not necessary. The free flap is useful because it uses the glabrous skin of the foot without any hand morbidity. It takes skin that is similar to the thumb, including the sensory qualities. However, due to differences in the preference of the surgeon and the burden of the anastomotic vessels, it cannot be said that any one of these is the best choice. It is possible that what I do well is not always good for others, and there may be techniques unfamiliar to me that are useful. Therefore, it is important to choose the most reasonable method according to patient's condition and the surgeon's preference.

## Nerve Repair

When sensory loss is solely caused by nerve trauma, it is best to suture the nerve. It is not difficult to nerve suture when there has been a sharp cut. But it may be necessary to remove some damaged nerve if the trauma is caused by compression or multiple instances of nerve damage. If a gap or tension on nerves occurs during the neurorrhaphy, a nerve graft is performed. If the nerve is not thick and the gap is relatively short, a nerve conduit may be used. However, nerve grafts are generally performed in large nerves.

After a sharp laceration injury, performing a nerve suture on the upper extremity of a peripheral nerve injury had better repair outcomes for the median and radial nerves than for the ulnar nerve. Secondary suture and graft repair outcomes were better for the median nerve than for the radial nerve and ulnar nerve [25]. The nerve restoration for a high median nerve injury is less than for a lower median nerve injury. If sensation is not restored after nerve repair, there are few options for surgical sensory restoration [4]. Restoring sensation of the thumb after radial nerve damage may not be necessary because sensory deficits from this injury are limited and sensation from the dorsal surface of the hand is less functionally important [26, 27].

## Pedicled Flap

### Third Finger Ulnar Side Cutaneous Island Flap Using Proper Digital Artery

This is a modification of the Littler flap that adds the sensory nerve [28]. It is mainly used for the ulnar side dorsolateral cutaneous tissue of finger 3 at the level of the middle phalanx. Sometimes the radial side of finger 4 is used. Usually the proper digital nerve is used as the sensory nerve. The vascular pedicle is dissected to the common palmar digital artery. Sometimes the vascular pedicle is extended to the superficial palmar arch. The ulnar side digital artery of finger 2 is ligated and cut for the rotation arc to the thumb [20]. For venous drainage, the vascular pedicle is elevated to include at least a 5 mm width of subcutaneous tissue.

Littler flaps are a useful method that can be used to reconstruct thumbs in institutions where microsurgery is burdensome or in the absence of microscopy equipment. However, this method involves donor site morbidities, including sensory loss, cold intolerance, and painful neuroma in some cases. There can also still be poorer sensory switching from the recipient site, residual paresthesia, and deterioration of the 2PD value over time [21]. To overcome allachesthesia and poor sensory switching, the simplest method is to cut the donor nerve and repair it to the recipient nerve [21]. A proper digital nerve or a dorsal branch of digital nerve is used for the flap [19, 20]. If the partial proper digital nerve is used rather than whole proper digital nerve, a nerve graft can be performed to prevent donor sensory loss morbidity [19]. However, if a partial proper digital nerve is used, pedicle elevation must be performed carefully and meticulously to prevent pedicle damage.

## Second Finger Dorsal Side Cutaneous Flap Using Dorsal Interosseous Artery

This method is the kite flap that includes the sensory nerve. The flap is mainly designed for the dorsum of finger 2 at the level of the proximal phalanx. If necessary, the donor area may extend to the middle phalanx. The pedicle is the first interosseous artery that branches from the radial artery that is past the snuffbox site. To allow for stable venous drainage, the pedicle should include more than 5 mm of subcutaneous tissue [29]. Sensory nerves usually include the superficial radial nerve. To further enhance the sensory ability of the thumb, the dorsal branch of the second finger might be elevated, including the proper digital nerve. After that, the donor proper digital nerve that is included in the flap undergoes neurorrhaphy to the proper digital nerve of the recipient thumb [29] (Fig. 13.5). In order to prevent allachesthesia, a superficial radial nerve that was originally distributed in the flap is cut and undergoes neurorrhaphy to the proper digital nerve on the dorsal branch of the recipient thumb [22].

## Free Flap

### Toe Pulp Free Flap

Sensory receptors of toe pulp are similar to those in the glabrous skin of the thumb and finger. Therefore, toe pulp can be the best choice for finger pulp reconstruction. Pulps from the second toe, the medial side of great toe, and the toe wrap-around flap are good candidates for a free flap reconstruction. The sensation recovery from these flaps is quite fast and has good results [30–33]. In the case of second toe pulp, primary repair of the donor site is possible even when about half of the pulp is harvested

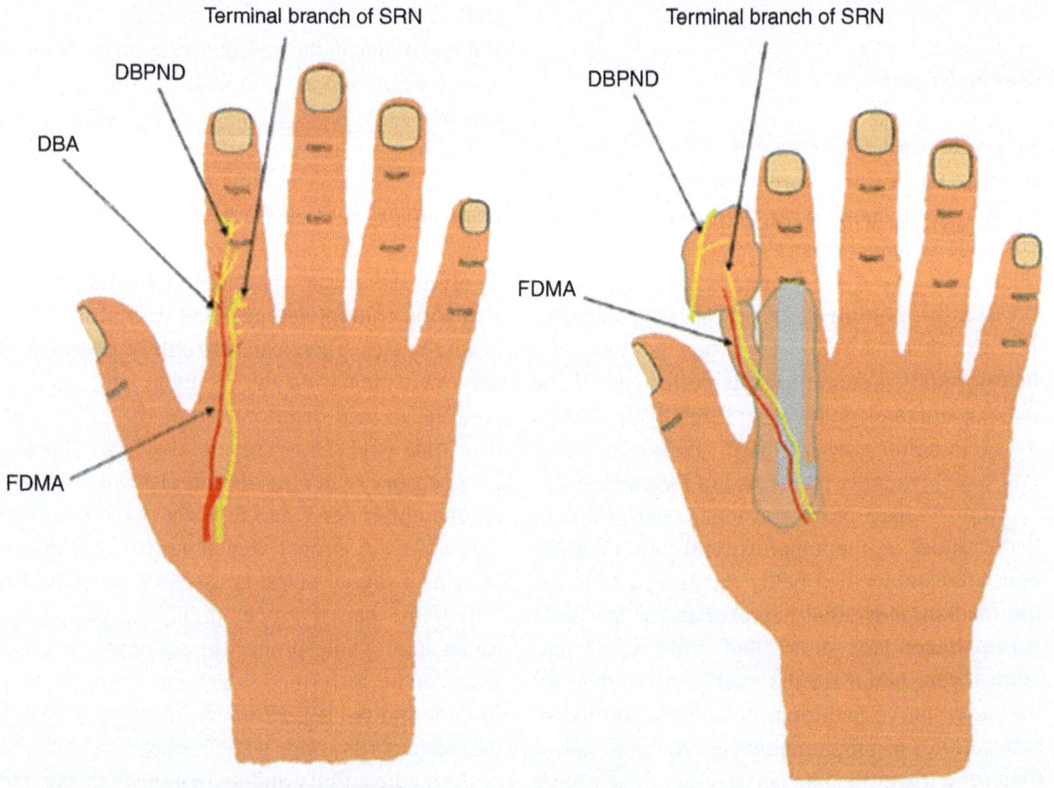


**Fig. 13.5** Modified kite flap, including the dorsal branch of the proper digital nerve. A superficial radial nerve is included with the first interosseous artery (from Wang et al. [29])

(Fig. 13.6). It is important to include the subcutaneous vein and surrounding subcutaneous tissue for venous drainage. Both the donor site and toe are reliable, and there are no gait problems if the flap size is less than half of the toe. The sensory recovery and aesthetic shape are also good [33, 34].

## Radial Artery Perforator Flap

This is the cutaneous flap that uses the perforator from the radial artery at wrist level, including the palmar cutaneous branch from the median nerve. It is used for defects that are relatively long and wide in volar areas on the thumb and finger. Basically, palmar skin has similar characteristics and concentration of sensory endings as glabrous skin [35]. The width of the flap is about 1.5 cm, and the length extends from the wrist crease to the proximal transverse crease. Primary repair is possible, and there is no need for carpal tunnel release during primary repair. A superficial perforator artery is branched within 1 cm, proximal to the radial styloid process. To ensure stable blood flow into the flap, the flap requires palmar cutaneous lesions over the scaphoid tubercle [23].

## Nerve Graft/Nerve Conduit

Nerve defects above the proper digital nerve are usually treated by a nerve graft. But for a proper digital nerve gap, a nerve conduit using a vein is also a common treatment. The results of these two procedures at proper digital nerve may be similar, due to the compensation from the other nerves. The use of a nerve conduit also prevents neuroma formation in the digital nerve [36].

A nerve defect concerns an actual amount of nerve tissue. In contrast, nerve gap is the distance between the proximal end and the distal end of "injured nerve." Therefore, a nerve gap might be

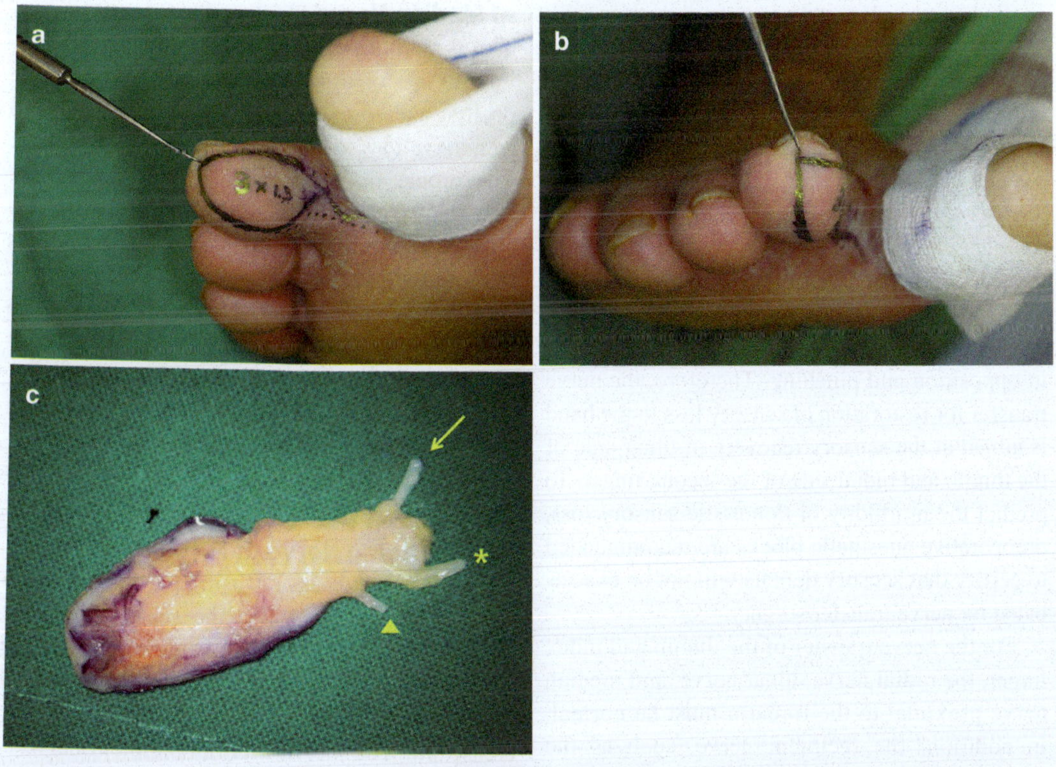


**Fig. 13.6** Second toe pulp harvest. (**a**) Second toe pulp for harvest is designated on the median side of the toe. (**b**) Half of the toe pulp is available for primary repair. Although vein skeletonization can be performed, subcutaneous tissue is included for venous drainage. (**c**) Base of the toe pulp flap. Artery (▲), vein (arrow), and plantar digital nerve (*)

considered more severe than a nerve defect. Harvest of a donor nerve is performed after the recipient site has been completely dissected or determined. The nerves of interest must be measured in the various postures of the extended state, and an extra 10–15% of nerve length is recommended for harvest. These considerations are necessary to ensure atraumatic technique. It is important to maintain moisture of the nerve during the harvest. The posterior interosseous nerve or the anterior interosseous nerve is used to replace the digital nerve. For an extremity nerve, the lateral or median antebrachial cutaneous nerve is appropriate. For an extremity nerve defect of the relatively thick brachial plexus, the sural nerve can be used.

## Nerve Transfer

Nerve transfer is the process of sacrificing normal nerve and reinnervating the normal nerve of the paralyzed area. This technique is mostly applied in the damage of the proximal nerves such as sensory loss region nerve repair, brachial plexus injury, and high median nerve injury rather than focal lesions. Nerve transfer is performed only if the functional/sensory loss of the recipient is more uncomfortable and severe than the loss of the donor site, whether it is motor neurons or sensory nerve. The most critical part of the sensory loss of the hand is the ulnar side of the thumb and the radial side of the second finger. This is because these areas are mainly contacted in opposition and pinching. Therefore, the nerve transfer for restoration of sensory loss in the hand is aimed at the sensory recovery of ulnar side of the thumb and radial side of the second finger. To predict the morbidity of donor site sensory loss, preoperative anesthetic blocks are recommended to certify that sensory deficits will not be exacerbated by nerve transfer surgery.

For the nerve transfer of the thumb and index finger, the radial nerve, ulnar nerve, and median nerve proximal to the forearm must be normal. In addition, the recipient nerve, such as the proper digital nerve of the thumb and the second finger to connect the transferred nerve, should be normal. For an effective nerve transfer, blood flow should be included in the transferred nerve as much as possible. Nerve transfer area should be soft, has abundant blood flow, and no scar [37]. To minimize tension, the donor and recipient nerve should be as long as possible [26].

In the nerve transfer, even if the nerve is sensated, it is remembered as the donor site sensory in the brain. Therefore, reeducation and rehabilitation are necessary. Through this process, the brain adapts to the sensory of the new domain. Usually, the sensation recovers within 3–6 months after the surgery. This process is quicker if the patient is younger and more intelligent. The better the patient is able to concentrate with motivation, the better the sensory rehabilitation. The first step is the localization of a stimulus. The second step is to recognize the stimulating object. This process is done with opened eyes at first and then later with closed eyes, repeatedly.

### Superficial Radial Nerve to First and Second Proper Digital Nerve of Median Nerve

This is mainly used for median nerve injury proximal to the forearm. The superficial radial nerve on first and second finger dorsum is neurotized (reinnervation) to the proper volar digital nerve. The proper digital nerve is performed on the ulnar side of the thumb and the radial side of the second finger (Fig. 13.7) [38]. The incision is made in the first web space, and a V-shaped incision is performed dorsally or palmar based. The entire first web space may be dissected. If the soft tissue of the first web space is not in good condition from scarring or trauma, it may be performed at the wrist level (Fig. 13.8) [37].

### Dorsal Ulnar Nerve to First and Second Proper Digital Nerve of Median Nerve

Superficial radial nerve is using the dorsal branch of the ulnar nerve. Since the transferred pivot point is far to the target site and the path of the nerve is long, it is technically difficult. It is passed through the subpalmar layer of the mid-palmar crease site. The location of the recipient nerve is similar to that of the superficial radial nerve (Fig. 13.9) [37].

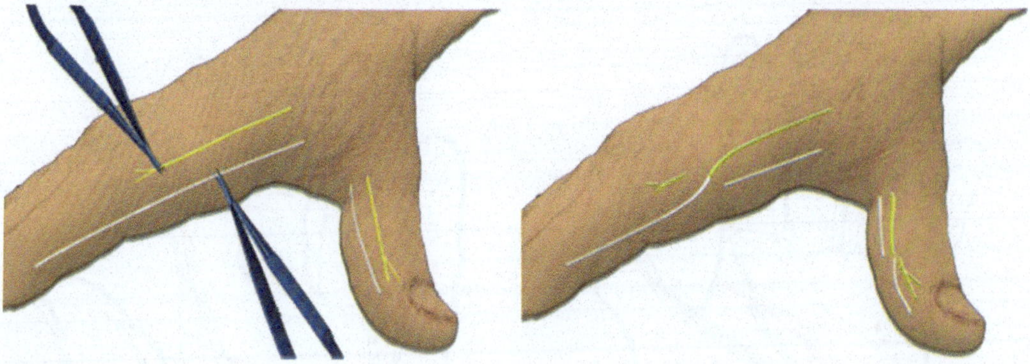

Fig. 13.7 The concept of nerve transfer from superficial radial nerve to proper digital nerve (from Bertelli and Ghizoni [38])

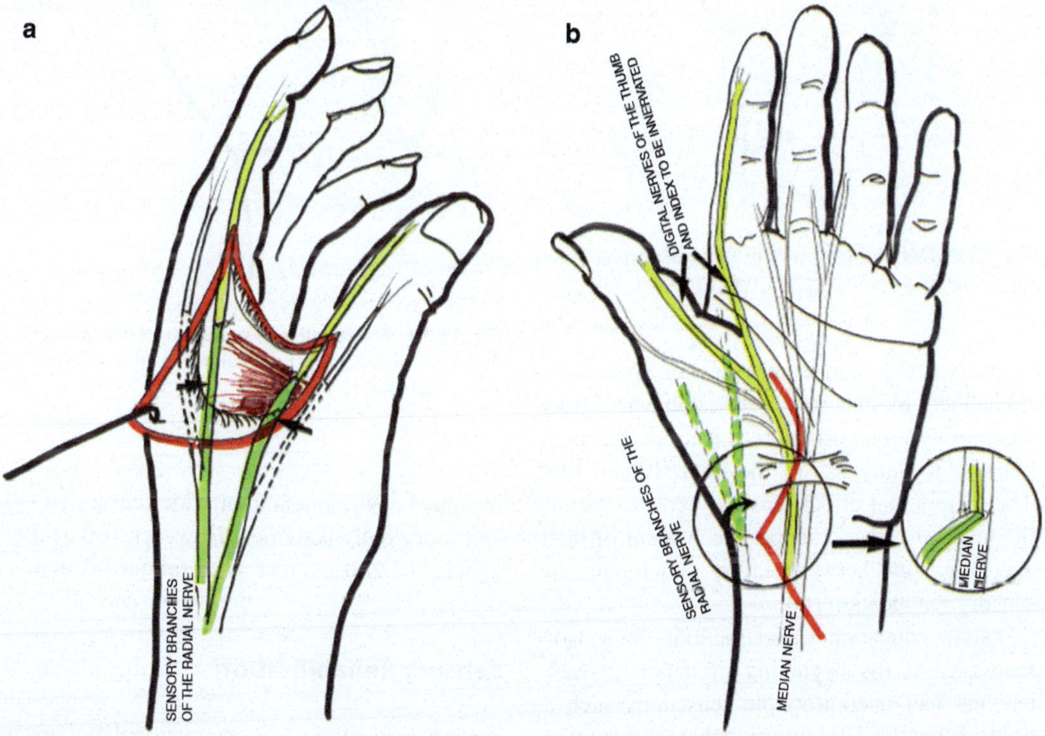


Fig. 13.8 Superficial radial nerve to first and second proper digital nerve of median nerve at first web space level (**a**) and wrist level (**b**) (from Brunelli [37])

### Fourth Web Space Proper Digital Nerve to the First and Second Proper Digital Nerve of the Median Nerve

Fourth web space proper digital nerve uses the nerves of the ulnar side of the fourth finger and the radial side of the fifth finger. The volar ulnar nerve is connected to the median nerve running to the thumb and index finger (Fig. 13.10) [37].

## Sensory Recovery, Education, and Rehabilitation

### Sensory Recovery and Education

The order of sensory recovery restoration is pain, temperature, and then touch [1]. Sensory

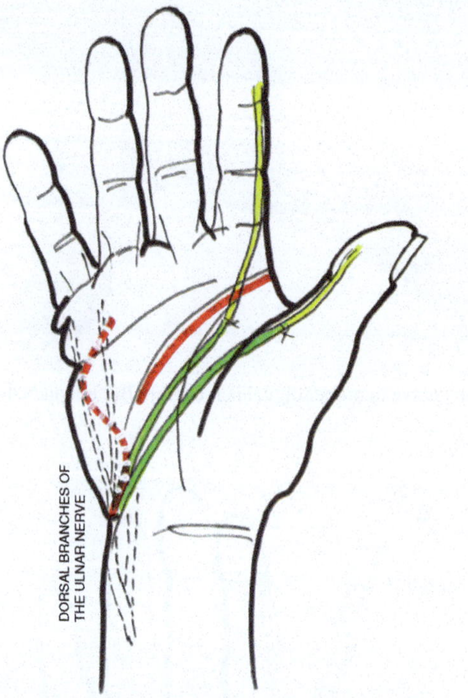


**Fig. 13.9** Dorsal ulnar nerve to first and second proper digital nerve of median nerve (from Brunelli [37])

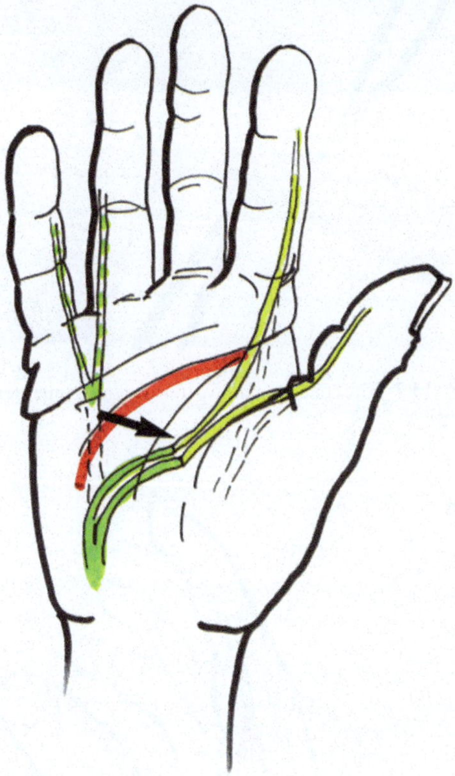

**Fig. 13.10** The fourth web space proper digital nerve to first and second proper digital nerve of median nerve (from Brunelli [37])

recovery is slow and requires several years and is influenced by the newly re-established fiber-receptor system, cortical reeducation, and attentiveness to daily use of the injured hand [39]. The factors that affect sensory recovery include the level of nerve damage, mechanism of damage, age, time between injury and repair, and sensory reeducation [40].

Patient education is also important for sensory recovery. At the beginning of nerve recovery, patients feel uncomfortable sensations such as tingling, but this is a good sign that the nerves are being regenerated. Therefore, it is good to explain the meaning of these symptoms to patients. The patients are also recommended to avoid cold or wind. Emotional stress and peripheral stimuli should be carefully controlled. Gloves can be helpful in cold weather. Because stimulation does not produce a response, injuries occur easily. Inadvertent stimulation may lead to wounds, secondary infection, and soft tissue defects in severe cases. The home program uses moisture cream and massage. It is also advisable to pick up beans in a quiet environment to provide sensory stimuli and to try daily activities. However, it is recommended to stop and rest when fatigue occurs.

## Sensory Rehabilitation

Sensory reeducation and occupational therapy are important for maintaining sensation and function [1]. Sensory reeducation is composed of two phases [39]. The early phase begins with reinnervation and the perception of feeling in the fingertip. Initially, it is performed using familiar objects, such as a pencil eraser, with the eyes open and then closed. The patient expresses whether she/he feels movement on the finger [41]. The late phase is performed when feelings of static, moving 2PD begins on the fingertips. Late-phase sensory reeducation includes the Moberg pickup test, locognosia exercises, and the identification of specific objects among similar objects, such as coins, keys, screws, or nuts [39, 42, 43].

## References


1. Halbert CF, Wei FC. Neurosensory free flaps. Digits and hand. Hand Clin. 1997;13:251–62.
2. Swartz WM. Restoration of sensibility in mutilating hand injuries. Clin Plast Surg. 1989;16:515–29.
3. Tecchio F, Zappasodi F, Melgari JM, Porcaro C, Cassetta E, Rossini PM. Sensory-motor interaction in primary hand cortical areas: a magnetoencephalography assessment. Neuroscience. 2006;141:533–42.
4. Ko JW, Mirarchi AJ. Late reconstruction of median nerve palsy. Orthop Clin North Am. 2012;43:449–57.
5. Jolley BJ, Stern PJ, Starling T. Patterns of median nerve sensory innervation to the thumb and index finger: an anatomic study. J Hand Surg Am. 1997;22:228–31.
6. Zaidenberg EE, Palumbo D, Martinez E, Pastrana M, Farias Cisneros E, Zaidenberg CR. Innervation of the interphalangeal joint of the thumb: anatomical study. J Hand Surg Eur Vol. 2018;43:631–4.
7. Bas H, Kleinert JM. Anatomic variations in sensory innervation of the hand and digits. J Hand Surg Am. 1999;24:1171–84.
8. Penfield W, Boldrey E. Somatic motor and sensory representation in the cerebral cortex of man as studied by electrical stimulation. Brain. 1937;60:389–443.
9. Sutherling WW, Levesque MF, Baumgartner C. Cortical sensory representation of the human hand: size of finger regions and nonoverlapping digit somatotopy. Neurology. 1992;42:1020–8.
10. Roux FE, Djidjeli I, Durand JB. Functional architecture of the somatosensory homunculus detected by electrostimulation. J Physiol. 2018;596:941–56.
11. Martuzzi R, van der Zwaag W, Farthouat J, Gruetter R, Blanke O. Human finger somatotopy in areas 3b, 1, and 2: a 7T fMRI study using a natural stimulus. Hum Brain Mapp. 2014;35:213–26.
12. Lundborg G, Rosen B. The two-point discrimination test--time for a re-appraisal? J Hand Surg Br. 2004;29:418–22.
13. Dellon AL. The moving two-point discrimination test: clinical evaluation of the quickly adapting fiber/receptor system. J Hand Surg Am. 1978;3:474–81.
14. Dellon AL, Kallman CH. Evaluation of functional sensation in the hand. J Hand Surg Am. 1983;8:865–70.
15. Dellon AL, Mackinnon SE, Crosby PM. Reliability of two-point discrimination measurements. J Hand Surg Am. 1987;12:693–6.
16. Ozcelik IB, Tuncer S, Purisa H, Sezer I, Mersa B, Kabakas F, et al. Sensory outcome of fingertip replantations without nerve repair. Microsurgery. 2008;28:524–30.
17. Woo SH, Kim JS, Seul JH. Immediate toe-to-hand transfer in acute hand injuries: overall results, compared with results for elective cases. Plast Reconstr Surg. 2004;113:882–92.
18. Woo SH, Yoo MJ, Paeng JW. Recent advances in immediate toe-to-hand transfer. J Hand Surg Asian Pac Vol. 2016;21:292–9.
19. Wang H, Yang X, Chen C, Wang B, Wang W, Jia S. Modified Littler flap for sensory reconstruction of large thumb pulp defects. J Hand Surg Eur Vol. 2018;43:546–53.
20. Hirase Y, Kojima T, Matsuura S. A versatile one-stage neurovascular flap for fingertip reconstruction: the dorsal middle phalangeal finger flap. Plast Reconstr Surg. 1992;90:1009–15.
21. Oka Y. Sensory function of the neurovascular island flap in thumb reconstruction: comparison of original and modified procedures. J Hand Surg Am. 2000;25:637–43.
22. Feng SM, Sun QQ, Cheng J, Wang AG, Li CK. Superficial radial nerve transection improves sensory outcomes in first dorsal metacarpal artery flaps. Plast Reconstr Surg. 2017;140:558–64.
23. Yang JW, Kim JS, Lee DC, Ki SH, Roh SY, Abdullah S, et al. The radial artery superficial palmar branch flap: a modified free thenar flap with constant innervation. J Reconstr Microsurg. 2010;26:529–38.
24. Lee TP, Liao CY, Wu IC, Yu CC, Chen SG. Free flap from the superficial palmar branch of the radial artery (SPBRA flap) for finger reconstruction. J Trauma. 2009;66:1173–9.
25. Murovic JA. Upper-extremity peripheral nerve injuries: a Louisiana State University Health Sciences Center literature review with comparison of the operative outcomes of 1837 Louisiana State University Health Sciences Center median, radial, and ulnar nerve lesions. Neurosurgery. 2009;65:A11–7.
26. Bertelli JA, Cavalli E, Mendes Lehn VL, Ghizoni MF. Sensory deficits after a radial nerve injury. Microsurgery. 2018;38:151–6.
27. Soldado F, Bertelli JA, Ghizoni MF. High median nerve injury: motor and sensory nerve transfers to restore function. Hand Clin. 2016;32:209–17.
28. Liu H, Regmi S, He Y, Hou R. Thumb tip defect reconstruction using neurovascular island pedicle flap obtained from long finger. Aesthet Plast Surg. 2016;40:755–60.
29. Wang H, Chen C, Li J, Yang X, Zhang H, Wang Z. Modified first dorsal metacarpal artery island flap for sensory reconstruction of thumb pulp defects. J Hand Surg Eur Vol. 2016;41:177–84.
30. Woo SH, Choi BC, Oh SJ, Seul JH. Classification of the first web space free flap of the foot and its applications in reconstruction of the hand. Plast Reconstr Surg. 1999;103:508–17.
31. Woo SH, Lee GJ, Kim KC, Ha SH, Kim JS. Immediate partial great toe transfer for the reconstruction of composite defects of the distal thumb. Plast Reconstr Surg. 2006;117:1906–15.
32. Wei FC, Chen HC, Chuang DC, Chen S, Noordhoff MS. Second toe wrap-around flap. Plast Reconstr Surg. 1991;88:837–43.

33. Lee DC, Kim JS, Ki SH, Roh SY, Yang JW, Chung KC. Partial second toe pulp free flap for fingertip reconstruction. Plast Reconstr Surg. 2008;121:899–907.
34. Wallace CG, Wei FC. Posttraumatic finger reconstruction with microsurgical transplantation of toes. Hand Clin. 2007;23:117–28.
35. Strauch B, Tsur H. Restoration of sensation to the hand by a free neurovascular flap from the first web space of the foot. Plast Reconstr Surg. 1978;62:361–7.
36. Alligand-Perrin P, Rabarin F, Jeudy J, Cesari B, Saint-Cast Y, Fouque PA, et al. Vein conduit associated with microsurgical suture for complete collateral digital nerve severance. Orthop Traumatol Surg Res. 2011;97:S16–20.
37. Brunelli GA. Sensory nerves transfers. J Hand Surg Br. 2004;29:557–62.
38. Bertelli JA, Ghizoni MF. Very distal sensory nerve transfers in high median nerve lesions. J Hand Surg Am. 2011;36:387–93.
39. Mavrogenis AF, Spyridonos SG, Antonopoulos D, Soucacos PN, Papagelopoulos PJ. Effect of sensory re-education after low median nerve complete transection and repair. J Hand Surg. 2009;34:1210–5.
40. Dellon AL. Sensory recovery in replanted digits and transplanted toes: a review. J Reconstr Microsurg. 1986;2:123–9.
41. Wei FC, Ma HS. Delayed sensory reeducation after toe-to-hand transfer. Microsurgery. 1995;16:583–5.
42. Marsh D. The validation of measures of outcome following suture of divided peripheral nerves supplying the hand. J Hand Surg Br. 1990;15:25–34.
43. Moberg E. Objective methods for determining the functional value of sensibility in the hand. J Bone Joint Surg Br. 1958;40-B:454–76.

# 14 Motor Loss

Jong-Pil Kim and Jae-Sung Yoo

The thumb motion in a human is facilitated through the coordination of intrinsic thenar and extrinsic musculatures. Therefore, it is noted that the thumb dynamically allows for precision pinching and power gripping movements. The most important function of the thumb is opposition to the index finger and to the other fingers [1–3]. The ability to oppose the thumb is necessary for both of the characteristic precision pinching and power gripping movements of the hand. Sterling Bunnell [4] defined opposition as "diametrically opposite the fingers with the thumb pulp facing the fingers and the thumb nail parallel to the volar surfaces of the fingers."

The opposition of the thumb is a complex motion made by coordination of (1) the abduction of the thumb from the palmar surface of the index finger, (2) the flexion of the metacarpophalangeal joint of the thumb, (3) the internal rotation or pronation of the thumb, (4) the radial deviation of the proximal phalanx of the thumb on the metacarpal, and (5) the motion of the thumb toward the fingers. When the thenar muscles are paralyzed, the balance of the hand is disrupted as well as loss of power to perform principal function of the thumb. That is, the thumb keeps an adducted position by the extrinsic musculatures such as extensor pollicis longus (EPL) and flexor pollicis longus (FPL), because these muscles are not opposed by the intrinsic muscles working for opposition and abduction. The hyperextended metacarpophalangeal (MCP) joint increases tension on the long thumb flexor tendon, that crosses the volar side of the joint, while the interphalangeal (IP) joint is flexed because of the FPL, which is unopposed by the paralyzed intrinsic muscles such as abductor pollicis brevis (APB) and adductor pollicis muscles (AP).

The prime muscle of thumb opposition is the APB, and both of the opponens pollicis (OP) and FPB also produce some opposition. Thus, any damage to the median nerve certainly can be the cause of a loss of thumb opposition. Of course, a noted injury to one of the three main nerves can cause a loss of thumb function and/or sensibility to that region. The ulnar nerve injury decreases thumb adduction force which is primarily provided by AP with the first dorsal interosseous (DI) [2]. In fact, the case of a radial nerve palsy also creates a disability in the thumb, which is predominantly loss of thumb extension and the consequent awkward flexed position.

J.-P. Kim (✉)
Hand and Microsurgery Division, Department of Orthopaedic Surgery, Dankook University College of Medicine, Cheonan, South Korea

Department of Kinesiology and Medical Science, Graduate School, Dankook University, Cheonan, South Korea
e-mail: kimjp@dankook.ac.kr

J.-S. Yoo
Hand and Microsurgery Division, Department of Orthopaedic Surgery, Dankook University College of Medicine, Cheonan, South Korea
e-mail: osarthro@dkuh.co.kr



S. H. Woo (ed.), *The Thumb*, https://doi.org/10.1007/978-981-10-4400-7_14

The tendon transfers to restore thumb motor function have the potential to greatly improve hand function, and the patient's well-being and ability to pursue a "normal" life. The principles of the tendon transfer surgery must be adhered to in all areas, regardless of whether the transfers are to restore median, ulnar, or radial nerve motor function.

## Principles of Restoration of Thumb Motor Function

The restoration of thumb function is divided into two separate stages: the opposition and the grasp. The restoration of opposition does not require a strong tendon transfer. Therefore, any tendons capable of moving the thumb can be used as an effective donor for opponensplasty, whereas a restoration of the power grasp which is mainly contributed by the key pinch usually requires a strong tendon transfer. However, if both functions are compromised and reconstructive surgeries are necessary, it should be noted that the restoring opposition is the first priority [5].

The thumb opposition depends primarily on function of its intrinsic muscles. Among them, the APB is the most important for opposition, because it rotates internally and abducts the thumb away from the index and also is known to be able to assist the EPL in extending the thumb. From these reason, most of investigators from Littler [6] to current clinicians [3, 7] emphasized restoration of APB function for restoration of thumb opposition using the procedure of a tendon transfer.

## Planning Tendon Transfer

The power grasp is not rarely significantly compromised in a low median nerve injury, where the lesion is distal to the origin of the anterior interosseous nerve, because the AP and the FPB which are innervated by the ulnar nerve are not impaired in that lesion [2]. Therefore, the restoration of opposition is enough for improving hand function in isolated low median nerve injury.

It is important to evaluate the functional deficit in the hand when there is significant functional impairment and a restoration of thumb function is required. For example, if the paralysis is secondary to a median nerve injury, the sensory deficit is far more disabling than the motor deficit in some patients. This is especially true in those patients who have isolated median nerve injury because they still can abduct their thumb though the action of the deep head of the FPB which has a dual inneration from both median and ulnar nerves [8].

## Evaluation of Donor Muscles

Several critical issues must be considered before the selection of the transfer donor can be made for the procedure [2]. First, the donor muscle must have adequate strength to perform its intended function in the patient. The strength of a muscle is graded from 0 to 5 on the MRC scale (Table 14.1) [9]. It is important to remember and consider that the muscle usually loses strength by one grade; therefore, the strength of the donor muscle must be at least 4 or 5 for a satisfactory tendon transfer [10]. Second, the donors must be expendable, and its absence must not result in considerable functional impairment after transfer, which means that the remaining muscles must have sufficient strength to account for the loss of the function that has been provided by the donor. Third, the synergy and the amplitude of excursion of its tendon also should be considered, because rehabilitation of a muscle whose tendon has been transferred is less difficult when the transfer is synergistic [10]. Finally, the amplitude of the excursion of the tendon should be sufficient for satisfactory function, although it may not be as great as that

**Table 14.1** Medical Research Council scale of muscle strength [9]

| Muscle function level | Grade |
|---|---|
| No contraction | 0 |
| Palpable contraction only | 1 |
| Moves joint but not against gravity | 2 |
| Moves joint against gravity | 3 |
| Moves joint against gravity and resistance | 4 |
| Normal strength | 5 |

of the tendon or tendons that is replaced. Among these, the most important points to remember in considering a donor muscle for transfer are its strength and expendability [11].

## Timing of Tendon Transfer

If the recipient site is injured, the tendon transfer should not be done until scar tissue on the recipient's site has been satisfactorily replaced by the healthy ones, because a transferred tendon must be surrounded by fat to prevent them from adhering to a raw bone or a subcutaneous scar. It is impossible for the thumb to have a greater range of active motion in a stiff joint; therefore, the maximum passive motion of all joints in the thumb must be preserved before a tendon transfer can be performed. In addition, any noted malalignment of bones must be corrected by osteotomy, or any necessary bone grafting must be accomplished before the proposed transfer. The other procedures to restore any loss of sensibility also must be proceeded to the tendon transfer.

The tendon transfer is the final step in rehabilitation of the hand, and therefore, transfers for thumb motion must be sufficiently delayed until it is recovered after neurorrhaphy of the peripheral nerve injuries. When intrinsic paralysis occurs after a median nerve laceration, a neurorrhaphy is the preferable procedure to utilize the tendon transfer, if the injury is within a 6-month time frame. For a more chronic injury of more than a 6-month time frame, the tendon transfer would be the appropriate option, because the motor end plates proceed to degeneration and their corresponding muscles undergo fibrosis.

## Restoration of Thumb Opposition

### Correction of Thumb Deformity

The failure to detect an established adduction contracture of the first web space is a common cause of failure in restoration of an opposition. Therefore, deformities or disabilities of the digit must be corrected before or during an opponensplasty procedure to restore the function of the thumb properly.

In a case of median nerve paralysis, the only functioning thumb motors are the EPL, EPB, and APL, which result in fixed adduction and external rotational deformity of the thumb [12]. This deformity often can be corrected with physiotherapy and splintage, but if these treatments are unsuccessful, the thumb requires a dorsal web space incision [13, 14]. Through this incision, the fascia over the AP and the first DI muscles can be released and divided by a subperiosteal stripping of the ulnar side of the first metacarpal. The dorsal web space skin can also be widened with a Z-plasty, skin graft, or flap [15–18]. In severe contractures, both of the rotational osteotomy at the base of the thumb metacarpal and the trapeziectomy can be required [19, 20]. For further severe deformity which cannot be corrected by osteotomy, the arthrodesis of the first MCP joint with a 15° of flexion, and slight internal rotation may be indicated. A tendon transfer for opposition still may be useful after such an arthrodesis because the more proximal joints may allow some motion. At the same time, the carpometacarpal joint of the thumb must be freely movable, unrestricted by contracture of the joint capsule or other structures of the thumb web.

### Donor for Transfer

The flexor digitorum sublimis (FDS) is likely the most well described and widely used as a donor to achieve the thumb opposition, with numerous variations in techniques of donor harvest, pulley construction, and tendon insertion (Table 14.2). Among the FDSs, the tendon of the ring finger is primarily selected in most cases, and the second choice is the FDS to the middle finger. The most important point for the selection of the FDS as a donor, however, is that the FDS must be strong enough to restore opposition of the thumb as a transfer and the flexor digitorum profundus (FDP) in the same digit must be strong enough alone to flex the finger satisfactorily. Therefore, this technique is not indicated in high median nerve lesion or combined median and ulnar nerve lesions.

**Table 14.2** Satisfaction rate of opponensplasty

| Transferred tendon | Satisfaction rate | Reported studies |
|---|---|---|
| EIP | 88% | Anderson et al. [44] |
| | 88% | Burkhalter et al. [45] |
| FDS | 75%<br>78% | Kraker et al. [46]<br>Jacobs and Thompson [47] |
| | 81% | Jensen [48] |
| Palmaris longus | 93% | Terrono et al. [21] |
| | 91%<br>85% | Foucher et al. [49]<br>Park et al. [50] |
| ADM | 80% | Wissinger and Singsen [51] |

The extensor indicis proprius (EIP) is also an acceptable donor, which is popularly used in high median nerve palsy and other circumstance when the FDS tendons of the ring and middle finger are not available. There is no risk of loss of grip strength, and it does not require the surgical creation of a pulley, as the surgical step that EIP transfer goes around the ulna typically results in a creation of an ideal vector to achieve opposition [7].

The palmaris longus (PL) can be used as a simple transfer of opposition, which is known as Camitz opponensplasty. The PL can be transferred with minimal donor site morbidity in addition to no functional deficit. Furthermore, the PL works synergistically with the APB. The PL transfer is usually performed for restoration of thumb function from the loss of opposition and abduction due to severe thenar atrophy in carpal tunnel syndrome, but the technique is not recommended in the cases with a traumatic median nerve injury [21].

The abductor digiti minimi (ADM), which is a predictably available donor, can be used to restore opposition when other extrinsic donors are not available. The ADM has a similar dimension as the APB, which also can help with cosmesis by restoring some of the bulk of the thenar eminence in severe atrophy or congenital absence of the thenar muscle.

The wrist extensors such as extensor carpi ulnaris (ECU) and extensor carpi radialis longus (ECRL) with a free tendon interposition graft are also used as the next choices, but it should be considered only if the other wrist extensors are strong and have not been or will not be transferred elsewhere. The EDM is rarely selected because its strength is not enough to restore thumb opposition, and it requires tendon grafting to reach the point of attachment on the thumb.

## Surgical Techniques

**Extensor indicis proprius (EIP) transfer** (Fig. 14.1). It should be kept in mind that anatomic variance of the EIP includes its congenital absence at this level in 0–4%, radial location relative to extensor digitorum communis (EDC) in 10%, and multiple slips in 3–14% of humans or cadaveric specimens [7, 22, 23]. A dorsal transverse incision is made proximal to the MCP joint of the index finger, and the EIP is identified just ulnar and deep to the extensor digitorum communis to the index finger. The EIP is transected just proximal to the sagittal bands, and the rem-

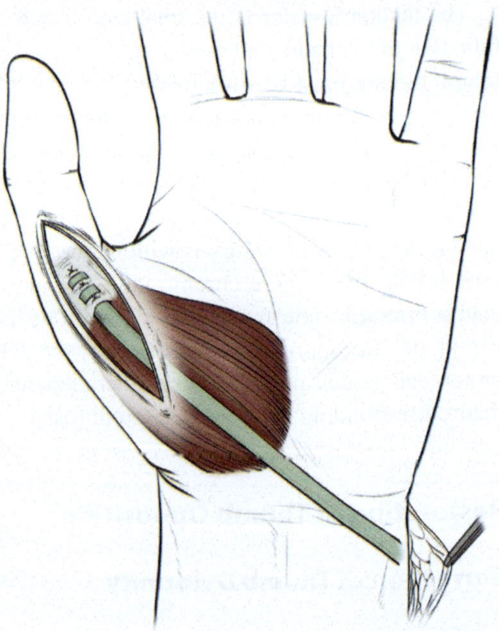

**Fig. 14.1** Extensor indicis proprius is delivered into a dorsoulnar wrist incision and passed through a subcutaneous tunnel around the wrist to an incision over the thumb metacarpophalangeal joint, and then it is sutured to the abductor pollicis brevis tendon

nant distal stump is sutured to the intact EDC to assist an even distribution of extensor strength across the MCP joint. Another incision is made proximal to the extensor retinaculum of the 4th compartment, where the musculotendinous junction of the EIP is identified. After the fascial attachments around the EIP are divided, the EIP is pulled proximally and withdrawn from this incision. Next, an oblique incision is made just proximal to the pisiform and distal forearm around the ulnar neck. And then the EIP is transferred to this incision through a subcutaneous tunnel. At this point, special care should be taken to avoid an iatrogenic injury to the dorsal cutaneous branch of the ulnar nerve. Next, a small incision is made on the dorsoradial aspect of the thumb MCP joint to expose the APB insertion. And the EIP is then subcutaneously passed over the ulna and the transverse carpal tunnel ligament and reached to the thumb MCP while ensuring that the tendon goes superficially to the FCU tendon. At this point, the ulna acts as a functional pulley for this tendon transfer. The transfer tendon is subsequently sutured into the APB insertion, with an appropriate tensioning that results in the thumb in maximal opposition with the wrist in 30° flexion [2].

Postoperatively, a thumb spica splint is applied for 4 weeks with the thumb and wrist held in a neutral position. The active assisted range of motion exercises starts at 4 weeks after surgery, and the resistive pinch and grip exercises start at 8–10 weeks. All activities except those that are requiring high demand can be allowed at 3–4 months.

**Flexor digitorum superficialis (FDS) transfer** (Fig. 14.2). The FDS is harvested through a 3–4 cm longitudinal incision on the radial border of the hypothenar muscle, which is overlying the A1 pulley of the ring or middle finger. Once the FDS is isolated, the proximal traction on the FDS typically with full flexion of the finger allows for the subsequent visualization of the bifurcation of FDS near to the Campers chasm, and the FDS is transected at this level. At this point, I do not recommend transecting near its insertion into the middle phalanx, because this technique has potential drawbacks, including the risk of devascularization of the vincular system in the FDS and the distinct possibility of the development of a swan neck deformity [24].

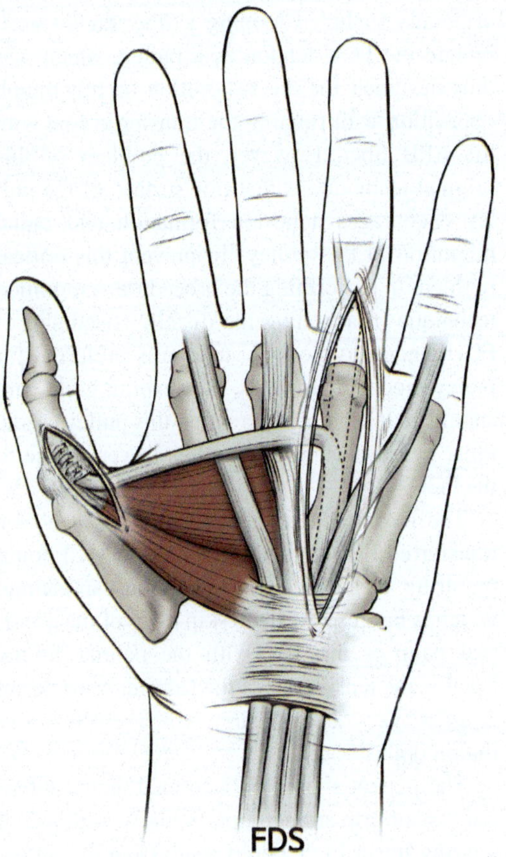


**Fig. 14.2** The window in the palmar fascia overlying the neck of the third metacarpal is used as a pulley, and the flexor digitorum superficialis transfer is attached to the abductor tubercle of the thumb

Once the donor FDS has been harvested distally, there are two options with regard to pulley formation: Royle-Thompson opponensplasty [25] and Bunnell's opponensplasty [4]. The Royle-Thompson procedure includes rerouting the FDS around the ulnar border of the palmar aponeurosis and transferring the FDS subcutaneously to the thumb. But this is not a favorite procedure to utilize, because the pulley is not fixed and migrated proximally [2]. Above all, a more crucial problem is that the vector of pull created with this technique is more suited to restore thumb flexion and abduction rather than the true opposition. The Bunnell's opponensplasty originally included looping a free tendon graft around the FCU tendon as a pulley, which was thus designed for the restoration of full thumb opposition with running the transfer in line with the APB fiber. However, the problem of this original technique is that raw surface of the pulley encourages adhesion formation and radial migration of this pulley. To prevent this critical problem in performing the procedure, a modified technique of attaching the distally based slip of FCU tendon to the ECU tendon is preferred for pulley reconstruction [2]. However, a great care should be taken during creating this pulley, as the ulnar neurovascular bundle lies in very close to the FCU.

The next steps is subcutaneous passage of a transferred FDS tendon to the thumb MCP joint, requiring a fairly aggressive blunt spreading, which is because the deep skin layer of the proximal palm is intimate with the palmar fascia. Finally, the tensioning of the transfer must be set as a passive wrist extension, which results in full thumb opposition.

The patient should be informed that a potential loss of grip strength, particularly with use of the ring finger FDS, could result from the pursuing of the procedure.

**Palmaris longus (PL) transfer (Camitz opponensplasty)** (Fig. 14.3). Before proceeding with this surgery, it should be confirmed whether the patients have a PL or not, because 15–20% of humans do not have the tendon [26, 27]. A skin incision is made starting with 2 cm proximal to the distal wrist crease with a zigzag fashion, running in line with the ring finger, and extending distally to the distal palmar crease. Since the PL is continuous distally with the pretendinous bands of the palmar aponeurosis, the PL can be free up enough length to reach the thumb, with a 1.0–1.5-cm-wide strip in continuity with the tendon. After an incision over the dorsoradial aspect of the thumb MCP joint is made, a subcutaneous tunnel is then created from an incision at the distal forearm incision to this incision. At this point, the palmar cutaneous branch of the median nerve, which runs radial to the PL and in the radial floor of the flexor carpi radialis sheath, must be preserved during the procedure. The transferred PL

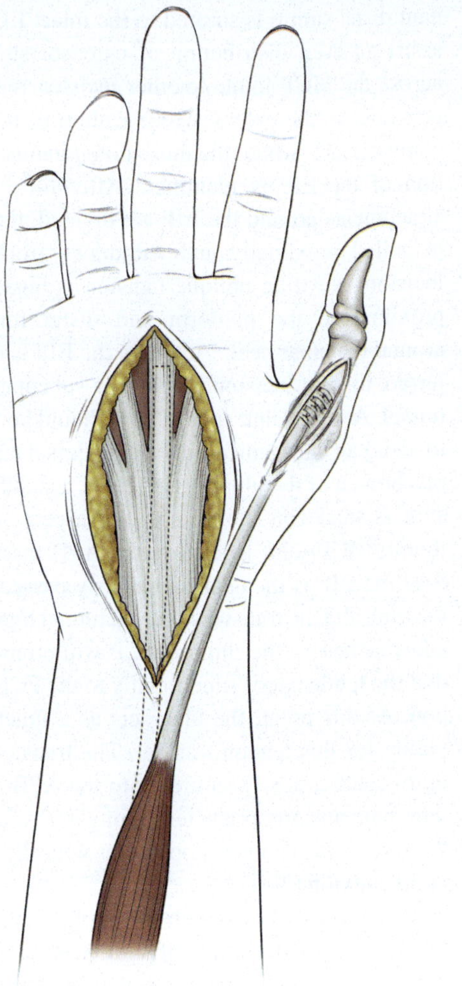

**Fig. 14.3** The palmaris longus is detached with a strip of palmar aponeurosis and attached to the abductor pollicis brevis insertion

is then sutured to the APB tendon with the thumb placed in passively full abduction while the wrist is held in a neutral position.

Several variations of a modified Camitz procedure, which is focusing on the incorporation and placement of a pulley, have been recently published [3, 28, 29]. Kang and colleagues [29] reported modified Camitz opponensplasty creating a transverse carpal ligament loop pulley in advanced carpal tunnel syndrome with good outcomes. However, there has been some debate about the necessity of performing a PL opponensplasty with the case of carpal tunnel syndrome, as a gradual recovery of thenar atrophy has been commonly noted after carpal tunnel release [28, 30].

**Abductor digiti minimi (ADM) transfer (Huber opponensplasty)** (Fig. 14.4) [31]. A midlateral incision is made on the ulnar border of the little finger and extended to a point just proximal to the pisiform. The insertion of the ADM into the proximal phalanx and extensor mechanism is meticulously incised, therefore maintaining as much length of the tendinous insertion as possible, ensuring an adequate length to reach the insertion site. And ADM is then meticulously separated from radially adjacent flexor digiti minimi and freed up from its originations including the pisiform, pisohamate ligament, and FCU, with a great care to preserve the neurovascular pedicle, which locates dorsoradially and just several millimeters distal from the pisiform [32, 33]. After a generous subcutaneous tunnel is created toward a second incision made over the APB insertion into the thumb, the ADM is subsequently passed through the tunnel. This step requires a turn through 180° on its longitudinal axis to reduce tension on neurovascular bundle supplying the ADM. Next, the thumb is placed in maximum opposition and the ADM is sutured appropriately. In some cases with an inadequate length, the transfer requires an augmentation with a free tendon interposition graft.

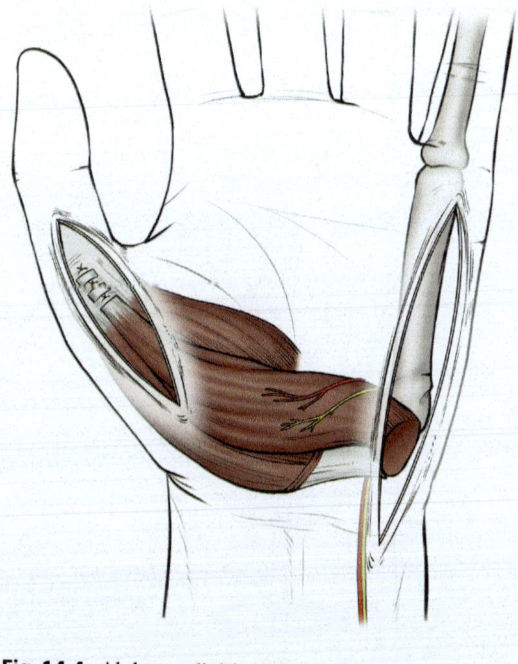

**Fig. 14.4** Abductor digiti minimi is detached with neurovascular structures while preserving an attachment to the flexor carpi ulnaris. The abductor digiti minimi is rotated on its long axis and passed subcutaneously and attached to the adductor pollicis brevis

## Restoration of Thumb Pinch

### Restoration of Thumb Adduction and Index Abduction

Adduction function of the thumb, which is primarily provided by adductor pollicis (AP), is as necessary for strong pinch as the abductor pollicis brevis (APB) is required for thumb opposition. Opposition is the refined, unique movement that places the tip of the thumb within the flexion arc of the fingers so that they can oppose, whereas adduction is the force that stabilizes the thumb in the desired position. If the AP is paralyzed, as noted in ulnar nerve palsy, a firm pinch between the pulps of the thumb and the flexed fingers is impossible (Froment sign). Although the FPL and EPL supports power of adduction, a loss of pinch power in ulnar nerve injury is estimated to 75–80% [34]. And their actions in the absence of the ulnar intrinsic eventually contribute to collapse of the thumb into a "Z-deformity," characterized by a hyperflexion of the IP joint and a hyperextension of the MCP joint of the thumb.

The aims of reconstructive surgery in the thumb with ulnar nerve palsy are the restoration of the adductor function which contributes to strong adduction of the thumb, active flexion of the extended MCP joint, and active extension of the flexed IP joint in order to regain power and precision function. Various tendon transfer techniques using the ECRB [35], FDS [36], EIP [37], or brachioradialis (BR) [36] have been devised to restore thumb adduction. However, such a transfer provides thumb adduction only.

If both of thumb adduction and opposition are absent and there is no other provision to restore adduction, a single tendon transfer to restore opposition should have its pulley located more distally to the pisiform, so that some adduction also is restored. On this point, the Royle-Thompson transfer is considered a better fit to this requirement, because a pulley of this technique is made by a step that the FDS of the ring finger is brought out in the palm distal to the deep transverse carpal ligament. The FDS transfer can also be used to restore both of abduction of the index finger and adduction of the thumb, via a procedure of splitting the FDS tendon and anchoring one slip to the tendon of the AP and the other to the insertion of the first dorsal interosseous (DI), as described by Omer [38].

In addition to restoring the adduction moment of the AP, it is important to determine whether the patient would benefit from the restoration of index finger abduction to augment pinch. That is because the stabilization of the index finger MCP joint for prevention of its drifting away from the thumb has a benefit to restore powerful pinch. Therefore, in the case of ulnar nerve palsy, the tendon transfer for restoration of thumb adduction can be combined with some procedures to restore abduction of the index finger. Several tendon transfers for restoration of index finger abduction have been described in the literature (Table 14.3) [39–42]. Although this transfer does not appreciably increase the pinch strength and it is not commonly performed, it can fairly support the index finger with stability and versatility [35]. I prefer to use accessory slip of the abductor pollicis longus (APL) via palmaris longus (PL) tendon graft. The EIP also can be used, but the result is unpredictable [43].

**Table 14.3** Surgical method and improvement of pinch strength

| Transferred tendon | Improvement of pinch strength | Reported studies |
|---|---|---|
| ECRB | 50% | Smith et al. [35] |
| ECRL | 73% (14–104%) | Fischer et al. [39] |
| Palmaris longus | Improvement (without comparison with contralateral side)<br>90% (71–107%) | Hirayama et al. [40]<br>Koh et al. [52] |
| EDM | 43% (35–52%) | Robinson et al. [41] |
| EPB and EPI | 62% (50–70%) | Alnot et al. [42] |
| ECRL, ECRB, and 4th FDS | 40% | Solonen and Bakalin [53] |

## Surgical Procedures of Thumb Adduction

**ECRB transfer** (Fig. 14.5). A dorsal transverse incision is made on the dorsum of the wrist, and the ECRB is released off the radial aspect of the third metacarpal base. After making a second incision proximal to wrist extensor retinaculum, the ECRB is then delivered out from this incision. A third incision is made between the dorsal aspects of the metacarpal base of the middle and ring fingers (third intermetacarpal space), followed by a creation of intermetacarpal space for passing the transfer tendon. Next, a longitudinal incision is

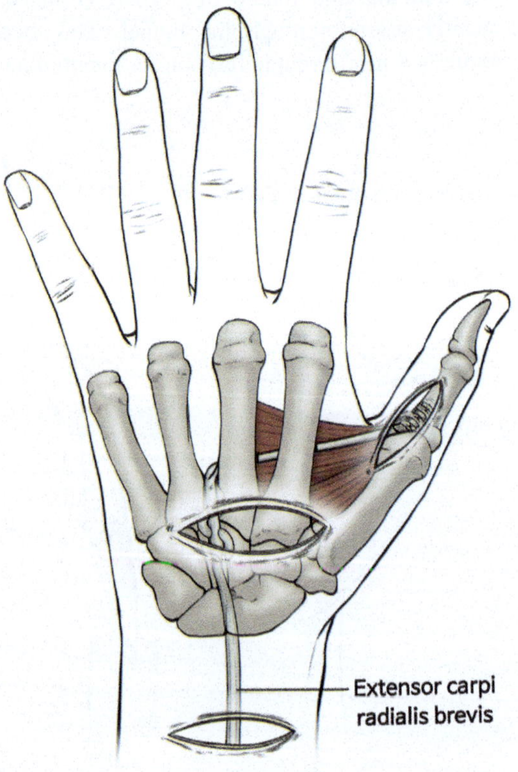


**Fig. 14.5** Extensor carpi radialis brevis is passed between the third and fourth metacarpals and across the palm to insert into the abductor tubercle of the first metacarpal

made on the ulnar base of the thumb MP joint, and a curved hemostat is then tunneled from this incision. After a palmaris longus tendon graft is harvested and sutured to the end of the ECRB through a Pulvertaft weave, this tendon is transferred to the AP tendon insertion by passing along with the transverse muscle belly of the AP and deep to the flexor tendons and neurovascular bundle. On this point, if the insertion of the transfer is made on the strong fascia over the abductor tubercle, it may improve pronation motion of the thumb for powerful pinch [36]. The appropriate tension includes that the thumb should be placed in adducted position while the wrist in neutral, and passively full abduction of the thumb should be possible with the wrist in extension. A thumb spica splint is applied for 4 weeks after surgery with the thumb in a neutral position and the wrist in a position of 30–40° of extension. Gentle active and active assisted range of motion exercises begin at 4 weeks and resistive pinch and grip at 8–10 weeks. All activities except those requiring high demand can be allowed at 3–4 months after surgery.

**FDS transfer**. The harvest procedure of the ring finger FDS is similar to the technique described earlier in the section of the FDS opponensplasty. Once the donor FDS has been harvested distally, it is then passed around the free distal edge of the superficial palmar fascia attaching onto the middle finger metacarpal, which forms a pulley of the transfer. After making an incision of ulnar side of the thumb MCP joint, the FDS is transferred subcutaneously toward the AP tendon insertion, followed by suturing them each other with the wrist in a 30° of extension and the thumb in an adducted position against the index finger.

**EIP transfer**. The EIP is detached from the extensor hood and pulled out proximally to the extensor retinaculum, as described earlier in the EIP opponensplasty. And then another incision is made between the middle and ring finger metacarpals. Through the space, the transfer is passed along the transverse muscle belly of the AP, deep to the flexor tendons and neurovascular bundle, and it is sutured to the AP at its insertion. Proper tension is achieved by suturing it with the wrist in a neutral and the thumb in an adducted position.

## Surgical Techniques of Index Abduction

**APL transfer** (Fig. 14.6) [43]. The APL is exposed through an incision over the insertion of the APL on the thumb metacarpal base. After one slip of the APL is detached from its insertion, the slip is retracted proximally out of the first extensor compartment and then passed subcutaneously toward the first dorsal interosseous (DI) tendon. This transfer may require necessity of tendon lengthening with a tendon graft. The transfer tendon is sutured to the DI tendon at its insertion with an appropriate tension, at which the index finger is abducted in a neutral position of the wrist.

**EIP transfer**. The EIP tendon is detached from the extensor hood and withdrawn into a transverse incision made on the wrist. The tendon is passed under the EDC and around the radial

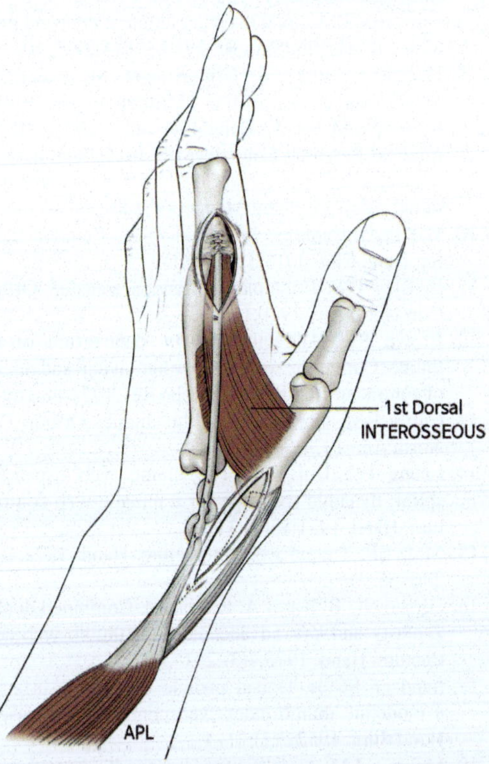


**Fig. 14.6** An accessory slip of the abductor pollicis longus is detached and attached into the tendon insertion of the first dorsal interosseous

border of the 2nd metacarpal, and then inserted into the first DI tendon, palmar to the rotation axis of the MCP joint.

## References


1. Kaplan EB, editor. Kaplan's functional and surgical anatomy of the hand. 3rd ed. Philadelphia: J.B. Lippincott; 1984.
2. Davis TRC, editor. Principles of tendon transfers of median, radial, and ulnar nerve. 7th ed. Philadelphia: Elsevier; 2017.
3. Naeem R, Lahiri A. Modified camitz opponensplasty for severe thenar wasting secondary to carpal tunnel syndrome: case series. J Hand Surg. 2013;38(4):795–8.
4. Bunnell S. Opposition of the thumb. J Bone Jt Surg Am. 1938;20:269–84.
5. Posner MA, Kapila D. Restoration of opposition. Hand Clin. 2012;28(1):27–44.
6. Littler JW, Li CS. Primary restoration of thumb opposition with median nerve decompression. Plast Reconstr Surg. 1967;39(1):74–5.
7. Chadderdon RC, Gaston RG. Low median nerve transfers (opponensplasty). Hand Clin. 2016;32(3):349–59.
8. Rowntree T. Anomalous innervation of the hand muscles. J Bone Joint Surg Br. 1949;31B(4):505–10.
9. Paternostro-Sluga T, Grim-Stieger M, Posch M, Schuhfried O, Vacariu G, Mittermaier C, Bittner C, Fialka-Moser V. Reliability and validity of the Medical Research Council (MRC) scale and a modified scale for testing muscle strength in patients with radial palsy. J Rehabil Med. 2008;40(8):665–71.
10. Wilbur D, Hammert WC. Principles of tendon transfer. Hand Clin. 2016;32(3):283–9.
11. Beasley RW. Principles of tendon transfer. Orthop Clin North Am. 1970;1(2):433–8.
12. Brown PW. Adduction–flexion contracture of the thumb. Correction with dorsal rotation flap and release of contracture. Clin Orthop Relat Res. 1972;88:161–8.
13. Curtis RM. Opposition of the thumb. Orthop Clin North Am. 1974;5(2):305–21.
14. Leung PC, Hui KM. The thumb web expanding splint: dynamic splintage for traumatic web contracture. Hand. 1981;13(3):311–7.
15. Mutz SB. Thumb web contracture. Hand. 1972;4(3):236–46.
16. Hirshowitz B, Karev A, Rousso M. Combined double Z-plasty and Y-V advancement for thumb web contracture. Hand. 1975;7(3):291–3.
17. Sandzen SC Jr. Dorsal pedicle flap for resurfacing a moderate thumb-index web contracture release. J Hand Surg. 1982;7(1):21–4.
18. Mahmoud M, Abdel-Ghani H, Elfar JC. New flap for widening of the web space and correction of palmar contracture in complex clasped thumb. J Hand Surg. 2013;38(11):2251–6.
19. Wang QR. [Correction of congenital adduction flexion deformity of the thumb by release of soft tissue contracture and rotating wedge osteotomy of the metacarpal bone]. Zhonghua Zheng Xing Shao Shang Wai Ke Za Zhi. 1988;4(3):193–4.
20. Goldner JL, Clippinger FW. Excision of the greater multangular bone as an adjunct to mobilization of the thumb. J Bone Joint Surg Am. 1959;41-A(4):609–25.
21. Terrono AL, Rose JH, Mulroy J, Millender LH. Camitz palmaris longus abductorplasty for severe thenar atrophy secondary to carpal tunnel syndrome. J Hand Surg. 1993;18(2):204–6.
22. Gonzalez MH, Weinzweig N, Kay T, Grindel S. Anatomy of the extensor tendons to the index finger. J Hand Surg. 1996;21(6):988–91.
23. Taylor J, Casaletto JA. Absence of extensor indicis tendon complicating reconstruction of the extensor pollicis longus. J Hand Surg Eur Vol. 2017;42(5):528–9.
24. Anderson GA, Lee V, Sundararaj GD. Opponensplasty by extensor indicis and flexor digitorum superficialis tendon transfer. J Hand Surg. 1992;17(6):611–4.
25. Thomas LI, Thompson TC, Straub LR. Transplantation of the external oblique muscle for abductor paralysis. J Bone Joint Surg Am. 1950;32A(1):207–17, illust.
26. Koo CC, Roberts AH. The palmaris longus tendon. Another variation in its anatomy. J Hand Surg. 1997;22(1):138–9.
27. Caughell KA, McFarlane RM, McGrouther DA, Martin AH. Developmental anatomy of the palmar aponeurosis and its relationship to the palmaris longus tendon. J Hand Surg. 1988;13(4):485–93.
28. Rymer B, Thomas PB. The Camitz transfer and its modifications: a review. J Hand Surg Eur Vol. 2016;41(6):632–7.
29. Kang SW, Chung YG, Lee JY, Jo WL. Modified camitz opponensplasty using transverse carpal ligament loop pulley in patients with advanced carpal tunnel syndrome. Plast Reconstr Surg. 2012;129(4):761e–3e.
30. Mondelli M, Reale F, Padua R, Aprile I, Padua L. Clinical and neurophysiological outcome of surgery in extreme carpal tunnel syndrome. Clin Neurophysiol. 2001;112(7):1237–42.
31. Schneider LH. Opponensplasty using the extensor digiti minimi. J Bone Jt Surg Am. 1969;51(7):1297–302.
32. Dunlap J, Manske PR, McCarthy JA. Perfusion of the abductor digiti quinti after transfer on a neurovascular pedicle. J Hand Surg. 1989;14(6):992–5.
33. Uysal AC, Alagoz MS, Tuccar E, Sensoz O, Tekdemir I. The vascular anatomy of the abductor digiti minimi and the flexor digiti minimi brevis muscles. J Hand Surg. 2005;30(1):172–6.
34. Goldner JL. Tendon transfers for irreparable peripheral nerve injuries of the upper extremity. Orthop Clin North Am. 1974;5(2):343–75.
35. Smith RJ. Extensor carpi radialis brevis tendon transfer for thumb adduction—a study of power pinch. J Hand Surg. 1983;8(1):4–15.

36. Edgerton MT, Brand PW. Restoration of abduction and adduction to the unstable thumb in median and ulnar paralysis. Plast Reconstr Surg. 1965;36:150–64.
37. Zweig J, Rosenthal S, Burns H. Transfer of the extensor digiti quinti to restore pinch in ulnar palsy of the hand. J Bone Jt Surg Am. 1972;54(1):51–9.
38. Omer GE. Tendon transfers for combined traumatic nerve palsies of the forearm and hand. J Hand Surg. 1992;17(6):603–10.
39. Fischer T, Nagy L, Buechler U. Restoration of pinch grip in ulnar nerve paralysis: extensor carpi radialis longus to adductor pollicis and abductor pollicis longus to first dorsal interosseus tendon transfers. J Hand Surg. 2003;28(1):28–32.
40. Hirayama T, Atsuta Y, Takemitsu Y. Palmaris longus transfer for replacement of the first dorsal interosseous. J Hand Surg. 1986;11(1):84–6.
41. Robinson D, Aghasi MK, Halperin N. Restoration of pinch in ulnar nerve palsy by transfer of split extensor digiti minimi and extensor indicis. J Hand Surg. 1992;17(6):622–4.
42. Alnot JY, Masquelet A. Restoration of thumb-index pinch by a double tendon transfer following ulnar nerve paralysis. Ann Chir Main. 1983;2(3):202–10.
43. Neviaser RJ, Wilson JN, Gardner MM. Abductor pollicis longus transfer for replacement of first dorsal interosseous. J Hand Surg. 1980;5(1):53–7.
44. Anderson GA, Lee V, Sundararaj GD. Extensor indicis proprius opponensplasty. J Hand Surg. 1991;16(3):334–8.
45. Burkhalter W, Christensen RC, Brown P. Extensor indicis proprius opponensplasty. J Bone Jt Surg Am. 1973;55(4):725–32.
46. de Kraker M, Selles RW, Zuidam JM, Molenaar HM, Stam HJ, Hovius SE. Outcome of flexor digitorum superficialis opponensplasty for Type II and IIIA thumb hypoplasia. J Hand Surg Eur Vol. 2016;41(3):258–64.
47. Jacobs BTT. Opposition of the thumb and its restoration. J Bone Joint Surg Am. 1960;42(A):12.
48. Jensen EG. Restoration of opposition of the thumb. Hand. 1978;10(2):161–7.
49. Foucher G, Malizos C, Sammut D, Braun FM, Michon J. Primary palmaris longus transfer as an opponensplasty in carpal tunnel release. A series of 73 cases. J Hand Surg. 1991;16(1):56–60.
50. Park IJ, Kim HM, Lee SU, Lee JY, Jeong C. Opponensplasty using palmaris longus tendon and flexor retinaculum pulley in patients with severe carpal tunnel syndrome. Arch Orthop Trauma Surg. 2010;130(7):829–34.
51. Wissinger HA, Singsen EG. Abductor digiti quinti opponensplasty. J Bone Jt Surg Am. 1977;59(7):895–8.
52. Koh S, Horii E, Hattori T. Flexor pollicis longus reconstruction using the palmaris longus in anterior interosseus nerve syndrome. Hand Surg. 2014;19(2):189–92.
53. Solonen KA, Bakalim GE. Restoration of pinch grip in traumatic ulnar palsy. Hand. 1976;8(1):39–44.

# Reconstruction of the Spastic Thumb

**15**

Sehun Kim and Hyun Sik Gong

## Spasticity of the Thumb

Spasticity is a motor disorder characterized by muscle hyperactivity or hypertony. It produces involuntary contraction of the involved muscles [1]. More specifically, Lance's widely accepted definition states: "Spasticity is a motor disorder characterized by a velocity-dependent increase in tonic stretch reflexes ("muscle tone") with exaggerated tendon jerks, resulting from hyperexcitability of the stretch reflex, as one component of the upper motor neuron syndrome" [2].

Spasticity usually occurs in patients with cerebral palsy, stroke, and brain damage [3]. Cerebral palsy is a term collectively referred to as a motor function disorder caused by a brain lesion that occurs before, during, or after birth, when the brain is still immature (up to the age of 2 years old) [4, 5]. There are various reasons for cerebral palsy: temporary lack of blood supply to the brain (anoxia), infection of the brain (encephalitis), vascular malformation in the brain, and bleeding inside the brain [6]. It has a nonprogressive nature [7].

In adults, stroke is the major cause of spasticity [3]. Vascular malformations or aging of the blood vessels (arteriosclerosis) may produce bleeding or thrombosis of some arteries within the brain, resulting in permanent damage to brain tissue [8, 9].

## Deformities in Spastic Thumb

The function of the hands of patients with spastic thumb is fairly limited [10–12]. The deformities of the hand are pronation of the forearm, flexion of the wrist and fingers, thumb-in-palm deformity, and swan neck deformity. Because the most important function of the hand requires the thumb, various treatments are performed to correct thumb-in-palm deformity.

In spastic hand, the thumb is often tight along the index finger or even flexed into the palm due to spasticity of two muscle groups: the intrinsic muscles (adductor pollicis, flexor pollicis brevis, first dorsal interosseous) which cause the web space to be closely tight and the extrinsic muscle (flexor pollicis longus) which causes the tip of the finger to flex. If this condition persists, it becomes difficult to extend the thumb, even if the muscles that extend the thumb are active [13]. Another reason for thumb deformity is an imbalance of forces between muscles [14]. The flexor and adductor muscles are spastic, and the force is too strong, and thus the relatively weak extensors do not overcome this force. In such cases, not only is the pinch between the thumb and the index finger impossible, but the thumb also gets in the way during grasping motions, thus

S. Kim · H. S. Gong (✉)
Department of Orthopedic Surgery, Seoul National University College of Medicine, Seoul National University Bundang Hospital, Seoul, South Korea
e-mail: hsgong@snu.ac.kr


S. H. Woo (ed.), *The Thumb*, https://doi.org/10.1007/978-981-10-4400-7_15

preventing the use of the hand. There are several classification systems of thumb-in-palm deformity [15].

## House Classification of Spastic Thumb

House et al. [15] classified the thumb-in-palm deformations into four types according to clinical features (Table 15.1). Type 1 is an isolated metacarpal adduction contracture, in which the main cause is stiffness of the adductor pollicis (Fig. 15.1a). Type 2 is a metacarpal adduction contracture with metacarpophalangeal joint flexion. Adductor pollicis and flexor pollicis brevis contracture can be thought to be the cause (Fig. 15.1b). Type 3 is accompanied by metacarpal adduction contracture and instability or hyperextension of the metacarpophalangeal joint (Fig. 15.1c). Type 4 is a metacarpal adduction contracture plus both metacarpophalangeal and interphalangeal joints flexion contracture. The interphalangeal joint flexion deformity is caused by the contracture of the flexor pollicis longus (Fig. 15.1d).

When the degree of contracture according to the movement of the wrist is checked, the muscles contributing to the deformation can be distinguished. If the intrinsic muscle such as the adductor pollicis or the flexor pollicis brevis is the main cause of deformation, the degree of contracture is constant irrespective of the movement of the wrist. On the other hand, if the extrinsic muscle such as the flexor pollicis longus mainly contributes to the deformation, the contracture is severe when the wrist is neutralized or extended, but the contracture improves if the wrist is fully flexed.

For thumb deformity, the House classification is widely used clinically as it is considered to be one of the most robust and has excellent clinical utility and reliability [16].

**Table 15.1** House classification of thumb-in-palm deformity

| Type | Description | Involved elements |
|---|---|---|
| I | Simple metacarpal adduction contracture | Spastic adductor and first dorsal interosseous |
| II | Metacarpal adduction contracture with MP flexion deformity | Spastic adductor, first dorsal interosseous, flexor pollicis brevis |
| III | Metacarpal adduction contracture with MP hyperextension and instability | Spastic adductor, first dorsal interosseous, extensor pollicis brevis |
| IV | Metacarpal adduction contracture, MP and interphalangeal deformities | Spastic adductor, first dorsal interosseous, flexor pollicis longus |

*MP* metacarpophalangeal

## Patient Assessment

The degree of finger deformation and the balance of the muscles causing deformation vary patient by patient. Careful and repetitive physical examination should therefore be performed before surgical treatment. Patients diagnosed with cerebral palsy should be able to cooperate with the medical staff, have some level of intellectual ability, and should have movement and sense.

Several evaluation tools have been proposed to evaluate the comprehensive function of hands. The House scale evaluates the use of the patient's hand in everyday life through a completed questionnaire from the patient and the caregiver and observation of the patient's hand use. The House scale can be used to evaluate the hand function in nine steps, so that small functional differences can be included in the evaluation (Table 15.2).

Patients with cerebral palsy have different paralytic states for each patient and thus undergo different surgical treatments. The MACS (Manual Ability Classification System) is used to comprehensively evaluate the function of the hand and compare it with other patients. MACS is a system for assessing the degree of use of the hand to manipulate things in daily life in patients with cerebral palsy. This system focuses on functions that can be performed with both hands rather than evaluating only the function of one hand (Table 15.3).

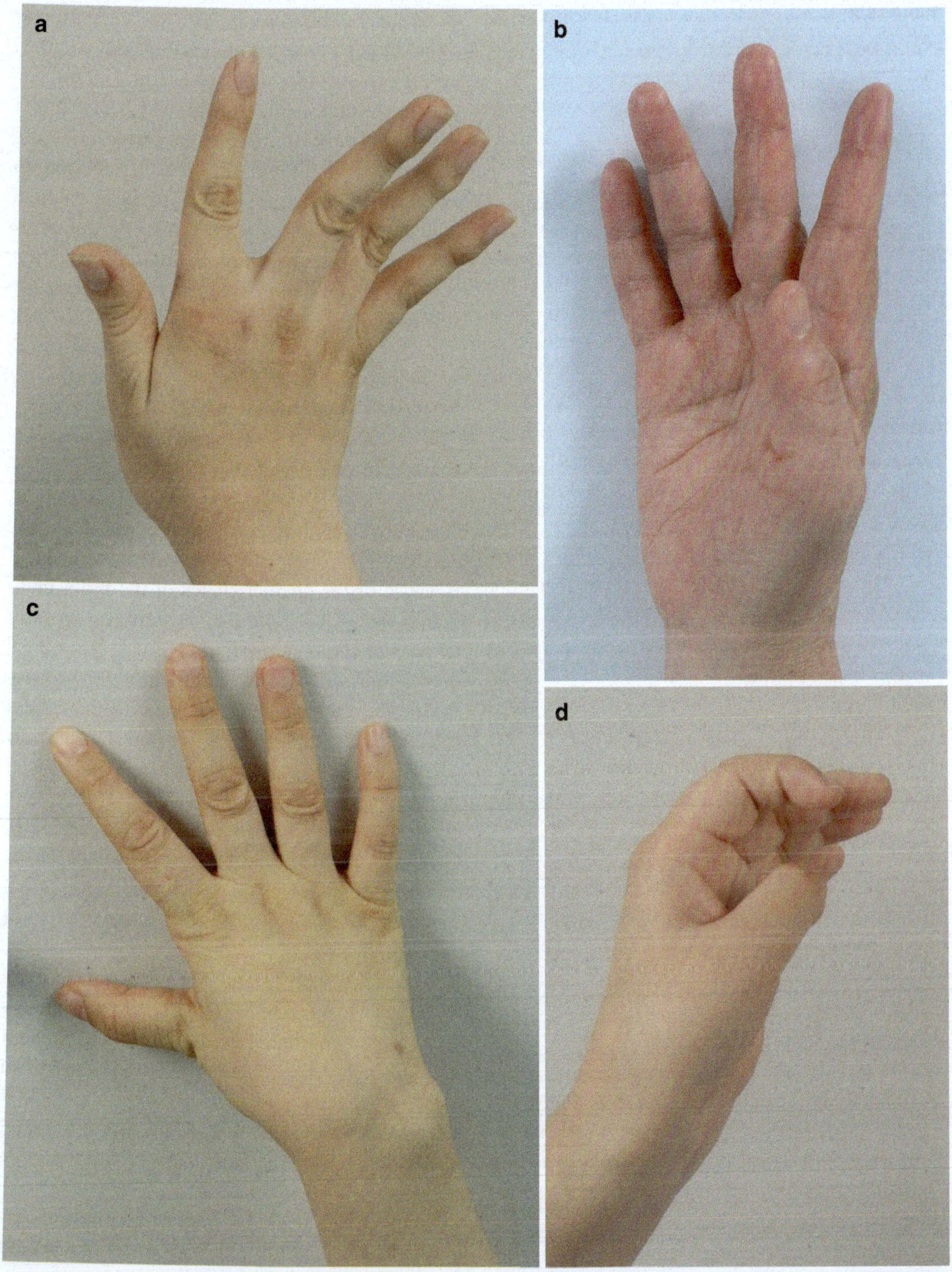


**Fig. 15.1** House classification of thumb-in-palm deformity. (**a**) Type 1: Simple metacarpal adduction contracture. (**b**) Type 2: Metacarpal adduction contracture and MP flexion deformity. (**c**) Type 3: Metacarpal adduction contracture combined with a MP hyperextension deformity or instability. (**d**) Type 4: Metacarpal adduction contracture combined with MP and IP flexion deformity

**Table 15.2** House classification of hand function

| Score | Designation | Activity level |
|---|---|---|
| 0 | Does not use | Does not use |
| 1 | Poor passive assist | Uses as stabilizing weight only |
| 2 | Fair passive assist | Can hold onto object placed in the hand |
| 3 | Good passive assist | Can hold object and stabilize for use by the other hand |
| 4 | Poor active assist | Can actively grasp object and hold it weakly |
| 5 | Fair active assist | Can actively grasp object and stabilize it well |
| 6 | Good active assist | Can actively grasp object, stabilize it well, and manipulate it against the other hand |
| 7 | Spontaneous use, partial | Can perform bimanual activities easily; occasionally uses the hand spontaneously |
| 8 | Spontaneous use, complete | Uses the hand completely independently, without reference to the other hand |

**Table 15.3** Manual Ability Classification System (MACS) of hand function

| Level | Description |
|---|---|
| I | Handles objects easily and successfully |
| II | Handles most objects but with somewhat reduced quality and/or speed of achievement |
| III | Handles objects with difficulty; needs help to prepare and/or modify activities |
| IV | Handles a limited selection of easily managed objects in adapted situations |
| V | Does not handle objects and has severely limited ability to perform even simple actions |

## Nonoperative Treatment

Nonoperative managements can be physical therapy [17], medical management, and botulinum toxin injections [18, 19]. Because of the characteristic of the plasticity of the brain, children inherently accept deficit and adapt to it in childhood [7, 20]. For example, children with hemiplegic use their affected arms to adapt to their normal arms. On the other hand, they also tend to ignore naturally, even if the affected arm is likely to have functional movement. They may end up "forgetting" it unless they are encouraged to use it. In this respect, exercise and occupational therapy have a significant impact on prognosis. Therefore, the upper limb must be managed early with exercise and occupational therapy, to develop its potential and fully use its capacity, even though limited. In addition to exercise, it is also possible to perform medical management such as muscle relaxant and anticonvulsant treatment. Botulinum toxin injection is also one of the effective treatment methods for spasticity [18].

## Surgical Treatment

### Principle of Surgical Treatment

The purpose of surgery is to improve function, not to regain completely normal function [15]. Because of the characteristics of the brain mentioned above, it is helpful to have surgery as early as possible. If the child's surgery is postponed until adolescence, the patient learns how to use the unaffected hand and relies on it. If the patient is undergoing surgery at a late age, more effort and time are needed to achieve a functional improvement than at an early age. This is also related to the plasticity of the brain [20]. Generally, the best age for performing surgery is around 6–12 years, since a clear evaluation of the function of the hands cannot be acquired until age 6 is reached.

The functional difference of the spastic hand has a fairly large range [10, 21]. Some patients use it almost normally, while others do not use it at all. In many stroke patients, the affected hand has little movement and sensory loss, and there is a tendency to neglect this. Some nonfunctional hands do not benefit from surgery in terms of functional enhancement.

In cases of spasticity due to head injury, surgery is usually performed at a time when recovery of motor and sensory nerves is no longer considered to be progressing. However, surgery may be needed early in some cases because symptoms may worsen continuously with appropriate conservative treatment.

## Surgical Methods Based on House Classification

Surgical methods based on House classification have been devised and include various elements [22]. It weakens the forces that cause deformation (release spastic intrinsic, adductor, and flexor muscles), strengthens the weak muscles (augment extensors and abductor muscles), and keeps the stability of the joint. In addition, the web space with contracture should be released.

### Weakening of Deforming Muscles

The spasticity of the thumb intrinsic muscle is observed in most patients with thumb-in-palm deformities. This is caused by the adductor pollicis (AP), flexor pollicis brevis (FPB), and first dorsal interosseous. The FPB is not involved if the metacarpophalangeal (MP) joint flexion is not severe. In this case, surgery can be performed to change the insertion of the AP proximally or to release it from the origin [15, 23]. If a voluntary movement of the AP is not possible, release can be performed at the insertion by proximal advancement rather than release at the origin. If a voluntary movement is possible, release at the origin by muscle slide or release at the myotendinous junction may be better for preserving the muscle strength. In type 4 deformity, fractional lengthening is performed for the spastic flexor pollicis longus (FPL).

### Augmentation of Weak Muscles

There are several ways to augment the extension and abduction of the thumb. Recently, it has been reported that transferring brachioradialis (BR) to extensor pollicis brevis (EPB) is more effective than transferring BR to abductor pollicis longus (APL) [24]. Extensor pollicis longus (EPL) rerouting or FPL abductorplasty can be performed to improve the extension of the thumb [25].

Rerouting of EPL is recommended when the EPL is strong and a good extension of the interphalangeal (IP) joint is possible with the wrist in neutral extension. EPL rerouting can help increase the power of the EPL. Additional BR to EPB transfer can be considered when EPL is not strong [26]. Imbrication of the APL and EPB tendons may be performed to augment the abduction and extension of the thumb in patients who are weak in EPL and cannot perform EPL rerouting.

### Stabilization of the Joint

Volar capsulodesis is performed when the thumb MP joint tends to hyperextend. Augmentation of the thumb extension and abduction leads to inadvertent hyperextension of the MP joint which makes the abduction of the thumb ineffective. Arthrodesis or chondrodesis may prevent hyperextension of the MP joint and may help to correct the thumb-in-palm deformity by limiting the flexion of the thumb [27].

The authors' preferred surgical methods for thumb-in-palm deformity are combinations of z-plasty lengthening of the first web, proximal advancement of the AP insertion, rerouting of the EPL, transfer of the BR to the EPB, and volar capsulodesis of the thumb MP joint [28, 29] (Fig. 15.2).

## Techniques

### Release of the Origin of Spastic Thumb Intrinsic Muscles

If selective and active control of AP and FPB is possible, release at the origin can be performed. The use of release at the origin rather than release at insertion can make the function of the hand better after surgery.

The palmar aponeurosis and distal half of the carpal tunnel are incised. When approaching, special care must be taken around the superficial palmar arch vessels and the recurrent branch of the median nerve and the sensory branch to the thumb. The flexor and lumbrical muscles running on the second and third fingers are retracted. The origin of the AP attached to the third metacarpal bone is exposed. The incision of the origin is performed from the distal to proximal part of the tendon while paying attention to the deep branch of the ulnar nerve. If the flexion contracture of the MP joint is accompanied, the origin of the FPB originating at the carpal bone located in the proximal portion of the MP joint can also be released (Fig. 15.3).

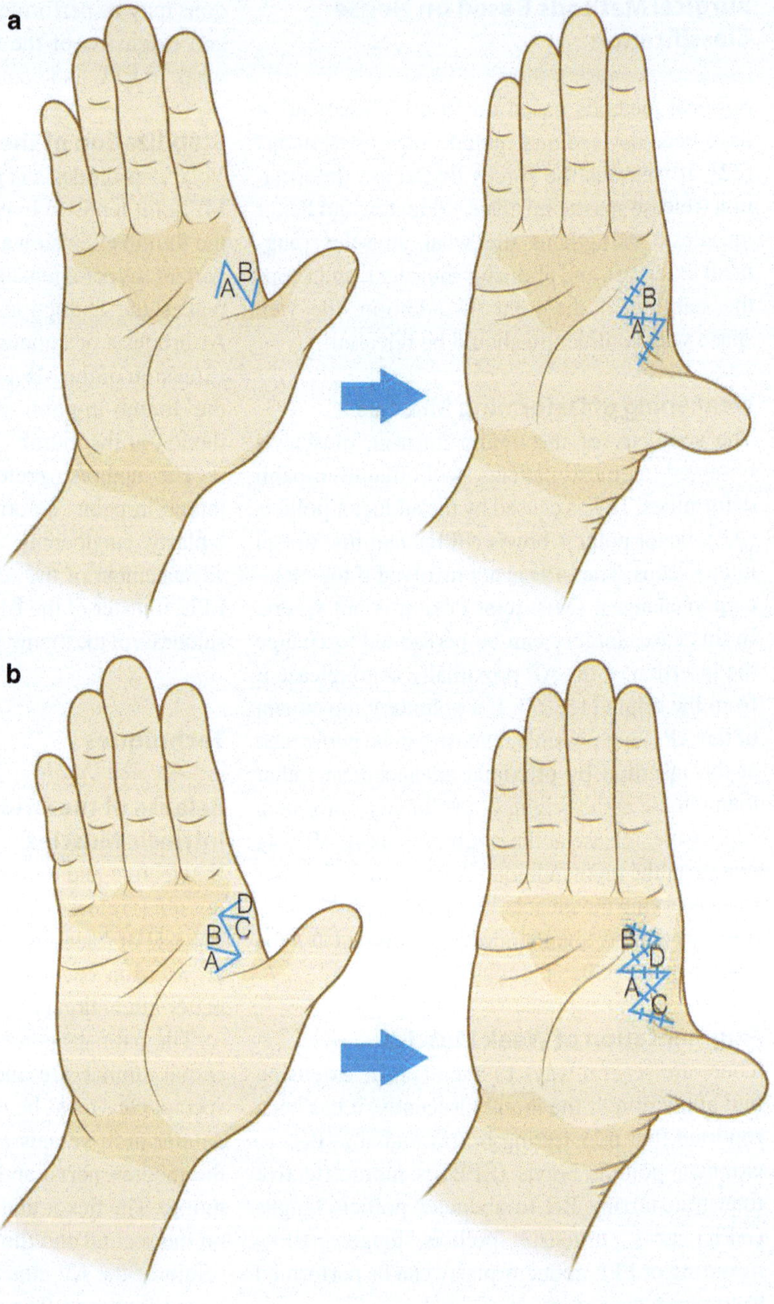


**Fig. 15.2** Z-plasty (**a**) or four-flap Z-plasty (**b**) for contracted first web space (Reproduced with the permission from Gunja publishing company)

### Release or Proximal Advancement of the Insertion of the Spastic Thumb Adductor

If the first web space is narrow and selective control of the AP is impossible, it is easier to release the insertion. If selective and active control of the AP is possible, the adduction power of the thumb may be much weaker after surgery, so lengthening or proximal advancement of AP tendon is required.

The first web space is incised by z-plasty. The AP tendons attached to the first metacarpal bone and sesamoid bone should be identified. The AP tendon is cut at the insertion, or the cut adductor tendon is advanced proximally by suturing it to the periosteum of the midportion of the first meta-

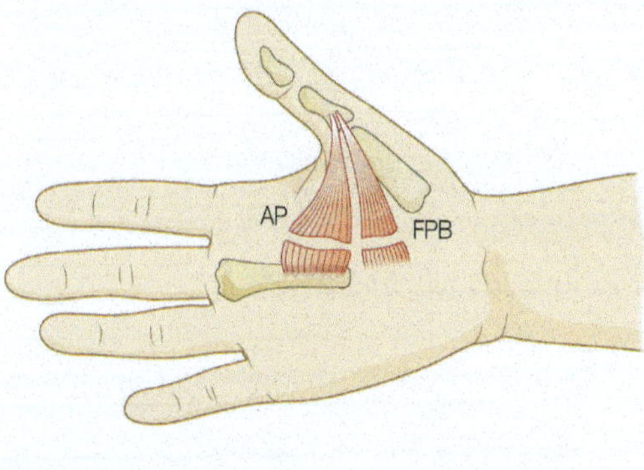


**Fig. 15.3** Release of the origin of spastic thumb intrinsic muscles (Reproduced with the permission from Gunja publishing company)

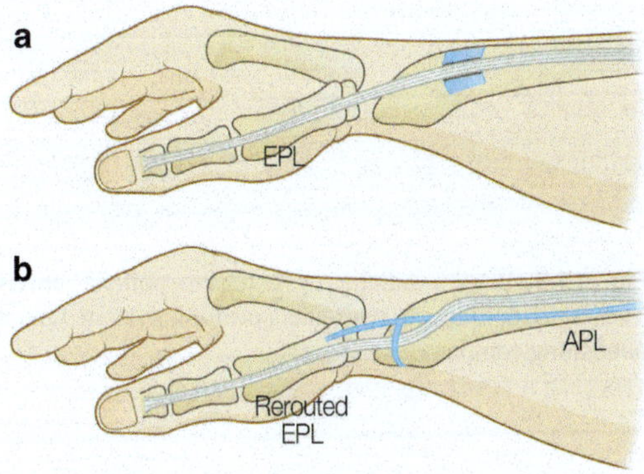


**Fig. 15.4** EPL rerouting. It functions as adductor muscle (**a**) before surgery but functions as abductor muscle (**b**) after surgery (Reproduced with the permission from Gunja publishing company)

carpal bone. The first metacarpal bone is fixed with a K-wire with as much extension and abduction of the carpometacarpal joint as possible.

## Lengthening of FPL

If the contracture of the thumb is severe when the wrist is extended but the contracture is not severe when the wrist is bent, FPL lengthening can be performed. If there is a contracture of the thumb only when the wrist is in neutral position, fractional lengthening can be performed. Z-lengthening can be performed in severe cases where the thumb is not fully extended even when the wrist is bent.

An incision is made in the forearm to expose the FPL. If fractional lengthening is to be performed, it is cut at the site of transition from the tendon to muscle with two sites at 1 cm intervals. If z-lengthening is to be performed, the required length is calculated based on the angle of the contracture. About 0.5 mm lengthening per contracture of 1° is considered necessary. The suture should be performed with the wrists in neutral position and the MP and IP joints flexed slightly.

## EPL Rerouting

If the thumb is severely adduced, EPL rerouting can be performed to eliminate its adductor function and act as an abductor. This procedure can be performed if the function of the EPL is intact and the active extension of the IP joint is possible with the wrist in neutral position. EPL rerouting should be accompanied by flexor and adductor release.

A longitudinal incision is made on the radial side of Lister's tubercle, and the EPL is exposed. The extensor retinaculum is incised to allow the EPL to move to the radial side. A longitudinal incision is made in the first dorsal compartment. Using APL, a pulley is created to wrap the EPL and to prevent it from returning to its original position. The first metacarpal bone is fixed with a K-wire in extension and abduction as much as possible (Fig. 15.4).

## BR to EPB Transfer

If EPL is weak, additional BR to EPB transfer can be performed.

A longitudinal incision is made in the 3–4 cm proximal region of the radial styloid. The insertion of BR is detached. The EPB tendon is cut in the proximal part, and the cut EPB is sutured to the BR using the weaving method. Sutures are performed in the flexion of the elbow and in the neutral position of the wrist (Fig. 15.5).

## FPL Abductorplasty

This operation can be performed when the adduction contracture of the thumb is mainly due to the rigidity of the FPL and the weakness of the APL. Patients with weak pinch power before surgery will lose the function of the FPL after this procedure. In addition, patients who already have MP joint fusion are not indicated for this operation because the IP joint will be tenodesed after undergoing this operation.

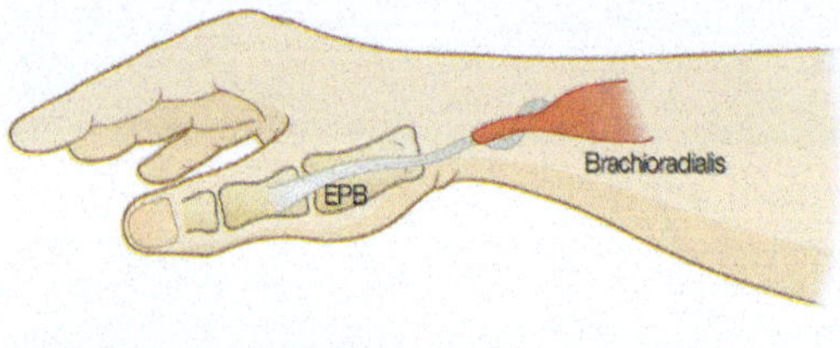


**Fig. 15.5** Brachioradialis to extensor pollicis brevis transfer (Reproduced with the permission from Gunja publishing company)

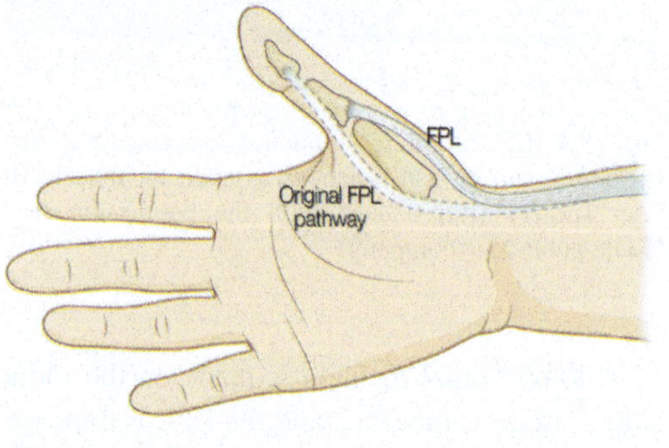


**Fig. 15.6** Flexor pollicis longus abductorplasty (Reproduced with the permission from Gunja publishing company)

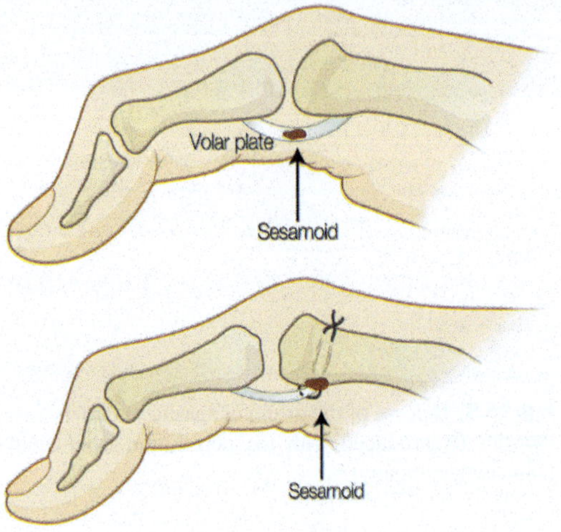


**Fig. 15.7** Metacarpophalangeal joint volar capsulodesis (Reproduced with the permission from Gunja publishing company)

The FPL is exposed by incising the lateral side around the IP joint of the thumb. The FPL is cut at the midportion of the proximal phalanx; the distal part of the cut FPL is attached to the proximal phalanx using the pullout suture or suture anchor method. At this time, the IP joint maintains 15–20 degrees of flexion. At the wrist, a longitudinal incision is made on the radial side of the FCR, and the proximal part of the cut FPL is pulled out. A subcutaneous tunnel is used to approach the posterior radial side of the MP joint. The proximal part of the cut FPL is attached to the posterior radial side of the MP joint capsule (Fig. 15.6).

### MP Joint Volar Capsulodesis

This operation can be performed when the MP joint is hyperextended. It can also strengthen the extension of the thumb in patients who have an unstable MP joint and may have hyperextension deformity after surgery.

The posterior radial side of the MP joint is approached. The accessory collateral ligament is incised, and the volar plate is exposed. The cartilage of the sesamoid bone attached to the volar plate is removed. The cortex is removed at the head-neck junction of the metacarpal bone to create a trough that can contact the sesamoid. After pulling the sesamoid bone into a proximal position to attach to the trough of the metacarpal bone, the sesamoid bone is fixed using a pullout suture with the MP joint flexed at 30°. The MP joint is fixed using a K-wire (Fig. 15.7).

### MP Joint Arthrodesis

This operation is performed when the instability of the MP joint cannot be stabilized by volar capsulodesis. Patients with IP joint fusion are not indicated for this procedure.

The joint between the EPL and the EPB is exposed using the dorsal side approach. Care should be taken not to expose the growth plate of the proximal phalanx. Only the cartilage of the joint is removed exposing the secondary ossification center. The MP joint is fixed using two K-wires with 10° of flexion.

## Outcomes of Treatment

The results of the upper limb reconstructive surgery for children with spastic hemiplegia are generally satisfactory. Functionally, the House scale improves by an average of 1.6–2.6 levels after surgery. Patients with active control of the thumb or who had a high MACS level before surgery could expect more improvement after surgery [30]. Patient satisfaction is also elevated after surgery from the aspect of appearance.

## References


1. Mukherjee A, Chakravarty A. Spasticity mechanisms—for the clinician. Front Neurol. 2010;1:149.
2. Lance J. Symposium synopsis. In: Feldman RG, Young RR, Koella KP, editors. Spasticity: disordered motor control. Chicago: Year Book; 1980. p. 485–500.
3. Burke D, Wissel J, Donnan GA. Pathophysiology of spasticity in stroke. Neurology. 2013;80: S20–S6.
4. Bax MC. Terminology and classification of cerebral palsy. Dev Med Child Neurol. 1964;6:295–7.
5. Bax MC, Flodmark O, Tydeman C. Definition and classification of cerebral palsy. From syndrome toward disease. Dev Med Child Neurol Suppl. 2007;109:39–41.
6. MacLennan AH, Thompson SC, Gecz J. Cerebral palsy: causes, pathways, and the role of genetic variants. Am J Obstet Gynecol. 2015;213:779–88.
7. Aisen ML, Kerkovich D, Mast J, Mulroy S, Wren TA, Kay RM, et al. Cerebral palsy: clinical care and neurological rehabilitation. Lancet Neurol. 2011;10:844–52.
8. Dirnagl U, Iadecola C, Moskowitz MA. Pathobiology of ischaemic stroke: an integrated view. Trends Neurosci. 1999;22:391–7.
9. Warach S, Gaa J, Siewert B, Wielopolski P, Edelman RR. Acute human stroke studied by whole brain echo planar diffusion-weighted magnetic resonance imaging. Ann Neurol. 1995;37:231–41.
10. Arner M, Eliasson AC, Nicklasson S, Sommerstein K, Hägglund G. Hand function in cerebral palsy. Report of 367 children in a population-based longitudinal health care program. J Hand Surg. 2008;33:1337–47.
11. Eliasson A-C, Krumlinde-Sundholm L, Rösblad B, Beckung E, Arner M, Öhrvall A-M, et al. The Manual Ability Classification System (MACS) for children with cerebral palsy: scale development and evidence of validity and reliability. Dev Med Child Neurol. 2006;48:549–54.
12. Dahlin LB, Komoto-Tufvesson Y, Sälgeback S. Surgery of the spastic hand in cerebral palsy: improvement in stereognosis and hand function after surgery. J Hand Surg Br. 1998;23:334–9.
13. Tonkin MA. Thumb deformity in the spastic hand: classification and surgical techniques. Tech Hand Up Extrem Surg. 2003;7:18–25.
14. Inglis AE, Cooper W, Bruton W. Surgical correction of thumb deformities in spastic paralysis. JBJS. 1970;52:253–68.
15. House JH, Gwathmey F, Fidler M. A dynamic approach to the thumb-in palm deformity in cerebral palsy. JBJS. 1981;63:216–25.
16. McConnell K, Johnston L, Kerr C. Upper limb function and deformity in cerebral palsy: a review of classification systems. Dev Med Child Neurol. 2011;53:799–805.
17. Bütefisch C, Hummelsheim H, Denzler P, Mauritz K-H. Repetitive training of isolated movements improves the outcome of motor rehabilitation of the centrally paretic hand. J Neurol Sci. 1995;130:59–68.
18. Brashear A, Gordon MF, Elovic E, Kassicieh VD, Marciniak C, Do M, et al. Intramuscular injection of botulinum toxin for the treatment of wrist and finger spasticity after a stroke. N Engl J Med. 2002;347:395–400.
19. Sampaio C, Ferreira JJ, Pinto AA, Crespo M, Ferro JM, Castro-Caldas A. Botulinum toxin type A for the treatment of arm and hand spasticity in stroke patients. Clin Rehabil. 1997;11:3–7.
20. Sterling C, Taub E, Davis D, Rickards T, Gauthier LV, Griffin A, et al. Structural neuroplastic change after constraint-induced movement therapy in children with cerebral palsy. Pediatrics. 2013;131:e1664–e9.
21. Novacheck TF, Trost JP, Sohrweide S. Examination of the child with cerebral palsy. Orthop Clin N Am. 2010;41:469–88.
22. Sakellarides HT, Mital MA, Matza RA, Dimakopoulos P. Classification and surgical treatment of the thumb-in-palm deformity in cerebral palsy and spastic paralysis. J Hand Surg. 1995;20:428–31.
23. Gob A. The treatment of spastic thumbs in palm deformity. Reconstr Surg Traumatol. 1972;13:51–7.
24. Roth JH, O'Grady SE, Richards RS, Porte AM. Functional outcome of upper limb tendon transfers performed in children with spastic hemiplegia. J Hand Surg Br. 1993;18:299–303.
25. Manske PR. Redirection of extensor pollicis longus in the treatment of spastic thumb-in-palm deformity. J Hand Surg. 1985;10:553–60.
26. Van Heest AE. Surgical technique for thumb-in-palm deformity in cerebral palsy. J Hand Surg Am. 2011;36:1526–31.
27. Szabo RM, Gelberman RH. Operative treatment of cerebral palsy. Hand Clin. 1985;1:525–43.
28. Carlson M. The treatment of thumb in palm deformity in cerebral palsy. Atlas Hand Surg. 2002;7:119.
29. Carlson MG, Athwal GS, Bueno RA. Treatment of the wrist and hand in cerebral palsy. J Hand Sur. 2006;31:483–90.
30. Gong HS, Chung CY, Park MS, Shin H-I, Chung MS, Baek GH. Functional outcomes after upper extremity surgery for cerebral palsy: comparison of high and low manual ability classification system levels. J Hand Surg. 2010;35:277–83.e3.

# Part VI

# Tumors

# Benign Tumors

# 16

Yang-Guk Chung

## Introduction

Bone and soft tissue tumors can arise at any site of our body. The hand and thumb are not exceptions. The hand and thumb have complex and diverse anatomic and functional characteristics, and consideration of those characteristics is necessary for proper management of tumors in this region. Masses arising in the hand and thumb include true tumors, bone protuberances, cysts, reactive granulomas, tenosynovial proliferations, foreign bodies, abscesses, and skin and facial lesions. The majority of tumors arising in the hand or thumb are benign. Ganglion cysts, epidermoid inclusion cysts, giant cell tumors of tendon sheath, and the palmar nodules of Dupuytren's contracture comprise the majority of the lesions. Although benign lesions are much more common in this region, the surgeons always consider the possibility of malignant lesions in managing processes because many malignant tumors may have benign appearances or growth behaviors [1]. Benign tumors and tumor-like lesions in the thumb are basically similar to those of the hand, so in this chapter, I will describe the benign tumors in the hand and thumb together.

Y.-G. Chung (✉)
Department of Orthopedic Surgery, Seoul St. Mary's Hospital, College of Medicine, The Catholic University of Korea, Seocho-gu, Seoul, South Korea
e-mail: ygchung@catholic.ac.kr

## Evaluation and Staging

Systematic orderly process of work-up for a definitive diagnosis is important to avoid potential disastrous consequences for the patients. Plain radiographs are warranted along with a detailed history and physical examination as an initial evaluation of any tumorous lesions. The age, sex, and location of lesion are important factors in diagnosis. Computed tomography (CT) scanning is the preferred imaging tool in bone tumors, and evaluation by magnetic resonance imaging (MRI) is the gold standard for soft tissue lesions. To establish or confirm the diagnosis, a histological evaluation of biopsied specimen is necessary. Ganglion cysts, subcutaneous lipomas, or epidermal inclusion cysts which have obvious imaging and clinical findings can be exempted for biopsy. Because most of the benign tumors do not metastasize to regional lymph node or chest, chest radiograph and CT scanning of the chest or abdomen are not necessary in routine evaluation protocol. One exception is the giant cell tumor of the bone, which can rarely metastasize to the lung. No specific laboratory study is helpful to establish the diagnosis.

The Musculoskeletal Tumor Society provided the staging system described by Enneking et al. [2]. Based on clinical, radiographic, and histological data, it categorizes the lesions according to their aggressiveness. Benign bone lesions are divided into latent, active, or aggressive ones depending on their radiographic appearances



S. H. Woo (ed.), *The Thumb*, https://doi.org/10.1007/978-981-10-4400-7_16

**Table 16.1** Enneking staging system for benign bone tumors [2]

| Stage | Definition | Behavior | Example |
|---|---|---|---|
| 1 | Latent | Remain static, heals spontaneously | Inactive simple bone cyst |
| 2 | Active | Progressive growth, limited by natural barriers | Nonossifying fibroma in children |
| 3 | Aggressive | Progressive growth, not limited by natural barriers | Giant cell tumor |

(Table 16.1). The American Joint Committee on Cancer (AJCC) staging system is a different one which is for the malignant bone or soft tissue sarcomas [3].

## Bone and Cartilage Tumors

### Enchondroma

Enchondroma is a benign hyaline cartilage neoplasm and is the most common primary bone tumor of the hand, up to 54% of all enchondromas involving the hand and wrist [4]. It develops from fragments of cartilage originated from the central physis. They favor the diaphysis of the small tubular bones of the hand, and most tumors are solitary. However, they involve more than one bones in Ollier's disease (multiple enchondromatosis) and Maffucci syndrome (multiple enchondromatosis associated with multiple soft tissue hemangiomas) (Fig. 16.1a–c).

Patients may be asymptomatic or present with pain related to actual or impending pathologic fracture caused by the expansile remodeling of the lesion. The majority of patients present within the second to fifth decades of life. Both sexes are equally affected.

Although malignant transformation is extremely rare in a solitary enchondroma, the incidence of secondary chondrosarcoma in patients with Ollier's disease was about 25% at the age of 40 years and almost a certainty in patients with Maffucci's syndrome [5]. Increased pain or development of pain in a previously asymptomatic lesion and rapid growth of an enchondroma may suggest malignant transformation. Radiographically, enchondromas form well-marginated tumors that vary from radiolucent to heavily mineralized. The characteristic mineralization patterns are punctate, flocculent, or ring and arc. In small tubular bones, enchondromas are frequently expansile and show endosteal scalloping and cortical thinning (Fig. 16.2). MRIs are helpful to evaluate the extents of tumors in the medullary space, which demonstrate the multilobulated, hyperintense enchondroma on fluid-sensitive sequences (Fig. 16.3a–c).

Histologically, enchondromas are white to blue-gray lobulated lesions with varying degrees of calcification. In the hand and thumb, a higher degree of cellularity and cellular atypia is acceptable for benign lesions as compared to other anatomic sites. Correlation with radiographic findings is necessary.

Differential diagnosis of enchondroma in the hand includes bone infarct, chondrosarcoma, chondroblastoma, nonossifying fibroma, fibrous dysplasia, and aneurysmal bone cyst.

A painless lesion can be observed through the regular radiographic follow-ups. For expansile lesions with thin cortexes, the potential for pathologic fracture should be considered, and an annual radiographic follow-up for 2-year period is reasonable to establish stability of the lesions. Surgical treatment is necessary in patients with a symptomatic lesion or a lesion at risk for pathologic fracture. If the radiologic imaging studies showed the characteristic features for benign enchondroma, no biopsy is necessary. In case of possible chondrosarcoma or other kind of neoplasm, open biopsy through a small window and establishment of the accurate histologic diagnosis are recommended. Because differentiation of benign enchondroma from a low-grade chondrosarcoma is difficult on frozen section for the cartilaginous tumors, it is prudent to defer the definite surgery after permanent section analysis of the biopsy specimen if there is concern regarding malignancy.

A thorough curettage through sufficient-sized bone window is the way of surgical treatment for

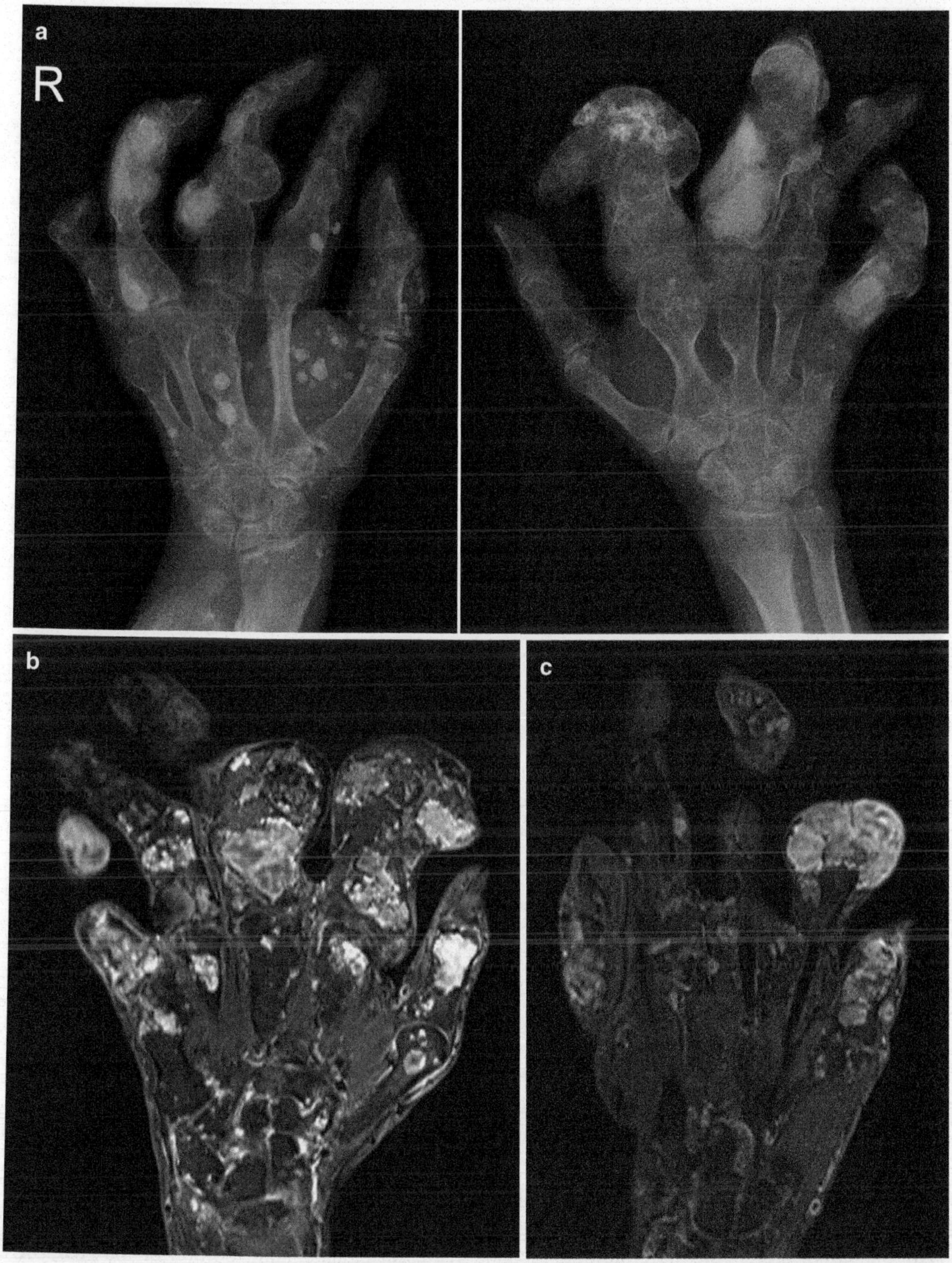


**Fig. 16.1** Plain radiographs of a 47-year-old female patient with Maffucci syndrome show multiple enchondromas with deformed thumbs and fingers (**a**). Phleboliths can be seen in the soft tissue of the right hand (**a**). MRIs of T1-weighted gadolinium-enhanced coronal view of right and left hands show marked deformities and large bulging mass formations with prominent bright heterogeneous enhancement which involve the proximal, mid, and distal phalanges (**b** and **c**)

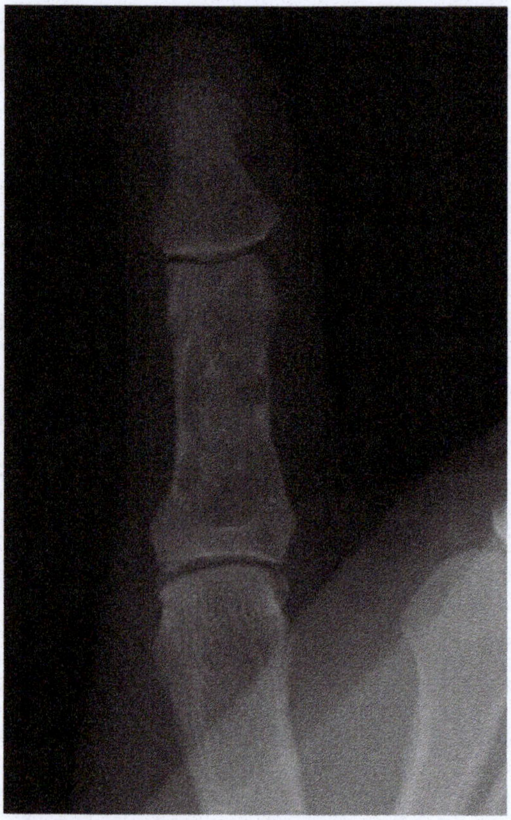

**Fig. 16.2** Right thumb AP view of patient with enchondroma shows central radiolucent bony lesion in the proximal phalange of the thumb with endosteal scalloping and punctate, flocculent matrix calcifications

benign enchondromas. The margin of excision can be extended with a high-speed burr, and electric cautery or chemical cauterization of the cavity with phenol or absolute alcohol may be helpful to reduce the recurrence rate. The bone defect is packed with autogenous iliac cancellous bone, allograft, or a synthetic bone substitute to heal (Fig. 16.4a–d) [6, 7]. Although there were reports that successful simple curettage of the lesion without intralesional bone graft [8, 9] and packing of bone defect with methyl methacrylate [10], the author prefers the more biologic reconstruction methods of autograft or allograft. In case of pathologic fracture, surgical treatment after fracture healing with initial immobilization was recommended because of lower complication rate than immediate curettage and bone graft (Fig. 16.5a–f) [11].

The reported recurrence rate of enchondroma after curettage was 2–15% [12]. There is a possibility of malignancy in recurred cases; a careful review of radiographs and histology is advised, and again a clinical and radiographic correlation is important.

## Aneurysmal Bone Cyst

Aneurysmal bone cyst (ABC) is a destructive, expansile, benign neoplasm of the bone composed of multiloculated blood-filled cystic spaces. It accounts for 5–6% of benign bone tumors, and fewer than 5% of aneurysmal bone cysts are localized to the hand [13]. Metacarpal lesions are more frequent than phalangeal or carpal lesions. It is most common during the first two decades of life (80%) with no sex predominance.

The clinical presentation may be a slowly enlarging bony lesion with or without pain. In the lesion close to a joint, there may be limitation of joint motion. Plain radiographs will demonstrate a central, expansile metaphyseal and epiphyseal lesion with cortical thinning. ABCs in the hand may be purely lytic, lack sclerotic margin, and appear more destructive (Fig. 16.6a–f) [14]. Differential diagnosis will be giant cell tumor of the bone, giant cell reactive granuloma, enchondroma, and telangiectatic osteosarcoma. Magnetic resonance imaging, which shows internal septa and the characteristic fluid-fluid level, may be useful for differential of lesions and evaluation of soft tissue extension [14]. The histology of ABCs is a blood-filled cyst with membranous lining on which shows fibrous tissues, foam cells, and giant cells similar to chronic inflammation. More solid areas can be seen and they may represent either a solid portion of the ABC or a component of a primary tumor such as giant cell tumor of the bone, osteoblastoma, chondroblas-

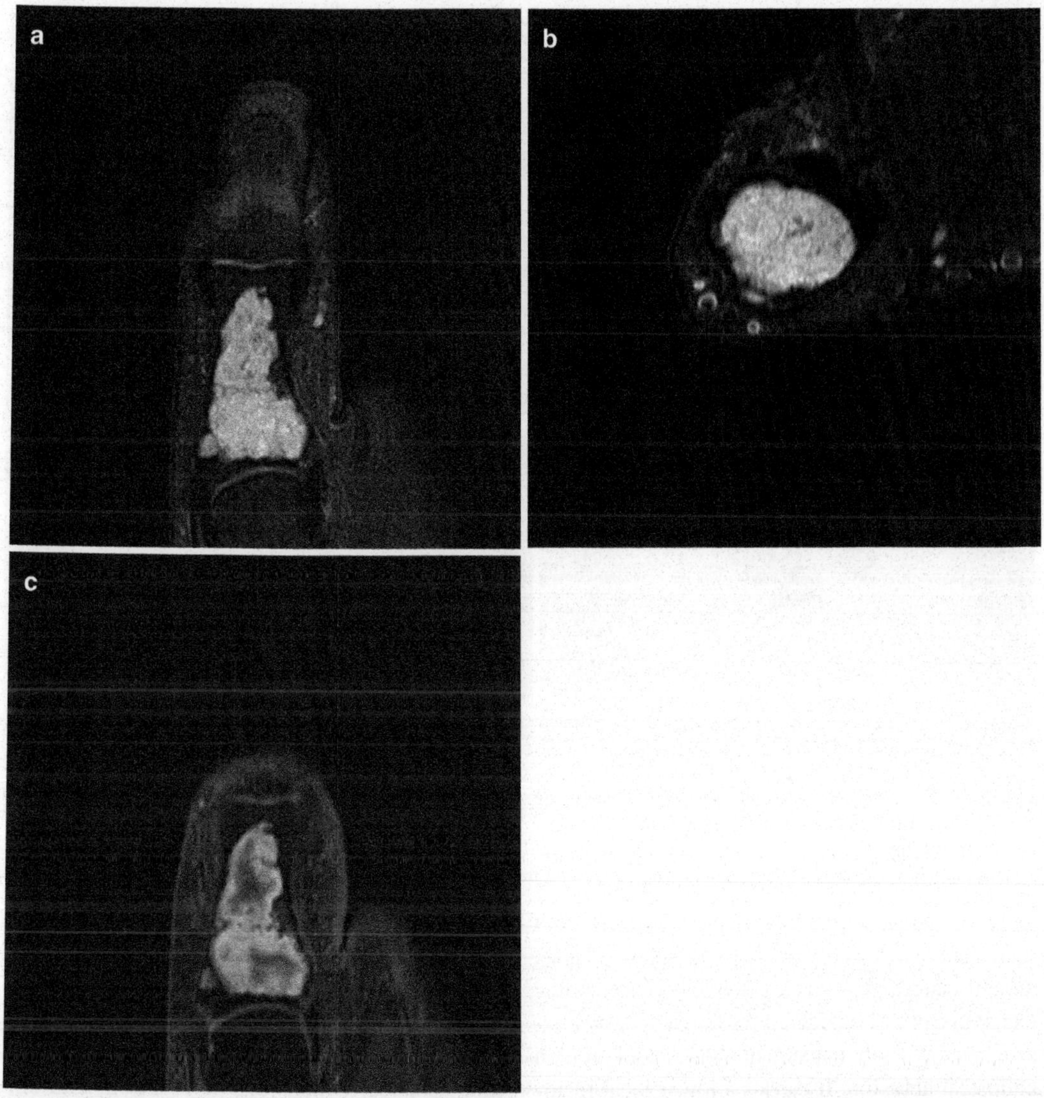


**Fig. 16.3** T2-weighted fat suppression coronal (**a**) and axial (**b**) images and T1-weighted fat suppression gadolinium-enhanced coronal MR (**c**) images on left hand of patient with enchondroma show lobulated high signal intensity intramedullary lesion with peripheral rim enhancement at proximal phalange of left thumb

toma, or fibrous dysplasia, which has undergone secondary ABC-like changes [15].

The standard treatment for ABCs is through extended curettage with adjuvant liquid nitrogen, high-speed burring, and electric or chemical cauterization, which reduce the recurrence rate to 12–18% [16, 17]. The bone defect site was filled with bone graft or bone cement. Creation of a large cortical window or "exteriorization" will be helpful to improve the visualization of the lesion and to facilitate treatment of the lesion cavity. The use of high-speed burr is indicated if there is sufficient bone stock provided. Liquid nitrogen can reduce the risk of local recurrence, but it is techni-

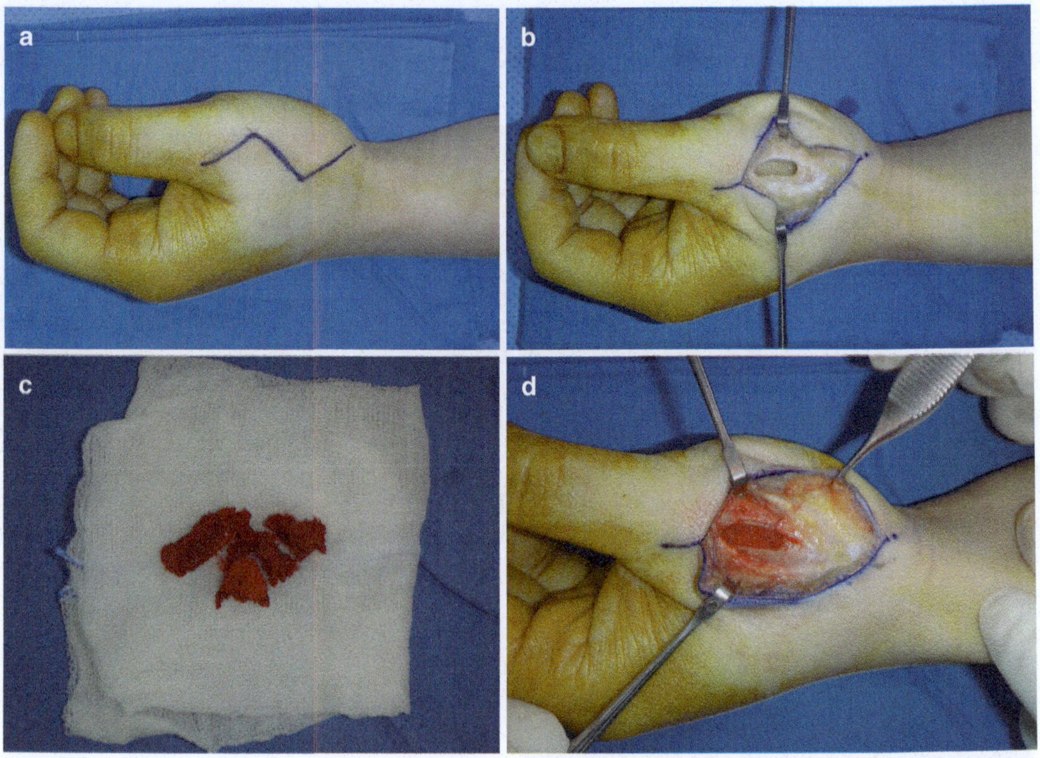


**Fig. 16.4** Extended curettage and bone graft. Through the zigzag incision (**a**) on the dorsum of first metacarpal bone, an elliptical bony window was made with power burr (**b**). The defect that remained after curettage was filled with autogenous cancellous iliac bone chips (**c** and **d**)

cally demanding and may be associated with increased risk of infection, fracture, joint collapse, and premature physeal closure [18]. Wide en bloc excision can be considered for large, very aggressive lesions with inadequate bone stock for an endosteal abrasion. It carries a lower local recurrence risk than curettage and bone grafting at the expense of greater morbidity [19]. Amputation may be necessary for very large destructive lesions, particularly ones in distal phalanx.

## Giant Cell Tumor

Giant cell tumors (GCTs) in the hand account for about 2% of all. It occurs most commonly in the third and fourth decades and has slight female predominance. Although GCT in the bone is basically a benign, locally aggressive lesion, it does have the potential to metastasize [20, 21]. Pain and swelling of the affected area are common clinical findings, and pain may be aggravated after pathologic fracture. Radiographically GCTs appear as radiolucent, eccentric, epiphyseal lesions with a lytic matrix. The matrix typically has no calcification. Cortical expansion, perforation, and soft tissue extension are common on plain radiograph (Fig. 16.7a–i).

Campanacci et al. [21] described a staging system based on plain radiographs. Lesion with normal contour and no perforation of cortex is considered stage I, active lesion with expanded cortex without perforation is stage II, and more aggressive lesion with perforated cortex and extension into surrounding soft tissues is stage III (Table 16.2).

GCTs of the bone in the hand are more aggressive with higher local recurrence and metastasis rates. The local recurrence risk after intralesional curettage was approximately 80% [22]. Reported metastasis rate was as high as

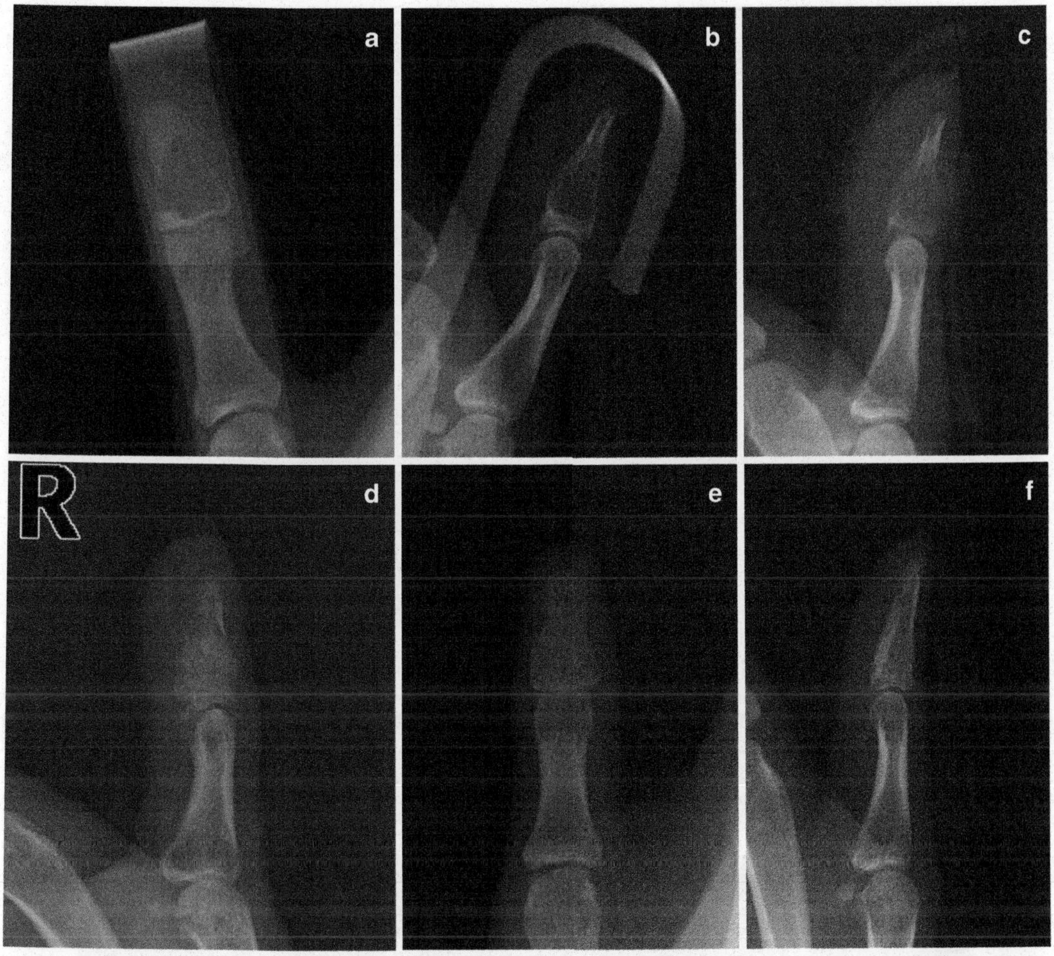


**Fig. 16.5** Plain radiographs of right thumb AP (**a**) and lateral (**b**) view of patient with enchondroma show linear fracture line through the radiolucent bony lesion. After 6-week splint immobilization, the bone union was obtained (**c**). The patient underwent a thorough curettage and bone graft (**d**). Postoperative 6-month radiographs revealed solid incorporation of grafted bone (**e** and **f**)

10%, and metastasis is seen more commonly after local recurrence. Because of this characteristics, aggressive treatments such as wide excision or amputation for patients with GCT of the bones of the hand are recommended as the best form of definite local treatment (Fig. 16.7a–i) [14]. There is a recent report [23] that three patients treated with curettage, cryosurgery, and cementation had no recurrence, which suggest that this technique may have a role for hand lesions without soft tissue extension (Campanacci stage I or II). Postoperatively, patients are followed up with hand and chest radiographs every 6 months for the first 2 years, then every year. Chest CT should be considered in those patients with local recurrence [14].

## Osteochondroma

Osteochondroma is a benign bony prominence capped with hyaline cartilaginous tissue. Patients are diagnosed in childhood mostly. Smaller lesions in hand and feet are affected in about 10% of cases. In the Mayo series, only 4% of osteochondromas involved the hand and wrist [4]. One characteristic feature of osteochondroma is

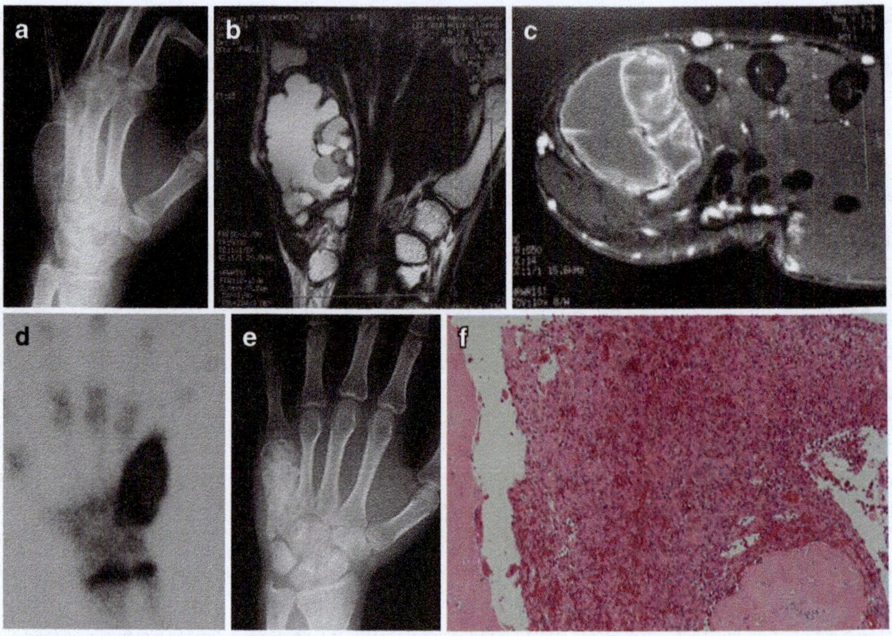

**Fig. 16.6** Plain radiograph of right hand demonstrates a central, markedly expansile multiloculated, radiolucent bony lesion with cortical thinning (**a**). MRIs show expansile multiloculated lesion with peripheral rim enhancement (**b** and **c**). Bone scintigraphy reveals hot uptake of radioisotopes (**d**). Extended curettage with debulking cortical modeling and autogenous iliac bone grafting were performed (**e**). Histological examination demonstrates that the hemorrhagic cyst wall lacks a distinct cell lining and is composed of blend spindle-shaped cells with scattered osteoclast-type giant cells and reactive woven bones (**f**)

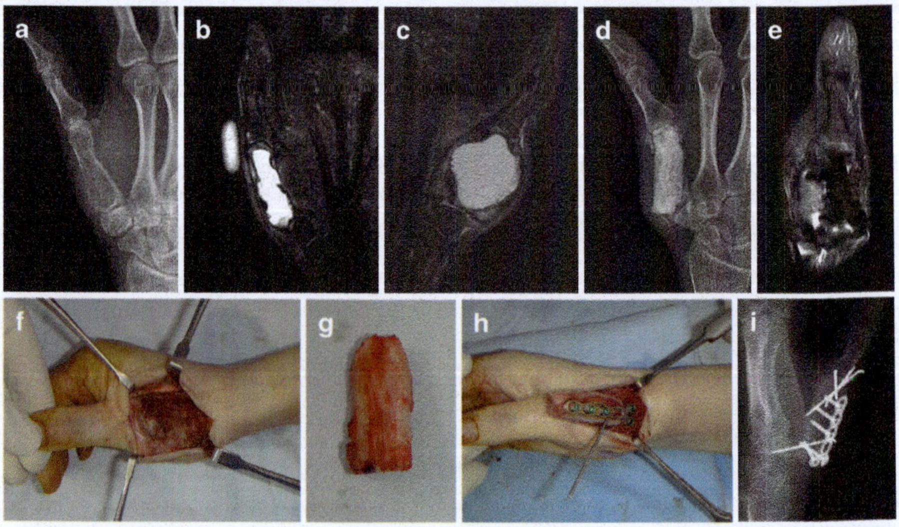

**Fig. 16.7** Plain right thumb lateral radiograph of a 35-year-old female patient showed slightly expansile, radiolucent bony lesion involving near whole first metacarpal bone (**a**). T2-weighted MR image demonstrated intraosseous lesion with thinned cortex, but there was no definite cortical perforation (**b**). Nine-month follow-up MRI showed markedly expansion of cortical bone (**c**). Plain radiographs at 3 years after extended curettage and cementation showed subluxation of cement block with destructive osteolytic changes of overlying cortical bone (**d**). MRI (T2, fat-suppressed sagittal) demonstrated recurrent GCT around the cement block (**e**). After wide en bloc resection of the first metacarpal bone, (**f**) a tricortical iliac bone block (**g**) was harvested and implanted into the bone defect site with arthrodesis of basal joint (**h**). Postoperative radiograph shows the reconstructed first metacarpal bone (**i**)

**Table 16.2** Campanacci staging system for giant cell tumors of the bone [21]

| Stage | % | Description | Treatment |
|---|---|---|---|
| Stage I (latent) | 15% | Confined totally by the bone<br>Asymptomatic<br>Inactive on bone scan<br>Histologically benign | Extended curettage with high-speed burr and adjuvant PMMA |
| Stage II (active) | 70% | Expanded cortex with no breakthrough<br>Symptomatic<br>If pathologic fracture, active on bone scan<br>Histologically benign | |
| Stage III (aggressive) | 15% | Rapidly growing mass<br>Cortical perforation with soft tissue mass<br>May metastasize<br>Symptomatic<br>Extensive activity on bone scan<br>Histologically benign | Wide resection and osteochondral allograft |
| Malignant | Very rare | Sarcomatous lesion contiguous with benign GCT | |

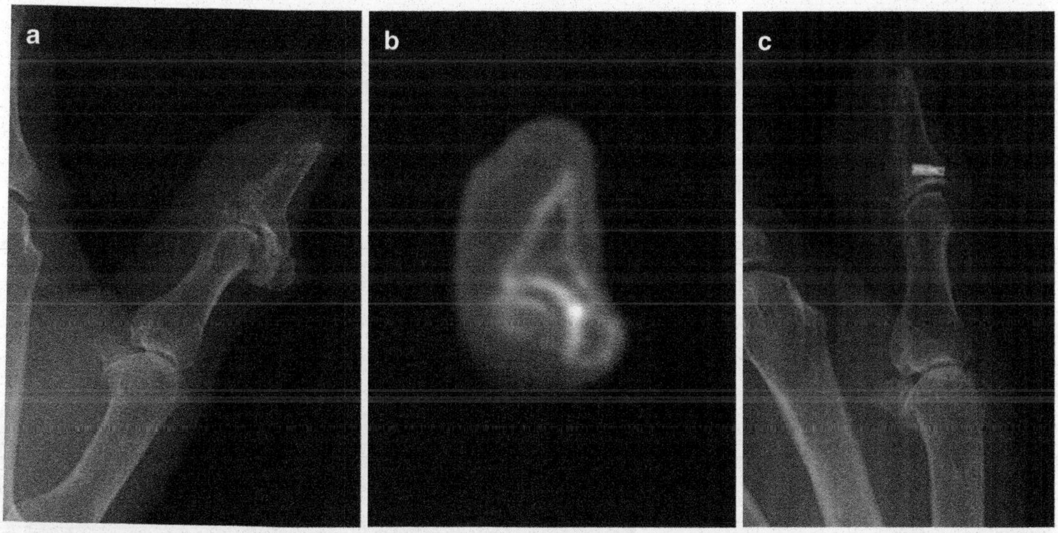


**Fig. 16.8** Plain right thumb lateral radiograph of an 83-year-old female patient showed protruded bony prominence on dorsal aspect of distal interphalangeal joint. CT scanning demonstrated the characteristic feature of osteochondroma, medullary continuity between the osteochondroma and the underlying parent bone (**b**). After excision of osteochondral tumor mass, the EPL tendon was attached to the base of distal phalangeal bone with suture anchor (**c**)

medullary continuity between the osteochondroma and the underlying parent bone (Fig. 16.8a–c). Because solitary osteochondroma in the hand is unusual, the patient with osteochondroma in the hand should be evaluated for multiple osteochondromatosis, an autosomal dominant inherited disease which can result in angular deformity of nearby joint. Symptoms may be related to irritation of the surrounding soft tissues. Sometimes juxta-articular lesions cause the deformity and limitation of joint motion. Growth of the osteochondroma should cease on physeal closure. Malignant transformation of a solitary osteochondroma is rare. Sudden growth of the lesion, irregular mineralization, and change of the lucent region of the lesion are signs for sarcomatous degeneration. Surgical excision can be considered for symptomatic lesions. A corrective osteotomy may be necessary to correct deformity of fingers associated with osteochondromas.

## Osteoid Osteoma

Osteoid osteoma is a benign bone-forming neoplasm characterized by a central nidus within the surrounding sclerotic bone. Approximately 10% of all benign bone tumors are osteoid osteoma, and about 5–15% of cases affect the wrist and hand. Patient with osteoid osteoma typically presents in the second to third decades of life with a significant, well-localized pain aggravating at night. Within the nidus abnormally high concentration of prostaglandin $E_2$ and $I_2$ has been demonstrated. This may be related to pain resolution with administration of aspirin or nonsteroidal anti-inflammatory drugs [24].

Swelling and loss of motion of in adjacent joints are common, and point tenderness over the region of the nidus and associated soft tissue edema are common physical findings.

Radiographically a radiolucent nidus is surrounded by a rim of dense reactive bone. The nidus is seldom larger than 1 cm in diameter. Osteoid osteoma usually arises within the cortex, but sometimes it has a intramedullary location. Bone scintigraphy and CT scanning are helpful to find nidus obscured by reactive bone or invisible in a radiograph [25]. Histologically the nidus is composed with abundant, loose, fibrovascular connective tissue between amorphous osteoid bars, intertwined with numerous osteoblasts and osteoclasts surrounding the bony trabeculae. The periphery is composed of reactive woven and trabecular bones.

In some cases, osteoid osteoma may be self-limiting. But its course is unpredictable and may be protracted. Curettage of nidus and bone graft can be helpful to relieve intolerable significant pain (Fig. 16.9). CT-guided percutaneous radiofrequency thermal ablation has proven to be an effective, reliable, minimally invasive technique [26]. After identification of nidus under the CT guidance, a radiofrequency probe is placed within it and then heated to 90 °C for 6 min [27]. However, there is little or no experience with RFA of osteoid osteoma in the small bones of the hand, and a little volume of cushion between the nidus and vital tissues is available. So open techniques are preferred ones for lesions in the hand and thumb region. If the nidus has not been excised completely, recurrences are more likely [28].

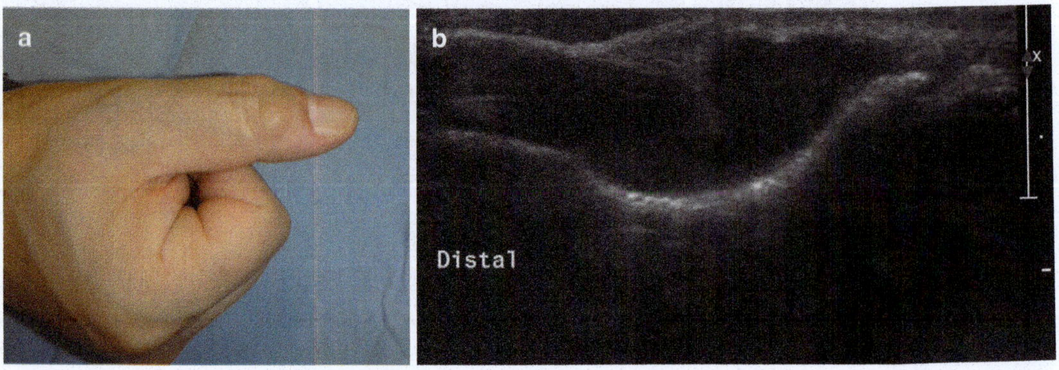


**Fig. 16.9** A clinical photograph of right thumb showed mucoid cyst on dorsoradial aspect of distal phalangeal joint with nail deformity (**a**). The pressure on the nail matrix by mucoid cyst can cause a longitudinal grooving of the nail. Ultrasonogram reveals mucoid cyst over the nail matrix (**b**)

## Soft Tissue Tumors

### Ganglion

Ganglion cyst is the most frequent soft tissue mass in the hand and thumb, compromising approximately 50% of hand tumors. They arise most frequently during the second through fourth decades in any location in the hand and wrist but are usually adjacent to joints or tendons [29].

The pathogenesis of ganglion cysts is unclear; one theory accepted widely until recently is that ganglions are arisen as a result of mucoid degeneration. Stretching of capsular and ligamentous supporting structures stimulates the production of mucin, which dissects through those supporting structures and forms capsular ducts and lakes that eventually coalesce into the main cyst [30]. It is a mucinous cyst attached to the adjacent underlying joint capsule, tendon, and tendon sheath with or without a small stalk. The fluid may enter into the cyst through a one-way check valve mechanism. At least 10% of cases have specific traumatic events, and repeated minor trauma may be an etiologic factor in their development [31].

Frequent locations are dorsal wrist, volar wrist, dorsal interphalangeal joint (mucinous cyst), and volar metacarpophalangeal joint (volar retinacular cyst). Patients generally complain of fluctuating mass due to connection between the cyst and joint capsule. The history, physical examination, positive transillumination test, and aspiration of mucinous material should allow a conclusive diagnosis. Malignant degeneration of ganglion cysts has never been reported; however malignant soft tissue tumors are frequently misdiagnosed as ganglion cysts. So care should be taken to differentiate.

Asymptomatic ganglions are managed with observation initially. Observation has been advocated in the pediatric population especially due to the high likelihood of spontaneous resolution [32]. Aspiration may provide long-term relief in 20–30% of patients with wrist ganglions. Patient assurance of its nonmalignant nature will be important in nonsurgical treatment.

Surgery is considered for cases with persistent symptoms. Complete open or arthroscopic excision of the ganglion including the entire stalk leading into joint space is essential to prevent recurrence. Recent comparative studies demonstrated the similar outcomes from the points of relative risks and benefits of open versus arthroscopic procedures [33, 34].

Volar retinacular ganglion which arises from the proximal annular ligament (A1 pulley) of the flexor tendon sheath is a small, firm, tender mass palpable under the MP flexion crease. The cyst is attached to the tendon sheath. A needle rupture and digital massage to disperse the cyst contents can delay or obviate the need for surgery. Ganglion is approached through the oblique or chevron incision over the mass. The mass can be traced to the tendon sheath and excised with a small portion of the surrounding margin of tendon sheath together.

A mucinous cyst, ganglion of the distal interphalangeal joint (interphalangeal joint of the thumb), generally occurs in association with degenerative arthritis between the fifth and seven decades. The pressure on the nail matrix can cause a longitudinal grooving of the nail (Fig. 16.9a, b). The 3–5-mm cyst typically lies to one side of extensor tendon and between the dorsal digital joint crease and eponychium. The radiographic evidences of osteoarthritic changes in the joint are usually seen. The cyst and osteophytes both should be excised to ensure a satisfactory result. Through the chevron incision over the IP joint, the cyst is mobilized, traced to the joint, and excised with the joint capsule. Osteophytes can be excised with a rongeur, and all soft tissue between the retracted extensor tendon and adjacent collateral ligaments on the affected side should be excised. Then with the joint extended and the extensor tendon retracted dorsally, the opposite side is explored, and the occult cysts or hypertrophied synovial tissue is excised also. Care for preservation of the insertion of extensor tendon and nail matrix should be taken. Instead of elliptical excision of thinned overlying skin, the fine separation and preservation of overlying skin with compression dressing can allow to avoid additional skin coverage procedures.

## Epidermal Inclusion Cyst

Epidermal inclusion cysts are the third most common type of tumor in the hand. They are keratin-filled cysts that often resulted from trauma when epithelial cells were introduced into the underlying subcutaneous tissues or bone. The cells grow slowly and produce a cyst lined with epithelial cells and filled with keratin material [31]. Most common locations are fingertip of left thumb and long finger in men in the third and fourth decades of life. It takes months or years following the trauma event to become clinically apparent.

Clinically it present as a slow-growing, well-circumscribed, firm, painless mass with slight mobility just underneath the skin. Sometimes they may be adherent to the overlying skin. In the fingertip, there may be bony erosion within the distal phalanx which may mimic a malignant or infectious process. Marginal excision is curative and recurrence rates are low. Malignant transformation has not been reported.

## Giant Cell Tumor of Tendon Sheath

Giant cell tumors of tendon sheath are the second most common soft tissue tumors in the hand. They are slow-growing benign soft tissue tumors and are more common in the fourth through sixth decades. They are usually painless, multilobular, fairly well circumscribed, more firm than ganglia, and often fixed to the underlying tissues including tendon and capsular structures. A sensory deficit may be present when the lesion occurs in proximity to the digital nerves. In some cases, the lesions can be locally aggressive and infiltrative into tendon substance and cause bony erosion. Plain radiographs will often demonstrate soft tissue mass, and if the mass is juxtacortical, erosion of underlying bone may occur (Fig. 16.10a–e). They have satellite lesions frequently, and it is one of the main courses of recurrence after marginal excision of giant cell tumors of tendon sheath. Preoperative evaluation using magnetic resonance imaging is recommended to detect the satellite lesions and evaluate the extent of involvement (Fig. 16.11a–e). Malignant transformation of giant cell tumors of tendon sheath in the hand has not been reported.

Complete marginal excision is the recommended treatment. During the surgical procedure, care must be taken to identify and protect the digital neurovascular bundles which can be displaced as well as enveloped by tumor masses. For the tumors arisen from the flexor sheath, a portion of the sheath is routinely excised at the site of tumor origin [29]. If the tumors are arisen from the joint, a capsulotomy should be performed, and inspect the joint space and debride any pigmented tissue remaining within the joint [35]. If extensive joint involvement or degenerative changes are seen, arthrodesis may be necessary after excision. The reported recurrence rates are 5–50% following a primary excision. Incomplete excision and the presence of satellite lesions are the main causes of recurrences [36]. To reduce the recurrence rate, it is important to carefully explore the surrounding tissues for satellite lesions. Radiation can be considered for multiple recurrent or aggressive lesions [37].

## Lipoma

Lipoma is one of the common benign soft tissue tumors of the hand. They can arise in the subcutaneous fat anywhere in the hand or can occur intramuscularly, involving thenar or hypothenar muscles. They may also arise within the deep spaces such as carpal tunnel, Guyon's canal, or the deep palmar space and can grow to substantial size to cause pressure effects [38].

The patients usually present with a slowly growing, painless mass. Physical examination shows a rubbery, flexible consistency and mobile mass without transillumination.

Plain radiography and computed tomography show a characteristic radiolucency of mature fat, which will be pathognomonic for lipoma [39]. Magnetic resonance imaging is diagnostic for lipoma. The T1-weighted image of a lipoma reveals high signal intensity in a well-circumscribed soft tissue mass [40].

An asymptomatic lipomatous mass with little or no growth can be observed regularly. For the symptomatic lesion, marginal surgical excision is recommended. The tumor is usually encapsulated and surrounded by a thin areolar tissue.

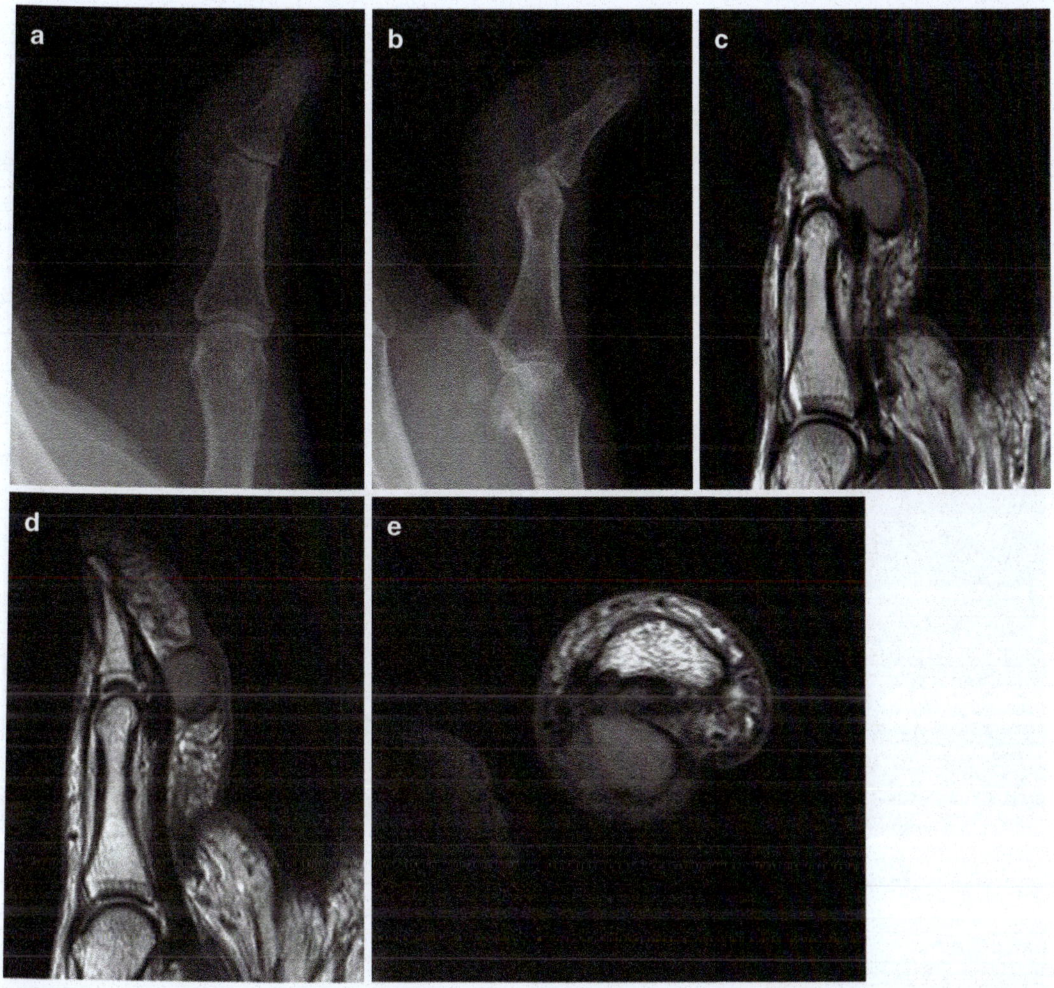


**Fig. 16.10** Plain radiographs (**a** and **b**) of patient with soft mass on voloulnar aspect of interphalangeal joint of the thumb show bony indentation at the base of distal phalanx. MR images (T2 weighted, sagittal, and axial, **c**, **d**, and **e**) demonstrate soft tissue mass, eroded cortical bone and subtendinous invasion

Even by blunt dissection, the mass shelled out from the surrounding tissue easily. Recurrence after marginal excision of lipoma is rare, and malignant transformation into liposarcoma is extremely rare.

## Angiolipoma

Angiolipoma is another benign tumor of adipose tissue composed of mature lipocytes mixed with proliferating endothelium-lined vascular sinuses.

It presents as a tender, painful lump and tends to be poorly encapsulated. Wide local excision with surrounding normal tissue will minimize the local recurrence rate. Malignant transformation of angiolipoma has not been reported.

## Nerve Tumor

Tumors origined from peripheral nerve tissues also can occur in the hand and thumb. Neurilemmoma and neurofibroma are the two common ones.

Neurilemmoma is the most common benign nerve tumors which originate from the Schwann cell and produce a slowly growing, well-circumscribed, eccentric lesion in the peripheral nerve. They are usually seen in middle-aged patients. They have a variety of clinical manifestations ranging from

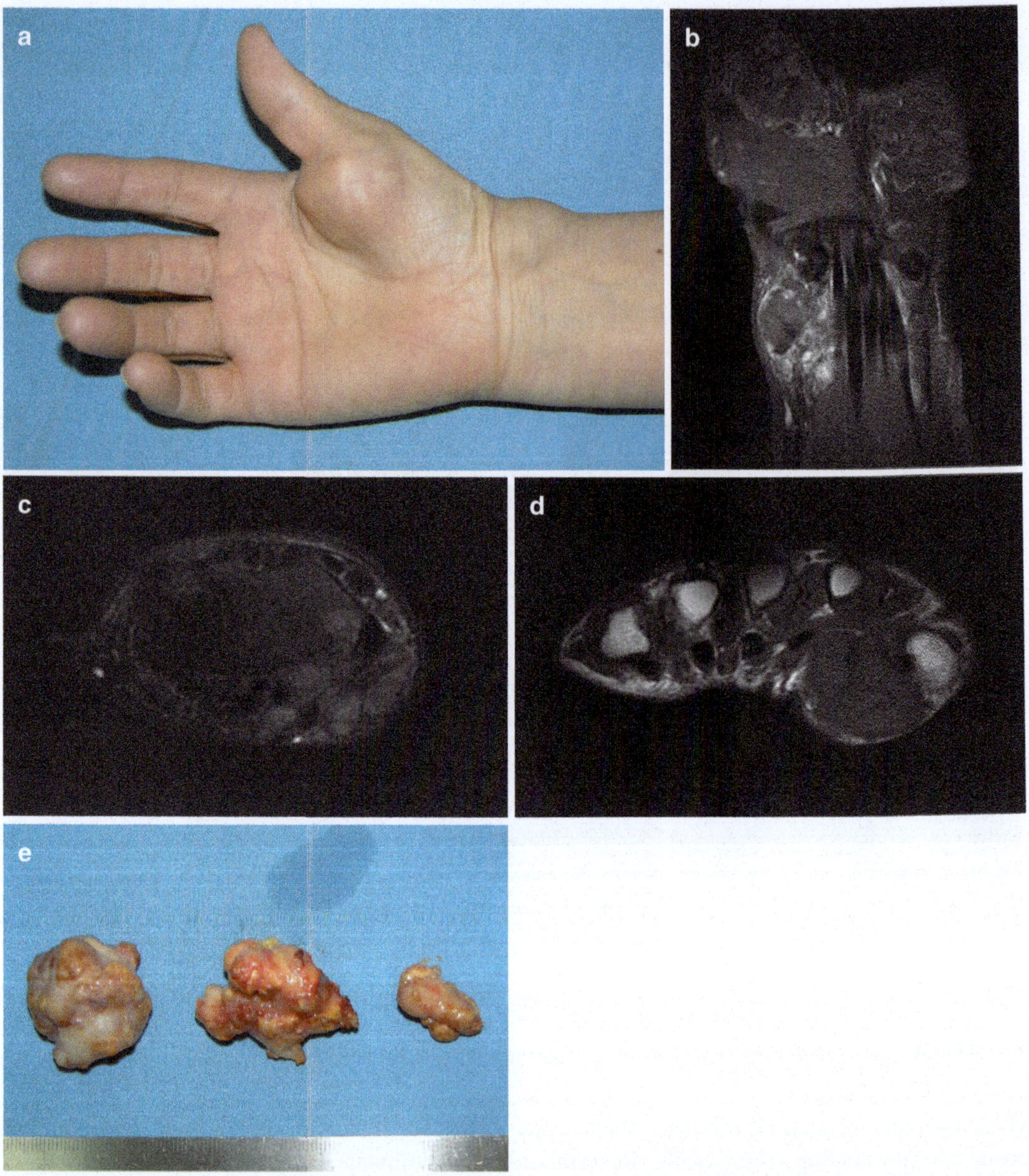

**Fig. 16.11** A 48-year-old female patient presented with protruding soft masses on thenar area (**a**). Magnetic resonance imaging showed multilobulated, elongated, and heterogeneously enhanced masses at the voloradial aspect of the right wrist with bony erosions. The lesion is extended to the palmar aspect of flexor tendons medially and also extended distally to the MP joint level (**b, c**, and **d**). Gross picture shows excised multilobulated masses with yellowish discoloration (**e**)

no symptom to pain and paresthesia. Percussion over the mass usually produces radiating pain in a specific nerve distribution (positive Tinel's sign). The lesion is often mobile in a transverse direction but not longitudinal direction. It is frequently misdiagnosed as a ganglion cyst, and magnetic resonance imaging is useful in delineating the lesion [41]. Neurilemmoma can be shelled out from the surrounding nerve, but interfascicular involvement may make the dissection more difficult. Optical magnification and microsurgical technique may be helpful to reduce the risk for postoperative neurologic deficit. Following excision, transient paresthesia may occur frequently, but the permanent neurologic deficits are unusual [42–44]. The incidence of postoperative neurologic deficit is approximately 5–15% [45]. In the majority of cases, the excision with intraneural fine dissection is curative and the recurrence is rare. There are rare reports of malignant transformation of neurilemmoma [46].

Neurofibromas are benign nerve tumors arising within nerve fasciculi. Symptoms and clinical findings are similar to those seen with neurilemmoma. Solitary lesion may be seen, but multiple neurofibromas are more common in the setting of neurofibromatosis. Because of the difficulty of separating neurofibromas from their associated nerves, they are typically more difficult to excise. Transection of the entering and exiting fascicles is usually required [47]. If the involved nerve has little functional importance the lesion can be excised otherwise, the nerve can be reconstructed. Postoperative neurologic deficit is more common than after excision of neurilemmomas. Surgical treatment of neurofibromas in patient with neurofibromatosis should be reserved for lesions that are growing or producing progressive symptoms. Plexiform neurofibromas in neurofibromatosis-1 have a high risk for progression to malignancy and can eventually degenerate to malignant peripheral nerve sheath tumors [48].

## Vascular Tumors

### Pyogenic Granuloma

Pyogenic granuloma occurs as a rapidly developing solitary pedunculated lesion with a friable, easily traumatized surface (Fig. 16.12) [49]. It is a polypoid form of capillary hemangioma occurring on the skin and mucosal surfaces. Previous history of injury or foreign body penetration is often accompanied. Hypertrophied, protuberant masses bleed with minimal trauma. Treatment options include electrocautery, laser treatment, and surgical excision. Surgical excision including narrow surrounding normal skin resulted in high success rate.

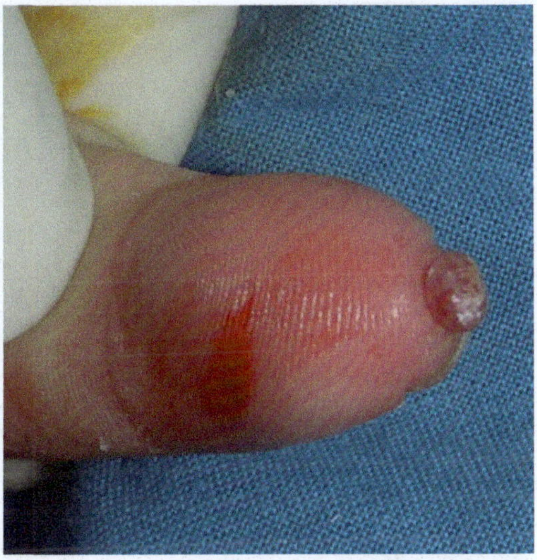

**Fig. 16.12** A clinical photograph shows a polypoid, friable, purple-red mass on the pulp tip of index finger. The lesion can be managed with complete excision including small amount of surrounding normal tissue

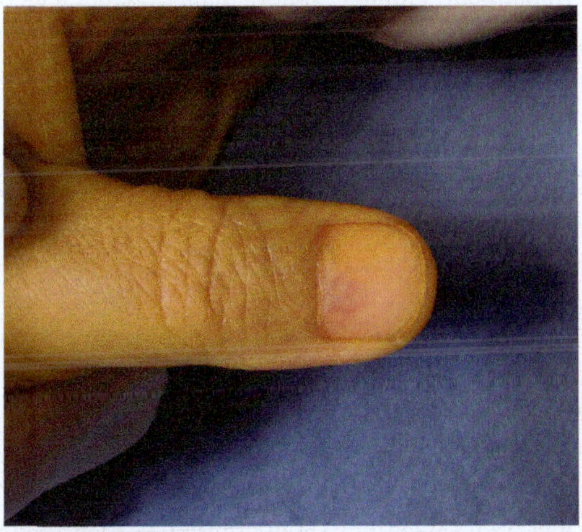

**Fig. 16.13** A clinical photograph of patient with pain and cold sensitivity of thumb shows a bluish discoloration of thumb nail, which suggests glomus tumor

### Glomus Tumor

The glomus body is a normal structure functioning as a thermoregulator, the anatomy of which is a specialized arteriovenous shunt that responds to local temperature changes. It is most numerous in the fingertips and under the nail beds. The classic symptom triads are pain, cold intolerance, and point tenderness over the lesion. A bluish discoloration overlying the mass may be a characteristic on physical examination (Fig. 16.13). MRI or ultrasonography is useful to localize masses (Fig. 16.14a–d). A thorough surgical excision is usually curative.

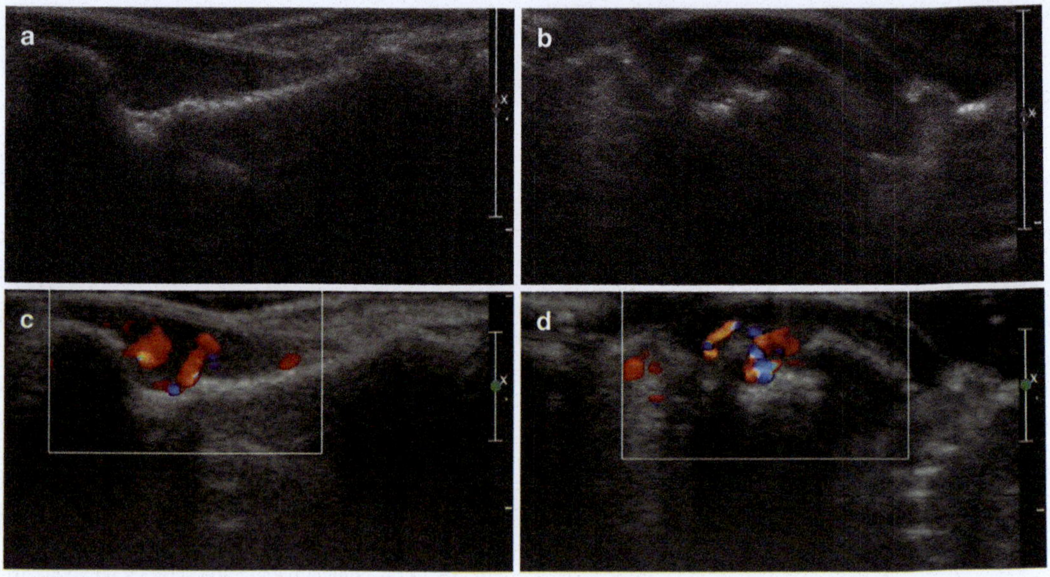


**Fig. 16.14** Ultrasonography of patient with glomus tumor demonstrated subungual mass (**a** and **b**) with arteriovenous signals on color Doppler examination (**c** and **d**)

Subungual glomus tumors can be enucleated without long-term nail deformity through transungal approach (Fig. 16.15a–f). Symptoms relieved immediately, and recurrence is uncommon if all the mass is excised [50].

## Hemangioma

Hemangiomas are noted within the first 4 weeks of life. Rapid cell proliferation and growth during 10–12 months of age resulted in maximum tumor size. Then slow growth begins to match the growth of the child. About 70% of hemangiomas have regressed by age 7 years. Symptomatic hemangiomas can be removed by marginal excision. Recent alternative treatments are cryosurgery, steroid, laser ablation, and embolization [51].

## Vascular Malformation

Vascular malformations are unusual in the hand and upper extremity. There are two types of malformation: low-flow and high-flow lesions. Low-flow malformations are subdivided further into capillary, venous, lymphatic, and combined types. Venous malformation is the most common and the excision of these is usually straightforward. A surgical approach preserving vascular supply and nerve function is warranted because the treatment of even recurred lesions will not be difficult.

The patients with a high-flow arteriovenous malformation are often severely symptomatic in terms of pain and disability. Proximal shunting of blood flow through a large arteriovenous fistula leads to distal ischemia, or even high-output congestive heart failure can develop in large lesions. Embolization may be helpful and ischemic digits are probably best amputated [52].

## Angioleiomyoma

Angioleiomyoma is a relatively common neoplasm, accounting 4–5% of benign soft tissue tumors. Lesions are common during the fourth to sixth decades of life and most often seen in the extremities, especially in the lower legs. It typically presents as a small, slowly growing circumscribed nodule located in subcutaneous layer, which is usually accompanied by pain and ten-

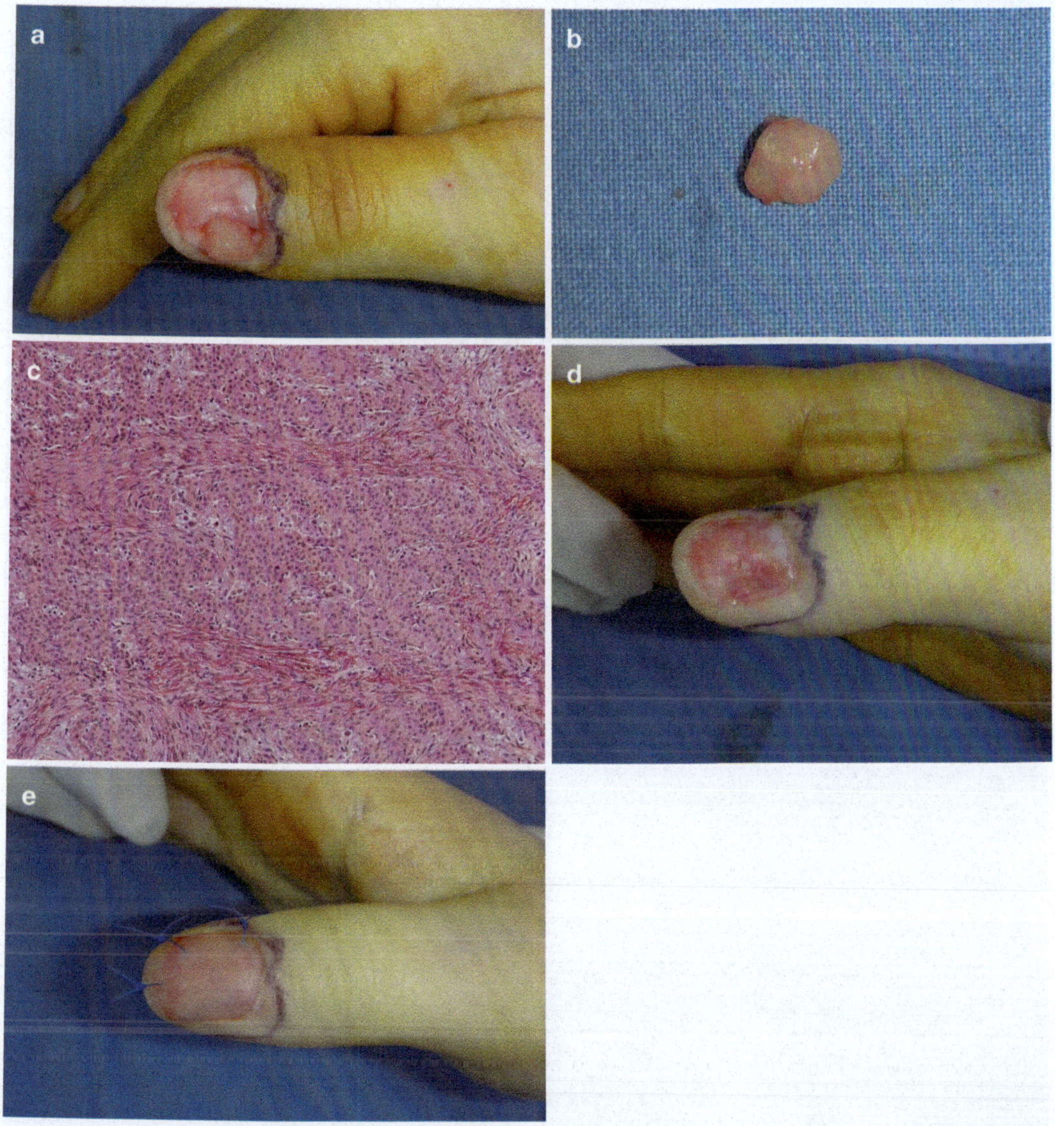

**Fig. 16.15** A 45-year-old female patient with glomus tumor. After temporal extraction of thumb nail, a longitudinal incision of nail bed exposed small rounded red-blue nodule (**a**). A gross picture (**b**) and histological examination (**c**, H&E stain, ×100) showed characteristic features of glomus tumors, nests of uniform, round glomus cells with well-defined cell membrane and surrounding capillary-sized vessels. The nail bed was best repaired with thin absorbable suture material (**d**), and the nail was repositioned to prevent desiccation of nail bed (**e**)

derness (Fig. 16.16a–d). MRI shows mixed hyperintense and isointense areas on T2-weighted images and strong enhancement after gadolinium infusion. Histologically angioleiomyoma is a benign soft tissue tumor composed of well-differentiated smooth muscle cells with intervening vascular channels [53]. Simple excision is curative and local recurrences are rare.

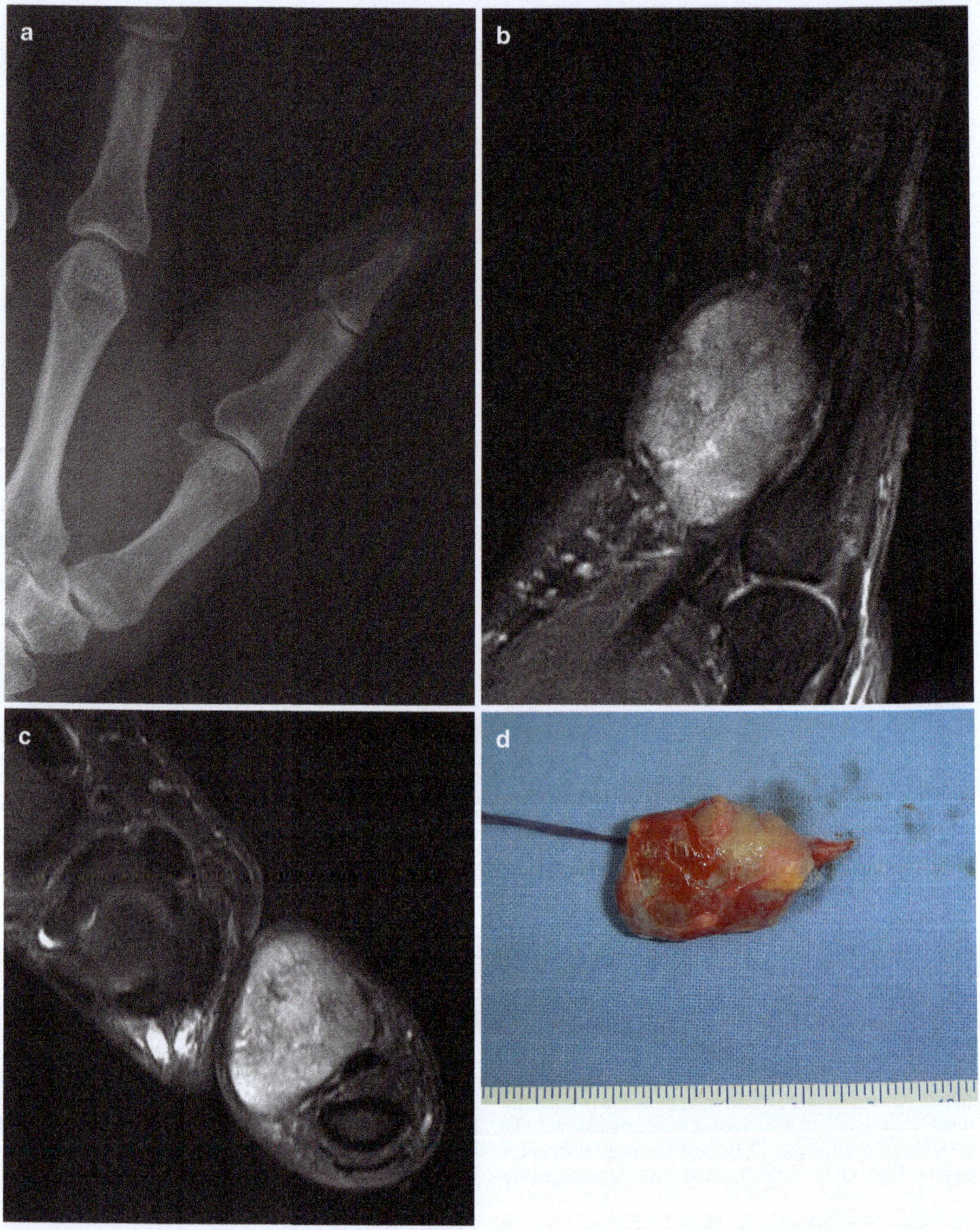


**Fig. 16.16** Plain radiograph of 55-year-old male patient shows a soft tissue mass shadow in proximal phalangeal area of the thumb (**a**). MR imagings demonstrated well-circumscribed, hyperintense mass in subcutaneous layer with heterogeneous enhancement (**b** and **c**). Gross picture of excised lesion showed a 5.2 cm-sized, thin capsulated, oval-shaped mass (**d**) and histological examination of which demonstrated the typical features of angioleiomyoma

## References


1. Murray PM. Soft tissue neoplasm: benign and malignant. In: Trumble T, editor. Hand surgery update 3. Rosemont, IL: American Society for Surgery of the Hand; 2003. p. 569–81.
2. Enneking WF, Spanier SS, Goodman MA. Current concepts review: the surgical staging of musculoskeletal sarcoma. J Bone Joint Surg. 1980;62A:1027–30.
3. Wunder JS, Healey JH, Davis AM, et al. A comparison of staging systems for localized extremity soft tissue sarcoma. Cancer. 2000;88:2721–30.
4. Unni KK, Dahlin DC. Dahlin's bone tumors: general aspects and data on 11,087 cases. 5th ed. Philadelphia: Lippincott-Raven; 1996.
5. Schwartz HS, Zimmerman NB, Simon MA, Wroble RR, Millar EAA, Bonfiglio M. The malignant potential of enchondromatosis. J Bone Joint Surg. 1987;69A:269–74.
6. Yasuda M, Masada K, Takeuchi E. Treatment of enchondroma of the hand with injectable calcium phosphate bone cement. J Hand Surg. 2006;31A:98–102.
7. Joosten U, Joist A, Frebel T, Walter M, Langer M. The use of an in situ curing hydroxyapatite cement as an alternative to bone graft following removal of enchondroma of the hand. J Hand Surg. 2000;25B:288–91.
8. Wulle C. On the treatment of enchondroma. J Hand Surg. 1990;15B:320–30.
9. Goto T, Yokokura S, Kawano H, Yamamoto A, Matsuda K, Nakamura K. Simple curettage without bone grafting for enchondromata of the hand: with special reference to replacement of the cortical window. J Hand Surg. 2002;27B:446–51.
10. Bickels J, Wittig JC, Kollender Y, et al. Enchondromas of the hand: treatment with curettage and cemented internal fixation. J Hand Surg. 2002;27A:870–5.
11. Ablove RH, Moy OJ, Peimer CA, Wheeler DR. Early versus delayed treatment of enchondroma. Am J Orthop. 2000;29:771–2.
12. Giles DW, Miller SJ, Rayan GM. Adjunctive treatment of enchondromas with $CO_2$ laser. Lasers Surg Med. 1999;24:187–93.
13. Athanasian EA, McCormack RR. Recurrent aneurysmal bone cyst of the proximal phalanx treated with cryosurgery: a case report. J Hand Surg. 1999;24A:405–12.
14. Athanasian EA. Aneurysmal bone cyst and giant cell tumor of the bone of the hand and distal radius. Hand Clin. 2004;20:269–81.
15. Nielsen GP, Fletcher JA, Oliveira AM. Aneurysmal bone cyst. In: Fletcher CD, Bridge JA, Hogendoorn PC, Mertens F, editors. WHO classification of tumors of soft tissue and bone. 4th ed. Lyon: International Agency for Research on Cancer; 2013. p. 348–9.
16. Marcove RC, Shrth DS, Takemoto S, Healey JH. The treatment of aneurysmal bone cyst. Clin Orthop Relat Res. 1995;311:157–63.
17. Gibbs CP Jr, Hefel MC, Peabody TD, Montag AG, Aithal V, Simon MA. Aneurysmal bone cyst of the extremities: factors related to local recurrence after curettage with a high-speed burr. J Bone Joint Surg. 1999;81A:1671–8.
18. Ramirez AR, Stanton RP. Aneurysmal bone cyst in 29 children. J Pediatr Orthop. 2002;22:533–9.
19. Borrelli J Jr, RR MC Jr. Aneurysmal bone cyst involving the long finger metacarpal in a child: a case report. J Hand Surg. 1994;19A:800–2.
20. Rock MG, Prichard DJ, Unni KK. Metastases from histologically benign giant-cell tumor of bone. J Bone Joint Surg. 1984;66A:269–74.
21. Campanacci M, Giunti A, Olmi R. Giant cell tumors of bone: a study of 209 cases with long-term follow up in 130. Ital J Orthop Traumatol. 1975;1:24–7.
22. Athanasian EA, Wold LE, Amadio PC. Giant cell tumor of the bones of the hand. J Hand Surg. 1997;22A:91–8.
23. Wittig JC, Simpson BM, Bickels J, Kellar-Graney KL, Malawer MM. Giant cell tumor of the hand: superior results with curettage cryosurgery and cementation. J Hand Surg. 2001;26A:546–55.
24. Greco F, Tamburelli F, Ciabattoni G. Prostaglandins in osteoid osteoma. Int Orthop. 1991;15:35–7.
25. Wilson Y, Fogelman I, Evans DM. Detection of an elusive osteoid osteoma using a registration bone scan. J Hand Surg. 1997;22B:801–4.
26. Barei DP, Moreau G, Scarborough MT. Percutaneous radiofrequency thermal ablation of osteoid osteoma. Oper Tech Orthop. 1999;9:72–8.
27. Rosenthal DI, Hornicek FJ, Torriani M, Gebhardt MC, Mankin HJ. Osteoid osteoma: percutaneous treatment with radiofrequency energy. Radiology. 2003,229:171–5.
28. Bednar MS, Weiland AJ, Light TR. Osteoid osteoma of the upper extremity. Hand Clin. 1995;11:211–21.
29. Nahra ME, Bucchieri JS. Ganglion cysts and other tumor related conditions of the hand and wrist. Hand Clin. 2004;20:249–60.
30. Carp L, Stout AP. A study of ganglion with special reference to treatment. Surg Gynecol Obstet. 1928;47:460–8.
31. Athanasian EA. Bone and soft tissue tumors. In: Wolfe SW, Hotchkiss RN, Pederson WC, Kozin SH, Cohen MS, editors. Operative hand surgery, vol. 2. 6th ed. Philadelphia: Elsevier; 2017. p. 1987–2035.
32. Wang AA, Hutchison DT. Longitudinal observation of pediatric hand and wrist ganglia. J Hand Surg. 2001;26A:599–602.
33. Edwards SG, Johase JA. Prospective outcomes and associations of wrist ganglion cysts resected arthroscopically. J Hand Surg. 2009;34A:395–400.
34. Kang L, Akelman E, Weiss AP. Arthroscopic versus open dorsal ganglion excision: a prospective, randomized comparison of rates of recurrences and residual pain. J Hand Surg. 2008;33A:471–5.
35. Moore JR, Weiland AJ, Curtis RM. Localized nodular tenosynovitis: experience with 115 cases. J Hand Surg. 1984;9A:412–7.
36. Glowacki KA, Weiss APC. Giant cell tumors of tendon sheath. Hand Clin. 1995;11:245–53.

37. Coroneos CJ, O'Sullivan B, Ferguson PC, et al. Radiation therapy for infiltrative giant cell tumor of the tendon sheath. J Hand Surg. 2012;37A:775–82.
38. Ingari JV, Faillace JJ. Benign tumors of fibrous tissue and adipose tissue in the hand. Hand Clin. 2004;20:243–8.
39. Enneking WF. Neoplasms of soft tissue. In: Enneking WF, editor. Clinical musculoskeletal pathology. 3rd ed. Gainesville: University of Florida Press; 1990. p. 422–49.
40. Azouz EM, Babyn PS, Mascia AT, Tuuha SE, Decarie JC. MRI of the abnormal pediatric hand and wrist with plain film correlation. J Comput Assist Tomogr. 1998;22:252–61.
41. Stull MA, Moser RP Jr, Kransdorf MJ, et al. Magnetic resonance appearance of peripheral nerve sheath tumors. Skelet Radiol. 1991;29:9–14.
42. Swada T, Sano M, Ogihara H, Omura T, Miura K, Nagano A. The relationship between preoperative symptoms, operative findings and postoperative complications in schwannomas. J Hand Surg. 2006;31B:629–34.
43. Park MJ, Seo KN, Kang HJ. Neurologic deficit after surgical enucleation of schwannomas of the upper limb. J Bone Joint Surg. 2009;91B:1482–6.
44. Kang JW, Lee YS, Kim CJ, Shin SH, Chung YG. Neurologic deficits after surgical enucleation of schwannoma in the upper extremity. J Korean Soc Surg Hand. 2017;22:41–8.
45. Siqueira MG, Socolovsjy M, Martins RS, et al. Surgical treatment of typical peripheral schwannomas: the risk of new postoperative deficits. Acta Neuroch (Wien). 2013;155:1745–9.
46. Alektiar KM, Leung D, Zelefsky MJ, et al. Adjuvant radiation for stage IIB soft tissue sarcoma of the extremity. J Clin Oncol. 2002;20:1643–50.
47. Donner TR, Voorhies RM, Kline DG. Neural sheath tumors of major nerves. J Neurosurg. 1994;81:362–73.
48. Ferner RE, Gutmann DH. International consensus statement on malignant peripheral nerve sheath tumors in neurofibromatosis. Cancer Res. 2002;62:1573–7.
49. Fleming ANM, Smith PJ. Vascular cell tumors of the hand in children. Hand Clin. 2000;16:609–24.
50. Phillips CS, Murphy MS. Vascular problems of the upper extremity: a primer for the orthopaedic surgeon. J Am Acad Orthop Surg. 2002;10:401–2.
51. Walsh JJ IV, Eady JL. Vascular tumors. Hand Clin. 2004;20:261–8.
52. Upon J, Coombs CJ, Mulliken JB, Burrows PE, Pap S. Vascular malformation of the upper limb: a review of 270 patients. J Hand Surg. 1999;24A:1019–35.
53. Hisaoka M, Quade B. Angioleiomyoma. In: Fletcher CD, Bridge JA, Hogendoorn PC, Mertens F, editors. WHO classification of tumors of soft tissue and bone. 4th ed. Lyon: International Agency for Research on Cancer; 2013. p. 120–1.

# Malignant Tumors

# 17

Sung Tack Kwon and Byung Jun Kim

## Basal Cell Carcinoma

### Introduction

Basal cell carcinoma (BCC) is the most common skin cancer, but the incidence of BCC of the hand is much lower than that of squamous cell carcinoma (SCC) at this area. BCCs are malignant epithelial neoplasms arising from the basal layer of the epidermis or pilosebaceous adnexa. Characteristic cells are observed that have a large basophilic nucleus with minimal cytoplasm. In any nest of cells, peripheral tumor cells are aligned with long axis perpendicular to the nest, showing a "picket fence" appearance. Excessive sun damage is the most common factor predisposing to the development of BCC. Although BCC is more common in adults, it can also occur in children, especially in those with certain syndromes (e.g., nevoid basal cell syndrome and Bazex syndrome). BCC is also associated with xeroderma pigmentosum, irradiation, burn scars, and chronic exposure to arsenic [1].

S. T. Kwon · B. J. Kim (✉)
Department of Plastic and Reconstructive Surgery, Seoul National University Hospital, Seoul, South Korea
e-mail: stk59@snu.ac.kr

### Clinical Manifestations

BCCs are generally observed as ulcerated lesions on the skin with elevated and pearly edges with erythema in middle-aged and older individuals. Specifically, circumscribed or diffuse lesions are primarily presented. BCCs of the hand usually occur in hair-bearing dorsal locations [2].

### Classification

BCCs are classified into circumscribed and diffuse types as previously described. Nodular and circumscribed lesions are generally less virulent than diffuse lesions. Moreover, diffuse BCCs have increased recurrence rate compared to circumscribed lesions because they extend deeply into the dermis further from the clinically visible or palpable border. More specifically, BCCs can be classified into five major types; fibroepithelioma, morpheaform, nodulo-ulcerative, pigmented, and superficial BCC [3]. Nodulo-ulcerative type is the most common form of BCC. It is dome-shaped with well-defined borders and often appears as a pink-red papule displaying a "pearly" appearance with telangiectasia. Although its growth pattern is circumscribed, nodular BCC may be poorly differentiated histologically. Superficial BCC has multiple foci that are actually connected with each other. Its



S. H. Woo (ed.), *The Thumb*, https://doi.org/10.1007/978-981-10-4400-7_17

extension beyond clinically visible borders makes it highly recurrent after surgical treatment.

## Differential Diagnosis

BCCs should be differentiated from factitious ulceration, eczema, actinic keratosis, psoriasis, and fungal infection. Nodular pigmented BCC may resemble melanoma in appearance which makes it more difficult to be distinguished.

## Treatment

Excision is commonly recommended as a treatment option. Surgical excision offers a greater than 90% cure rate [4]. For a less than 1 cm in diameter nodular lesion, a 2-mm surgical margin may be sufficient. For lesions up to 2 cm, however, a 3–5-mm margin is more appropriate. In this case, the deep margin should extend into a subcutaneous fat. Lesions greater than 2 cm and those with aggressive growth patterns (e.g., morpheaform and superficial "multicentric" BCC) may require 10-mm resection margins [5]. Curettage and electrodessication is the technique for treating BCC but is limited for primary lesions less than 1 cm in diameter. This technique is appropriate for lesions of the hand extremity. Cryosurgery can be applied to well-defined lesions [6]. However, neuropathy is a potential risk of cryosurgery due to uncontrolled depth of freeze. For this reason, cryosurgery should not be applied on digits and around the ulnar nerve at the elbow. Cure rate for curettage, electrodessication, and cryosurgery for small lesions has been reported to be as high as 97%. However, these techniques have an inherent disadvantage of lacking a microscopic verification of complete tumor removal.

## Prognosis

BCC arises without a precursor lesion and is usually slow growing, locally destructive, and recurrent. However, it is not clinically aggressive and metastasis is rare [7]. Regular follow-up is indicated to identify recurrences and new lesions.

# Squamous Cell Carcinoma

## Introduction

SCC is known as the most common malignant tumor of the hand [8]. In general, SCC is a skin-colored or pink lesion that is usually found on the dorsal surface of the hand. SCC can occur from premalignant lesions (actinic keratosis), in situ variant (Bowen's disease), or de novo [9].

## Clinical Presentation

SCC appears with a various range of clinical presentations, including (1) small, firm, and pigmented lesions of carcinoma in situ (Bowen's disease); (2) ulcerated lesions with surrounding induration; (3) exophytic and large tumor mass with hyperkeratosis, (4) wartlike lesions, especially in the periungual area; and (5) nodular lesions in a burn scar. Although early Bowen disease has low risk to become an invasive cancer, the larger the lesions, the greater the possibility of developing into a metastatic disease [10] (Fig. 17.1). SCC lesions can also progress into aggressive lesions, such as in the case of Marjolin's ulcer, a malignant neoplasm arising in a burn, radiation scar, or other chronic wounds. Generally, SCC requires a long time before its occurrence; however, in some cases, SCC development has been reported as early as 6 weeks after a burn [11].

## Risk Factors

Risk factors of SCC include solar radiation, ionizing radiation, chronic inflammation, exposure to chemicals (e.g., arsenicals), certain disease states (e.g., xeroderma pigmentosum, Bowen's disease, leukoplakia, and epidermodysplasia verruciformis), human papillomavirus, Caucasian race, and smoking [12]. Immunocompromised

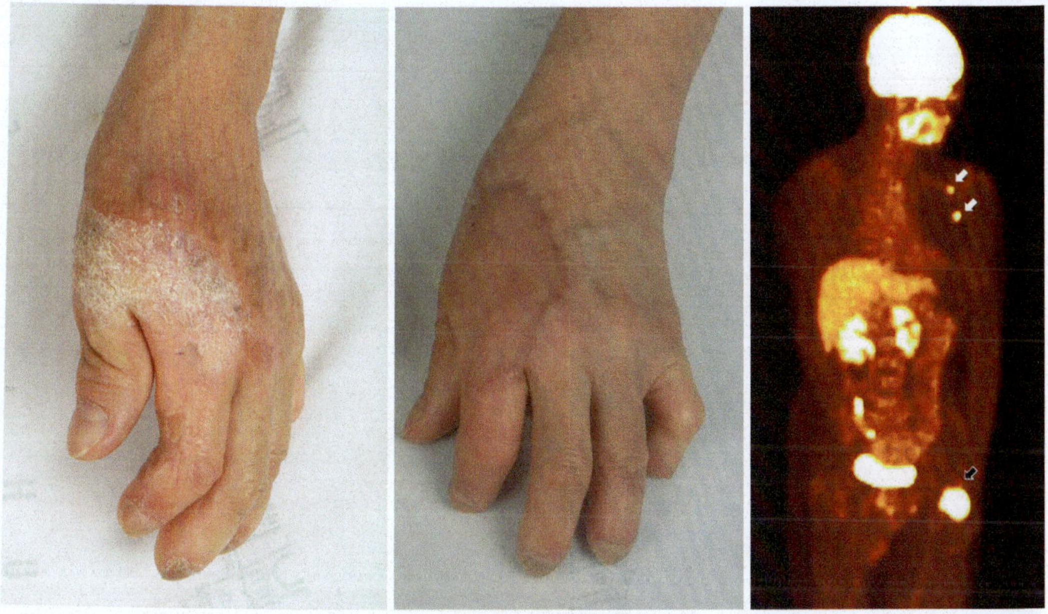

**Fig. 17.1** Squamous cell carcinoma on the left hand dorsum (left) that was treated with wide excision and skin graft (middle). This patient presented with axillary lymph node metastasis on diagnosis (right). White arrows indicate axillary lymph node metastasis, and black arrow stands for primary lesion on the left hand

patients, especially those with renal and heart transplants, are 65% more susceptible to develop SCC compared with those who are healthy. These patients may also have multiple lesions and more aggressively behaving SCCs. Histological evaluation of the primary tumor is important in predicting the prognosis of SCC. High grade of differentiation ratio (grade 3 and 4), tumor size greater than 2 cm, tumor depth extension into the subcutaneous layer (or greater than 4 mm), perineural invasion, and paronychia are high-risk factors associated with tumor recurrence and metastasis [13].

## Treatment

Complete surgical excision with an adequate margin is the main treatment of choice; however, in low-risk SCCs, alternative treatment options can include cryotherapy, electrodessication, curettage, or photodynamic therapy. Safety margin including 5-mm normal tissue results in complete tumor removal in 95% of cases [14]. Generally, the excision margin for low-risk lesions is 4 mm, and for high-risk SCCs, it is at least 6 mm and extends into the subcutaneous fat or even fascia. Mohs micrographic surgery may be indicated for high-risk lesions, such as recurrent tumors, perineural invasion, poorly differentiated and deeply penetrating tumors, and in areas where tissue conservation is desired (e.g., on fingers) [15]. In cases of large or recurrent SCC, especially with bone involvement, amputation at the distal joint may be required [16]. Following wide excision of SCCs, resulting defects are generally closed directly, but large wounds can be reconstructed with skin graft or various flap operations (Fig. 17.2) [17]. Sentinel lymph node biopsy aids the decision-making process regarding lymph node dissection in the treatment of SCC. If the result of a sentinel lymph node biopsy is positive, an appropriate lymph node dissection is recommended.

## Prognosis

Within the first 5 years after SCC development, metastasis is detected in 5% of patients. It is

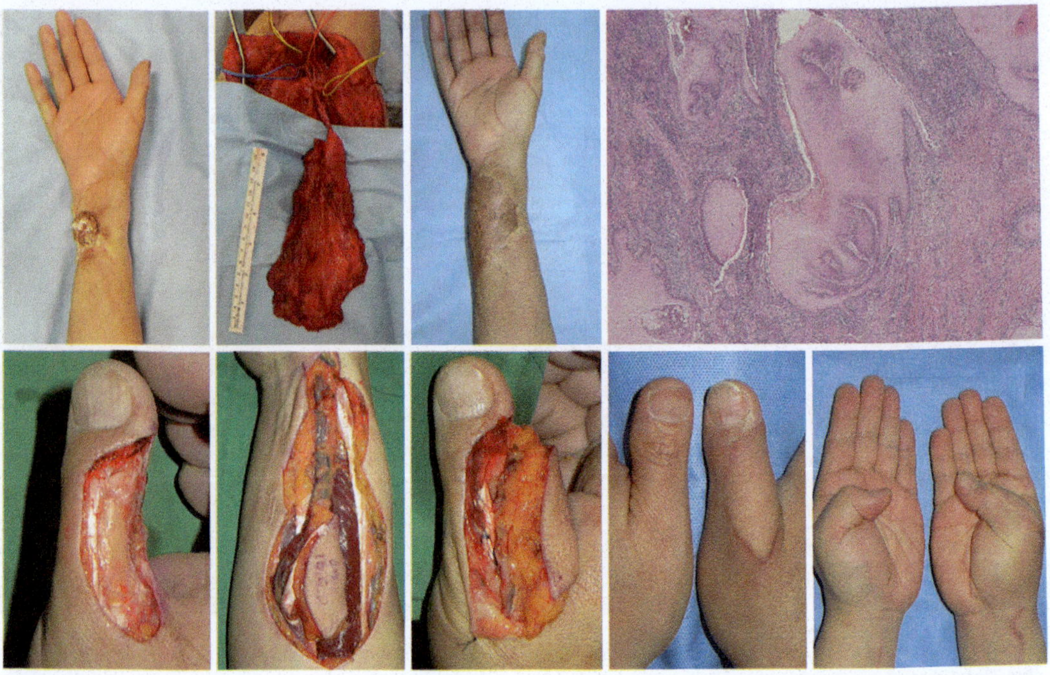

**Fig. 17.2** Various reconstruction methods after wide excision of the squamous cell carcinoma; serratus anterior fascia free flap with split-thickness skin graft (upper) and reverse radial forearm tendocutaneous island flap (lower). Histology showed the invasion of squamous cells with recruitment of inflammatory cells (hematoxylin and eosin stain × 40) (The lower case photos courtesy of Dr. Woo SH)

estimated that 2–5% of upper extremity SCCs metastasize to axillary nodes. The mortality rate for SCC of the hand is higher than that of other anatomic sites [8]. Factors affecting recurrence and metastasis include tumor size and thickness, histologic differentiation, site of the primary tumor, immune status of the host, carcinoma arising from scar tissue (Marjolin's ulcer), and neurotropic SCC [18]. Five-year survival rate decreases to 40% in the presence of axillary node metastases. However, since the incidence of lymph node metastasis is low, elective node dissection or sentinel lymph node biopsy has no advantage in treating SCC, unless nodes are clinically enlarged [19]. SCCs show slower invasion than cutaneous malignant melanomas and, hence, do not easily invade deeper tissues. Superficial dermis and epidermis lack lymphatic drainage, making SCC less likely to spread via lymphatics. Long-term follow-up after treatment of SCCs is critical to assess for recurrence or metastatic spread because metastasis can be found occasionally, even up to 10 years after the primary resection of the tumor.

## Malignant Melanoma

### Incidence

The incidence of cutaneous melanoma has been rapidly increased during the last decades compared with other malignant neoplasms, while melanoma of the hand shows relatively stable pattern of incidence [20]. Public medical education on the significance of early detection of melanoma has greatly contributed to the increase of the percentage of cases diagnosed at early stage. However, melanoma shows high rate of recurrence or metastasis even after curative treatment. Melanoma of the hand is known to have poorer prognosis compared with melanoma of other areas of the body [21].

## Clinical Presentation

Melanoma can arise from normal-shaped melanocytes, congenital nevi, and atypical pigmented lesions. Half of melanomas develops de novo, unrelated to preexisting melanocytic lesions [3]. However, it is not easy to distinguish malignant lesions from other benign pigmented lesions. Cutaneous melanoma shows a visible change over months to years, and the patients may be unaware of the lesions. Therefore, careful physical examination and meticulous history taking are very important. A general rule that warrants medical attention is the ABCD mnemonic that stands for asymmetry, border irregularity, color change, and diameter greater than 6 mm. Some investigators have added "E" for elevation or evolution of the lesion or "F" for family history. Signs of bleeding, ulceration, itching, or unusual sensation are associated with cutaneous melanoma. The growth patterns of melanoma are superficial spreading, lentigo maligna, nodular, and acral lentiginous. Among them, acral lentiginous type, which accounts for most melanoma cases of the hand, is predominant in darkly pigmented races, such as Asians and Blacks rather than Caucasians (Fig. 17.3).

## Diagnosis

Meticulous clinical examination and patient history are the most important factors in the diagnosis of melanomas. Dermoscopy, which magnifies the pigmented lesions with handheld dermatoscope, is a noninvasive and useful method to differentiate between benign and atypical pigmentations. Dermoscopy can increase the diagnosis accuracy by approximately 10%, and various algorithms can increase the sensitivity and specificity over 80% by adopting a scoring system [22].

Diagnosis is confirmed by incisional or excisional biopsy. Breslow thickness is measured in millimeter as a distance from the granular layer of the epithelium to the deepest portion of melanocytic invasion. Importantly, Breslow thickness is correlated with lymphatic invasion and the risk of distant metastasis.

Clinically palpable ipsilateral axillary lymph nodes should be meticulously evaluated, and elective lymph node dissection is recommended in patients with positive results. For occult lymph nodes, retrospective studies have revealed the benefit of elective lymph node dissection in the treatment of intermediate-thickness cutaneous melanoma (1–4 mm) [23]. Sentinel lymph node is the first node where lymphatic drainage occurs in an orderly manner and melanoma metastasize to; hence, sentinel lymph node biopsy is widely used to facilitate diagnosis and treatment of lymph node metastasis [24]. Sentinel lymph node biopsy has demonstrated an ability to reduce the morbidity of lymphedema in breast cancers or melanomas and has shown a good negative predictive value [25]. Melanomas thicker than 1 mm, with ulceration, high mitotic rate, lymphatic invasion, and microsatellites have shown a 14% risk of occult metastatic disease [26]. Therefore, sentinel lymph node biopsy is recommended for patients with melanomas with intermediate thickness or with greater than 25% risk of lymph node metastasis [27].

In melanomas with invasion depth more than 4 mm, the risk of nodal metastasis is very high (60–80%). In high-risk patients, general metastatic workups should be performed to exclude any nodal or distant metastasis. Since the lung is the most common site of distant metastasis, chest radiography is recommended for screening and postoperative follow-ups. Ultrasonography is useful in screening axillary lymph nodes and liver state. Laboratory evaluation, including evaluation of alkaline phosphatase and lactic dehydrogenase (LDH) levels, is also recommended to identify advanced stage melanomas. In highly suspicious patients for distant metastasis, chest computed tomography and positron emission tomography can be performed.

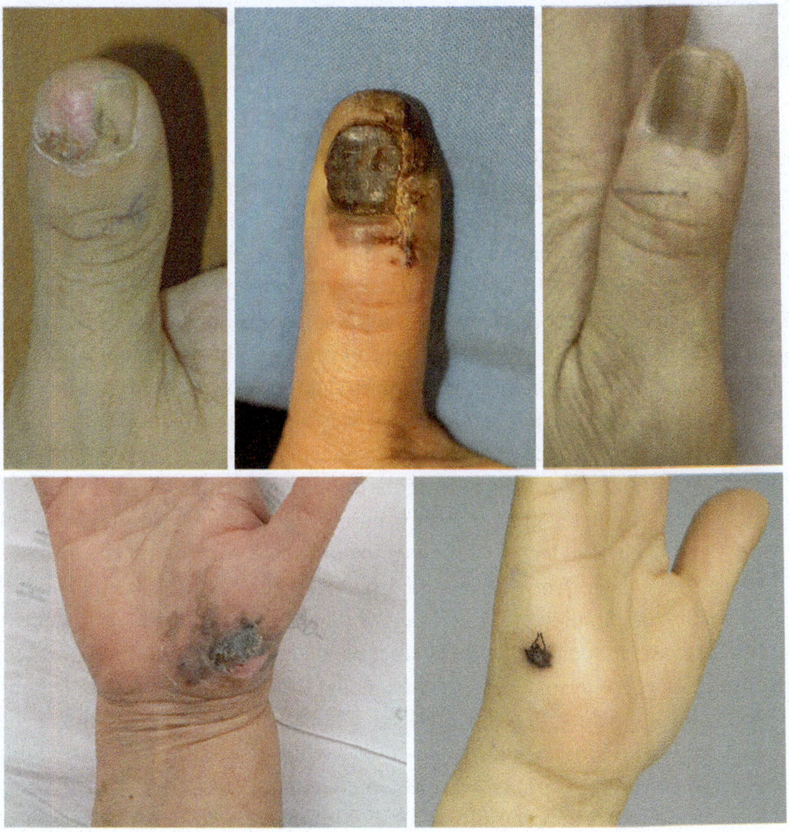

**Fig. 17.3** Various cases with malignant melanoma on the hands or thumbs (subungual melanomas)

## Staging

The TNM staging system, developed by the American Joint Committee on Cancer (AJCC), is the most commonly used method to determine clinical and pathologic stage of cutaneous melanoma. In the recently revised 8th edition, T1 is subcategorized into T1a, including non-ulcerated melanomas less than 0.8 mm in thickness, and T1b, including melanomas 0.8–1.0 mm in thickness with or without ulceration or less than 0.8 mm with ulceration. Furthermore, tumor mitotic rate is no longer a staging criterion for T1 tumors. As the N category also becomes more complicated in the 8th edition, stage III grouping is subdivided into four rather than three subgroups (A, B, C, and D). Lastly, the M category becomes more elaborate as central nervous system metastasis is re-categorized as M1d, and elevated LDH level is applied as a prognostic factor in each M subcategory. For example, brain metastasis with elevated LDH level is classified as M1d [1].

## Treatment

Wide excision of the primary tumor along with subcutaneous tissue (usually not including muscle fascia) is a mainstream between many surgeons. The appropriate extent of surgical margin is recommended according to the tumor thickness (Table 17.1). For the in situ lesions, 0.5–1-cm surgical margin is enough to achieve a curative surgery. Tumors less than 1-mm invasion can be treated with 1-cm margins, while invasion depth more than 2 mm needs a 2-cm safety margin. This guideline has been suggested by the

**Table 17.1** Recommended safety margin of cutaneous malignant melanomas based on the tumor depth (Breslow thickness)

| Tumor depth (Breslow thickness) | Excision margin |
|---|---|
| In situ | 0.5–1 cm |
| 0–1 mm | 1 cm |
| 1–2 mm | 1–2 cm |
| 2–4 mm | 2 cm |
| >4 mm | 2–3 cm |

WHO randomized trial and the Intergroup Melanoma Surgical Trial.

An early study has demonstrated an increased 5-year survival rate following elective lymphadenectomy for clinically occult lymph nodes compared to delayed lymphadenectomy for clinically palpable nodes [28]. However, a recent long-term randomized control study has presented no increase in the melanoma-specific survival of patients who had immediate completion of lymph node dissection after positive results from frozen section biopsy [29].

Melanoma is considered relatively radioresistant, but radiation therapy can provide effective treatment modality in some clinical settings. Primary curative radiotherapy can be attempted for localized inoperable mucosal melanoma. Adjuvant radiotherapy is effective in reducing the risk of recurrence in primary tumors or regional lymph node metastasis [30]. Radiotherapy can also be used for palliation, to reduce signs and symptoms related to melanoma [31].

Classical cytotoxic chemotherapy (e.g., dacarbazine and cisplatin) has resulted in regression of disseminated melanoma in very few patients with no evidence of long-term survival gain. Conventional immunotherapies, such as interleukin-2 and interferon, are still useful for limited indications but are ineffective in the majority of patients because of drug-related general toxicity. Ipilimumab is an immune checkpoint inhibitor that activates immune system by targeting a cytotoxic T-lymphocyte-associated antigen (CTLA-4). Pembrolizumab is an anti-programmed cell death (PD-1) immunotherapeutic agent. In patients with *BRAF* gene mutation, which can accelerate tumor cell growth, a BRAF inhibitor (Zelboraf) has been approved for prescription by the Food and Drug Administration. Recent clinical trials have shown a long-term survival gain following the combination of these agents [32]. Ongoing clinical trials and genetic studies will provide further data on these agents, showing a long-standing remission of melanoma.

## Subungual Melanoma

Subungual melanoma, arising beneath the nail plate, should be categorized as a single separate entity of acral lentiginous melanoma due to its unique anatomical location and poor prognosis. Subungual melanoma represents around 2% of all the cutaneous melanoma but shows a high prevalence in Black populations (15–20%) or Asians. Subungual melanoma can occur from any nail matrix of fingers or toes, but the thumb and the great toe are the most frequent sites of tumor development. The patients show pigmented strip-like lesions in the early stage, and they sometimes accompany nail deformity, pain, bleeding, and ulceration as the tumor progresses. To rule out benign pigmented nail bands, investigators have presented the ABCDEF mnemonic that suggests a malignant melanoma. This mnemonic stands for age greater than 40 years; African American; band width greater than 3 mm; border irregularity; change; digit involvement in the thumb, hallux, or index finger; extension onto the surrounding skin; and family history [33]. Hutchinson's sign, which is the extension of the pigmented lesion onto the nail fold or hyponychium, strongly suggests a malignant lesion [34]. The poor prognosis of subungual melanoma is believed to be due to its delayed diagnosis. Subungual lesions are easily misdiagnosed as subungual hematoma, fungal infection (onychomycosis), inflammatory lesion, or other benign pigmented lesions (e.g., melanonychia). Moreover, a recent history of minor trauma of fingers or toes can mask the malignancy, and amelanocytic subungual melanoma can make diagnosis even more difficult. Therefore, a failure of subungual hematoma to disappear in several months commonly precipitates a biopsy of the nail matrix. Accurate diagnosis of subungual melanoma can be delayed for more than 2 years, and, hence, more than 1/4 of patients have metastasis [35].

Complete surgical excision is the treatment of choice. Disarticulation of the involved finger at the distal interphalangeal joint (DIPJ) or amputation proximal to the DIPJ level is usually performed. The extensor tendon and flexor digitorum profundus tendon are anchored with balanced tension to prevent quadriga effect. Volar soft tissue is spared to cover the defect as fillet flap. However, conventional amputation can deteriorate hand function especially when it comes to the thumb. Aesthetically displeasing figure can make the patients socially withdrawn. Glat et al. described the first web space deepening technique using Z-plasty to improve the function of an amputated thumb [23]. Functional surgery can be performed to preserve function and cosmesis of hands (Fig. 17.4). Indication for functional surgery in subungual melanoma has not yet been clearly established. However, early lesion (melanoma in situ or invasion depth less than 1 mm) is usually accepted for functional surgery. A wide excision with 5–20-mm safety margin including the periosteum is performed. The defect is reconstructed with a secondary healing, skin grafts, cross finger flap, or thin flaps, such as venous free flap and superficial circumflex iliac artery perforator free flap [17]. Toe tissue can be transferred to the amputated digit to restore hand function in the invasive subungual melanoma lesions (Fig. 17.5).

General metastatic workup is required as aforementioned. Clinically palpable ipsilateral axillary lymph nodes should be meticulously evaluated in the intermediate tumor depth, and elective lymph node dissection is recommended following positive results. However, the Breslow thickness is hard to be applied in the subungual melanoma due to the lack of the granulosum layer in the nail matrix. The thickness of the nail matrix down to the periosteum has been found to be less than 2 mm in a cadaver study [36]. The overlying nail plate and bony structure underneath can affect the growth and progression of subungual melanoma. Further studies are required to determine the unique anatomy and the clinical relevance of the nail bed. The authors suggest that a

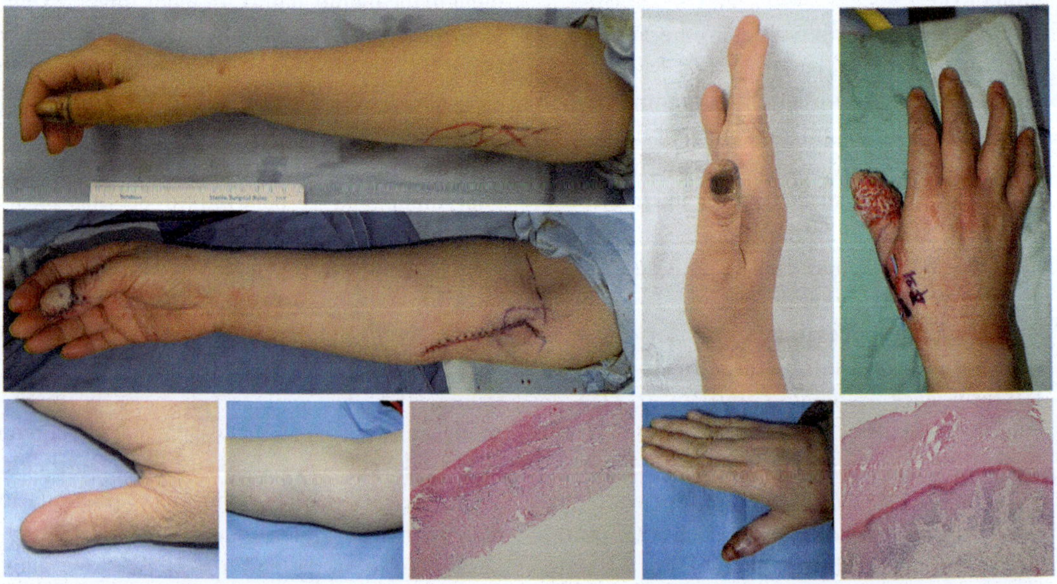

**Fig. 17.4** Functional surgery can be performed to restore hand function and appearance in early stage subungual melanoma. Sixty-eight-year-old female patient had wide excision of the subungual melanoma on her right thumb. The defect was covered with venous free flap. Photos taken 1-year postoperatively showed good postoperative results in both recipient and donor sites. Histology revealed melanoma in situ without invasion of the tumor cells (hematoxylin and eosin × 100) (left). Fifty-year-old female patient showed in situ subungual melanoma that extended to the volar skin. Following wide excision, the circumferential defect was reconstructed with serratus anterior fascia free flap and skin graft. Postoperative 6-month photo showed acceptable functional and aesthetic results. Histology revealed melanoma in situ without invasion of the tumor cells (hematoxylin and eosin × 100) (right)

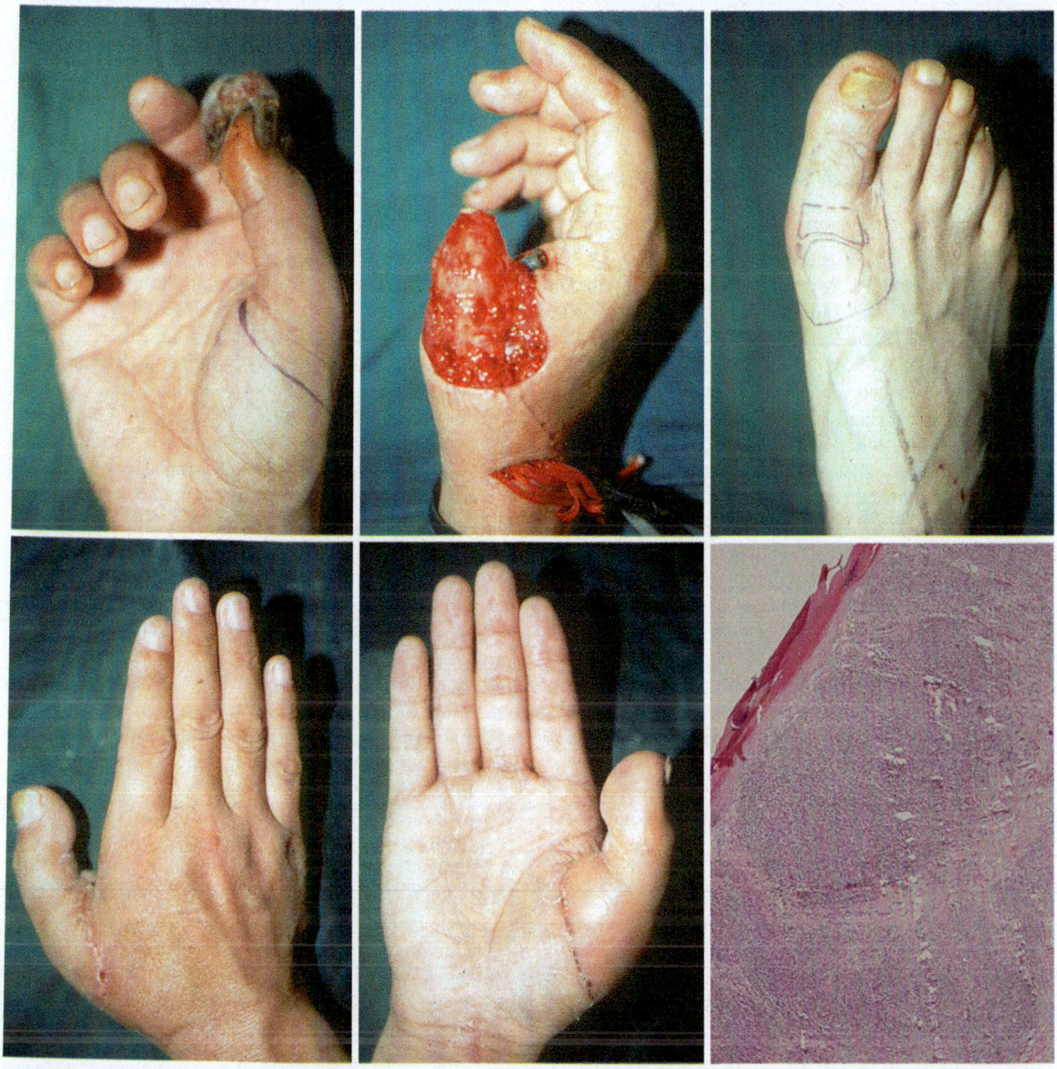

**Fig. 17.5** Fifty-eight-year-old male patient was diagnosed with malignant melanoma on his right thumb. The amputated thumb was reconstructed with ipsilateral great toe which showed good functional and aesthetic results in 1-year follow-up. Histology showed the invasion of melanocytes with severe recruitment of inflammatory cells (hematoxylin and eosin stain × 40) (Photos courtesy of Dr. Jin Suk Byun)

separate treatment guideline should be established for subungual melanoma in the future.

The prognosis of subungual melanoma is poor irrespective of races. According to Klausner et al., the 5-year overall survival rate for subungual melanoma was 28–30%, and the 10-year overall survival rate was 0–13% [37]. In the Asian group, the 5-year overall survival rate for subungual melanoma was 41%, which was 30% lower than that for other cutaneous melanomas [38].

## References


1. Kirkham N. Tumors and cysts of the epidermis: pseudocarcinomatous hyperplasia. Lever's histopathology of the skin. Philadelphia: Lippincott-Raven; 1997. p. 717–9.
2. Jacobs GH, Rippey J, Altini M. Prediction of aggressive behavior in basal cell carcinoma. Cancer. 1982;49:533–7.
3. Plate A-M, Steiner G, Posner MA. Malignant tumors of the hand and wrist. J Am Acad Orthop Surg. 2006;14:680–92.

4. Ilyas EN, Leinberry CF, Ilyas AM. Skin cancers of the hand and upper extremity. J Hand Surg. 2012;37:171–8.
5. Dubin N, Kopf AW. Multivariate risk score for recurrence of cutaneous basal cell carcinomas. Arch Dermatol. 1983;119:373–7.
6. Kuijpers DI, Thissen MR, Berretty PJ, Ideler FH, Nelemans PJ, Neumann MH. Surgical excision versus curettage plus cryosurgery in the treatment of basal cell carcinoma. Dermatol Surg. 2007;33:579–87.
7. Hv D, Stevens PJ. Metastatic basal cell carcinoma: report of five cases and review of 170 cases in the literature. J Am Acad Dermatol. 1984;10:1043–60.
8. Schiavon M, Mazzoleni F, Chiarelli A, Matano P. Squamous cell carcinoma of the hand: fifty-five case reports. J Hand Surg. 1988;13:401–4.
9. Anadolu-Brasie R, Patel A, Patel S, Singh A, Nouri K. Squamous cell carcinoma of the skin. In: Nouri K, editor. Skin cancer, vol. 104. New York: McGraw-Hill; 2008.
10. Fink JA, Akelman E. Nonmelanotic malignant skin tumors of the hand. Hand Clin. 1995;11:255–64.
11. Love RL, Breidahl AF. Acute squamous cell carcinoma arising within a recent burn scar in a 14-year-old boy. Plast Reconstr Surg. 2000;106:1069–71.
12. Belinkie SA, Swartz WM, Zitelli JA. Invasive squamous cell carcinoma of the carpus: malignant transformation of epidermis dysplasia verruciformis. J Hand Surg. 1986;11:273–5.
13. Goepfert H, Dichtel WJ, Medina JE, Lindberg RD, Luna MD. Perineural invasion in squamous cell skin carcinoma of the head and neck. Am J Surg. 1984;148:542–7.
14. Brodland DG, Zitelli JA. Surgical margins for excision of primary cutaneous squamous cell carcinoma. J Am Acad Dermatol. 1992;27:241–8.
15. Dika E, Fanti PA, Patrizi A, Misciali C, Vaccari S, Piraccini BM. Mohs surgery for squamous cell carcinoma of the nail unit: 10 years of experience. Dermatol Surg. 2015;41:1015–9.
16. Krull E. Epidermoid carcinoma of the subungual and periungual tissues. In: Krull E, Zook EG, Baran R, Haneke E, editors. Nail surgery: a text and atlas. Philadelphia: Lippincott, Williams & Wilkins; 2001. p. 297–304.
17. Park JU, Kim K, Kwon ST. Venous free flaps for the treatment of skin cancers of the digits. Ann Plast Surg. 2015;74:536–42.
18. Stadelmann WK, Javaheri S, Cruse CW, Reintgen DS. The use of selective lymphadenectomy in squamous cell carcinoma of the wrist: a case report. J Hand Surg. 1997;22:726–31.
19. Reschly MJ, Messina JL, Zaulyanov LL, Cruse W, Fenske NA. Utility of sentinel lymphadenectomy in the management of patients with high-risk cutaneous squamous cell carcinoma. Dermatol Surg. 2003;29:135–40.
20. Olson JJ, Jaques DP, Coit DG, Hwu W-J. Staging work-up and post-treatment surveillance of patients with melanoma. Clin Plast Surg. 2000;27:377–90, viii
21. Day CL Jr, Sober AJ, Kopf AW, et al. A prognostic model for clinical stage I melanoma of the upper extremity. The importance of anatomic subsites in predicting recurrent disease. Ann Surg. 1981;193:436.
22. Argenziano G, Soyer HP, Chimenti S, et al. Dermoscopy of pigmented skin lesions: results of a consensus meeting via the Internet. J Am Acad Dermatol. 2003;48:679–93.
23. Glat PM, Spector JA, Roses DF, et al. The management of pigmented lesions of the nail bed. Ann Plast Surg. 1996;37:125–34.
24. Cochran A. The Augsburg Consensus. Techniques of lymphatic mapping, sentinel lymphadenectomy and completion lymphadenectomy in cutaneous malignancies. Cancer. 2000;89:236–41.
25. Balch CM, Soong S-J, Murad TM, Ingalls AL, Maddox WA. A multifactorial analysis of melanoma: III. Prognostic factors in melanoma patients with lymph node metastases (stage II). Ann Surg. 1981;193:377.
26. Mraz-Gernhard S, Sagebiel RW, Kashani-Sabet M, Miller JR III, Leong SP. Prediction of sentinel lymph node micrometastasis by histological features in primary cutaneous malignant melanoma. Arch Dermatol. 1998;134:983–7.
27. Ali-Salaam P, Ariyan S. Lymphatic mapping and sentinel lymph node biopsies. Clin Plast Surg. 2000;27:421–9, ix
28. Balch CM. The role of elective lymph node dissection in melanoma: rationale, results, and controversies. J Clin Oncol. 1988;6:163–72.
29. Faries MB, Thompson JF, Cochran AJ, et al. Completion dissection or observation for sentinel-node metastasis in melanoma. N Engl J Med. 2017;376:2211–22.
30. Vongtama R, Safa A, Gallardo D, Calcaterra T, Juillard G. Efficacy of radiation therapy in the local control of desmoplastic malignant melanoma. Head Neck. 2003;25:423–8.
31. Horvat A, Kovač V, Strojan P. Radiotherapy in palliative treatment of painful bone metastases. Radiology and Oncology. 2009;43:213–24.
32. Wolchok JD, Chiarion-Sileni V, Gonzalez R, et al. Overall survival with combined nivolumab and ipilimumab in advanced melanoma. N Engl J Med. 2017;377:1345–56.
33. Levit EK, Kagen MH, Scher RK, Grossman M, Altman E. The ABC rule for clinical detection of subungual melanoma. J Am Acad Dermatol. 2000;42:269–74.
34. Yun SJ, Kim S-J. Hutchinson's Nail Sign. N Engl J Med. 2011;364:e38.
35. Briggs JC. Subungual malignant melanoma: a review article. Br J Plast Surg. 1985;38:174–6.

36. Kim JY, Jung HJ, Lee WJ, et al. Is the distance enough to eradicate in situ or early invasive subungual melanoma by wide local excision from the point of view of matrix-to-bone distance for safe inferior surgical margin in Koreans. Dermatology. 2011;223:122–3.
37. Klausner JM, Inbar M, Cutman M, et al. Nail-bed melanoma. J Surg Oncol. 1987;34:208–10.
38. Park K, Blessing K, Kernohan NM. Surgical aspects of subungual malignant melanomas. The Scottish Melanoma Group. Ann Surg. 1992;216:692.

# Part VII

# Bone and Soft Tissue Reconstruction

# 18 Soft Tissue Reconstruction

Seong Eon Kim and Hyun Tae Lee

The thumb is the shortest but the most important finger. It is responsible for 40% of the hand function. The essential function is opposition, that is, the thumb moves to other fingers to make pad to pad pinch. To generate a normal opposition, the thumb must have suitable length with pliable and sensate soft tissue. The external appearance of the thumb with the normal nail is also very important due to its noticeable position. Thumb defect is classified into four groups by Lister [1]: (1) acceptable length but poor soft tissue coverage, (2) subtotal amputation with uncertainty in length, (3) total amputation with basal joint, and (4) total amputation without basal joint. Most of the soft tissue defects that require flap coverages are classified as Group I. The goals of the reconstructions in Group I are length, sensory, and appearance. Among them, the most important one is sensory recovery that comprises 40% of reconstruction goals [2]. To achieve the goals, thumb soft tissue defects should be covered with sensate nonpainful flap with normal nail appearance.

The soft tissue defects of the thumb can occur by machinery compression, burn, knife injury, and various inflammations. Many options are available for thumb soft tissue reconstruction, including local flap, distant flap, and free flap. Factors that affect the choice of option include patient's age, dominant hand, sex, occupation, and desire where the donor site is. Surgeon's familiarity with a specific flap is also an important factor in flap choice.

## Palmar Advancement Flap

In 1964, Moberg described palmar advancement flap for resurfacing of thumb pulp defects [3]. Palmar advancement flap is based on both neurovascular bundles in the thumb. It permits coverage for defects as large as 1.5 cm in longitudinal diameter [4]. This flap is considered a standard option for thumb tip defects because it provides immediate sensibility and glabrous skin while preserving thumb length [5]. Postoperative appearance is acceptable, and donor site morbidities are minimal. Palmar advancement flap may result in complication such as flexion contracture of interphalangeal joint and limiting thumb extension. However, such complications are rare unless the joint is arthritic or has been injured [6].

Because the dorsum of the thumb has its own blood supply from dorsal branches of the radial artery, palmar advancement flap can be elevated safely without compromising arterial perfusion of dorsal skin or perionychium [7]. The thumb interphalangeal joint can be flexed up to 45°. Therefore, sufficient flap advancement is possible.

Indications of palmar advancement flap are the presence of thumb pulp defect of longitudinal diameter less than 1.5 cm (Fig. 18.1).

S. E. Kim (✉) · H. T. Lee
Department of Plastic and Reconstructive Surgery, Pohang SM Christianity Hospital, Pohang-si, Gyeongsangbuk-do, South Korea


S. H. Woo (ed.), *The Thumb*, https://doi.org/10.1007/978-981-10-4400-7_18

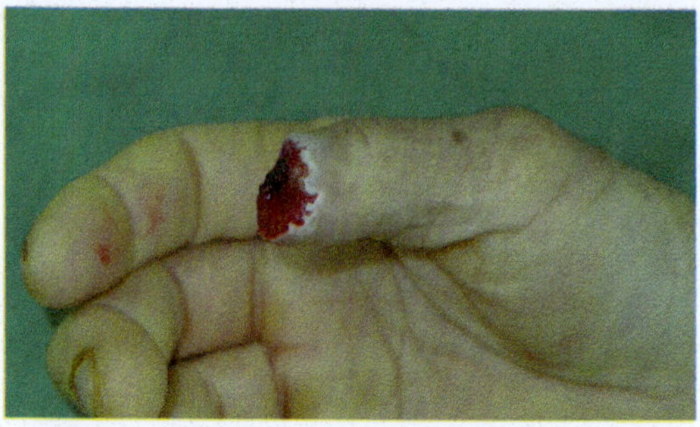

**Fig. 18.1** Palmar advancement flap. Transverse distal thumb amputation with distal phalanx exposed

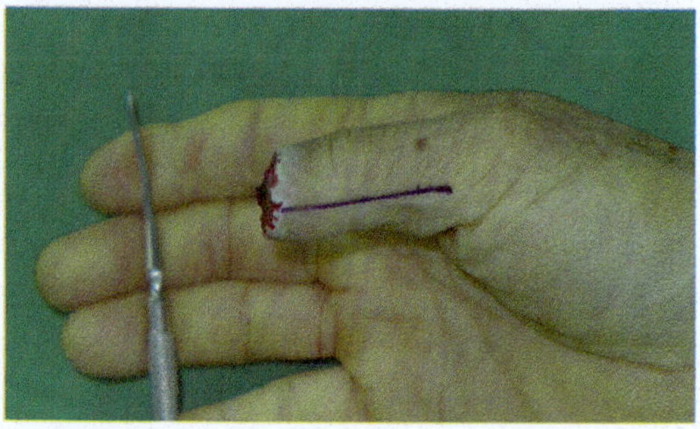

**Fig. 18.2** Incision along both midaxial lines from the defect to the MP joint crease

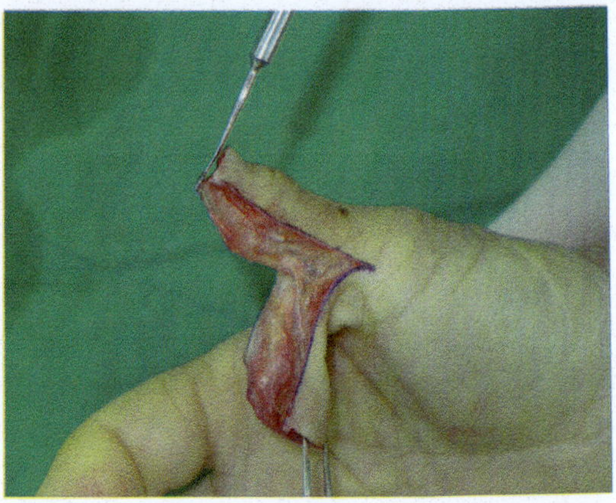

**Fig. 18.3** Proximal refection of the advancement flap. Flap is elevated superficial to the sheath of the flexor tendon

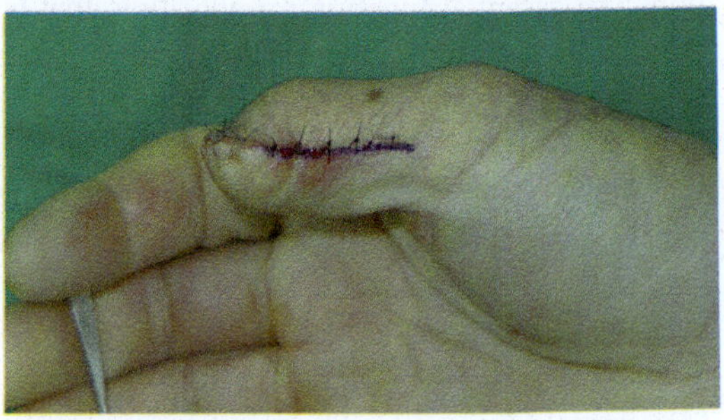

**Fig. 18.4** Wound coverage with palmar advancement flap. Distal tip of the flap is trimmed for well-rounded shape

## Operative Technique

Under tourniquet control, thorough debridement of necrotic tissue is carried out. Incisions are made on both radial and ulnar mid-lateral lines of the thumb from the injury to the proximal thumb crease (Fig. 18.2). The palmar flap is elevated superficial to the flexor tendon sheath (Fig. 18.3). One should include both neurovascular bundles with subcutaneous tissue within the flap. After flap elevation, any tension is checked by advancing the flap tip over the defect site. If there is difficulty in advancing the flap, one can extend the mid-lateral incision proximally onto the thenar eminence, flex the interphalangeal joint, or elevate the flap as island by transverse incision at the flap base with a full-thickness skin graft to the secondary defect. The distal edge of the flap is trimmed to give a rounded tip. It is then sutured to the distal end of the defect (Fig. 18.4).

## Reverse Homodigital Dorsal Radial Flap

Reverse homodigital dorsal radial flap described by Moschella et al. [8] is a useful option for extensive thumb defects. This reverse-flow flap is elevated from the dorsal radial side of the first metacarpal area. It is pedicled on the dorsal radial digital artery of the thumb which has constant communication with palmar circuit [8, 9].

This flap does not require sacrifice of major vessels. Donor site morbidity is low. The surgical technique is also relatively simple. A definite advantage of dorsal radial flap is that this flap can be raised within the thumb independently from another digit. In multiple digital trauma, dissecting vessels of adjacent finger is frequently unreliable. These vessels could be reserved for reconstruction of another digit. However, the lack of sensory resurfacing is an inherent drawback of the flap [10]. In cases of coverage of a dorsal defect of the thumb, sensory deficit is not a serious concern. However, in thumb pulp reconstruction, particularly the ulnar side, sensate flap should be considered [11].

At the anatomical snuffbox, the dorsal radial artery originates from the radial artery. The vessel passes under the extensor pollicis brevis tendon to the middle third of the proximal phalanx and takes a straight direction along the radial side of the thumb in a subcutaneous plane. At the middle third of the proximal phalanx, the pivot point of the flap, the dorsal radial artery has constant communication with palmar circuit.

The wide arc of rotation makes this flap suitable for distal palmar and dorsal defect of the thumb (Fig. 18.5). Radial defects of the proximal and distal phalanx can also be managed with this flap. The dorsal radial flap can be raised as large as 5 × 4 cm in size [12], which makes this flap a useful local option for covering large thumb defects.

## Operative Technique

Preoperatively, Doppler examination is conducted to trace the dorsal radial artery and define the pivot point of the flap in the middle third of the proximal phalanx. A skin island is designed over the dorsoradial side of the first metacarpal bone centered on the dorsal radial artery (Fig. 18.6). The skin island should be designed to be slightly larger than the original defect at appropriate position considering the arc of rotation. Flap elevation is executed under tourniquet hemostasis and loupe magnification. The first incision is made on the proximal half of the skin island. The proximal skin margin is incised down to the paratenon to make certain that the arterial pedicle is included in the flap (Fig. 18.7). A branch of the superficial radial nerve that is located close to the dorsal radial artery should be included in the flap. The rest of the skin margin is then incised. At the distal limit of the skin island, one should incise the skin superficially to avoid injury to the pedicle. A lazy-S or zigzag skin incision and subdermal dissection are performed over the flap pedicle to the middle point of the proximal phalanx. With a

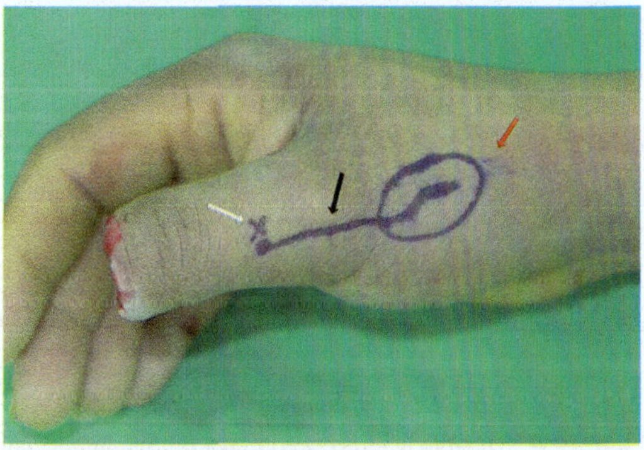

**Fig. 18.6** Preoperative design. A skin flap outlined over the dorsoradial side of the first metacarpal bone is centered on the dorsal radial artery (black arrow). White arrow, pivot point; red arrow, extensor pollicis brevis

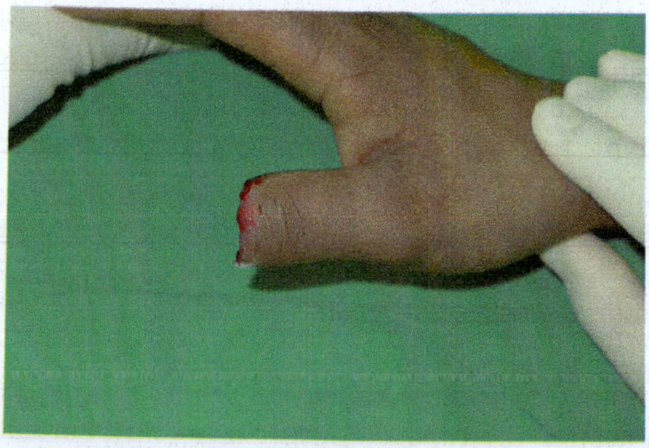

**Fig. 18.5** Reverse homodigital dorsal radial flap. Transverse distal thumb amputation

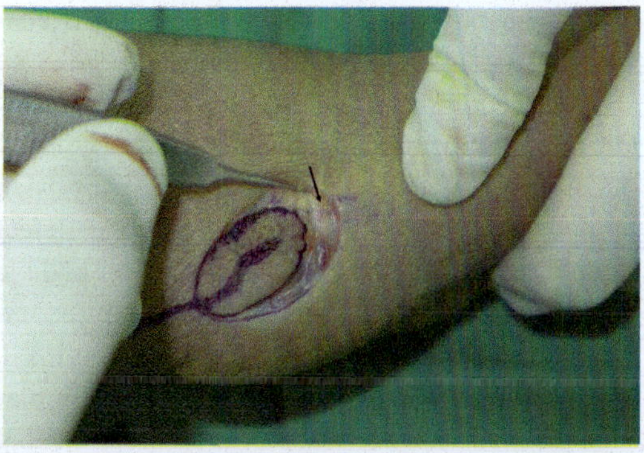

**Fig. 18.7** The dorsal radial artery (black arrow) is included in the flap

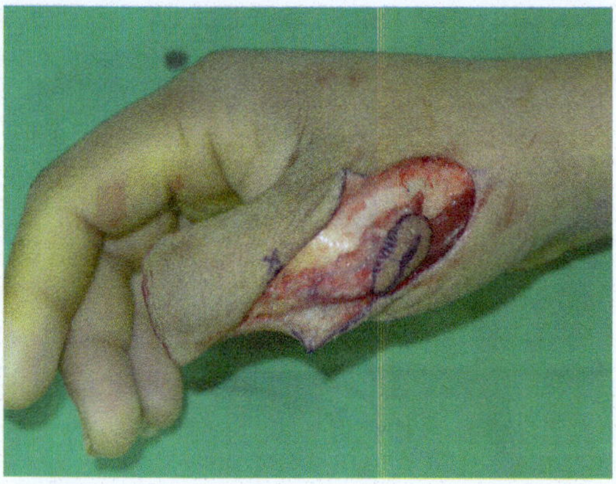

**Fig. 18.8** The flap is elevated. Visible vein and a certain quantity of subcutaneous tissue are incorporated to the flap pedicle

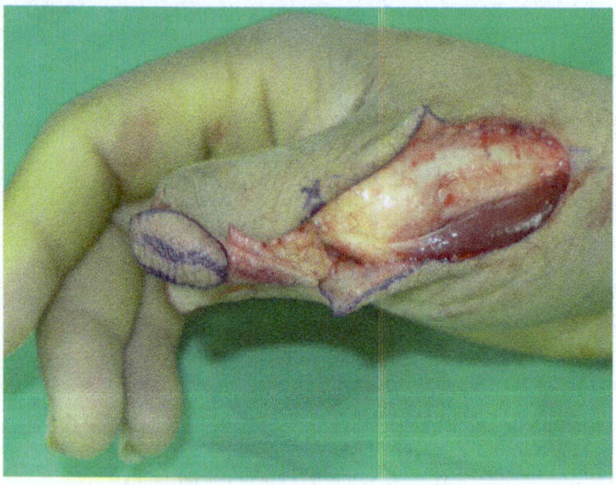

**Fig. 18.9** The flap is transferred to the thumb defect. The skin bridge is incised and raised for flap transfer

proximal to distal direction, the pedicle is divided en bloc around the axis of the flap in the epiparatendinous plane. The pedicle should incorporate a certain quantity of subcutaneous tissue and visible vein for sufficient venous drainage (Fig. 18.8). The dissection should not exceed beyond the middle third of the proximal phalanx to preserve communication with the palmar circuit. Any skin bridge between the pivot point and the defect should be incised and elevated to prevent pedicle compression. Tunneling of the flap is not recommended. After the flap is completely mobilized, the tourniquet is released to confirm flap circulation (Fig. 18.9). Once viability is assured, the flap is rotated and sutured to the defect (Figs. 18.10 and 18.11). Any tension or compression to the

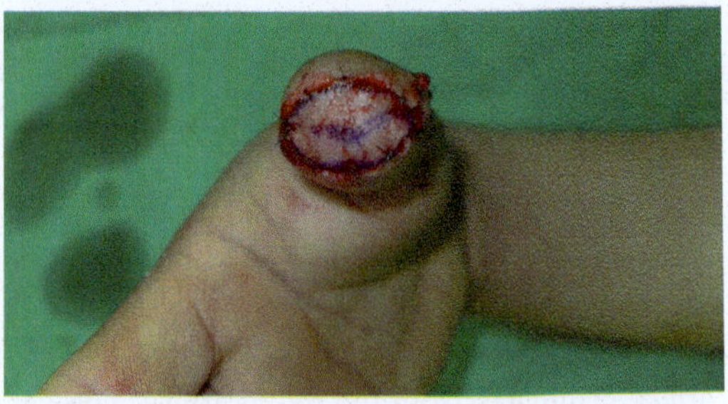

**Fig. 18.10** Skin defect covered with a reverse homodigital dorsal radial flap

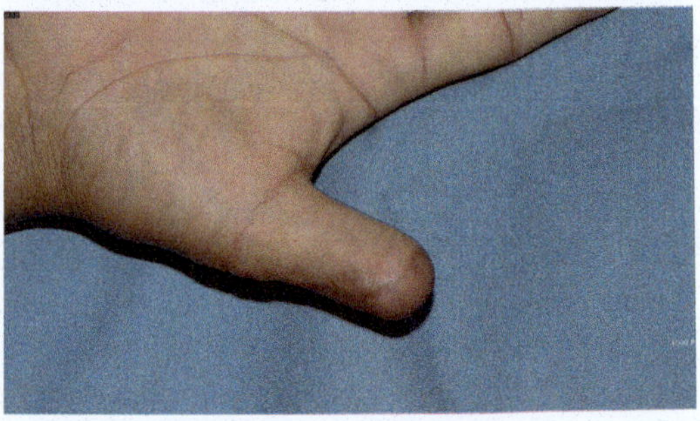

**Fig. 18.11** Six months after the operation

pedicle must be avoided to prevent flap congestion. Skin grafting or secondary intention healing can be applied to the pedicle. For donor site, primary closure is possible in most cases. But, a full-thickness skin graft might be necessary in some cases (Fig. 18.12).

## Cross-Finger Flap

Cross-finger flap has been used widely for coverage of the thumb and other digits. For the thumb, this heterodigital flap is generally raised from the dorsum of the index proximal phalanx with radially based. It can be particularly suitable for thumb defects because of thumb opposability, which allows the dorsal skin from the index finger to be transposed to the thumb with the thumb sitting in a comfortable position [13]. Several innervated modifications have been described to improve the protective sensation of cross-finger flap for fingertip reconstruction [14, 15], but satisfactory sensibility can be acquired with conventional technique in the long term [16].

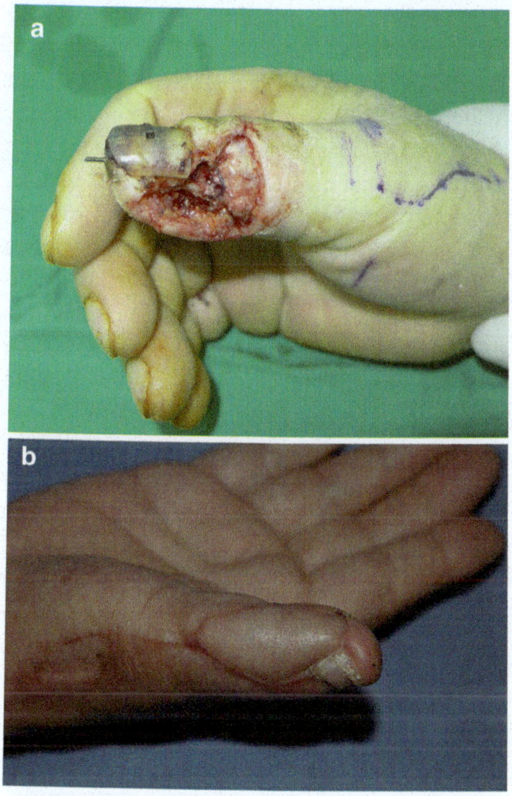


**Fig. 18.12** (**a**) A 57-year-old man sustained a bone exposure skin defect on the radial thumb. (**b**) Three months after the skin defect was resurfaced with a reverse homodigital dorsal radial flap

Cross-finger flap is reliable and can provide durable coverage with sufficient padding. Regarding disadvantages of the flap, it requires a secondary procedure for flap division. It also needs immobilization of the thumb and the index finger.

Cross-finger flap can be used for intermediate-sized pulp defect of the thumb when palmar advancement flap is not applicable.

## Operative Technique

A pattern of thumb defect is made and placed at the dorsum of the index proximal phalanx. The thumb is adducted toward the radial side of the index finger to locate the flap base at appropriate level along the radial midaxial line. After that, a skin flap slightly larger than the original defect is outlined. The width of the flap should be broader enough to prevent

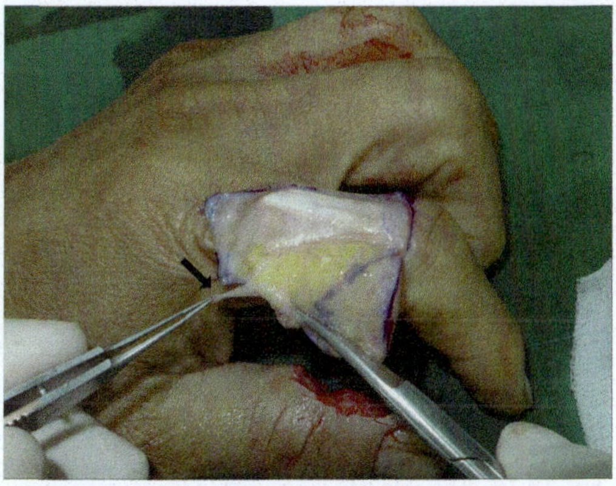

**Fig. 18.13** Innervated cross-finger flap. Flap elevation in a plane of supraparatenon layer. Dorsal sensory branch of the radial nerve to the index proximal phalanx is isolated (black arrow)

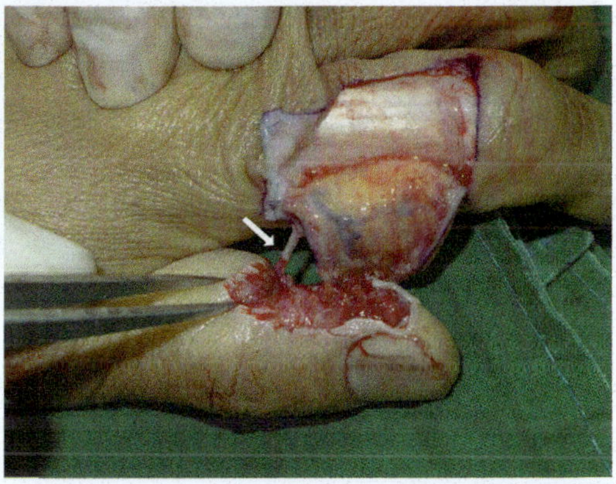

**Fig. 18.14** Isolated dorsal sensory branch of radial nerve is coapted to the ulnar digital nerve of the thumb (white arrow)

undue tension on the flap base. However, the ulnar edge of the flap should not extend to the midaxial line. Flap borders are incised through the skin and the subcutaneous layer under tourniquet control. Dorsal veins encountered during flap incision should be coagulated with bipolar cautery and divided. The flap is raised in a plane superficial to the extensor paratenon from ulnar to radial direction (Figs. 18.13 and 18.14). When dissecting at the base of the flap, caution is needed to avoid injury to dorsal branches of radial digital artery that supplies the flap [17]. Once the flap is completely elevated to its base, the thumb is adducted against the index finger to confirm flap position. The size of donor defect to be covered by a full-thickness skin graft is then measured.

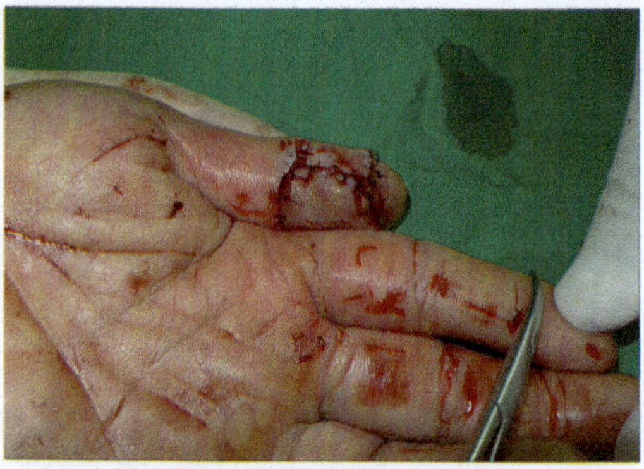

**Fig. 18.15** The skin flap is secured to the thumb defect

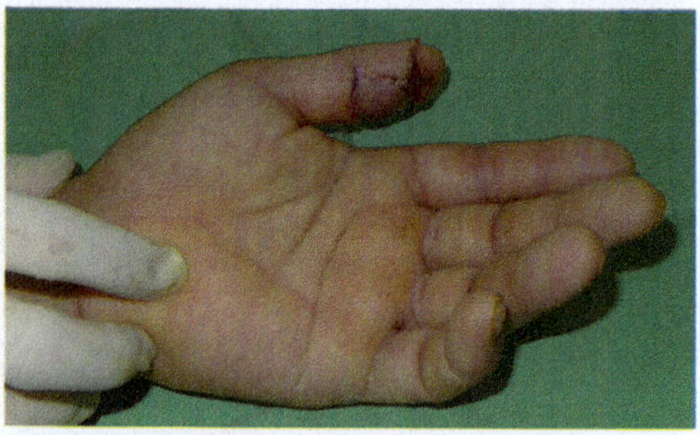

**Fig. 18.16** Division of the flap 3 weeks later

A full-thickness skin graft is harvested from the medial arm or lateral groin. Its width should be broader than the original donor defect to cover the base of the reflected flap. After the tourniquet is released, meticulous hemostasis is achieved, and a full-thickness skin graft is sutured to the donor site. The flap is reflected, followed by its suture to the thumb defect (Fig. 18.15). A full-thickness skin graft is secured with a tie-over dressing.

After 2–3 weeks, the flap can be divided safely (Fig. 18.16). Raw surface after flap division can be inset by marginal trimming and partial elevation of the wound edge. Secondary intention healing is also possible.

## First Dorsal Metacarpal Artery Island Flap

The first dorsal metacarpal artery (FDMA) island flap was described by Foucher and Braun in 1979 [18]. They described the detailed anatomy of the FDMA and demonstrated that it could be raised as a pure island flap which they named "kite flap." [18] Since then the FDMA flap has been widely applied for resurfacing of thumb defects. The FDMA flap is created from the dorsum of the adjacent index finger carrying the FDMA with its concomitant veins and terminal dorsal sensory branch of the radial nerve. It is considered as a workhorse flap for innervated distal thumb reconstruction due to its certain advantages [4].

The FDMA flap provides immediate sensation to the pulp of the thumb without complicating microsurgical techniques [19]. The FDMA flap is notably practical for older patients, in whom nerve coaptation may yield unfavorable sensory recovery and prolonged immobilization which might result in long-term stiffness [4]. However, in common with other pedicled neurovascular flaps, the dual-location phenomenon and the cortical reorientation can be disadvantages [20]. In addition, frequent hair growth on dorsum of the index finger and visible scar at grafted donor are drawbacks of the FDMA flap.

In the first intermetacarpal space, the FDMA originates from the radial artery just distal to the extensor pollicis longus tendon before the radial artery passes between the heads of the first dorsal interosseous muscle [21]. It courses distally parallel to the radial aspect of the second metacarpal bone within the fascia overlying the first dorsal interosseous muscle. The FDMA is divided into radial branch to the thumb, intermediate branch to the interosseous muscle, and ulnar branch to the index finger. The latter runs along the groove which is between the ulnar head of the first dorsal interosseous muscle and the second metacarpal bone. It terminates near the metacarpophalangeal joint and then ramifies into small branches that supply the skin of the dorsum of the proximal index finger. The sensory branch of the radial nerve to the index finger runs parallel with the FDMA in the superficial layer of subcutaneous tissue. This branch usually terminates at the distal third of the proximal phalanx and supplies the dorsal skin [18, 20].

Defects on proximal phalanx and proximal parts of the distal phalanx of the thumb are best indications for the FDMA flap (Fig. 18.17) [20].

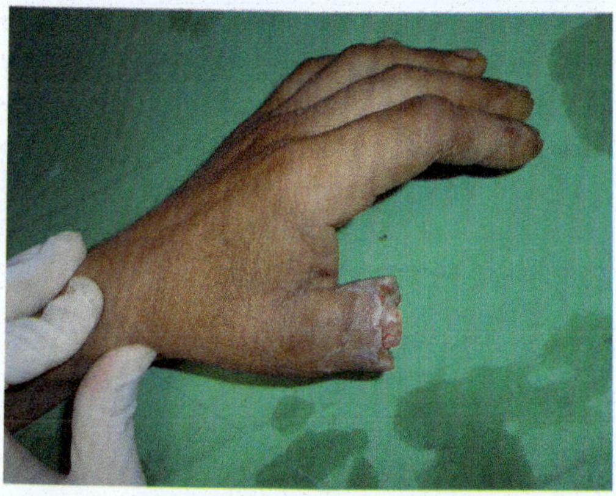

**Fig. 18.17** FDMA flap. Distal thumb amputation at IP level

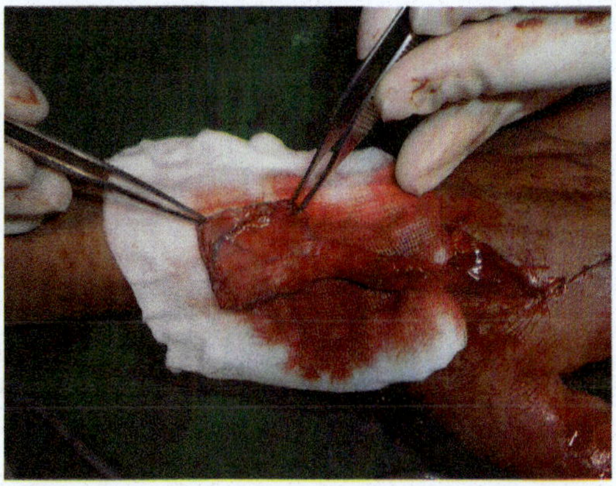

**Fig. 18.18** FDMA flap is elevated through zigzag incision on the first intermetacarpal space. For FDMA, a dorsal sensory branch of the radial nerve and a superficial dorsal vein are incorporated. The donor defect is covered by a full-thickness skin graft and secured with tie-over dressing

## Operative Technique

Before operation, the course of the FDMA is traced by Doppler examination from the radial aspect of the second metacarpal base to the index MP joint. The skin island is designed over the proximal phalanx of the index finger. The extent is limited from the MP joint to the PIP joint to prevent scar contracture. For a defect of the distal tip, the skin island should be positioned at the distal part of the proximal phalanx. The width of the flap can extend from mid-lateral line to mid-lateral line. A lazy-S or zigzag line is drawn from the proximal base of the skin flap proximally to the apex of first web between bases of the first and second metacarpal bones; this represents pivot point of the flap. Dissection is performed under tourniquet control. Skin flaps over the flap pedicle are incised and elevated in subdermal layer to develop an adipofascial pedicle. The sensory branch of radial nerve and superficial veins can be identified without difficulty. Both should be included in the pedicle. The skin island is then incised and raised in a plane just superficial to the paratenon. Dissection is generally commenced from the distal to proximal and from ulnar to radial direction. At the radial border of the MP joint, the skin flap should be carefully raised to prevent unintended injuries to terminal branches of the FDMA to the subdermal plexus. The flap pedicle is dissected by incising the periosteum at the ulnar margin of the second metacarpal bone and fascia of the ulnar head of the first dorsal interosseous muscle at the radial margin. The FDMA artery does not have to be visualized. Instead, a wide strip of fascia and subcutaneous tissue ensure flap viability. Once dissection is completed to the pivot point, the tourniquet is deflated, and the vascular flow of the flap is assessed (Fig. 18.18). The flap is then transferred into the defect of the thumb through a subcutaneous tunnel (Fig. 18.19). The dorsal donor site of the index finger is then closed with a full-thickness skin graft (Fig. 18.20). A case of FDMA flap in 27-year-old male patient had skin defect on his thumb at the level of MP joint is presented (Fig. 18.21).

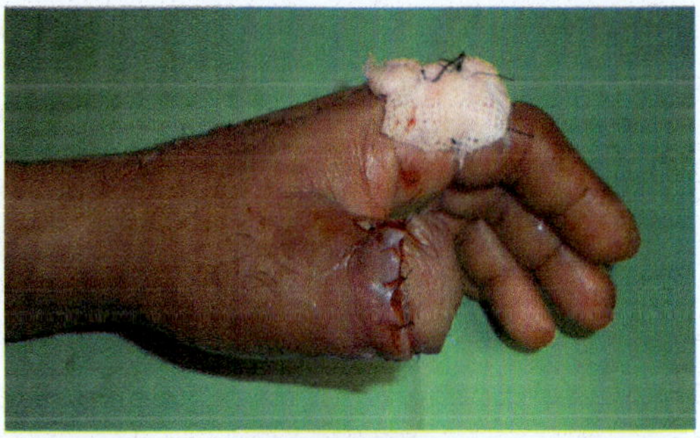

**Fig. 18.19** Flap is transferred through subcutaneous tunneling

## Free Pulp Flap

To conduct normal daily function of the thumb, the pulp must have nonpainful, scarless, and sensate glabrous skin which is a unique structure present only in the palm and plantar area. For thumb pulp defect caused by trauma, burn, tumor, or infection, reconstructive plan should focus on fulfilling the normal condition of the pulp. From this point of view, a flap from the lateral side of the great toe is the best choice for pulp reconstruction. The medial surface of the second toe can be another donor site for pulp reconstruction. However, its utility is restricted by its small flap size and poor sensory recovery compared to the lateral side of the great toe [22, 23]. Indications of free pulp flap are acute loss of the pulp, unstable skin after previous pulp reconstruction, post-traumatic distal insensibility with pulp atrophy, and distal neuroma with impossible condition of nerve anastomosis [24]. Arterial supply of the pulp area is from the lateral plantar digital artery which is the continuation of the first dorsal metatarsal artery. Sensory innervation is from the lateral plantar digital nerve. The venous pedicle is from dorsal veins on the great toe which drain into the great saphenous vein (Fig. 18.22).

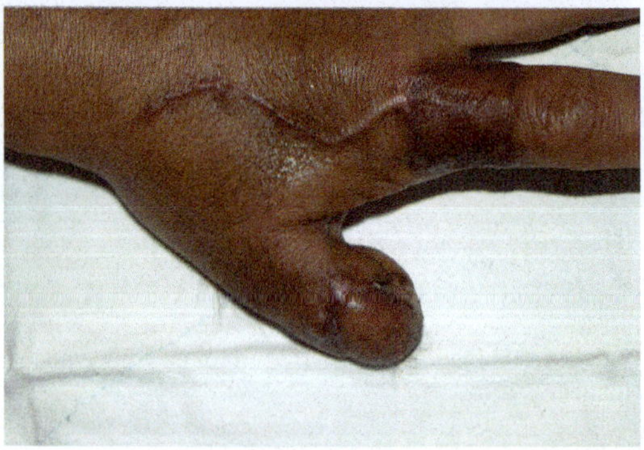

**Fig. 18.20** Three months after the procedure

## Operative Technique

### Recipient Site Preparation

After adequate debridement, recipient thumb is prepared through volar zigzag incision, and subdermal dissection is performed to preserve volar veins that will be the recipient veins using No. 15 blade (Fig. 18.23). If one is not familiar with

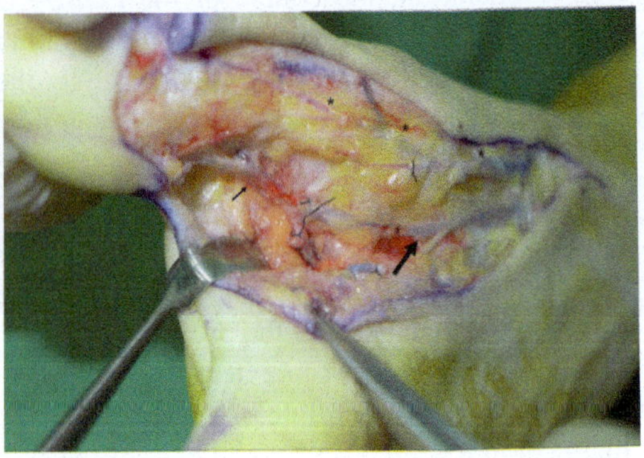

**Fig. 18.22** Surgical anatomy of the vascular pedicle of pulp flap. The lateral plantar digital artery (small arrow). The first dorsal metatarsal artery (large arrow). Dorsal vein (asterisks)

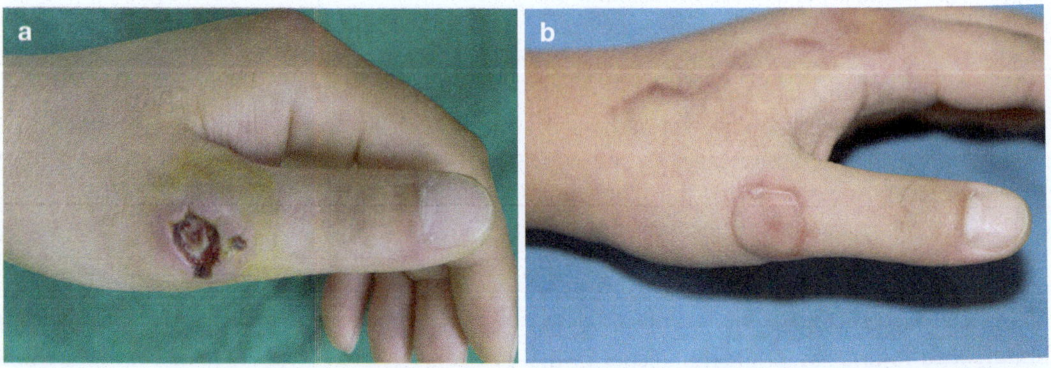


**Fig. 18.21** (**a**) A 27-year-old man with skin defect on his thumb dorsal side at the level of MP joint by infection after tenorrhaphy. (**b**) Six months after the defect was covered by FDMA flap

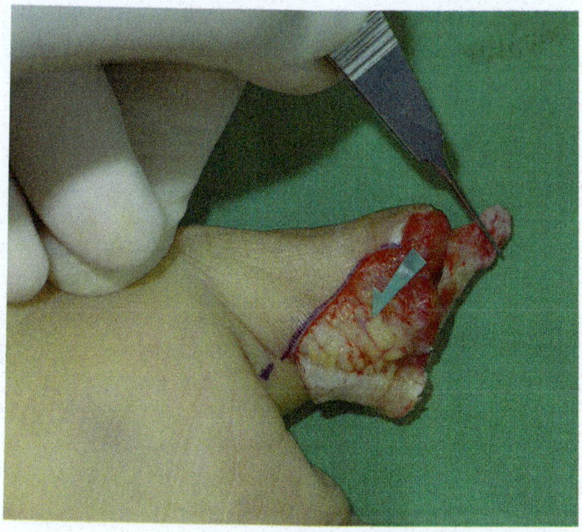

**Fig. 18.23** To preserve the volar vein, subdermal dissection with No. 15 blade is required. Green arrow—volar vein

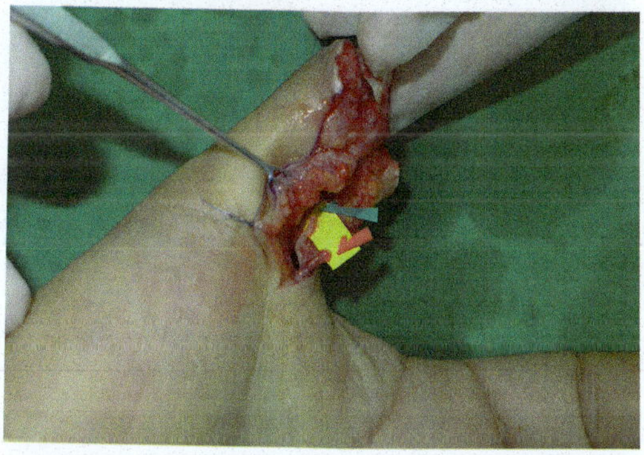

**Fig. 18.24** After volar vein identification, the dissection is continued for the ulnar artery (green arrow) and the ulnar digital nerve (red arrow)

volar veins, dorsal veins can be substituted. However, longer venous pedicle and additional incision are required. After securing volar veins, the dissection is continued to isolate the ulnar digital artery and nerve. Arterial ejection and healthy nerve fascicle should be confirmed (Fig. 18.24). Using the digital artery as a recipient artery has several advantages. It reduces donor site morbidity by minimal dissection, avoids anatomic variation of the first dorsal metatarsal artery, and shortens operation time. However, microanastomosis is performed at digital level with small vessels. Therefore, microvascular technique is very demanding. Recently, this short vascular technique, in which vascular anastomosis is performed at digital level, has been successfully used in partial toe transfer even in children [25].

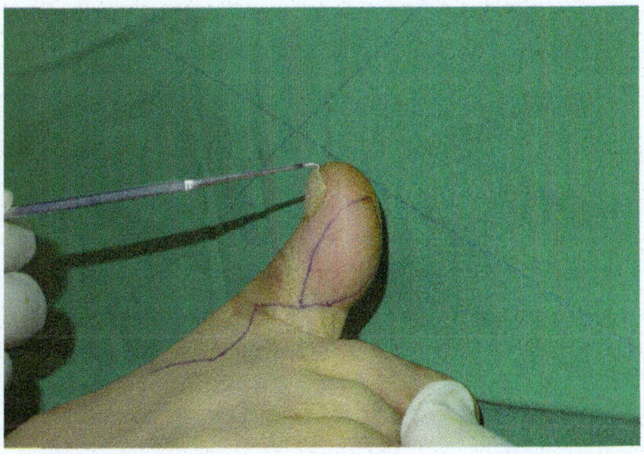

**Fig. 18.25** Using surgical pattern, the defect area is marked on the lateral side of the great toe without invading the paronychium or the web space

## Donor Site Design and Flap Dissection

Donor leg is elevated, and electric tourniquet is turned on to 300 mmHg without squeezing. Using a surgical pattern, a defect area is designed on the lateral side of the contralateral great toe without invading the lateral paronychium or web space (Fig. 18.25). A zigzag dorsal extended incision is also drawn. The first surgical approach is to isolate the venous pedicle. Skin-only incisions are performed on the dorsal surface of the flap and proximal extended incision line. Under 3.5× loupe magnification, careful subdermal dissection from the proximal and dorsal flap margin is started with No. 15 blade. It is continued to the dorsal surface of the great toe (Fig. 18.26). This procedure is very tedious because veins are very small and fragile. After sizable dorsal vein isolation, the dissection proceeds to deep plane to explore the lateral plantar digital artery and nerve (Fig. 18.27). By gentle dissection, the lateral plantar digital artery can be found with ease at web space level. Dissection is then proceeded proximally to the junction of the medial plantar digital artery of the second toe (Fig. 18.28). Since the lateral plantar digital artery is acceptable as a donor artery with reliable results, no further proximal dissection is required. However, if needed, the dissection can proceed proximally to the first dorsal metatarsal artery. After identifying the artery, the dissection

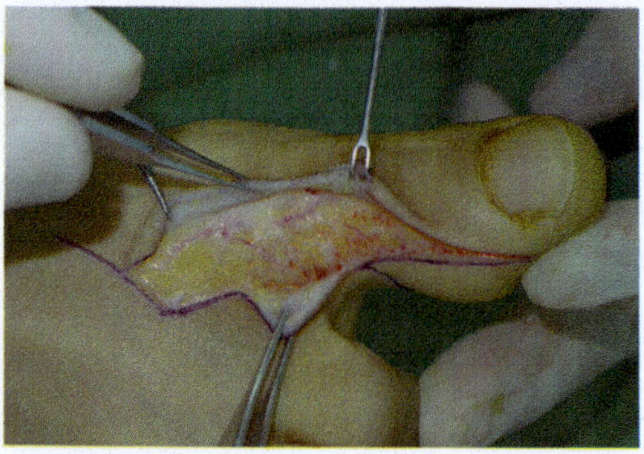

**Fig. 18.26** Multiple veins of the flap dorsal side draining to dorsal vein are small and fragile (small arrows). Subdermal dissection continues to the sizable dorsal vein carefully (large arrow)

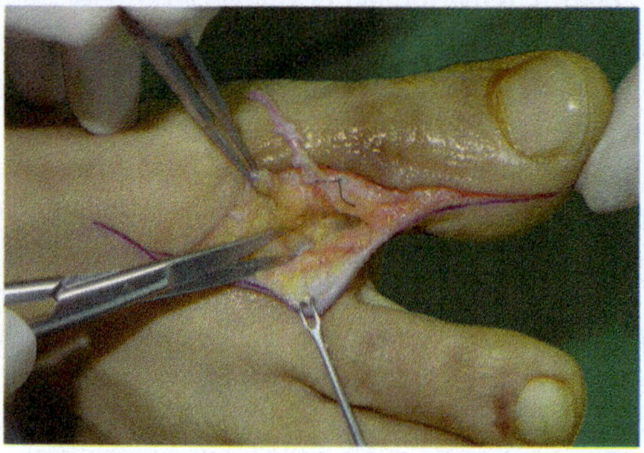

**Fig. 18.27** After securing the dorsal vein (arrow), the dissection is deepened toward the plantar side to isolate lateral plantar digital artery and nerve

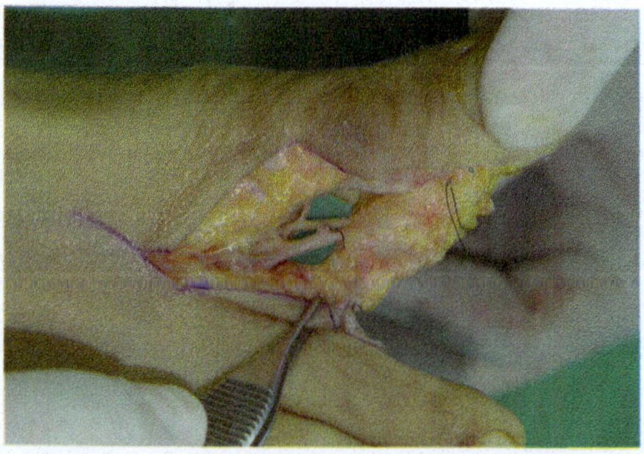

**Fig. 18.28** Lateral plantar artery (large arrow) and nerve (small arrow)

continues to the plantar surface. The lateral plantar digital nerve can be found easily and dissected proximally considering coaptation level with the recipient digital nerve.

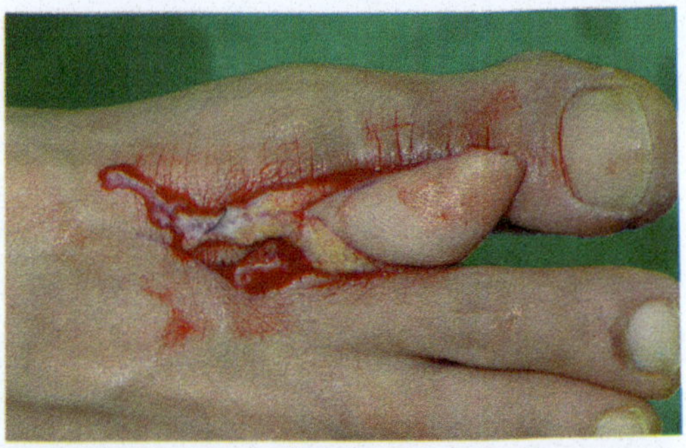

**Fig. 18.29** The pulp flap is elevated by only attaching the lateral digital artery. The tourniquet is turned off. Flap circulation and venous outflow are observed for more than 20 min to release vascular spasm

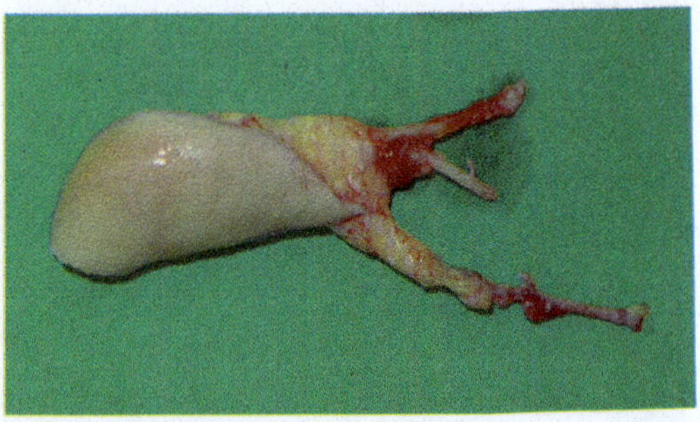

**Fig. 18.30** The flap is elevated and ready for transfer. The lateral digital artery of the great toe is shown in red arrow. The lateral digital nerve is shown in yellow arrow. The dorsal vein is shown in blue arrow

The flap elevation can be started from dorsal to plantar and distal to proximal directions with care to include all the preserved pedicles. During the flap off from underlying tissue, the collateral branch of the lateral plantar digital artery which is branched at the level of the proximal phalangeal neck should be identified and ligated. After complete elevation of the flap except the lateral plantar digital artery, the tourniquet is turned off. Flap circulation and venous outflow are observed for more than 20 min to prevent vascular spasm (Fig. 18.29). After that, the lateral plantar digital artery is resected, and the flap is ready for transfer to the recipient site and performing microprocedure (Fig. 18.30). The lateral plantar digital artery anastomoses to the ulnar digital artery of the thumb within digital level. In venous anastomosis, one can choose the volar or dorsal vein of the thumb as a recipient vein. The volar vein is technically dif-

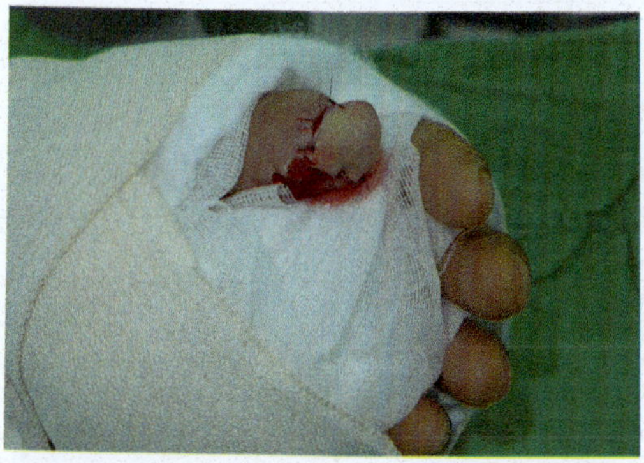

**Fig. 18.31** After complete bleeding control, gentle light dressing is applied to permit easy flap monitoring

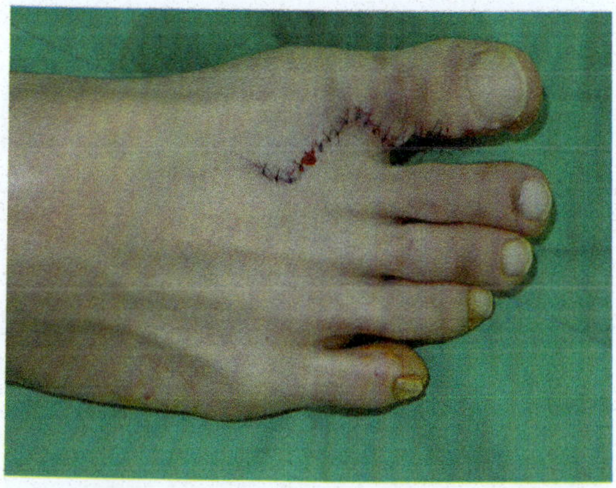

**Fig. 18.32** Donor site primary closure is possible. If impossible, split-thickness skin graft is applied to minimize donor site scar

ficult in microanastomosis due to its small size and thin vascular wall. However, it provides handiness without further dissection. In addition, the anastomosis is carried out in the same operative field. Although the dorsal vein is larger in diameter with thicker venous wall than the volar vein, subcutaneous tunneling and longer venous pedicle are required to reach the thumb dorsal side.

The lateral plantar digital nerve is coapted to the ulnar digital nerve of the thumb at the shortest length from the flap edge without tension. Complete bleeding control and tension-free suture are very important to avoid the pedicle compression (Fig. 18.31). Primary closure of the donor site is possible (Fig. 18.32). If it is difficult, split-thickness skin graft should be applied to eliminate raw surface that accelerate wound healing and reduce donor site scar.

## Complications

### Flap Necrosis

Flap necrosis can be fatal. It results in serious damage to both patients and surgeons. Close postoperative monitoring is important to detect any vascular compromise. In any type of vascular compromise, reexploration is mandatory as soon as possible. Leech is also helpful in venous obstruction which is difficult to get over by reexploration.

### Flap Bulkiness

If there are some bulkiness on the pulp flap, it can be corrected by simply excision of redundant skin and fat without interfering with flap sensory or circulation after several months.

### Delayed Donor Site Healing

The great toe wound at the donor site may be delayed than the recipient site due to decreased blood flow and dependent position. The patient should rest in a bed with restricted walking for 2 weeks.

## Radial Artery Superficial Palmar Branch Free Flap: Modified Free Thenar Flap

To reconstruct the large volar thumb skin defect involving the thumb pulp, a free thenar flap is a useful option (Fig. 18.33). The first report of the free thenar flap innervated by the lateral antebrachial cutaneous nerve based on radial artery superficial palmar branch (RASP) was in 1993 by Kamei et al. [26] Since then, several studies have reported about free flaps from the thenar region with constant nerve innervation and vascular supply. In 2010, Yang et al. [27] reported a modified free thenar flap with constant innervation from the palmar cutaneous branch of the median nerve (PCMN) through fresh cadaver study. It was named RASP flap. Lee et al. [28] reported clinical results of the finger soft tissue reconstruction with RASP flap of 125 patients. Based on their report, the mean two-point discrimination of RASP flap was 12 mm in neurorrhaphy group and 13 mm in

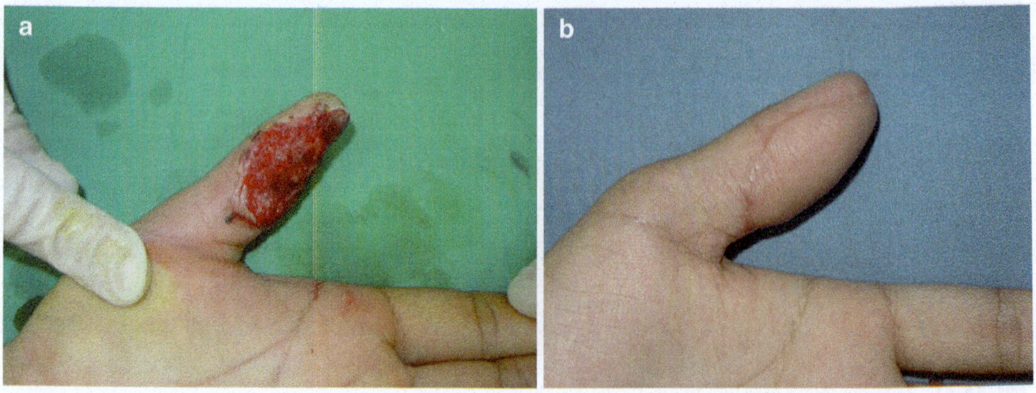


**Fig. 18.33** (**a**) A 45-year-old male showed subtotal pulp defect on his left thumb by crushing injury. (**b**) A postoperative photograph at 6 months after the reconstruction

non-neurorrhaphy group. They concluded that the sensory recovery was not significantly different between the two groups. RASP flap can be considered for the large thumb volar skin defect in patient who does not want to take a flap from toes.

RASP constantly supply 4 × 3 cm palmar skin over the abductor pollicis brevis and the opponens pollicis [29]. The artery is branched from the radial artery at the proximal wrist. It continues its course beneath the flexor retinaculum. As the artery passes over the scaphoid tubercle through subcutaneous level, the perforators sprout and supply the thenar skin. The mean diameter is 1.4 mm and sometimes larger than 2 mm. The venous system consists of venae comitantes and the superficial palmar vein. For safety, two venous systems should be included in the flap.

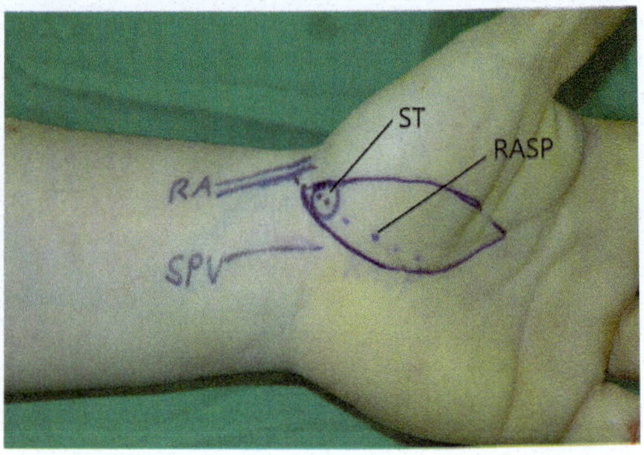


**Fig. 18.34** Preoperative flap design. *RA* radial artery; *ST* scaphoid tubercle; *RASP* radial artery superficial palmar branch; *SPV* superficial palmar vein

## Operative Technique

After thorough debridement in the recipient site, exploration for the recipient artery and the volar vein is accomplished through extended incision and subdermal dissection as in previously described free pulp flap. In the donor site, usually the ipsilateral wrist, the course of RASP is followed and marked distally from the scaphoid tubercle using a Doppler ultrasound device. An elliptical-shaped flap is designed on the proximal wrist containing the scaphoid tubercle proximally and the RASP. Not invading of the ulnar border to the thenar crease can hide the donor site scar. The superficial palmar vein which traverses the flap is marked (Fig. 18.34). The incision starts from the radial and proximal flap margin. The dissection is performed toward the radial artery keeping in mind that the RASP is branched from 1 cm proximal level of the radial styloid process and the distal wrist crease (Fig. 18.35) [29]. After identifying the RASP and venae comitantes, complete incision is then made preserving the superficial palmar vein. The distal portion of the flap is then elevated from the palmar fascia and continued proximally (Fig. 18.36). In the thenar region, subfascial dissection is preferred; the branch of the RASP to the thenar muscle is secured and ligated (Fig. 18.37). During dissection of the flap ulnar side, the PCMN can be located on the ulnar side of the flexor carpi radialis which comes up from the superficial transverse carpal ligament at the distal wrist crease level (Fig. 18.38) [27]. The

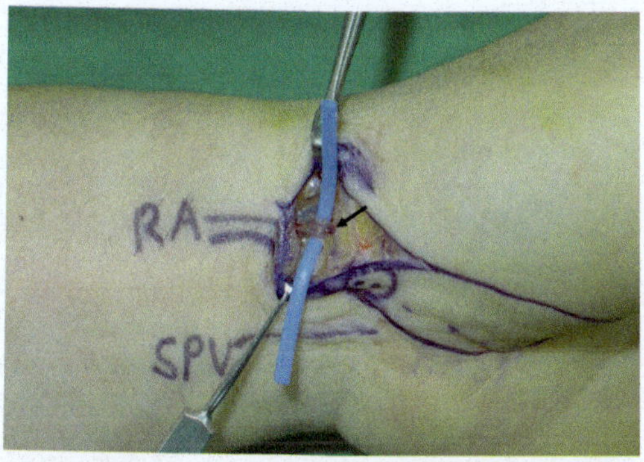


**Fig. 18.35** Through radial and proximal flap incision, the radial artery palmar branch and venae comitantes (arrow) are isolated at 1 cm proximal level of the radial styloid process

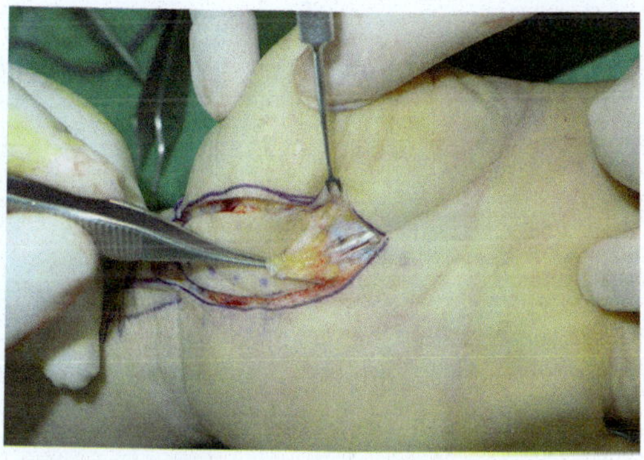

**Fig. 18.36** The flap dissection is begun from the distal portion while preserving the palmar fascia

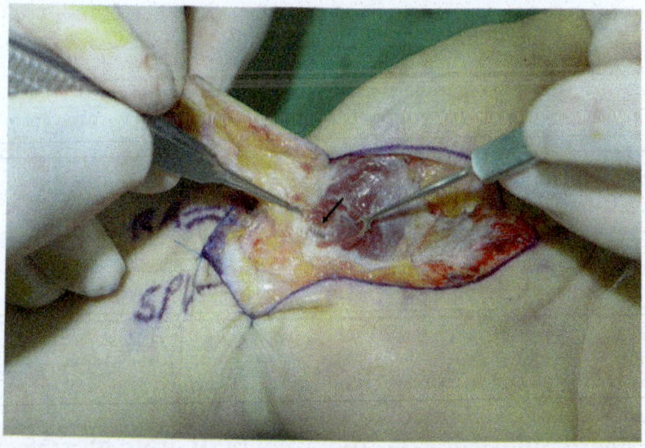


**Fig. 18.37** In the thenar region, subfascial dissection is performed to preserve perforators of the RASP. During the dissection, the branch of the RASP to the thenar muscle (arrow) is isolated and ligated

dissection is proceeded toward the scaphoid tubercle where the perforators of the RASP are sprouted. In this area, the dissection should be done carefully to avoid injury to the perforators. The flap is elevated with intact RASP

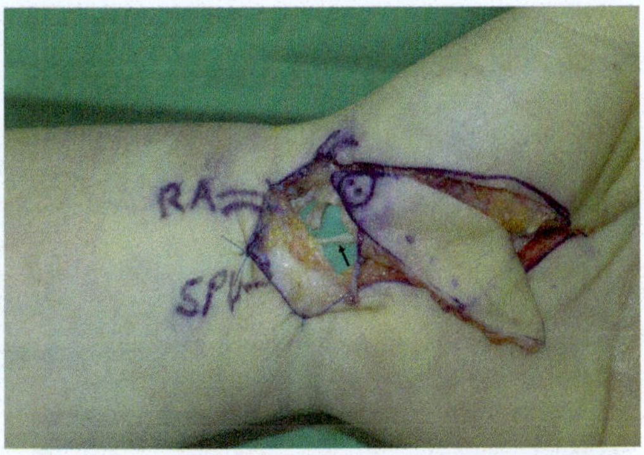


**Fig. 18.38** On the flap ulnar side, the palmar cutaneous branch of the median nerve (arrow) can be located on the ulnar side of the flexor carpi radialis

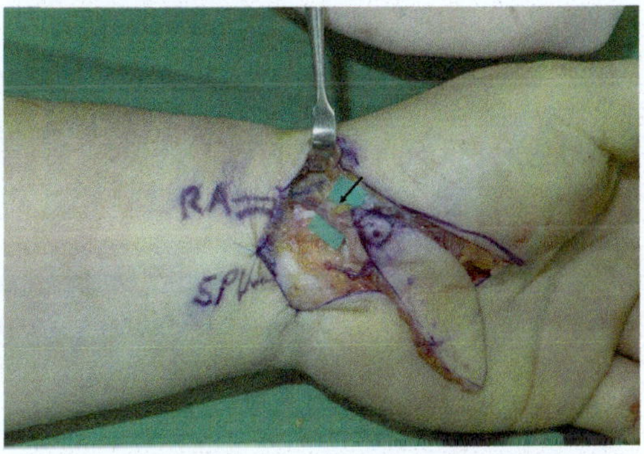


**Fig. 18.39** The flap is elevated with superficial palmar branch (arrow) of the radial artery intact

(Fig. 18.39). The tourniquet is then released. The flap circulation should be observed for more than 20 min. The RASP is severed and the flap is positioned to the recipient area. Microanastomosis procedure is then started between the RASP and the ulnar digital artery of the thumb. Vein anastomosis is carried out using the venae comitantes or the superficial palmar vein depending on the position of the recipient volar vein. Donor site primary closure is possible if the flap width is less than 2 cm.

## Complications

### Wrist Pain

Some patients complain about wrist pain after the operation. It could last for several months. In most cases, the pain subsides without any wrist morbidity.

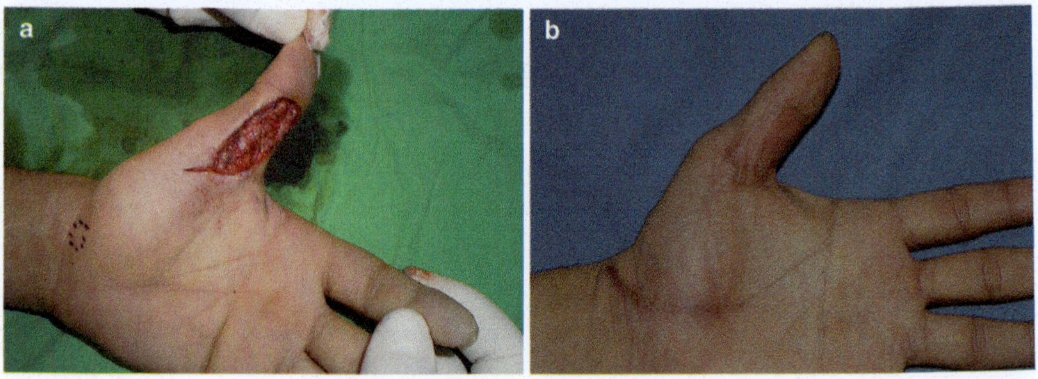


**Fig. 18.40** (**a**) A 33-year-old man with a skin defect on his thumb volar side by contact burn. (**b**). A photograph at 6 months after the skin defect was covered by the radial artery superficial palmar branch flap. Note an inconspicuous scar on the wrist

### Donor Site Scar

Donor site scar is less conspicuous. Most patients well tolerate donor site scar (Fig. 18.40).

### Flap Bulkiness

The RASP flap is very thin. However, when swelling subsides, the flap looks bulky. A flap debulking procedure can be performed after several months.

## Nail Reconstruction with Partial Toe Transfer

The nail is composed of the nail bed, nail fold, eponychium, paronychium, and hyponychium. These compositions are also called nail unit. The nail bed is also divided into the germinal and the sterile matrix. The germinal matrix, located proximally, is responsible for 90% of nail production. The rest is produced from the sterile matrix. Functionally, the nail protects and stabilizes the distal digit and transmits sensations to the proximal nail bed. It is esthetically very important, especially in children and women [30]. For substantial thumb nail defect usually manifested as onycho-osteo-cutaneous defect (Fig. 18.41), partial great toe transfer including the nail, distal phalanx, and pulp is ideal. Its result is excellent functionally and esthetically. The best indication is subtotal loss of the nail unit in dorsal oblique amputation of the thumb [31].

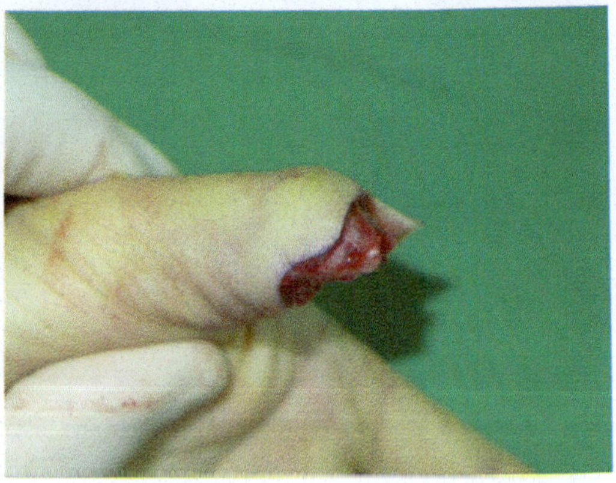

**Fig. 18.41** Thumb nail defect is usually accompanied with distal phalanx and pulp defect

### Operative Technique

The surgical anatomy and dissection technique are nearly the same as the free pulp transfer. As a donor site, the ipsilateral great toe is preferred to place the donor artery and nerve on the ulnar side of the thumb. When carrying out partial toe transfer for the nail reconstruction, the flap should include the dorsal part of lateral pulp to contain arterial supply (Fig. 18.42). In case of whole toe

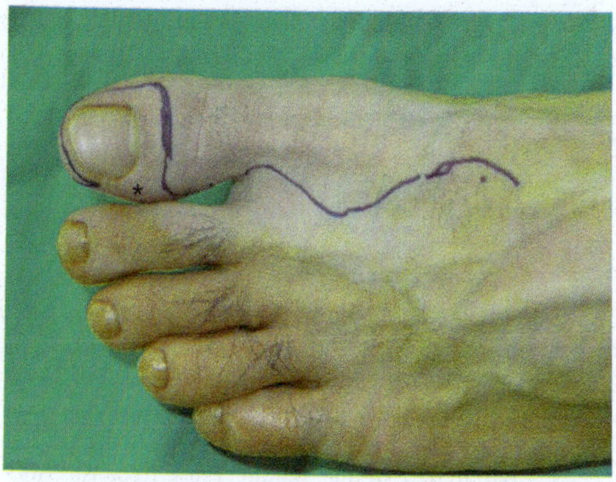

**Fig. 18.42** Design of the partial toe transfer for the nail reconstruction. The flap should include the dorsal part of lateral pulp (asterisk) to contain arterial supply

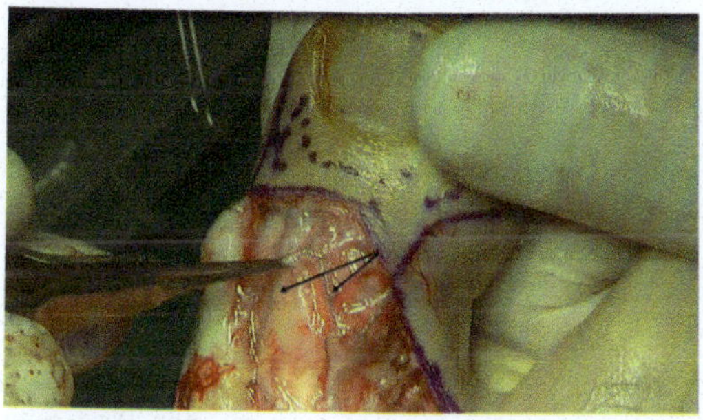

**Fig. 18.43** Multiple large dorsal veins are available (arrows) when the entire germinal matrix is included in the partial toe transfer

nail transfer, containing the entire germinal matrix, the venous pedicle dissection is relatively simple by using the large dorsal veins (Fig. 18.43). In partial toe nail transfer excluding the germinal matrix, the venous dissection is tedious because small and fragile veins need to be handled from the lateral side of the great toe as described in free pulp transfer (Fig. 18.26). After isolating the venous pedicle, dissection is continued to plantar direction to identify the lateral digital artery and nerve. After soft tissue dissection, the part of distal phalanx should be incorporated as required length to prevent nail deformity. This procedure is carried out with a small electric saw with care to prevent the pedicle injury (Fig. 18.44). Longer than 20 min after tourniquet release, the flap is transferred, and bone

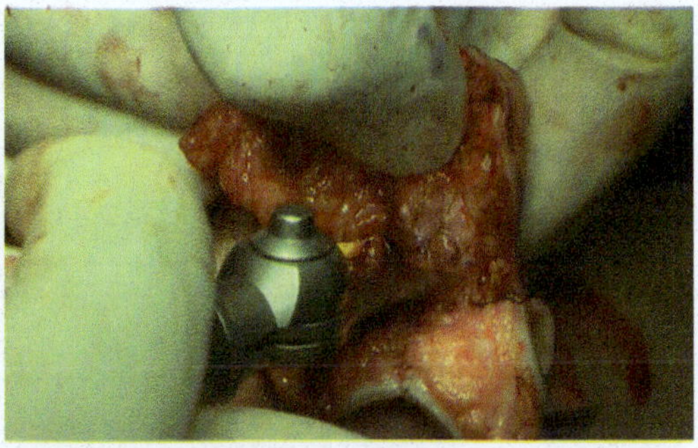

**Fig. 18.44** To prevent nail deformity, part of the distal phalanx of the great toe is incorporated using an electric saw

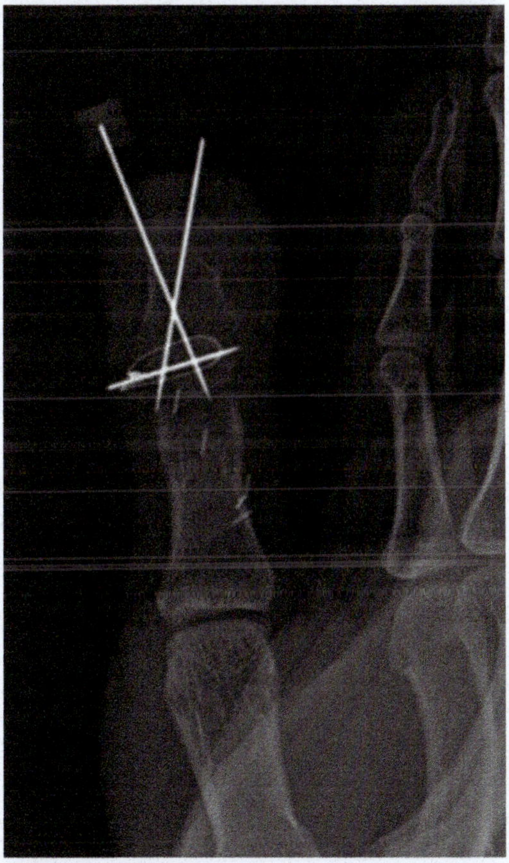

**Fig. 18.45** The toe nail with distal phalanx is transferred, and bone fixation is performed with K-wire or wiring

fixation is performed first with K-wire or wiring (Fig. 18.45). Microvascular procedures are the same as those in the free pulp transfer. A case of

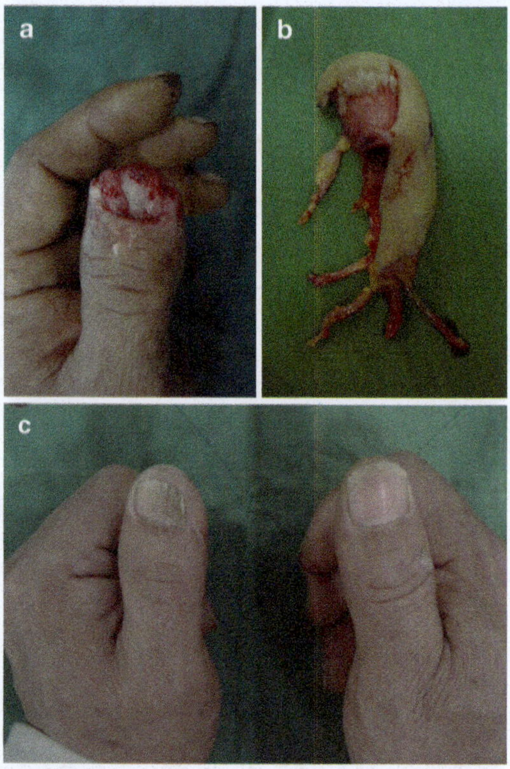


**Fig. 18.46** (**a**) A 53-year-old male patient has left thumb tip amputation with the sterile matrix defect. (**b**) Appearance of elevated free partial great toe flap. (**c**) Postoperative view at 6 months after the operation

partial toe transfer in 53-year-old male patient had left thumb tip amputation with the steril matrix defect is presented (Fig. 18.46).

## References

1. Tang JB, Elliot D, Adani R, Saint-Cyr M, Stang F. Repair and reconstruction of thumb and finger tip injuries: a global view. Clin Plast Surg. 2014;41(3):325–59.
2. Lister G. The choice of procedure following thumb amputation. Clin Orthop Relat Res. 1985;195:45–51.
3. Moberg E. Aspects of sensation in reconstructive surgery of the upper extremity. J Bone Joint Surg. 1964;46A:817–25.
4. Germann G, Sauerbier M, Rudolf KD, Hrabowski M. Management of thumb tip injuries. J Hand Surg Am. 2015;40(3):614–22.
5. Germann G, Rudolf KD, Levin SL, Hrabowski M. Fingertip and thumb tip wounds: changing algorithms for sensation. aesthetics, and function. J Hand Surg Am. 2017;42(4):274–85.
6. Pederson WC. Nonmicrosurgical coverage of the upper extremity. In: Wolfe SW, Hotchkiss RN, Pederson WC, Kozin SH, editors. Operative hand surgery. 6th ed. Philadelphia: Churchill Livingstone; 2011. p. 1645–720.
7. Foucher G, Delaere O, Citron N, Molderez A. Long-term outcome of neurovascular palmar advancement flaps for distal thumb injuries. Br J Plast Surg. 1999;52(1):64–8.
8. Moschella F, Cordova A, Pirrello R, Brunelli F. Anatomic basis for the dorsal radial flap of the thumb: clinical applications. Surg Radiol Anat. 1996;18(3):179–81.
9. Moschella F, Cordova A. Reverse homodigital dorsal radial flap of the thumb. Plast Reconstr Surg. 2006;117(3):920–6.
10. Bao QY, Xiao CW, Peng F, Han D, Wang T, Gu YD. Restoration of thumb sensibility with innervated reverse homodigital dorsoradial flap. Reconstr Microsurg. 2014;30(1):15–20.
11. Brunelli F, Vigasio A, Valenti P, Brunelli GR. Arterial anatomy and clinical application of the dorsoulnar flap of the thumb. J Hand Surg Am. 1999;24(4):803–11.
12. Hrabowski M, Kloeters O, Germann G. Reverse homodigital dorsoradial flap for thumb soft tissue reconstruction: surgical technique. J Hand Surg Am. 2010;35(4):659–62.
13. Woon CY, Lee JY, Teoh LC. Resurfacing hemipulp losses of the thumb: the cross finger flap revisited: indications, technical refinements, outcomes, and long-term neurosensory recovery. Ann Plast Surg. 2008;61(4):385–91.
14. Wilkinson TS. Reconstruction of the thumb by radial nerve innervated cross-finger flap. South Med J. 1972;65(8):992–4.
15. Cohen BE, Cronin ED. An innervated cross-finger flap for fingertip reconstruction. Plast Reconstr Surg. 1983;72(5):688–97.
16. Peacock E. Reconstruction of the thumb. In: Flynn JE, editor. Hand surgery. Baltimore: Williams & Wilkins; 1966.
17. Strauch B, de Moura W. Arterial system of the fingers. J Hand Surg Am. 1990;15:148–54.
18. Foucher G, Braun JB. A new island flap transfer from the dorsum of the index to the thumb. Plast Reconstr Surg. 1979;63(3):344–9.
19. Chang SC, Chen SL, Chen TM, Chuang CJ, Cheng TY, Wang HJ. Sensate first dorsal metacarpal artery flap for resurfacing extensive pulp defects of the thumb. Ann Plast Surg. 2004;53(5):449–54.
20. Muyldermans T, Hierner R. First dorsal metacarpal artery flap for thumb reconstruction: a retrospective clinical study. Strategies Trauma Limb Reconstr. 2009;4(1):27–33.
21. El-Khatib HA. Clinical experiences with the extended first dorsal metacarpal artery island flap for thumb reconstruction. J Hand Surg Am. 1998;23(4):647–52.
22. Foucher G, Merle M, Maneaud M, Michon J. Microvascular free partial toe transfer in hand

reconstruction: a report of 12 cases. Plast Reconstr Surg. 1980;65(5):616–27.
23. Buncke HJ, Rose EH. Free toe-to-fingertip neurovascular flaps. Plast Reconstr Surg. 1979;63(5):607–12.
24. El-Gammal TA, Wei FC. Microvascular reconstruction of the distal digits by partial toe transfer. Clin Plast Surg. 1997;24(1):49–55.
25. Dautel G, Corcella D, Merle M. Reconstruction of fingertip amputations by partial composite toe transfer with short vascular pedicle. J Hand Surg. 1998;23B(4):457–64.
26. Kamei K, Ide Y, Kimura T. A new free thenar flap. Plast Reconstr Surg. 1993;92(7):1380–4.
27. Yang JW, Kim JS, Lee DC, Ki SH, Roh SY, Abdullah S, Tien HY. The radial artery superficial palmar branch flap: a modified free thenar flap with constant innervation. J Reconstr Microsurg. 2010;26(8):529–38.
28. Lee SH, Cheon SJ, Kim YJ. Clinical application of a free radial artery superficial palmar branch flap for soft-tissue reconstruction of digital injuries. J Hand Surg. 2017;42E(2):151–6.
29. Omokawa S, Ryu J, Tang JB, Han J. Vascular and neural anatomy of the thenar area of the hand: its surgical applications. Plast Reconstr Surg. 1997;99(1):116–21.
30. Endo T, Nakayama Y. Microtransfers for nail and fingertip replacement. Hand Clin. 2002 Nov;18(4):615–22.
31. Del Piñal F, Moraleda E, de Piero GH, Ruas JS, Galindo C. Onycho-osteo-cutaneous defects of the thumb reconstructed by partial hallux transfer. J Hand Surg Am. 2014;39(1):29–36.

# Replantation and Revascularization

# 19

Dong Ho Kang, Young Woo Kim, Ho Jun Cheon, and Hee Chan Ahn

## Introduction

The thumb contributes 50% to the overall function of the hand. Because the thumb is critical for gripping actions and fine prehension, the management of trauma and partial or total reconstruction of the thumb is an important issue in hand surgery. Replantation of an injured body part usually offers a result that is superior to any other type of reconstruction. The decision to attempt, and techniques involved in, a replantation procedure is often extremely challenging. The replantation of these parts involves more than microsurgery; it also involves successful repair of tendons and bone injuries to provide the patient with the quickest recovery and best functional outcome.

After the coaptation of blood vessels was first performed by Dr. Alexis Carrell in 1902, modifications followed in techniques for suturing and instrumentation and their applications. In 1962, Dr. Malt and McKhann performed the first replantation of a completely severed arm in a 12-year-old boy in Boston [1]. In 1963, Chen and colleagues performed the first successful replantation of an amputated hand in Shanghai, China [2]. In 1968, the first replantation of an individual digit, a thumb, was achieved by Drs. Komatsu and Tamai in Japan [3]. As centers became increasingly more familiar with the technique and as experience around the globe expanded, replantations of increasing complexity were performed.

## General Considerations in Replantation

### Emergency Management

Specific management of the amputated thumb should include collection of all amputated parts in the field, regardless of the degree of contamination or quality of tissue. These parts should be wrapped in a sponge saturated with saline, placed in a plastic bag, and subsequently placed in a bag of ice or on a bed of ice. The goal is to cool the part but avoid freezing of the tissue. The bag should be labeled with the patient's demographic information and transported with the patient to the hospital setting. The amputated stump should be treated with pressure dressings and elevation to control bleeding. Tourniquets should be avoided as well as attempts at ligation of blood vessels in the field, if possible.

D. H. Kang · Y. W. Kim (✉) · H. J. Cheon
H. C. Ahn
W Institute for Hand and Reconstructive Microsurgery, W Hospital, Daegu, South Korea


S. H. Woo (ed.), *The Thumb*, https://doi.org/10.1007/978-981-10-4400-7_19

## Patient Selection

Thumb replantation should be attempted irrespective of amputation level and injury patterns as function is severely compromised without opposition and prehensile function. Contraindications for replantation include medical instability that would make lengthy surgical intervention excessively risky, multiple level injuries, and mentally unstable patients.

## Mechanism of Injury

Perhaps the most predictive indicator for success with replantation is the mechanism of injury. O'Brien followed by several others demonstrated significantly higher success rates with replantation of guillotine versus avulsion amputations [4]. It may be unrealistic to expect to successfully replant a severely crushed and mangled body part. Avulsion injuries with traction along the neurovascular bundles create intimal tears and disruption of small branches to the skin. Small hematomas seen in the skin along the course of the neurovascular bundle result in the "red line sign," which symbolizes that the injury occurring to the neurovascular bundle was so detrimental that replantation is often fraught with poor success. Even though the anastomosis may be patent, there is no flow of arterial blood to the skin (Fig. 19.1). Another mark of injury to the vessels of an amputated digit is the "ribbon sign". This demonstrates torsion and stretch on a vessel. The vessel resembles a ribbon that has been stretched and curled for decoration on a wrapped gift. Vessels that have the ribbon sign often are not amenable to sustaining blood flow, because of intimal injury to the vessel. Replantation attempts in digits with the ribbon sign require vein grafting proximal and distal to this zone of injury.

## Ischemic Time

The recommended ischemic times for reliable success with replantation are 12 h of warm and 24 h of cold ischemia for the thumb. The minimization of ischemic time is more critical in replantation of parts containing the muscle, such as those proximal to the digit.

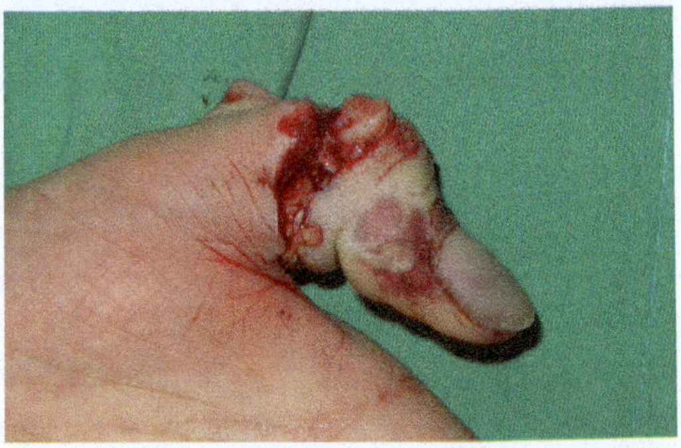

**Fig. 19.1** Red line sign demonstrates ecchymosis along the neurovascular bundles which is a poor prognostic indicator for replantation

## Other Preoperative Preparatory Evaluation

Before surgery, radiographs of the amputated parts and the stump should be performed to determine the levels of injury and suitability for replantation. Both parts should be photographed for documentation. An informed consent should be obtained, discussing the pros and cons with the patient and family regarding the failure rates, length of rehabilitation, and realistic expectations for recovery of sensation, mobility, and function. The preoperative preparation of the patient should also include prophylactic antibiotics, updating the patient's tetanus if indicated, fluid resuscitation to prevent hypotension critical in major limb replants, warming the patient to prevent hypothermia and vasoconstriction/spasm, Foley catheter insertion for volume monitoring, and protection for pressure points as these can be long operations risking pressure sore complications.

## Surgical Techniques of Thumb Replantation

### Surgical Anatomy

In digits, neurovascular bundles are located on the mid-lateral line, but in the thumb, neurovascular bundles are placed just both lateral to the volar midline (Fig. 19.2). There are two proper digital arteries that provide the major blood supply in the thumb. They are located in the dorsolateral aspect of the digital nerves and travel along both lateral sides to the flexor pollicis longus tendon between the volar Grayson ligament and the dorsal Cleland ligament. The ulnar digital artery of the thumb has a greater diameter than that of the radial digital artery. The diameter of the thumb digital arteries at the proximal phalanx is 1.0–1.5 mm and that of the terminal branch at the thumb tip is 0.2–0.3 mm [5].

### Surgical Procedure

The sequence of repair is dependent on the surgeon's preference, but the usual sequence is as follows:

1. Debridement and preparation
2. Bone shortening and fixation
3. Extensor tendon repair
4. Flexor tendon repair
5. Arterial repair
6. Nerve repair
7. Vein repair
8. Skin closure and coverage

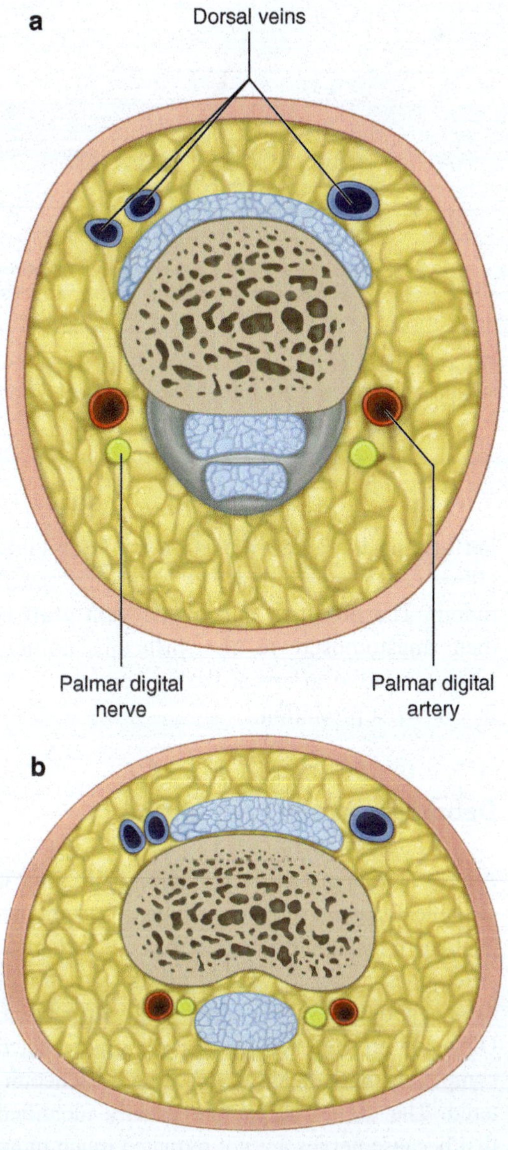


**Fig. 19.2** Cross section of the digit (**a**) and thumb (**b**) at the mid-shaft level of the proximal phalanx. Compared with digit, neurovascular bundles of the thumb are located just both lateral to the volar midline

### Positioning

The patient is placed in a supine position on an operating table. To expose the ulnar digital artery of the thumb in volar aspect, the wrist must be placed in a supination position. With this position, thumb prevents a good operation field vision, and the proximal artery is hidden in a deeper position. The hand should be placed in an extremely supinated position to repair the ulnar digital artery. In case of ulnar artery reconstruction with interpositional vein graft between princeps pollicis artery and ulnar digital artery, the distal anastomosis of the vein graft is performed on the back table before bone fixation and tendon repair (Fig. 19.3).

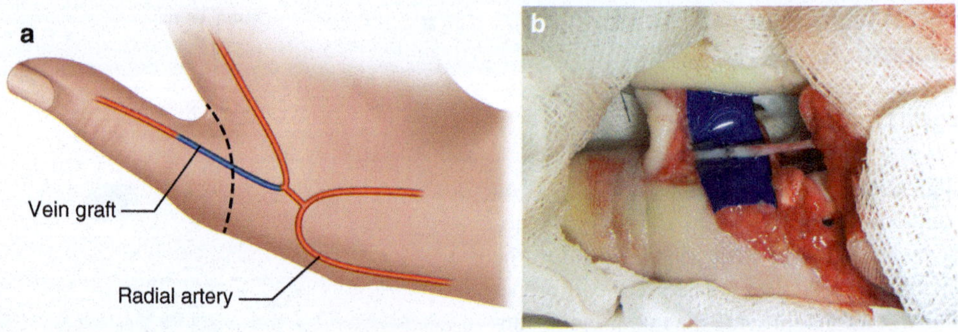


**Fig. 19.3** (**a**) Schematic view of artery reconstruction with interpositional vein graft between princeps pollicis artery and ulnar digital artery. (**b**) Interpositional vein graft from the volar wrist is anastomosed for arterial reconstruction

Performing the anastomosis on the back table allows easy positioning of the amputated thumb. The proximal end of the vein graft is then anastomosed to the princeps pollicis artery or radial artery at the anatomical snuff box in wrist pronation.

## Debridement and Preparation

A two-team approach is preferable here, and if possible, the parts should continue to be kept in a cool and moist condition until they are replanted. After massive sterile solution irrigation, debridement is performed under microscopic inspection. Dirty and crushed soft tissue margin is resected completely until healthy soft tissue is encountered. The digital nerves are usually identified first because nerves are not retracted much more than artery and are easier to find. As the nerve is pulled to midline, search for the retracted artery at the dorsolateral aspect of the nerve. If an additional incision is needed, application of a bilateral mid-lateral incision is preferable to expose the volar neurovascular bundle and prevent scar contracture of the skin. Both the palmar and dorsal flaps can be reflected as needed. After identification of arteries, nerves, and veins, tag with small hemo-clips or 8-0 nylon sutures. The tagging material should be placed as close to the end of structures as possible to avoid additional damage.

If the veins are difficult to isolate, the surgeon can delay the identification of vein until after the repair of arteries. After artery repair, engorgements of veins make them more prominent and easy to find. Once one vein is located, continue the dissection in the same subdermal plane to identify other veins.

Any attached tissue of an incomplete amputation should not be cut or harmed. This narrow connection may enhance a venous drainage especially in segmental amputation. Before the bone fixation, the retracted flexor pollicis longus tendon end must be found and tagged with a nylon suture or fixed at the proximal pulley with a needle to prevent proximal retraction. Every attempt should be made to repair all structures primarily, and any amputated parts which are not being replanted should not be discarded, as these are an excellent source for grafts.

## Bone Shortening and Fixation

The damaged bones in both the amputated part and the proximal stump are removed with a rongeur or saw with caution to prevent iatrogenic soft tissue damage, and consideration of the level and geometry of amputation is necessary. Bone surfaces should be smooth to achieve complete bony contact and a clean margin. Bone shortening may guarantee primary repair of the artery, vein, and nerves without graft as well as easy approximation of the soft tissue. The amount of shortening depends partly on the mechanism of injury. Crushing injuries usually need more resection than guillotine injuries. Bone shortening of the finger about 5–10 mm in length makes no definitive functional problem [6]. In case of thumb replantation, excessive shortening should be avoided to get appropriate hand function. Especially in multiple digit amputation, length of the thumb is more essential to oppose other digits. The bone resection should be performed mainly at the amputated part, because if the replantation fails, the remaining thumb length should be as long as possible.

A one or two longitudinal K-wire fixation technique is usually used to fix the distal phalanx level amputation. In proximal phalanx level amputation, a longitudinal or cross K-wire fixation is the preferred method. Temporary K-wires which cross this joint should be removed within 2–3 weeks after replantation to prevent joint stiffness of the interphalangeal joint. Remaining fixation devices should be maintained until solid bone union has been obtained. In the case of IP joint disarticulation, if the articular cartilage is severely damaged and joint function cannot be restored, arthrodesis is the preferred method of fixation (Fig. 19.4). With arthrodesis, shortening

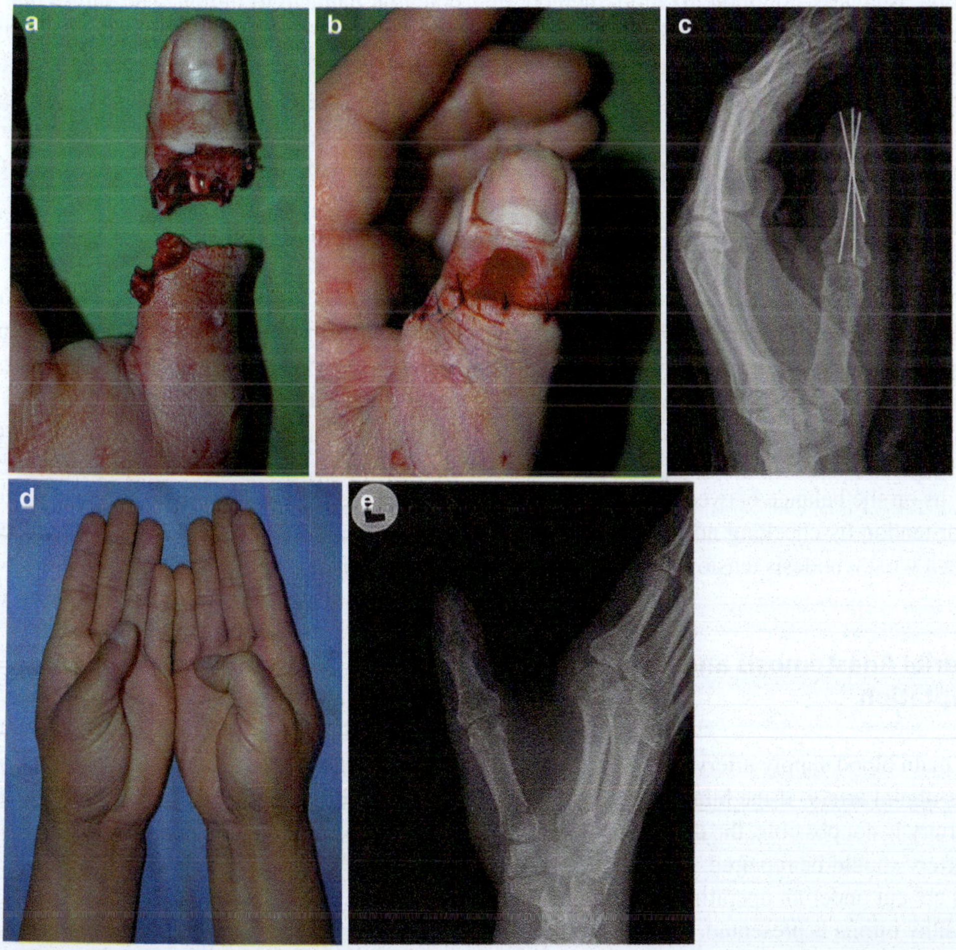


**Fig. 19.4** (**a**) Preoperative view of complete amputation at interphalangeal joint of the left thumb. (**b**) Immediate postoperative view. (**c**) Postoperative radiograph shows three K-wire fixation for the arthrodesis of the interphalangeal joint. (**d, e**) Postoperative view and radiograph

of the bone facilitates neurovascular anastomoses without tension. In amputation proximal to the IP joint, besides K-wire fixation, interosseous wiring and plate and screw can be used to fixate the bone, although these techniques may take time and result in additional dissection of the adjacent periosteum and soft tissue. A 90-90 or three 90-90 intraosseous wiring allows for early range of motion, is not so time-consuming, and needs less dissection of soft tissue than plate and screw fixation. Drill holes for passing a 24-gauge wire are placed dorsal to palmar or radial to ulnar orientation at both proximal and distal sides of fracture of proximal phalanx. Compared with plate and screw fixation, intraosseous wiring has the advantage of high union rate. Plate and screw fixation is a less common fixation method in thumb amputations as a plate is bulky, tendon adhesions are increased, and more dissection is required.

## Tendon Repair

The order of the tendon repair is the surgeon's choice, but extensor tendon is usually repaired first. Extensor tendon is repaired with an interrupted or horizontal mattress suture technique. After extensor tendon repair, the flexor tendon is repaired using a six-strand nonabsorbable core suture technique or modified Becker method with a focus on the balance between the extensor and flexor tendon by checking normal cascade or by using a wrist tenodesis tension technique.

## Arterial Anastomosis and Nerve Coaptation

The main blood supply artery to the thumb is the ulnar digital artery. If the bilateral repair of digital artery is not possible, the dominant ulnar digital artery should be repaired. The injured arterial ends are cut under an operating microscope until a healthy intima is presented. It is very important to check for strong pulsatile bleeding from the proximal end. If adequate blood flow is not obtained, evaluate the proximal vessel for all reversible causes of vasoconstriction including hypotension, hypovolemia, acidosis, pain, or cold environment. If vasospasms persist even after irrigating the lumen with warm heparinized solution, vessel dilatation and irrigation of the proximal vessel with 2% lidocaine solution is recommended. If this fails, more proximal artery should be explored for good pulsatile flow through the extended incision proximally.

Arterial anastomoses are performed with 9-0, 10-0, or 11-0 interrupted nylon sutures. Tension-free anastomosis between normal intimas is the most important factor in successful anastomosis. Arterial clamp should have less than 30 g of closing pressure and should be limited to no more than 30 min of application time to prevent potential damage to intima. The suture bite size should be one or two times the thickness of the arterial wall. Care must be taken to avoiding damage to the intima of the artery. During the artery anastomosis, repeatedly check the integrity of the intima and verify that no adventitia overhangs the lumen, the back wall is not captured, and that tension-free anastomosis has been achieved.

The digital nerve ends are examined under microscopic inspection and resected until mushroom-like sprouting of fascicles is apparent. The fascicles are topographically aligned, and epineurial repair is performed with two or three 8-0 or 9-0-sized monofilament nylon sutures. If tension-free repair is impossible, primary autogenous nerve graft is a good way to recover the thumb's sensory abilities. Donor sites are terminal branch of posterior interosseous nerve at the dorsum of the wrist and ipsilateral medial antebrachial cutaneous nerve. A gap less than 1 cm can be connected with interpositional vein conduit or artificial nerve conduit. Any amputated digits that are not candidates for replantation are also an excellent source of nerve graft.

## Venous Anastomosis

The diameter of dorsal vein is greater and a repair position of wrist pronation is preferable over wrist supination. Two or three dorsal vein anastomoses are performed to obtain sufficient venous drainage. When repairing the veins, each bite should be two or three times the thickness of the vein wall, and anastomosis with fewer sutures than that of artery due to the lower blood pressure in the vein. If there is no appropriate proximal vein to repair or an excessive gap exists, vein graft to a more proximal vein or index finger dorsal vein can be transposed to the thumb dorsal distal vein. In cases of combined defect of soft tissue and artery or vein, venous flap is a good option for resurfacing soft tissue as well as vessel. It can be harvested from the volar aspect of the wrist as skin flap including one or two veins.

In case of the amputation in distal phalanx level with no available distal vein, using the arteriovenous fistula may facilitate the outflow to reduce congestion. With very distal amputation, continuous venous external bleeding with stab incision on pulp or nail bed for 3–7 days will reduce venous congestion. Medicinal leeches (*Hirudo medicinalis*) can be used to maintain continuous external bleeding.

## Skin Closure and Dressing

The skin should be closed loosely after careful hemostasis. Even small postoperative hematomas can compress the vascular repair. If sufficient bone shortening has been performed, volar soft tissue can be repaired completely without excessive tension, but insufficient dorsal soft tissue coverage occurs often. If the repaired dorsal veins lack local coverage, a split- or full-thickness skin graft should be applied. The hand is placed in a soft and bulky dressing and should not be circumferential. Plaster splint extending above the elbow and the tip of the repaired digit is left exposed for postoperative monitoring.

## Postoperative Care

The patient should be kept in a warm room, preferably above 22 °C (72 °F). Usually the hand is elevated, but the level of elevation should be adjusted for changes in vascular status. If arterial insufficiency happens, the replanted digit changes to a white or pale color, capillary refilling is slow or nonexistent, and the skin becomes low in surface temperature, and is flaccid from low turgor. In this case, the hand is lowered. If venous congestion is present (dark red or purple color, briskly capillary refill, low surface temperature or firm skin turgor), the hand is raised.

Postoperative monitoring of replanted thumb is performed for 7 days. There is a preference for leaving the dressing in place nowadays unless excessive bleeding from the wound occurs and makes a blood cast that would restrict venous drainage and prompt an early dressing change. The patient is maintained in bed rest for the first 3–5 days, the room kept dark with minimal stimulation, and the patient is restricted from nicotine and caffeine.

Our standard protocol for prevention of thrombosis is a low dose of heparin at 1000 μ/h for 5–7 days, and enteric-coated aspirin (325 mg daily) is initiated and maintained for 3 weeks. When vasospasm is suspected, the factor that causes the patient discomfort should be identified and addressed first. Arterial spasm usually occurs within 24 h after anastomosis, but venous thrombosis usually occurs during the first 72 h following replantation. Once any arterial or venous problem is confirmed, the surgeon must carry out an immediate reexploration. Thrombectomy and reanastomosis of the vessel are the only ways to save the thumb.

# Special Conditions

## Distal Amputation

Distal amputation of the thumb is defined as distal to flexor pollicis longus insertion. In Tamai zone 1 thumb amputation, the distal transverse palmar arch and its branches run just superficial to the insertion of FPL tendon and bone. Among the terminal branches of arteries located along the center of pulp, central artery usually has the widest diameter and may appear when compressing the pulp gently. This central artery branch is

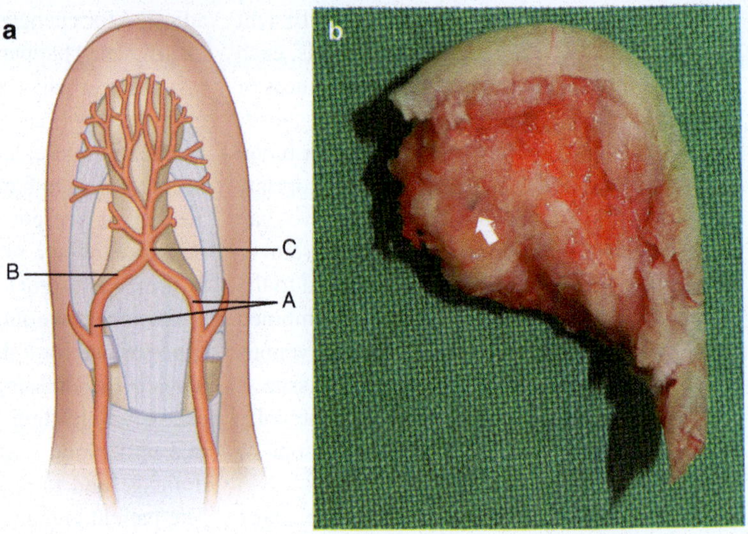


**Fig. 19.5** (a) Schematic view of the arterial anatomy of the thumb tip. Both proper digital arteries (**A**) form the distal transverse arch (**b, B**) and then central branch (**C**). (**b**) The central branch is often larger than other side branches; the white arrow indicates the central branch of transverse arch

the most reliable branch to restore circulation (Fig. 19.5). This portion includes specialized structures such as nail plate, nail matrix, distal phalanx bone, pulp tissue, and glabrous skin with fingerprints. Preservation of these structures should be a priority when treating amputation injury. Microvascular replantation is the treatment of choice except for such cases as severe soft tissue injuries in an amputated part or in irreparable cases.

Even in such cases as very distal amputations where replantation seems to be difficult, one must use operating microscopy to look for digital artery which might be repairable (Fig. 19.6). If arterial repair is deemed possible, after tagging vessels with 9-0 sutures, bone fixation should be performed first. After repairing digital artery with 10-0 or 11-0 nylon sutures, check if there are any remaining repairable digital veins. If there is no available vein, artery repair only and continuous external venous drainage may guarantee the survival of the replanted part [7, 8]. Venous congestion can be treated by continuous bleeding via a stab incision on the fingertips and topical administration of heparinized saline at the incision site to maintain bleeding. If any repairable nerves are found, repair them likewise. Even if severe avulsion makes nerve repair impossible, one can predict good sensory recovery.

## Avulsion and Degloving Amputation

Avulsion or degloving injuries are a very separate category of thumb amputations, having a worse prognosis for replantation success than local crush or guillotine-type injuries. In avulsion amputations, soft tissue injuries often occur more proximally than do skeletal injuries. These are subjected to high-traction-torsional force injuries caused by farm machinery, industrial belt, reins of a horse, or high-speed leisure activities like a waterskiing rope or a motorcycle chain. In 1980, success rate of thumb replantation was reported as 73.5% in 67 cases of amputation and 42.9% in avulsion amputation [9]. In 39 patients with thumb avulsion, success rate was also achieved in 26% [10].

The red line sign of the soft tissue and the ribbon sign of the avulsed vessels are recognized as indicators of damaged vessels, and their presence is suggestive of a poor prognosis for replantation. However, hand surgeons should try to find available vessels of the injured thumb for replantation. There is no better alternative of the thumb reconstruction than replantation or revascularization.

Degloving amputation is usually caused by crushing, shearing, and avulsing the soft tissue envelope, resulting in severe macroscopic and microscopic damage to the digital vessels and

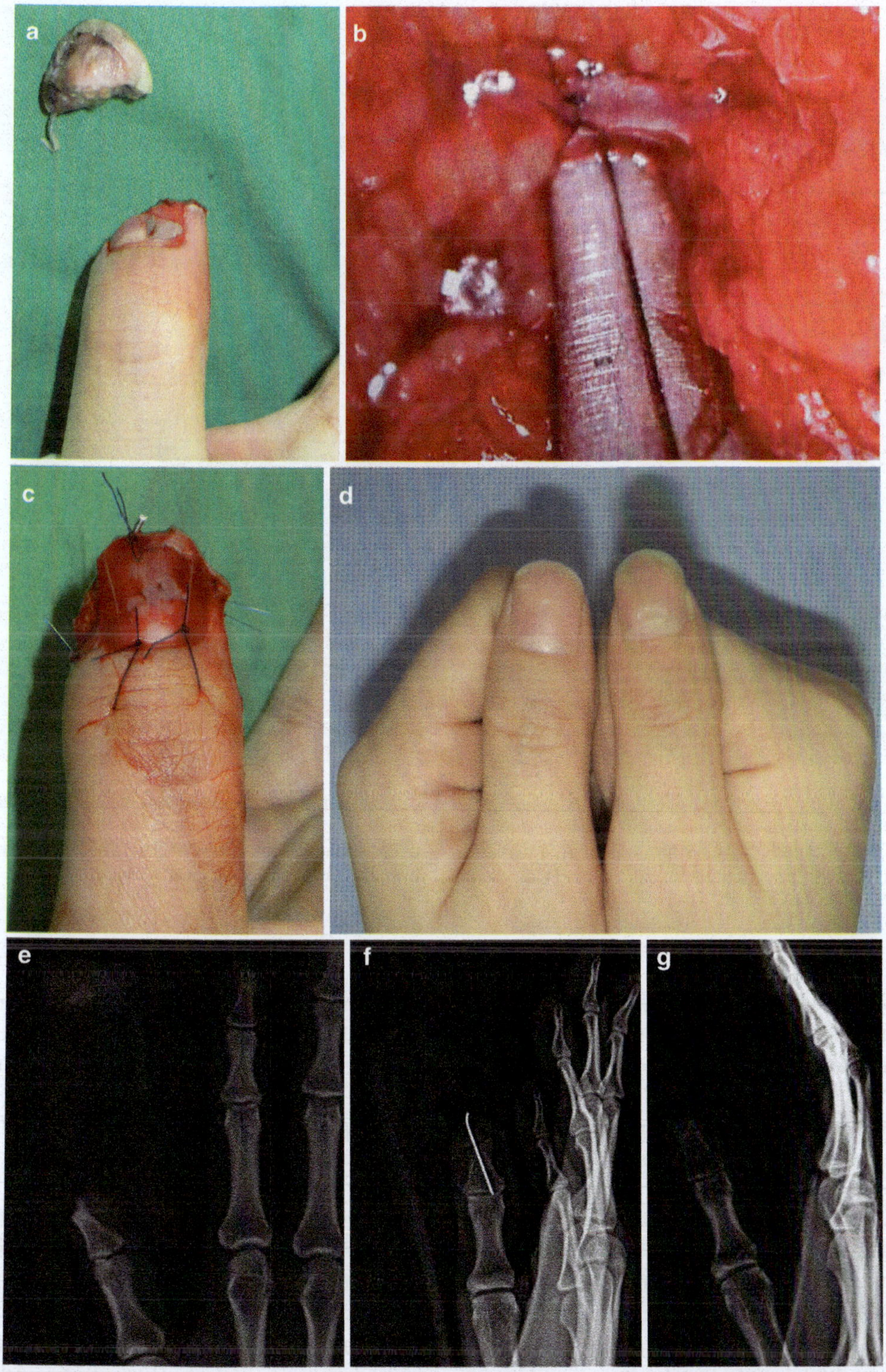


**Fig 19.6** (**a**) Preoperative view of the very distal amputation of right thumb. (**b**) After K-wire fixation, one central digital artery is microanastomosed. (**c**) Immediate postoperative view. External bleeding was maintained for 5 days through the slit incision on the pulp tip. (**d**) Postoperative appearance, 1 year later. (**e–g**) Preoperative, immediate postoperative, and radiograph 1 year later

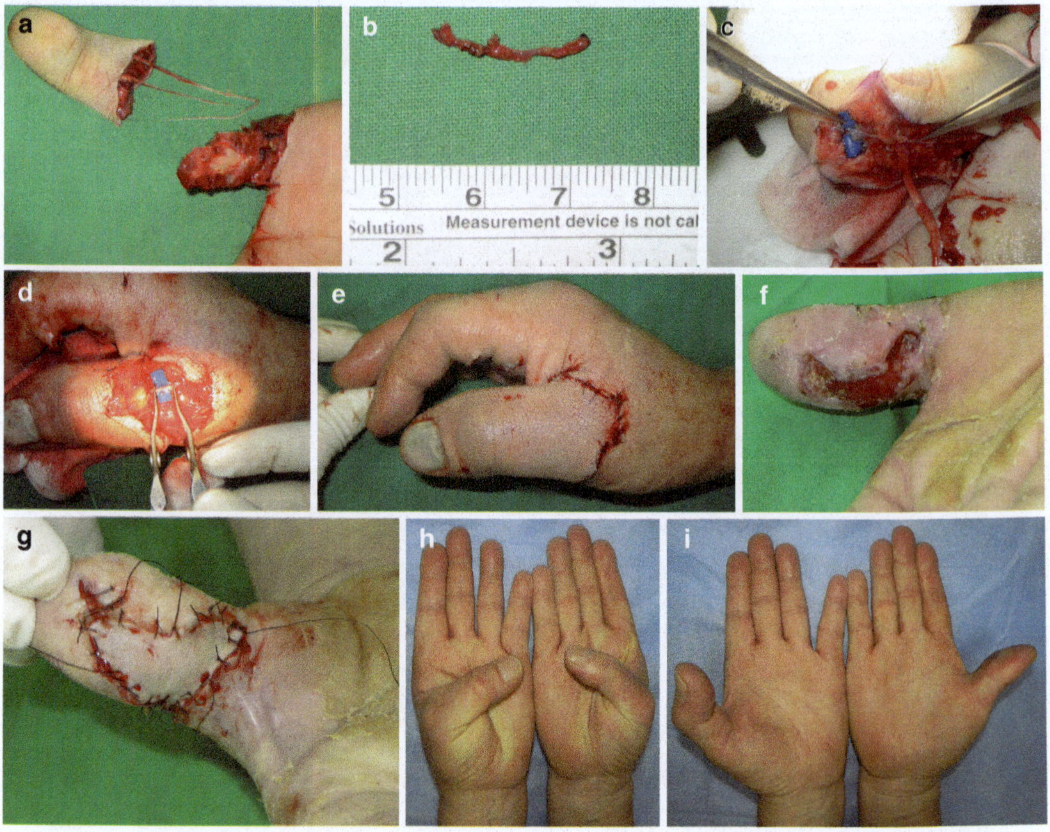


**Fig. 19.7** (**a**) A 61-year-old male with a degloving amputation of the soft tissue envelope at the metacarpophalangeal joint of the right thumb. (**b**) Vein graft is harvested from the volar aspect of the distal wrist. (**c**) Ulnar digital artery is reanastomosed to central digital artery with 2.5 cm vein graft. (**d**) One dorsal vein is repaired. (**e**) Immediate postoperative view. (**f**, **g**) Full-thickness skin graft is applied to cover the skin defect of the volar aspect. (**h**, **i**) Postoperative appearance, 38 months later

nerves (Fig. 19.7). Even after successful replantation, there is always accompanying partial skin necrosis, and a risk of having poor functional results remains. Because digital arteries are ruptured or avulsed around thumb tips, it is not easy to find healthy digital artery at the amputation level. Through the mid-lateral or volar zigzag incision on the amputated part, terminal digital artery should be dissected and found using an operative microscope. Direct anastomosis between ruptured ends of the arteries is always impossible. Interpositional vein graft or digital artery transfer from the index finger is a good option to overcome this problem. If there is no available vessel to anastomosis in the amputated part, degloved soft tissue is used as a full-thickness skin graft after defatting. Eventually where soft tissue is necrosed, various flaps including radial artery superficial palmar branch flap, radial forearm flap, venous flap, or metacarpal artery perforator flap are helpful to achieve appropriate length and appearance of the thumb.

In cases of avulsed flexor and extensor tendons from musculotendinous junction, tendon reconstruction is very complex. In clearly avulsed injury, avulsed tendons are repositioned into the viable muscle belly after radical debridement of avulsed muscle portion (Fig. 19.8). Another option for tendon reconstruction is primary transfer of the tendons from the 3rd or 4th flexor digitorum sublimus and extensor indicis proprius.

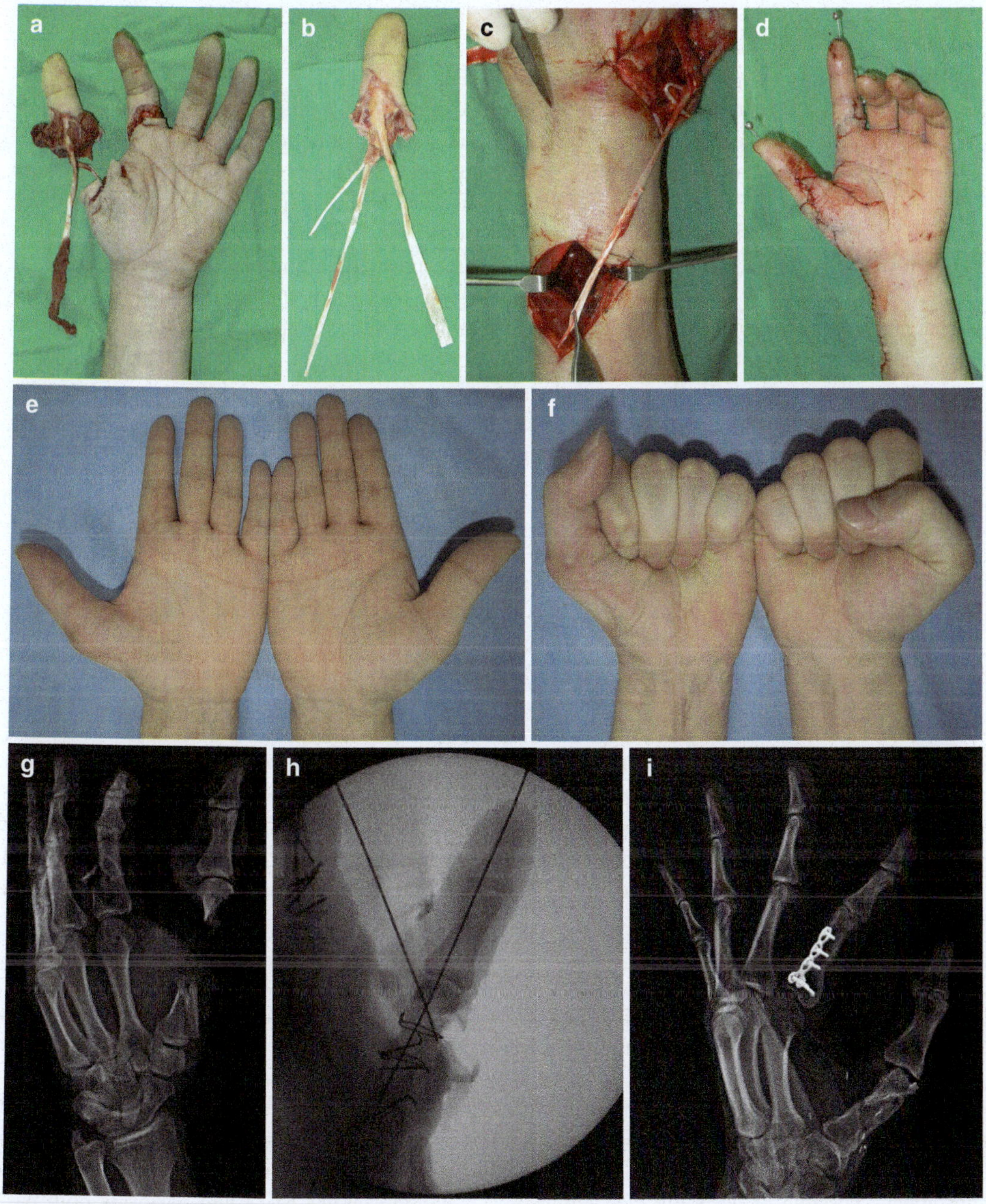


**Fig. 19.8** (**a**) Avulsion amputation of the left thumb and incomplete amputation of the index. (**b**) Muscle portion of the flexor and extensor tendons was clearly debrided. (**c**) Both flexor and extensor tendons are reattached to the viable muscle belly by interweaving suture at the proximal forearm. (**d**) Immediate postoperative view. (**e**, **f**) Postoperative appearance about 12 months demonstrates active motion of the interphalangeal joint. (**g**–**i**) Radiographs of the preoperative, intraoperative, and postoperative view

However, decision of the primary tendon transfer should be very carefully considered regarding replantation failure or possibility of infection. For the delayed reconstruction, artificial tendon insertion is recommendable. It usually takes 3 months for the secondary tendon graft.

## Segmental Amputation

Segmental amputation is also recognized as a contraindication for replantation. However, any replantation or surgery with the injured thumb parts should be attempted considering the effect on the overall function of the hand. Even though the thumb is stiff and has no sensation, it can act as the post for opposition with remnant digits. In segmental amputation, any attached tissue of segmental portion should not be cut or debrided because the narrow and small connection of soft tissue plays a major role in venous drainage between the amputation segments (Fig. 19.9). Before bone fixation, retracted flexor and extensor tendon end must be found and tagged with a nylon suture or fixed at the proximal pulley with a needle to prevent proximal retraction. All amputated structures should be repaired primarily with bone shortening or debridement of the injured portion of the amputated parts.

## Transpositional Replantation

Transpositional replantation of the thumb refers to the transposition and replantation of any digit to the thumb which plays a more significant role in the function of the hand. Replantation of all the amputated digits on their orthotopic positions is not always possible or desirable, depending on the quality of the available parts and stumps [11]. In the case of multiple finger amputations, the thumb should be reconstructed first, followed by the amputated long or ring finger, so that function of opposition, pinch, and grip can be restored [12]. However, if the degree of crushing in the thumb is judged to be so severe that replantation is not possible, perform thumb transpositional replantation using one of the other amputated fingers which degree of crushing is minimum and whose length is similar to that of the thumb (Fig. 19.10) [13]. If there are no digits for transpositional replantation, one should consider secondary reconstruction such as toe transfer. For the latter secondary option, it is important not to cut the remaining phalanx or metacarpal bone more but to cover the defect with flap. Transpositional thumb replantation remains a useful alternative for the treatment of multiple digit amputations, particularly in patients with severely damaged non-replantable amputated digits.

## Rehabilitation

Rehabilitation treatment of post-thumb replantation varies depending on the surgeon and the patient's condition such as level of amputation, characteristics of injury, condition in the microanastomosis of neurovascularity, and patient age. In addition, different surgeons have reported various times and methods of rehabilitation. The authors do not perform any special rehabilitation to stabilize vascularity for 5 days, but gentle motion is started on postoperative day 2, 3 within the confines of the splint. The patient keeps bed rest by keeping and maintaining the splint in a functional position on the dorsal side of the wrist and thumb.

When the blood flow and wounds are stabilized around 1 week after surgery, a passive exercise of the thumb begins. If it is difficult for the patient to start the passive exercise with the other hand, a rehabilitation therapist helps with the process of passive exercise. From 2 weeks, the patient keeps the thumb actively exercised with a dynamic exercise brace and performs both passive and active exercises. Massage and stretching on the replantation assists thumb movement as it gives flexibility to the soft tissues and joints.

The movement of elbows and wrists is unconstrained, and the passive and active exercise is performed since 2 weeks after the operation. A thumb brace should be used when not performing rehabilitation therapy. Rehabilitation therapy is carried out for around 3 months by increasing the

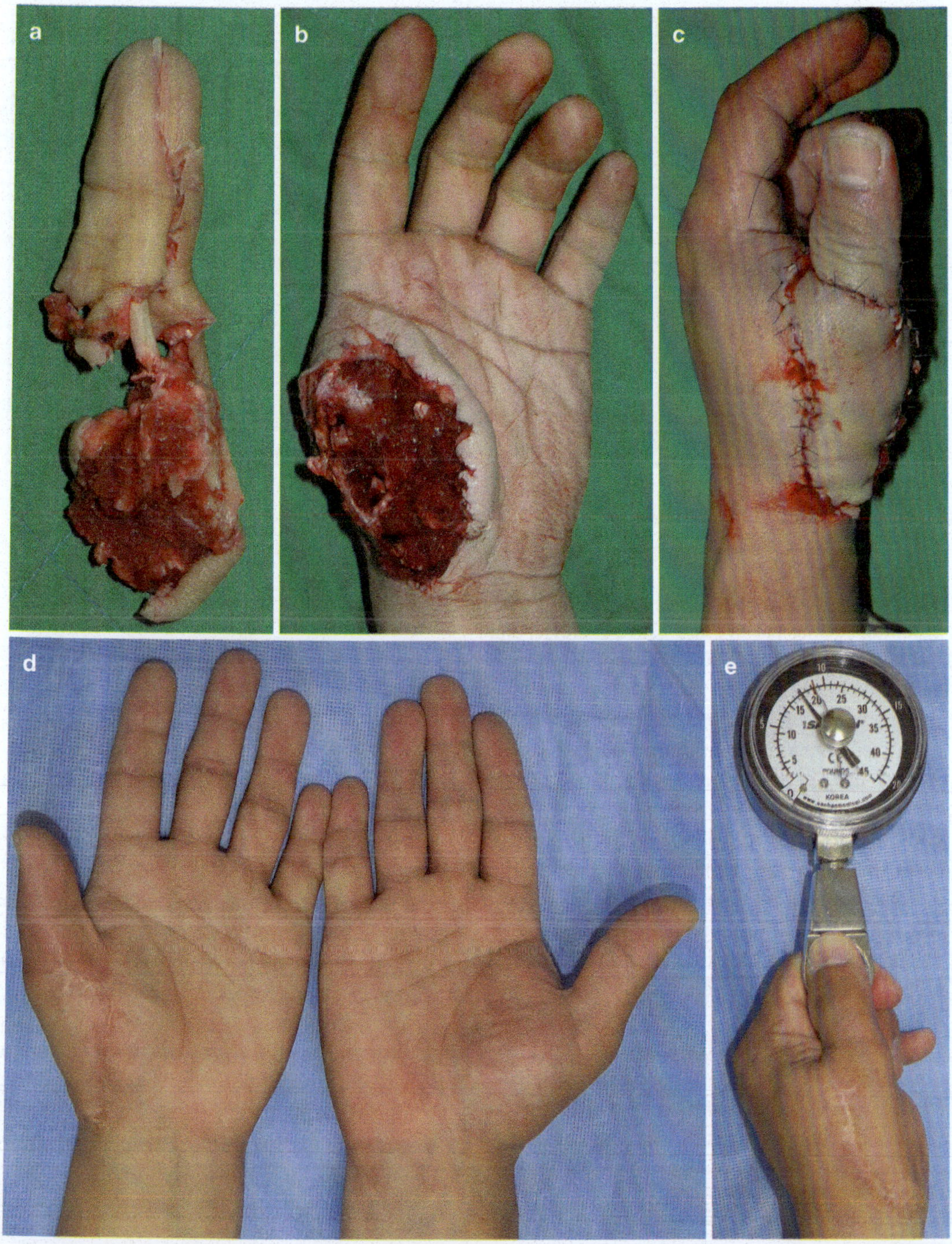


**Fig. 19.9** (**a**, **b**). A 37-year-old male had segmental amputation and crushing injury of the left thumb at the metacarpal shaft. (**c**) Two Kirschner wires are used for longitudinal fixation from the distal phalangeal bone to metacarpal base. Both flexor and extensor tendon are repaired, and the first metacarpal artery is anastomosed to the distal segment of ulnar side digital artery, and then princeps pollicis artery is microsutured to communicating artery branch at the metacarpal neck of the proximal segment. Very narrow skin bridge provides venous drainage between the amputation segments. (**d**, **e**) Postoperative appearance about 34 months later. Key pinch is 17 lbs, which is 85% of the contralateral side. (**f–h**) Radiographs of the preoperative, immediate postoperative, and 34 months later postoperative view

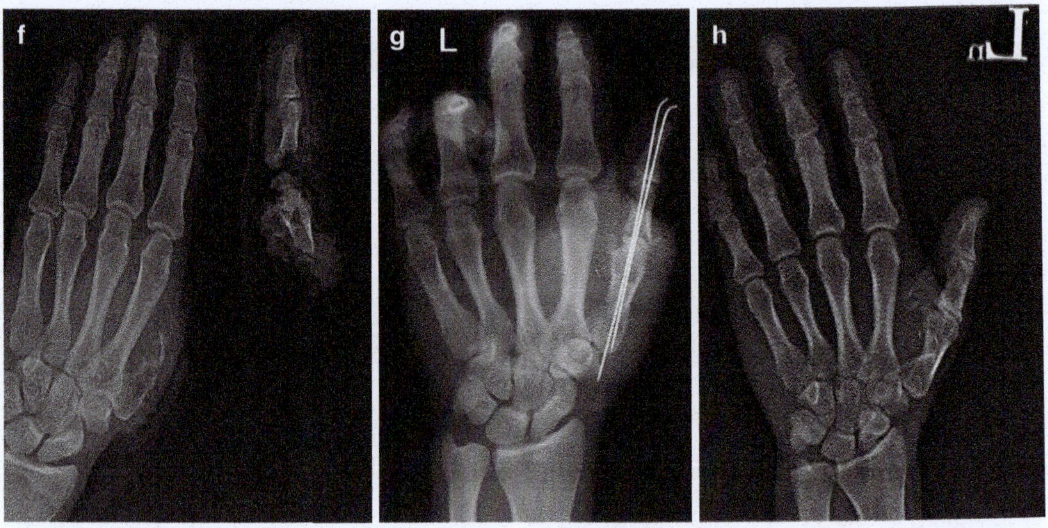


**Fig. 19.9** (continued)

range of motion of the thumb, performing rehabilitation such as passive and active exercise, and massaging/stretching to prevent tendon adhesion and joint contracture.

Depending on the degree of recovery after thumb replantation, the secondary reconstruction surgery may be performed on the bone, joints, and soft tissues. If the bone problems such as bone defect, nonunion, and malunion are present, corrective osteotomy, bone grafting, and a stable internal fixation should be performed. In the case of contracture and limitation of motion due to tendon adhesion and scarring after physical rehabilitation, tenolysis, scar contracture release, and joint manipulation are performed. Tendon graft and tendon transfer can be planned when the tendon defect is severe, or it is impossible to reconstruct by itself. Tendon grafts are mainly palmaris longus. EIP tendon transfer is mainly used for EPL reconstruction, and 3rd or 4th FDS transfer is used for FPL reconstruction.

For soft tissue defects, reconstruction of soft tissue can be performed by the skin graft or performing various flaps. Sensory recovery of the thumb is a very important factor in function. Neurolysis, neuroma excision, and nerve graft can be performed when there is a nerve problem. If thumb sensation is unsatisfactory or absent, sensory recovery can be restored by using the heterodigital neurovascular island flap or free sensory flap.

## Outcomes

In review of 52 consecutive isolated thumb replantation cases, the overall thumb survival rate was 92% [11]. Pinch and grip strengths were significantly worse after crush or avulsion injuries and injuries requiring joint intervention. Grip strength was also found to be negatively associated with increasing zone of injury. The need for secondary surgery is strongly related to zone of injury, with zone I injuries requiring the least one of secondary surgery. Patients with drug/alcohol abuse record and higher numbers of comorbid conditions had lower odds of replant success [12, 14]. Treatment in training hospitals and hospitals with a higher volume of thumb replantation increased the possibilities of replant survival. The risk-adjusted replantation success rate in high-volume hospitals was 12% higher than in low-volume hospitals. Regionalization of digit replantation procedures to high-volume centers can achieve the highest rate of successful revascularization.

Thumb function, sensory recovery, and appearance of thumb are assessed at 3 and 6 months postoperatively. The power of the thumb is assessed by key pinch, tip pinch, and opposition. Recovery of sensation will vary depending on damage severity and nerve repair and is based on the two-point discrimination test.

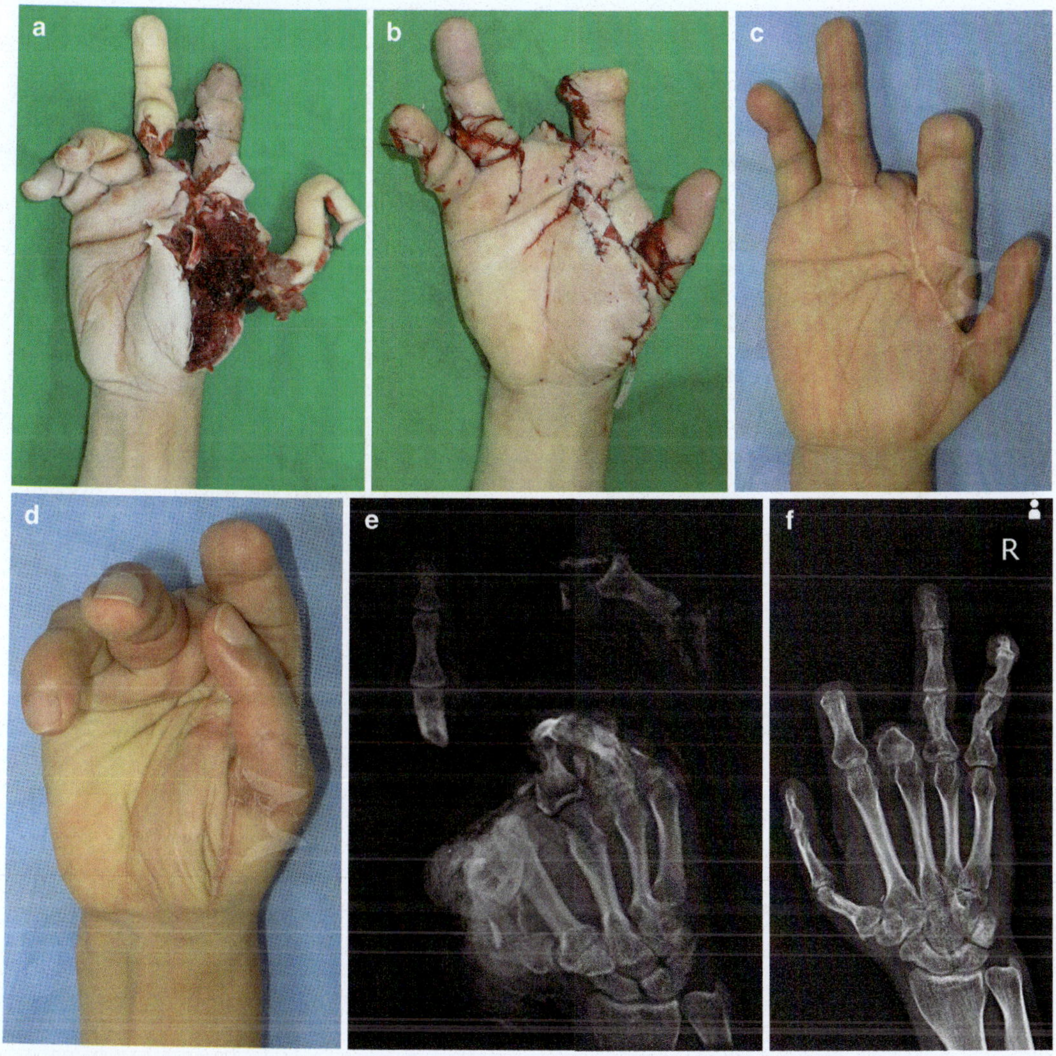


**Fig. 19.10** (**a**) Multiple digit amputation of the right thumb, index, and long finger with comminuted phalangeal fractures. (**b**) Immediate postoperative view. The thumb is seriously crushed and is not available for replantation. The amputated long finger is transposed to the thumb. (**c**, **d**) Postoperative view, 6 months later. The patient was able to pinch and grip using the reconstructed thumb, while the metacarpophalangeal joint is fused. (**e**, **f**) Preoperative and postoperative radiograph

In addition, cosmetic satisfaction is assessed by the appearance such as soft tissue atrophy, deformity, and scars. After 6 months of rehabilitation, we decide whether to perform the secondary procedure depending on the degree of the function, appearance, and sensory recovery.

The functional outcomes of thumb replantation, such as range of motion, appearance, and sensation, are inconsistent but still acceptable. More favorable outcomes are expected in younger patients, guillotine-type injuries, and patients with more distal level of amputation. Recovery of sensation is related to function, and better results are again evident in younger patients. The average two-point discrimination in replanted thumb is 10 mm. Sensation in avulsion and crushing injuries results in poorer outcomes. Range of motion is correlated with level of amputation and type of injury. Active interphalangeal joint motion in the thumb was an average of 30°. Although bone shortening, joint stiffness, and tendon adhesion may occur after replantation, a thumb that maintains length can restore favorable appearance and function.

## References


1. Malt RA, McKhann C. Replantation of severed arms. JAMA. 1964;189:716–22.
2. Chen CW, Chien YC, Pao YS. Salvage of the forearm following complete traumatic amputation: report of a case. Chin Med J (Engl). 1963;82:633–8.
3. Komatsu S, Tamai S. Successful replantation of a completely cut-off thumb: case report. Plast Reconstr Surg. 1968;42:374–7.
4. O'Brien B, Miller GDH. Digital reattachment and revascularization. J Bone Joint Surg. 1973;55A:714–23.
5. Hattori Y, Doi Y, Sakamoto S, et al. Fingertip replantation. J Hand Surg. 2007;32A:548–55.
6. Richard M, Lewis RG, Levin S. Wiesel's operative techniques in orthopedic surgery. Philadelphia: Lippincott Williams and Wilkins; 2011. p. 2888–99.
7. Huang HF, Yeong EK. Surgical treatment of distal digit amputation: success in distal digit replantation is not dependent on venous anastomosis. Plast Reconstr Surg. 2015;135:174–8.
8. Erken HY, Takka S, Akmaz I. Artery-only fingertip replantations using a controlled nailbed bleeding protocol. J Hand Surg. 2013;38A:2173–9.
9. Schlenker JD, Kleinert HE, Tsai TM. Methods and results of replantation following traumatic amputation of the thumb in sixty-four patients. J Hand Surg Am. 1980;5:63–70.
10. Bieber EJ, Wood MB, Cooney WP, et al. Thumb avulsion: results of replantation/revascularization. J Hand Surg Am. 1987;12:786–90.
11. Agarwal JP, Trovato MJ, Agarwal S, et al. Selected outcomes of thumb replantation after isolated thumb amputation injury. J Hand Surg Am. 2010;35:1485–90.
12. Mahmoudi E, Chung KC. Effect of hospital volume on success of thumb replantation. J Hand Surg Am. 2017;42:96–103.
13. Schwabegger AH, Harpf C, Rumer A, et al. Transpositional replantation of digits. Case reports. Scand J Plast Reconstr Surg Hand Surg. 1999;33:243–9.
14. Mahmoudi E, Huetteman HE, Chung KC. A population-based study of replantation after traumatic thumb amputation, 2007-2012. J Hand Surg Am. 2017;42:25–33.

# 20 Non-microsurgical Reconstruction

Sae Hwi Ki

The thumb is known to play a role in about 40% of hand function. The deformity or loss of the thumb thus causes a large dysfunction of the hand and dissatisfaction in a person's life. In the case of traumatic amputation of the thumb, we know that replantation is the best way to restore its function. However, there may be difficulty with successful replantation due to severe damage, severe contamination, or no amputee. Sometimes, the replantation procedure may be delayed or ignored due to accompanying severe injuries [1]. There are also other causes of thumb loss with congenital anomalies such as hypoplastic thumb, constriction ring syndrome, etc.

Before thumb reconstruction, the surgeon should know the patient's needs, hand dominance, occupation, hobbies, goals, and psychological status as well as the patient's history and physical examination results. In addition to this, identifying the remaining bones, tendons, muscles, nerves, and vessels after injury of the hand helps to establish a reconstruction plan. The following should be considered important when reconstructing the thumb: (1) the appropriate length of the thumb, (2) its stability, (3) the proper position to contact the next digit, (4) the sense but nontender tip of the thumb, and (5) its proper mobility and strength.

Littler said that "It is not the full length of the thumb, nor its great strength and movement, but rather its strategic position relative to the fingers and the integrity of the specialized terminal pulp tissue, which determines prehensile status" [2]. Following his assessment, it is important not only to reconstruct the thumb with proper stability and mobility but also to reconstruct it in harmony with the remaining fingers in the reconstruction plan of the thumb [3].

Due to recent advances in microsurgical procedure, various toe-to-finger surgical methods have been developed, and applied and have shown good results [4]. The author has also achieved good results in replanting toe to finger. However, if difficult conditions to use microsurgical techniques exist, such as poor operating room conditions, or patients experienced microsurgical reconstruction failure in a previous surgery, the use of conventional non-microsurgical reconstruction techniques is necessary [5].

While soft tissue reconstruction (Chap. 18) and microsurgical reconstruction (Chap. 21) will be discussed later, this chapter will introduce how to reconstruct the thumb to adequate length and adequate soft tissue coverage using non-microsurgical reconstruction methods.

S. H. Ki (✉)
Department of Plastic and Reconstructive Surgery, Inha University Hospital, Incheon, South Korea



S. H. Woo (ed.), *The Thumb*, https://doi.org/10.1007/978-981-10-4400-7_20

## Classification

There are several classifications to classify thumb defect caused by traumatic amputation. Of these, Lister has classified thumb defect into four stages: (1) acceptable length, (2) subtotal amputation, (3) total amputation with the basal joint preserved, and (4) total amputation with the basal joint destroyed [6]. Campbell-Reid classified thumb defect into the following four stages: (1) amputation distal to the metacarpophalangeal joint leaving an adequate stump, (2) amputation of the thumb distal to or through the metacarpophalangeal joint leaving a stump of inadequate length, (3) amputation through the metacarpal with preservation of some functional thenar muscles, and (4) amputation at or near the carpometacarpal joint [7] (Fig. 20.1a). Muzaffar et al. classified thumb defects into three stages as follows: IPJ distal, MPJ, and proximal defects [8] (Fig. 20.1b).

Although the classification of several scholars is slightly different, a common view is "The thumb reconstruction method and result depend on whether the thenar muscle has been preserved, and whether the thumb basal joint which determines the mobility of the thumb and the wide mobile range has been preserved." If the functions of the basal joint and thenar muscle are preserved, a method of reconstructing the function of the thumb is selected according to the remaining length of thumb among the following various methods.

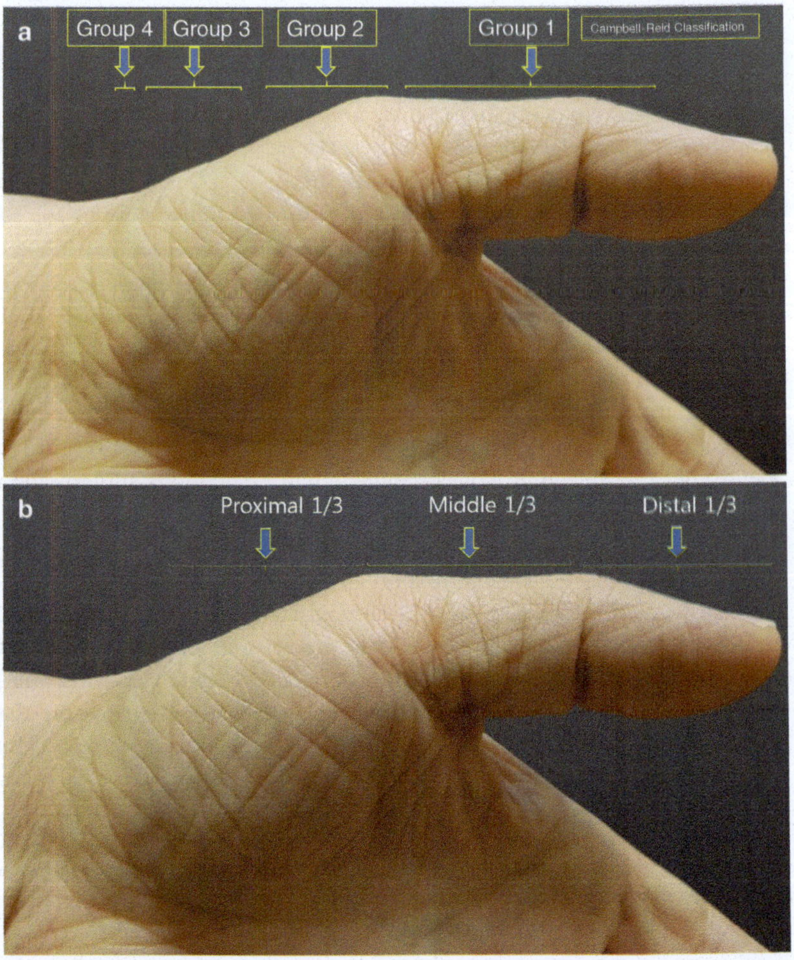


**Fig. 20.1** (**a**) Campbell-Reid classification of the traumatic thumb loss. Group 1: Amputation distal to the metacarpophalangeal joint leaving an adequate stump. Group 2: Amputation of the thumb distal to or through the metacarpophalangeal joint leaving an inadequate stump. Group 3: Amputation through the metacarpal with preservation of some thenar muscles. Group 4: Amputation at or near the carpometacarpal joint together with loss of the thenar muscles. (**b**) Muzaffar classification of the traumatic thumb loss

## Reconstruction Methods

### No Reconstruction

If the remaining length of thumb is acceptable and the soft tissue is adequately covered, no reconstruction is necessary. If the patient wants a cosmetic improvement, they can wear a cosmetic prosthetic or have a full thickness skin graft (FTSG) to act as camouflage [9].

### First Web Deepening Method

The first-web deepening procedure can be performed in case of amputation at the distal part of the proximal phalanx, because patients have difficulty in grasping large objects, a limitation on the fine pinch, and a reduced hand span. This method requires that the proximal half of proximal phalanx should remain to prevent web contracture after surgery. There are several methods to perform web deepening using local flaps, distant flaps, and free flaps depending on the condition of the surrounding tissue (Fig. 20.2a, b).

With local flap, Z-plasty, multiple Z-plasty, dorsal rotation flap, etc. can be used. With regional flap, Foucher flap based on the first dorsal metacarpal artery with a superficial radial nerve, groin flap, reverse radial forearm flap, posterior interosseous flap, etc. can be used [10–12]. A full thickness skin graft (FTSG) can be used (Fig. 20.2c, d).

### Osteoplastic Reconstruction (Fig. 20.3a, b)

Osteoplastic reconstruction consists of three components: skeletal reconstruction, soft tissue covering, and sensory flap for the pulp. For skeletal reconstruction, one of iliac bone, ulna, or radius (in case of reverse radial forearm flap) can be selected depending on the size of bone defects [13]. In the case of iliac bone graft, a tricortical bone is harvested from the lateral side of the iliac crest to obtain a rigid cortex. The fixation of the grafted bone is fixed at the distal portion of the stump (distal portion of the proximal phalanx or metacarpal bone). Several bone fixation methods can be used depending on the size of residual bone of the distal stump and the condition of the surrounding wound. Plate and screw fixation can be performed for early movement [14] (Fig. 20.3b).

In the case of using a reverse radial forearm flap, skeletal reconstruction using radius and flap reconstruction can be performed simultaneously. Therefore, it is advantageous that reconstruction of the thumb can be done quickly and bone resorption rate is less after surgery. However, there is a problem of leaving a graft scar on the forearm.

As in conventional methods of soft tissue reconstruction, groin flaps are often used. The groin flap is an axial flap based on the superficial circumflex artery that passed parallel to 2 cm above the inguinal ligament. Therefore, it should be designed considering the direction of this vessel. Recently, when the reconstruction is used with SCIP (superficial circumflex iliac artery perforator), thin flap can be made initially, so there is no need for additional thinning for debulking. After calculating the length and radius of a bone after skeletal fixation, the groin flap is designed. Then, it should be dissected to suprafascial layer over the muscle to elevate the flap. Elevated flaps wrap the bone in tube form. The division of groin flap should be performed 2–3 weeks after surgery, and staged thinning is performed according to the thickness of the flap.

For sensibility of the thumb tip, the neurovascular island flap is performed immediately or a few months after osteoplastic surgery [15]. The ulnar side of the middle finger for this flap is mainly selected, and its size is suitable as a 3 cm-long flap with an elliptical shape, but it can be made bigger or smaller as needed. The flap is harvested from the volar side and the first third on the dorsal side around the distal interphalangeal joint, and FTSG is performed on the donor site. The vascular pedicle should be transferred to the thumb tip with a sufficient length without tension, even if the thumb is in the position of maximal stretch [2]. Osteoplastic reconstruction can reconstruct the thumb quickly and safely without

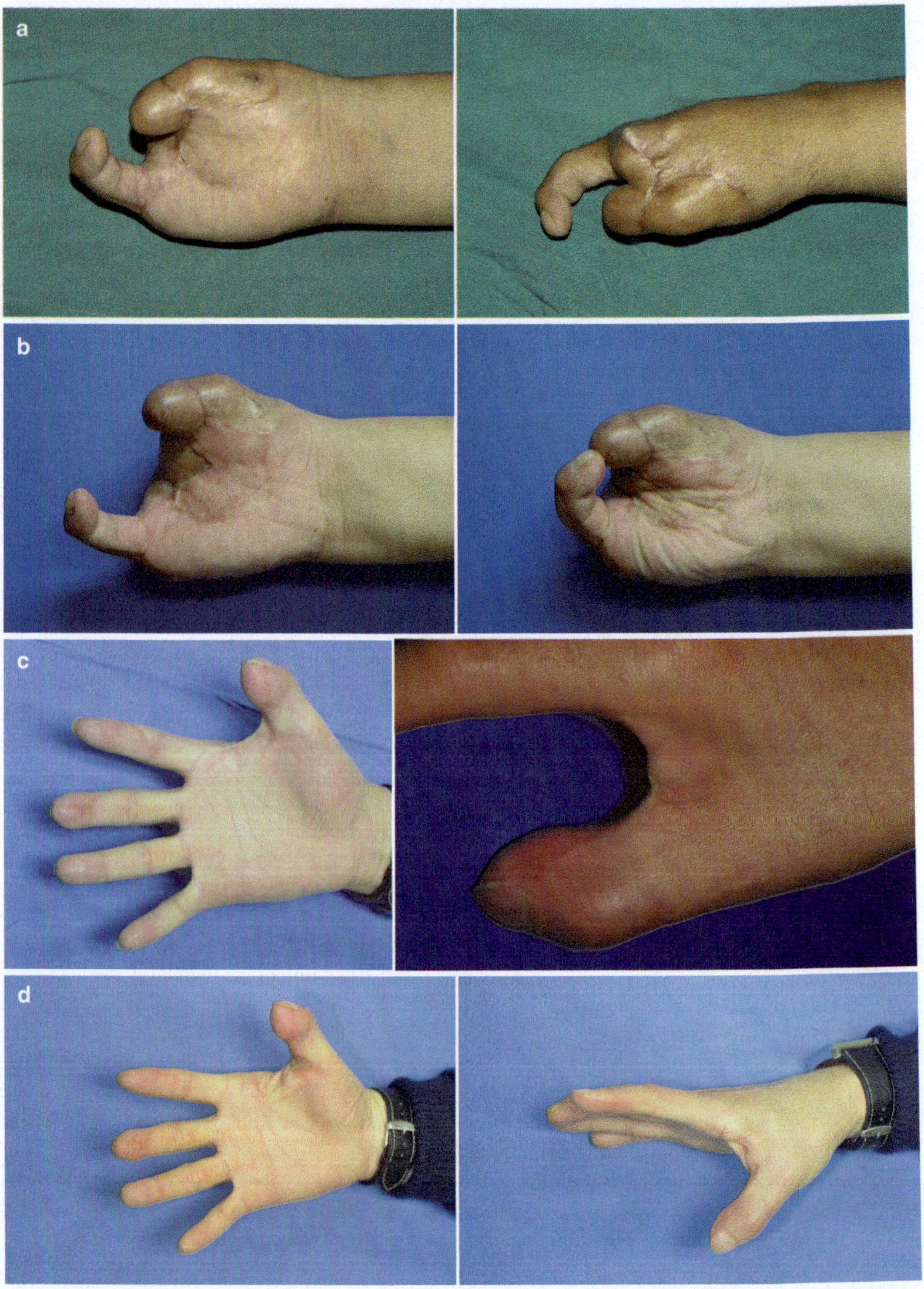


**Fig. 20.2** (**a**) First-web contracture after crushing amputation of the thumb and hand. Left: palmar view; right: dorsal view. (**b**) First-web contracture release with lateral arm flap. Left: palmar view; right: dorsal view. (**c**) First-web scar contracture after crushing injury of the thumb and first web. Left: palmar view; right: dorsal view. (**d**) First-web contracture release with full-thickness skin graft. Left: palmar view; right: dorsal view

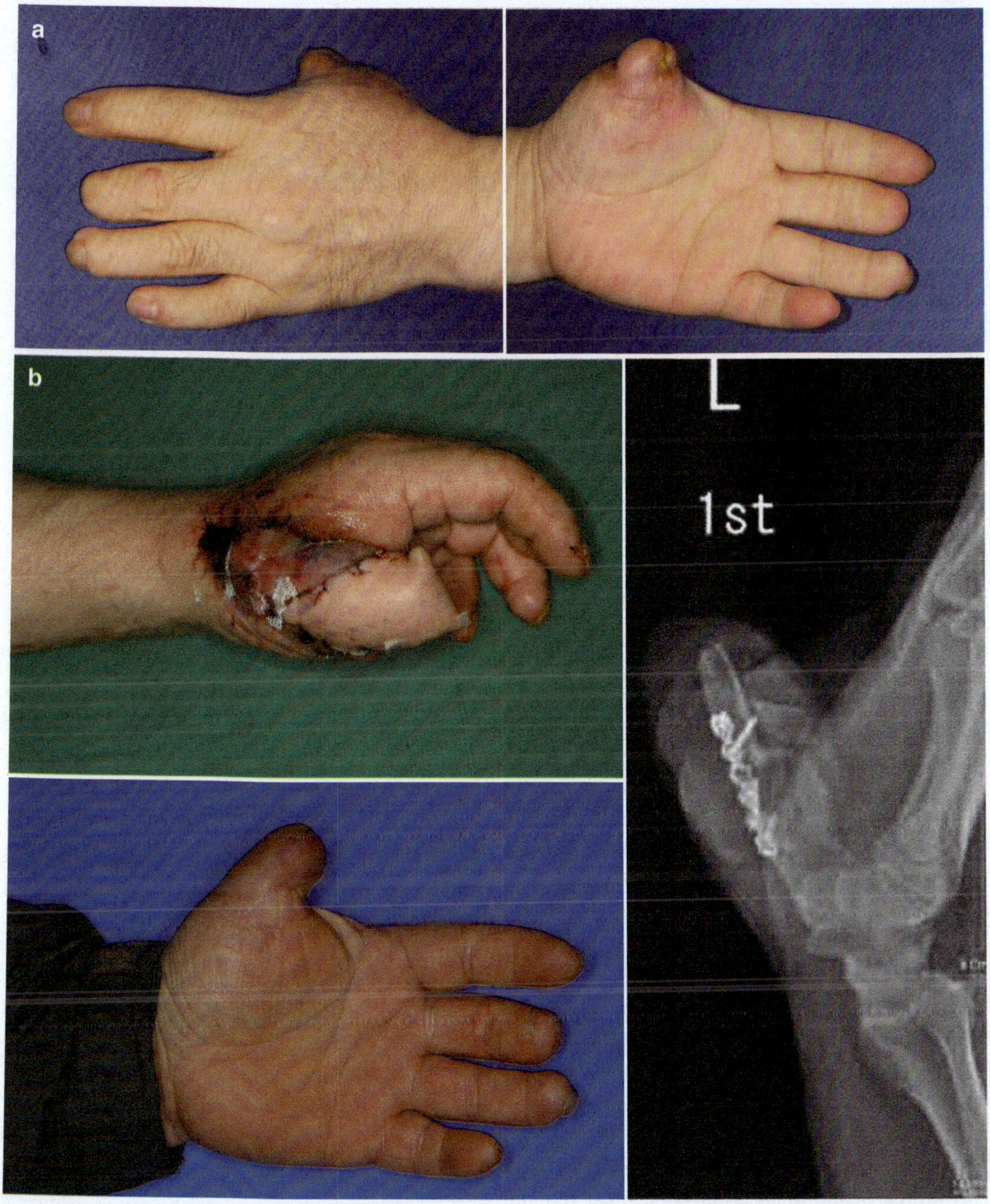


**Fig. 20.3** Osteoplastic thumb reconstruction. (**a**) Traumatic thumb loss at metacarpophalangeal joint. Left: dorsal view; right: palmar view. (**b**) Osteoplastic thumb reconstruction with lateral arm osteocutaneous flap. Upper: initial postoperative view; Right: bone fixation with plate and screw between the metacarpal bone and donor bone; Lower: follow-up postoperative finding after 2 years (Courtesy of Dr. JS. Kim, Gwang Myung, Korea)

sacrificing other fingers and also can restore sensation. However, multiple surgical steps are needed, and bone resorption progresses over time, resulting in thinning of the bone. In addition, there is the disadvantage that the reconstructed thumb is bulky.

## On-Top Plasty

If the defect on the thumb occurs with the damage of other fingers, on-top plasty can be performed using the remaining amputated index, in the form of pollicization or spare-part surgery [16]. On-top plasty is an especially good option for proximal phalanx level amputation. In patients with impaired index MP joint (metacarpophalangeal joint), if the arc of rotation of the digital artery is difficult, a method of transferring the dorsal metacarpal artery as the vascular base has been known [17]. On-top plasty using the index metacarpal results in a narrowing of the palm because the metacarpal width is reduced and then a decrease in grasping power. Therefore, this method should be used with caution in patients involved in manual labor [18].

## Distraction Osteogenesis

Distraction osteogenesis is another option when the toe-to-finger procedure is likely to be difficult or the donor toe is limited. The main advantage of using this method is to maintain native innervation. Before distraction osteogenesis, it is necessary to predict the condition of the soft tissue on the bone stump after lengthening. This procedure can extend length by about 3 cm, but at least two thirds of the metacarpal bone must remain (Fig. 20.4a).

Before the osteotomy, the pin for the distraction device should be fixed on the proximal and distal sites of metacarpal bone. Metacarpal bone through the dorsal incision should be exposed and the distraction device applied. Osteotomy is then performed on diaphysis (Fig. 20.4b). Bone lengthening could be 1 mm per day until the desired length (Fig. 20.4c). Until bone consolidation, the lengthening device should be maintained (Fig. 20.4d, e). Although ossification is rapid in children, secondary bone graft is needed if lengthening is performed quickly or in older patients. When secondary bone graft may be needed in the distraction gap, the treatment period becomes longer [19, 20]. Additional bone grafts are harvested from the iliac crest, ulna, and radius [14].

## Pollicization

It is very difficult to choose the reconstruction method of the thumb when the CMC joint (carpometacarpal joint) is damaged or amputation has occurred near the CMC joint (Fig. 20.5a).

Index pollicization is a method that can obtain the appropriate length of the new thumb and wide web space reconstruction using the index finger at the same time. In addition, index pollicization can replace new CMC joint using the index MP joint, and opposition reconstruction can be performed simultaneously in a patient with the loss of thenar muscle. For this reason, it is used in thumb reconstruction in patients with amputation at the CMC joint. In the case of children with thumb hypoplasia or aplasia, it is the choice of treatment for thumb reconstruction [21–23].

### Skin Incision

Various skin incision methods can be used. It should be designed considering the newly created first web and new position of the thumb after mobilization of the index (Fig. 20.5b, c).

After skin incision, caution should be taken in vein preservation, a critical surgical procedure.

### Soft Tissue Dissection

Through the palmar fascia, a neurovascular pedicle is dissected from the index-long finger web space to the index finger. After ligating the branch to the long finger, the common digital artery is dissected proximally. The radial side nerve of the long finger is dissected and preserved. The A1 pulley and the transverse metacarpal ligament

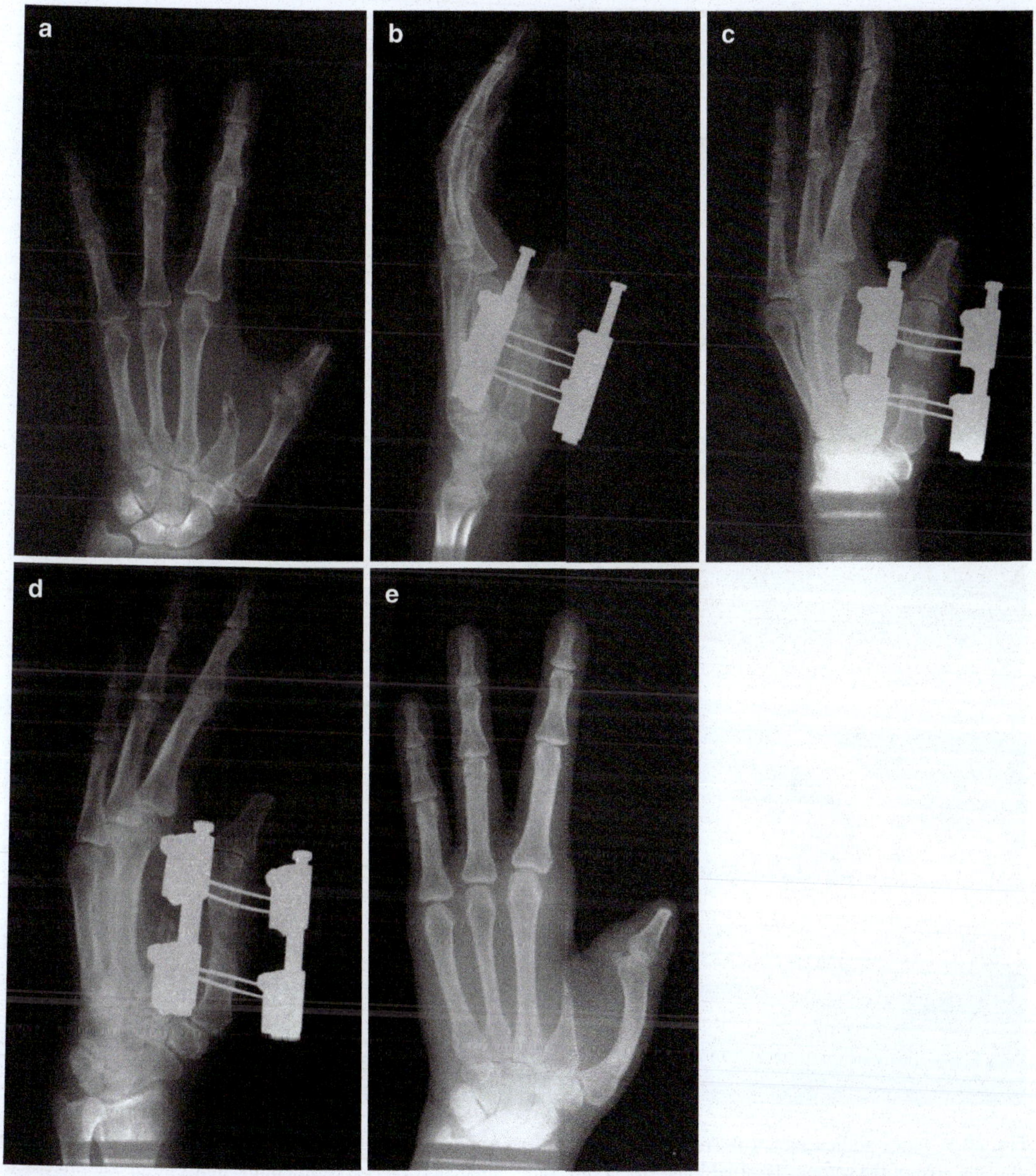


**Fig. 20.4** Distraction osteogenesis. (**a**) Traumatic thumb loss at distal area of the proximal phalanx. (**b**) Application of the thumb lengthening device (after osteotomy of the diaphysis). (**c**) 1 mm serial lengthening per day. (**d**) Periosteal bone formation on lengthening gap. (**e**) Final results (Courtesy of Dr. JS. Kim, Gwang Myung, Korea)

located below the neurovascular pedicle are identified and divided. The volar and dorsal interosseous muscles attached to the index finger are dissected and divided. The distal aponeurosis of these muscles should be left for later reinsertion and secure fixation.

## Skeletal Manipulation

After soft tissue dissection, the periosteum of the exposed metacarpal bone is stripped, and osteotomy is performed at two sites. At the distal site, transverse osteotomy is performed in the epiphysis below the metacarpal head, while

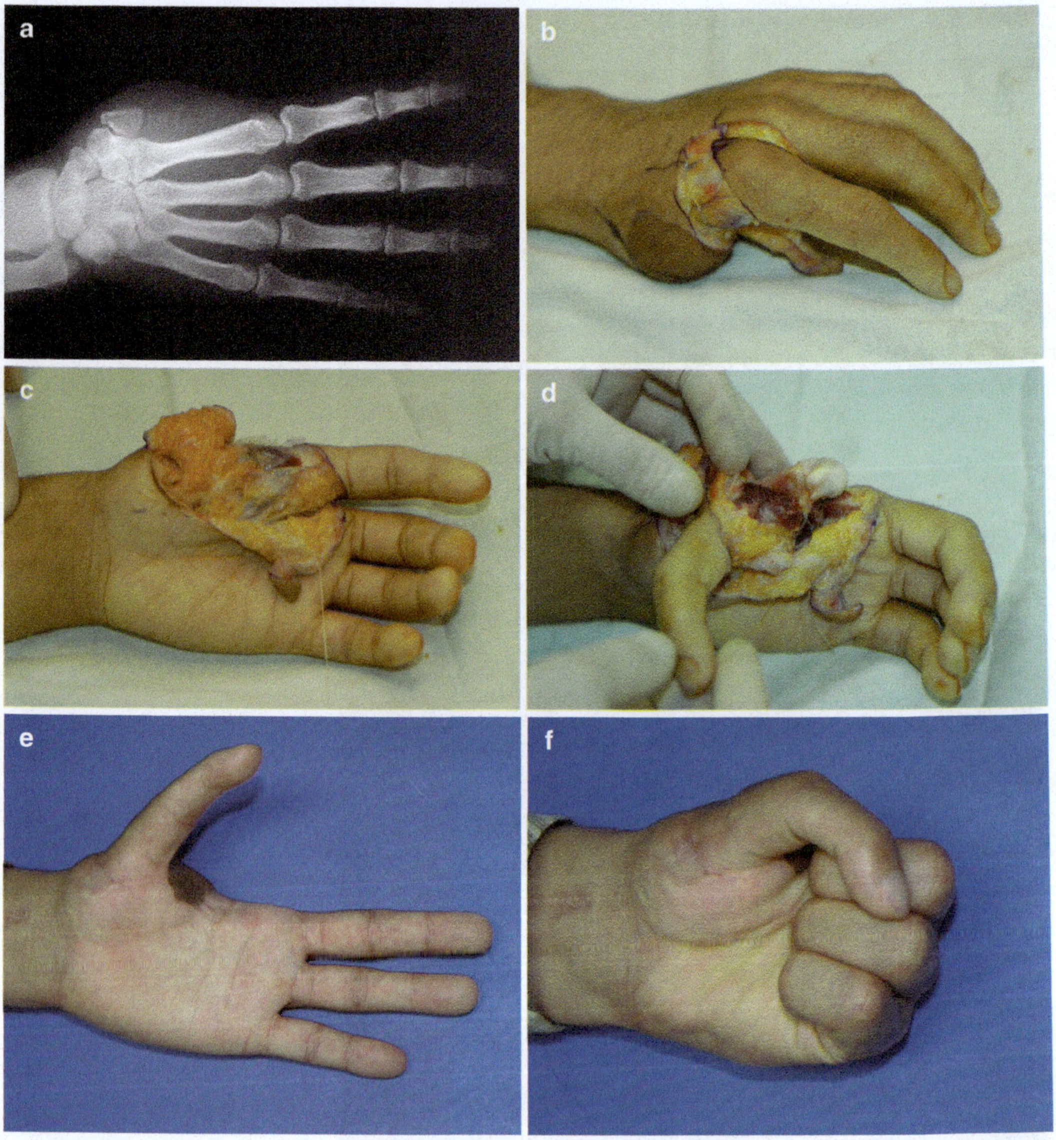


**Fig. 20.5** Index pollicization. (**a**) Traumatic amputation at distal area of the carpometacarpal joint. (**b**) Triangular skin flap on the dorsal side of the index. (**c**) Palmar side incision. (Radial side flap is placed radial side of neothumb; ulnar side flap is placed on the first web). (**d**) Angle of the neothumb: pronation 100°, flexion 35°, and abduction 25°. (**e**) Result of the index pollicization: extension (**f**) Result of the index pollicization: flextion and opposition (Courtesy of Dr. JS. Kim, Gwang Myung, Korea)

at the proximal site, dorsally oblique osteotomy is performed near the metacarpal base. It should be recorded because the same length of extensor shortening needed should match the length of the metacarpal bone removed. The distal metacarpal head is fixed at the proximal metacarpal base in the pronation position. Finally, the angle of neothumb is made to be as follows: pronation 100°, flexion 35°, and abduction 25°. Bone fixation is performed using suture or K-wire with this position maintained (Fig. 20.5d).

### Extrinsic Tendon Rebalancing

Extensor shortening is performed according to the length of skeletal shortening. After separating the extensor indicis proprius and common extensor, extensor indicis proprius replaces the function of extensor pollicis longus, and the common extensor replaces the function of abductor pollicis longus. In the case of trauma, suture should be performed using the tendons remaining in the proximal site. Flexor tendon shortening is not required in the case of hypoplastic thumb.

### Intrinsic Tendon Balancing

The first volar interosseous muscle is positioned to replace the function of adductor pollicis, and it is sutured to the lateral band of the proximal phalanx. Dorsal interosseous muscles are positioned to replace the function of abductor pollicis brevis.

### Skin Closure

Based on the location of the positioned neothumb, dorsal skin is mainly placed on the first web space. The palmar skin is placed on the radial side of neothumb. Residual tissue or adipofacial tissue may be used for thenar eminence prominence (Fig. 20.5e).

In performing index pollicization, surgeons have to consider problems in the severity of the injured index finger. The index radial side becomes a new first web space after pollicization, but if scar tissue is present due to previous damage, it is hard to cover with healthy skin flap. Also, when bare bone or critical structure after pollicization is exposed, flap is recommended over skin graft for coverage. Reverse posterior interosseous artery flap, reverse radial forearm flap, or free flap is the most commonly used.

Another problem is that, in most cases, the radial digital artery of the index finger is damaged during the index mobilization, and the ulnar digital artery alone is responsible for the arterial blood supply. Fortunately, the ulnar digital artery is the dominant artery of the index finger, so a sufficient blood supply is available. If there is a scar or vein injury to the finger dorsum, an alternative source for adequate venous drainage after finger mobilization should be planned. If volar vein is used, it should be of sufficient length together with a strip of volar skin. In case of complete loss of the thenar muscle or loss of long flexor or extensor tendon, tendon graft or tendon transfer may be needed after pollicization.

## Other Factors Affecting Selection Reconstruction Options

When the patient cannot accept the loss of a toe in toe-to-finger transfer, the surgeon is unfamiliar with microsurgical reconstruction, or it is difficult to apply microsurgery because of various other conditions, non-microsurgical reconstruction can be performed. Patient factors including age, medical comorbidities, cultural difference, and dominant hand can also affect the decision of the surgical methods. Another important factor in choosing a reconstruction method is cosmetic acceptance, whether or not nail reconstruction needs to be included. Therefore, if the patient requests nail reconstruction, it is more desirable to select the pollicization or toe-to-finger method.

## Summary

Following the development of microsurgical technique, the microreconstructive method is the best option among the various thumb reconstruction methods. However, the thumb can also be reconstructed using non-microsurgical reconstruction methods depending on the remaining length of the thumb and the condition of the basal joint (in patients who cannot accept the loss of a toe) and where microsurgical reconstruction cannot be performed.

## References

1. Del Piñal F, Pennazzato D, Urrutia E. Primary thumb reconstruction in a mutilated hand. Hand Clin. 2016;32(4):519–31.

2. Littler JW. Finger pollicization for traumatic loss. In: McCarthy J, editor. Plastic surgery: the hand, vol. 8. Philadelphia: Saunders; 1990. p. 5135–52.
3. Vedder NB, Friedrich JB. Thumb reconstruction: non-microsurgical techniques. In: Chang J, Neligan PC, editors. Plastic surgery, vol. 6. 3rd ed. Amsterdam: Elsevier; 2013. p. 282–94.
4. Wei FC, El-Gammal TA, Lin CH, Chuang CC, Chen HC, Chen SH. Metacarpal hand: classification and guidelines for microsurgical reconstruction with toe transplants. Plast Reconstr Surg. 1997;99:122–8.
5. Michon J, Merle M, Bouchon Y, Foucher G. Functional comparison between pollicization and toe-to-hand transfer for thumb reconstruction. J Reconstr Microsurg. 1984;1(2):103–10.
6. Lister G. The choice of procedure following thumb amputation. Clin Orthop Relat Res. 1985;195:45–51.
7. Campbell-Reid DA, McGrouther DA. Pollicization. In: Campbell-Reid DA, McGrouther DA, editors. Surgery of the thumb. London: Butterworths; 1986. p. 92–105.
8. Muzaffar AR, Chao JJ, Friedrich JB. Posttraumatic thumb reconstruction. Plast Reconstr Surg. 2005;116:103–22.
9. Lazar A, Abimelec P, Dumontier C. Full thickness skin graft for nail unit reconstruction. J Hand Surg Br. 2005;30(2):194–8.
10. Foucher G, Braun JB. A new island flap transfer from the dorsum of the index to the thumb. Plast Reconstr Surg. 1979;63:344–9.
11. Muyldermans T, Hielmer R. First dorsal metacarpal artery flap for thumb reconstruction; a retrospective clinical study. Strategies Trauma Limb Reconstr. 2009;4(1):27–33.
12. El-Khatib HA. Clinical experiences with extended first dorsal metacarpal artery island flap for thumb reconstruction. J Hand Surg [Am]. 1998;23:647–52.
13. Segu SS, Athavale SN, Maniunath P. Osteoplastic reconstruction for post traumatic thumb amputations around metacarpophalangeal joint. J Clin Diagn Res. 2015;9(8):11–3.
14. Matev IB. Thumb reconstruction through metacarpal bone lengthening. J Hand Surg [Am]. 1980;5(5):482–7.
15. Littler JW. Neurovascular skin island transfer in reconstructive hand surgery. Edinburgh: E&S Livingstone; 1960.
16. Bravo CJ, Horton T, Moran SL, Shin AY. Traumatized index finger pollicization for thumb reconstruction. J Hand Surg [Am]. 2008;33:257–62.
17. Pet MA, Ko JH, Vedder NB. Reconstruction of the traumatized thumb. Plast Reconstr Surg. 2014;134:1235–45.
18. Ozer K. Pollicization of the second metacarpal based on dorsal metacarpal arteries. J Hand Surg [Am]. 2016;41(9):317–21.
19. Friedrich JB, Vedder NB. Thumb Reconstruction. Clin Plast Surg. 2011;38:697–712.
20. Zimmerman R, Sailer R, Pechlaner S, Gabl M. Functional outcome with special attention to the DASH questionnaire following callus distraction and phalangization of the thumb after traumatic amputation in the middle one third. Arch Orthop Trauma Surg. 2003;123(10):521–6.
21. Amir H, Taghinia AH, Upton J. Index finger pollicization. J Hand Surg [Am]. 2011;36:333–9.
22. Graham D, Bhardwaj P, Sabapathy SR. Secondary thumb reconstruction in a mutilated hand. Hand Clin. 2016;32(4):533–47.
23. Brunelli G, Brunelli G. Reconstruction of traumatic absence of the thumb in the adult by pollicization. Hand Clin. 1992;8(1):41–5.

# 21 Microsurgical Reconstruction

Sang Hyun Woo

## Introduction

Microsurgical reconstruction with toe-to-hand transfer is the last and definitive option for the thumb resulting from traumatic amputations, congenital anomalies, or tumor ablation. In 1966, Buncke et al. successfully performed toe-to-thumb transfer on a rhesus monkey, proving the feasibility of this procedure in primates [1]. Since the first toe-to-thumb procedures were performed by Cobbett in 1967 [2], toe transplantation for thumbs has been established as the gold standard in replacing mutilated or unreplantable thumbs. The purposes of the toe-to-thumb transfer are restoration of the basic hand function in pinch or grasp, improving hand function in strength or length, providing more acceptable cosmesis, and facilitating wound coverage in acute defect. Toe-to-hand transfer frequently causes patients significant psychological stress as it requires prolonged anesthesia, and the patient may see the operation as the loss of a toe rather than the saving of a thumb. The operation is also stressful to surgeons as it demands a high level of microsurgical skill to yield aesthetically and functionally acceptable thumbs.

When thumb defects are to be reconstructed, sensation, stability, adequate length, and cosmesis of the thumb must be carefully considered and the most appropriate donor site chosen, in order to obtain the best functional and aesthetic results. Using the great toe and its adjacent structures as the donor is ideal because they have the best anatomical similarity to the thumb [3]. Currently, efforts are directed toward minimizing the morbidity at the donor site while improving the functional and aesthetic results in the reconstructed thumb [4, 5]. The reconstructive surgeon wishing to replace missing absent thumbs with toes now has a wide range of options for selection in order to achieve optimum results. This chapter outlines the current experience of toe-to-thumb transplantations, drawing from our experience of more than 300 cases over a 20-year period at W Hospital in Korea.

## Indications

There are three big major categories of thumb loss: congenital absence, defect after malignant tumor resection, and loss due to trauma. Regarding congenital total absence of the thumb, most hand surgeons still consider pollicization to be the best option [6]. The indications for toe transfers for congenital deformities of the thumb continue to evolve as surgeons become more comfortable with microsurgical techniques in young children. In general, toe-to-thumb transfer has been performed for congenital absence of the thumb, transverse arrest, longitudinal deficiency, congenital constriction ring syndrome, and symbrachydactyly [7]. The recommended age of the child at the time of operation is around 24 months. Partial defect or inadequate thumb can be reconstructed with partial great toe transfer at any age (Fig. 21.1).

S. H. Woo (✉)
W Institute for Hand and Reconstructive Microsurgery, W Hospital, Daegu, South Korea


S. H. Woo (ed.), *The Thumb*, https://doi.org/10.1007/978-981-10-4400-7_21

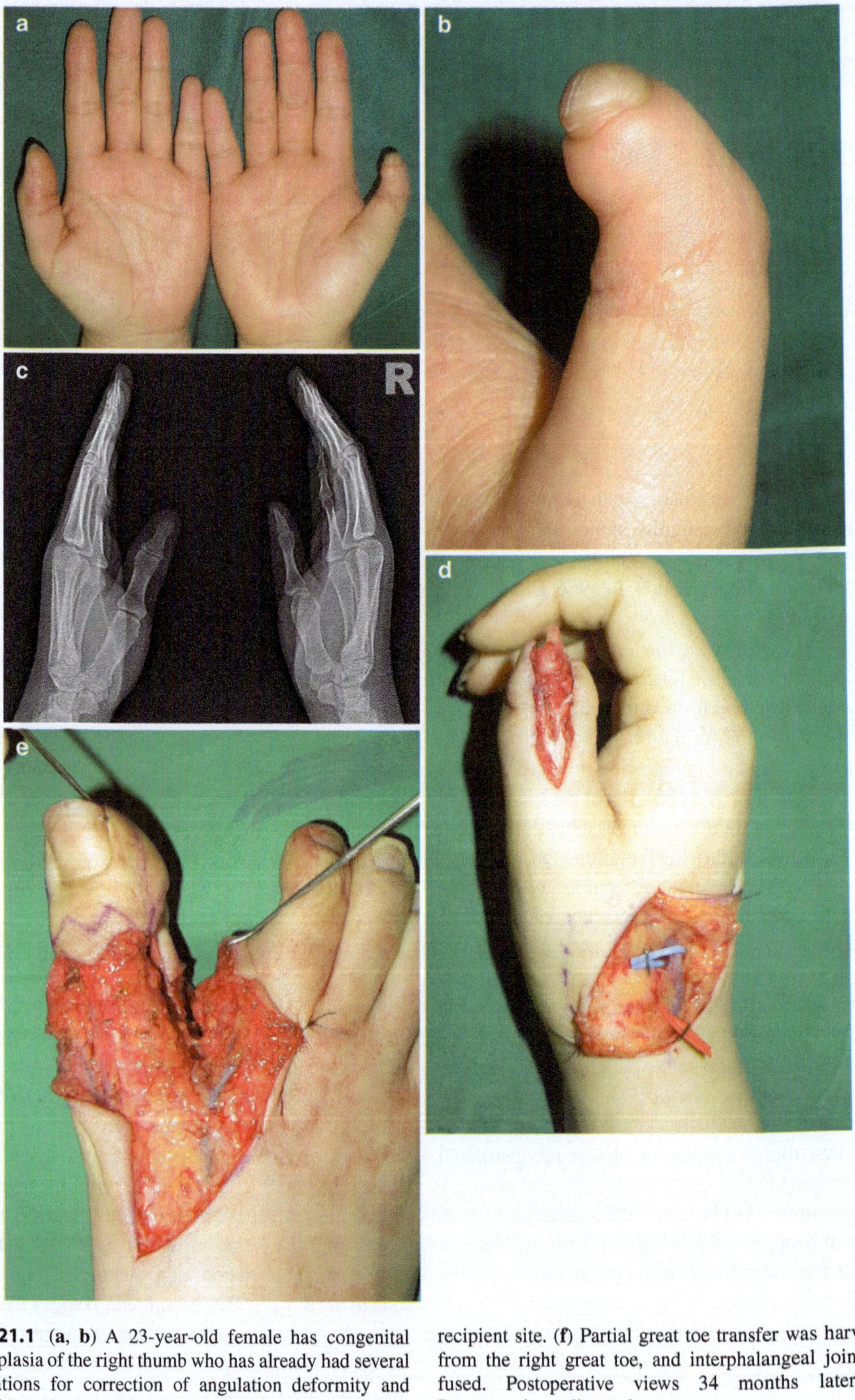


**Fig. 21.1** (**a**, **b**) A 23-year-old female has congenital hypoplasia of the right thumb who has already had several operations for correction of angulation deformity and atrophic pulp and small nail. (**c**) Preoperative radiograph of the both thumb. (**d**, **e**) Intraoperative view of donor and recipient site. (**f**) Partial great toe transfer was harvested from the right great toe, and interphalangeal joint was fused. Postoperative views 34 months later. (**g**) Postoperative radiograph

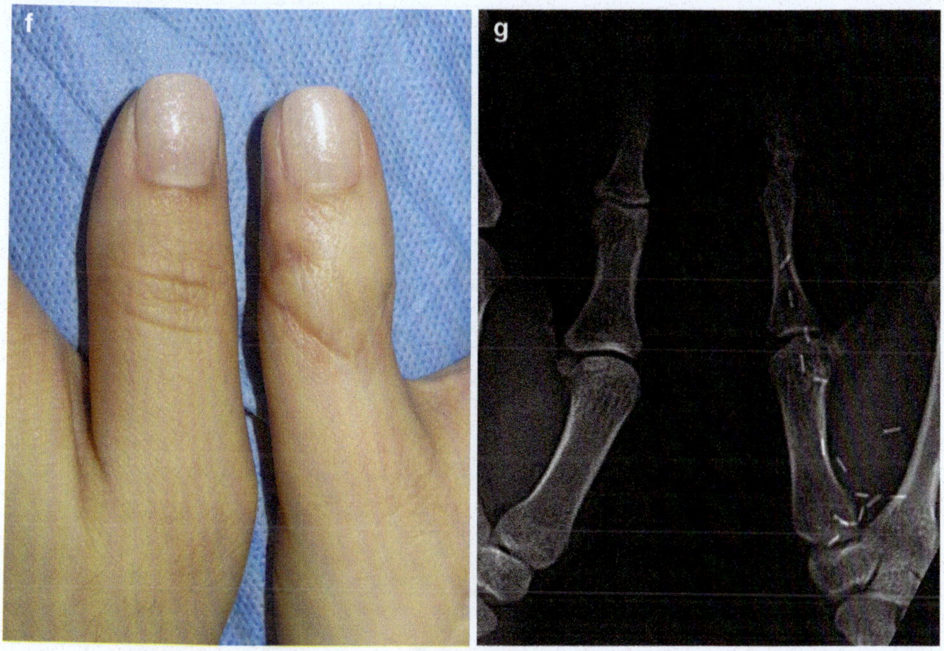

**Fig. 21.1** (continued)

In reconstruction of the thumb after malignant tumor resection, timing of the reconstruction always continues to be debated. Traditionally, reconstruction is deferred until all potential risk for tumor recurrence has passed and there is no evidence of tumor recurrence. In late reconstruction, this leaves patients functionally debilitated from several months to several years. Nguyen et al. [8] recommended that conservative resection is warranted because resection level does not influence outcome when histologically free margins are obtained. Most tumor recurrences are distant metastases rather than a local recurrence, and the elapsed time to recurrence is often long. Immediate great toe-to-thumb transfer may be considered after an adequate oncologic resection of aggressive benign or malignant tumors [9]. For those who are hesitant to proceed with reconstruction without confirmation of negative final pathology, consideration might be given to dressing the wound for a few days before reconstruction until final pathology is obtained (Fig. 21.2).

Traumatic loss of the thumb can result from a wide variety of injury mechanisms, including industrial, nonindustrial, and environmental factors. This type of traumatic loss is the most common indication for microsurgical thumb reconstruction. There are still modifying operative techniques to improve functional and aesthetic results of the new thumb and to decrease morbidity of the donor site. We modified amputation level according to Morrison et al. [10] This chapter mainly focused on a logical approach to microvascular reconstruction of the thumb after traumatic loss according to the amputation level (Figs. 21.3 and 21.4).

## Preoperative Considerations

When the patient with amputation or composite defect of the thumb arrives at the emergency room, thumb reconstruction strategy should be established by an experienced surgeon. According to the financial and physical conditions of the patient and contamination of the wound, timing of definitive reconstruction should be decided. In case of delayed or elective reconstruction, adequate or even some redundant skin cover over the

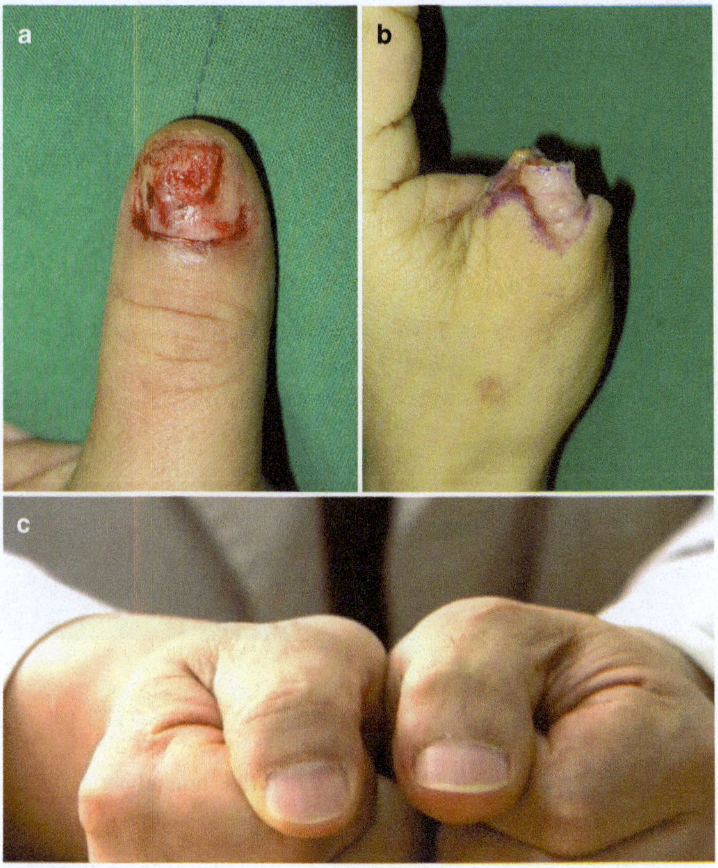


**Fig. 21.2** (**a**, **b**) A 48-year-old male has subungual melanoma of the left thumb. The patient, a cardiothoracic surgeon, wants to have immediate reconstruction after tumor resection. There was no sign or symptoms of local or distant metastasis. To prevent recurrence, amputation at the mid-shaft level of the thumb and great toe transfer was dome. (**c**) After 10 years postoperation, sensory and range of motion of the thumb are almost normal without any secondary operation

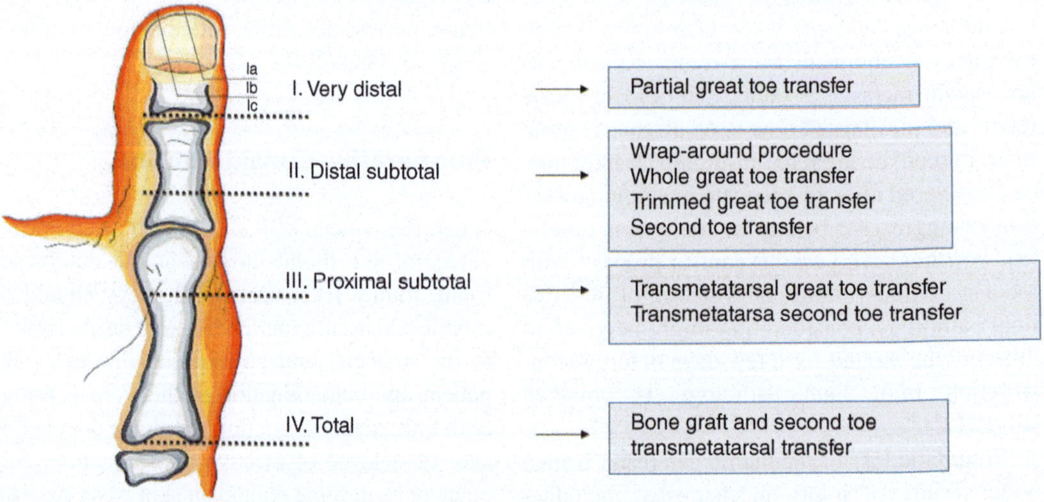


**Fig. 21.3** Reconstructive options according to amputation level of the thumb

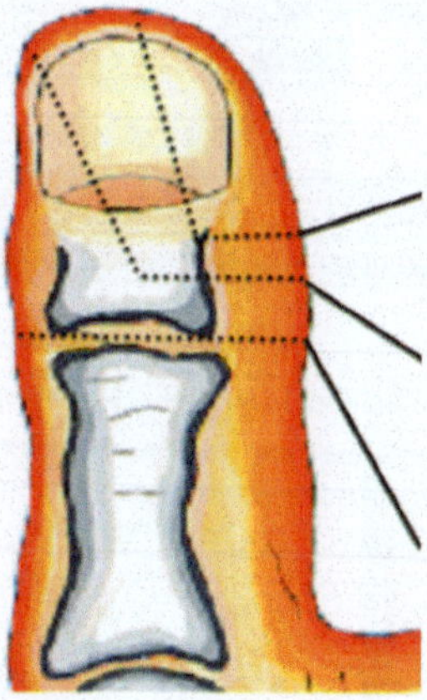


**Fig. 21.4** Reconstructive options according to very distal amputation of the thumb

stump of the hand is required. Immediate pedicled groin flap can cover the lateral aspect of transplanted toes, protect the pedicle, or form a web space in the hand. It also allows less skin to be harvested from the foot, allowing direct closure of the donor site (Fig. 21.5).

The treatment of patients with thumb loss requires careful evaluation of the problem and the patient, sound judgment in regard to the treatment plan, and excellent surgical technique to secure a favorable outcome. The patient should be an appropriate candidate for microvascular thumb reconstruction because this procedure requires significant physical demands for prolonged anesthesia on the patient and needs intensive postoperative care and rehabilitation. Careful consideration must be given to the patient's past medical history as well as psychological problems. The patient should not have been smoking in the month prior to operation, and a urine nicotine level can be checked within 24 h of surgery.

One of the most challenging obstacles to success of toe transfer is the great amount of anatomical variations of the FDMA (Fig. 21.6a) [11]. The study of color Doppler imaging can be used to quantitatively measure the intravascular blood flow and anatomical location of the FDMA (Fig. 21.6b). The incidence superficial to first dorsal interosseous muscle is about 50, 40% or less of intramuscular, and less than 10% of first plantar metatarsal artery dominant [12, 13]. The recent study by Hou et al. [14] newly classified the anatomical pattern of the FDMA, and the most common type is found in the space between the dorsal interosseous muscle and the first metatarsal bone. Because color Doppler imaging is noninvasive, convenient, safe, and cheap, preoperative angiography is no longer a routine procedure, only being recommended where patients had a medical history of, or physical examination results suggesting, lower-extremity peripheral vascular disease, were older than 50 years of age, or were known to suffer cardiovascular disease. If a surgeon knows the anatomical variation of the FDMA preoperatively, dissection time may be shortened. If the artery is dominant at the plantar side, dissection should start from the first web space to the plantar side (Fig. 21.6c).

Preoperative hand function must be considered to determine what functional needs the transferred toe has to supply. Key and tip pinch strength and strength of grasp are measured with appropriate instrumentation. Thumb range of motion including flexion, extension, opposition, and both palmar and radial abduction and adduction must be assessed. Sensibility can be assessed by subjective measurement of light touch and two-point discrimination and by Semmes-Weinstein monofilament testing.

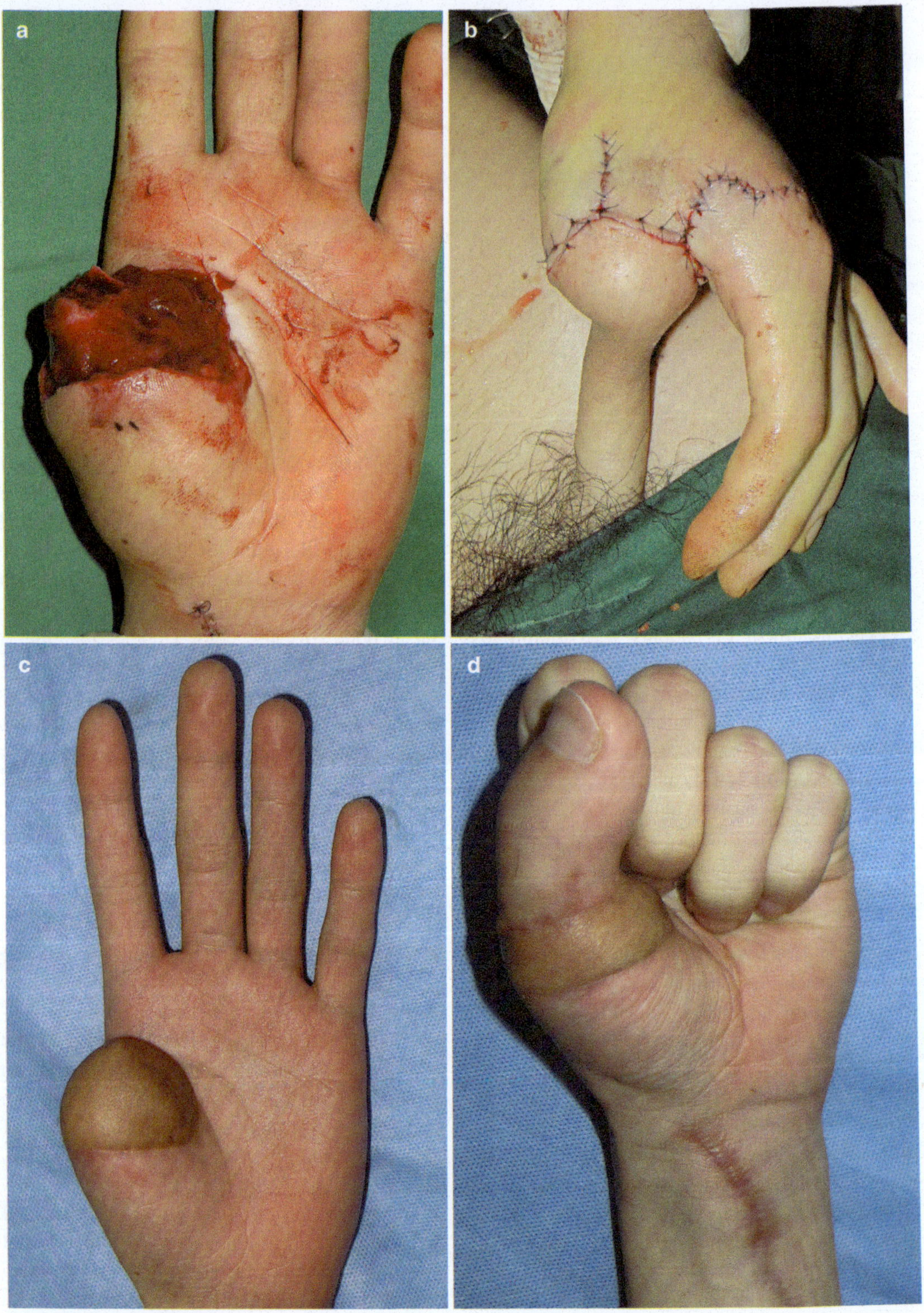


**Fig. 21.5** (**a**) A 34-year-old male has complete amputation and crushing injury by press machine. (**b**) Pedicled groin flap covered open wound of the thumb and the first web space. (**c–e**) After 6 months later, great toe transfer was performed

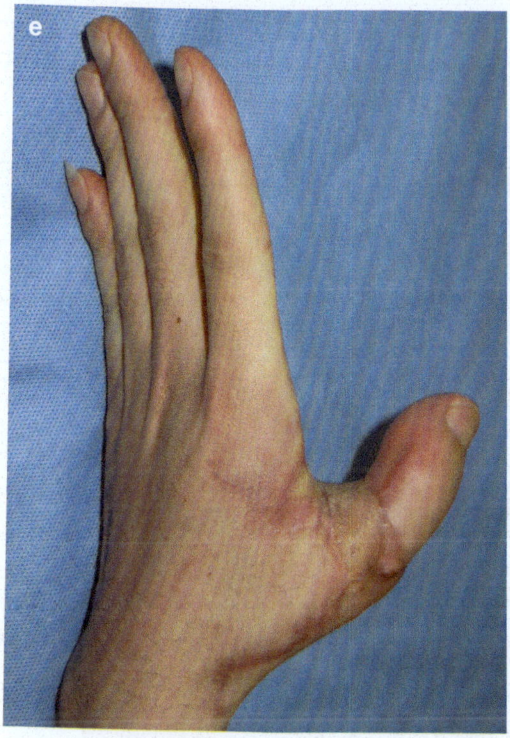


**Fig. 21.5** (continued)

## Reconstruction According to Amputation Level

### Level I. Reconstruction at Very Distal Defects Distal to or at IP Joint

The distal part of the thumb is composed of the nail bed and plate with adjacent dorsal skin, pulp, and distal phalangeal bone, and reconstruction of composite defects of the distal thumb to its original function and appearance is very challenging. This level of amputation does not cause any disability or functional impairment, and some patients may not feel the necessity for reconstruction, depending on their lifestyle, customs, or cultural background. However, in patients with a high demand for better aesthetic appearance and a more refined function of the thumb, a procedure to make the thumb as natural as possible is needed. The amputation level of the distal thumb can be subdivided into three levels (Fig. 21.4).

#### Operative Procedure

Dissection of the distal part of the great toe is very tedious because the pulp tissue should be freed from the distal phalangeal bone for trimming of its tip. Also, it is difficult to dissect the slender digital artery distal to the IP joint of the great toe. Thus, in most cases, a larger skin flap with a V-shaped lateral pulp area is harvested. Using a retrograde approach [15] on the first web space of the foot, a composite flap pedicled on the FDMA or dorsal digital artery is harvested. The artery is skeletonized by a radical resection of adventitia, and the vein is dissected with the perivenous tissues. Digital nerves of the great toe are also harvested to coapt with the corresponding structures of the thumb. The composite flap always includes a partial distal phalangeal bone whether the distal phalangeal bone of the recipient site had a bone defect or not. The venous network on the medial aspect of the great toe is more reliable than the first web space. There is usually a prominent branch of the great saphenous vein proximal to the medial nail fold on the tibial aspect of the great toe (Fig. 21.7a). This vein should be included in the flap to prevent necrosis of the remnant skin flap. On the dorsum of the great toe, the subdermal venous plexus should be preserved to close the donor site. In most cases, the donor site is repaired primarily without tension. Sometimes, a cross-toe flap or skin graft from the plantar aspect is performed to resurface the donor defect in cases of failed primary repair.

After fixation of the harvested toe flap to the distal phalangeal bone of the thumb using Kirschner wires, key skin sutures are placed. In addition, a temporary Kirschner wire is used to block joint motion, promote bone fusion, and provide stability, preventing kinking of anastomosed vessels.

In cases of partial nail bed transfer, meticulous repair of the nail beds between the great toe and the thumb is performed using 6-0 Vicryl or chromic catgut suture, and an artificial nail plate or extracted nail is placed over the repaired nail bed for compression and protection. Secure repair of the nail bed between the great toe and thumb is essential to prevent nail fold deformities like

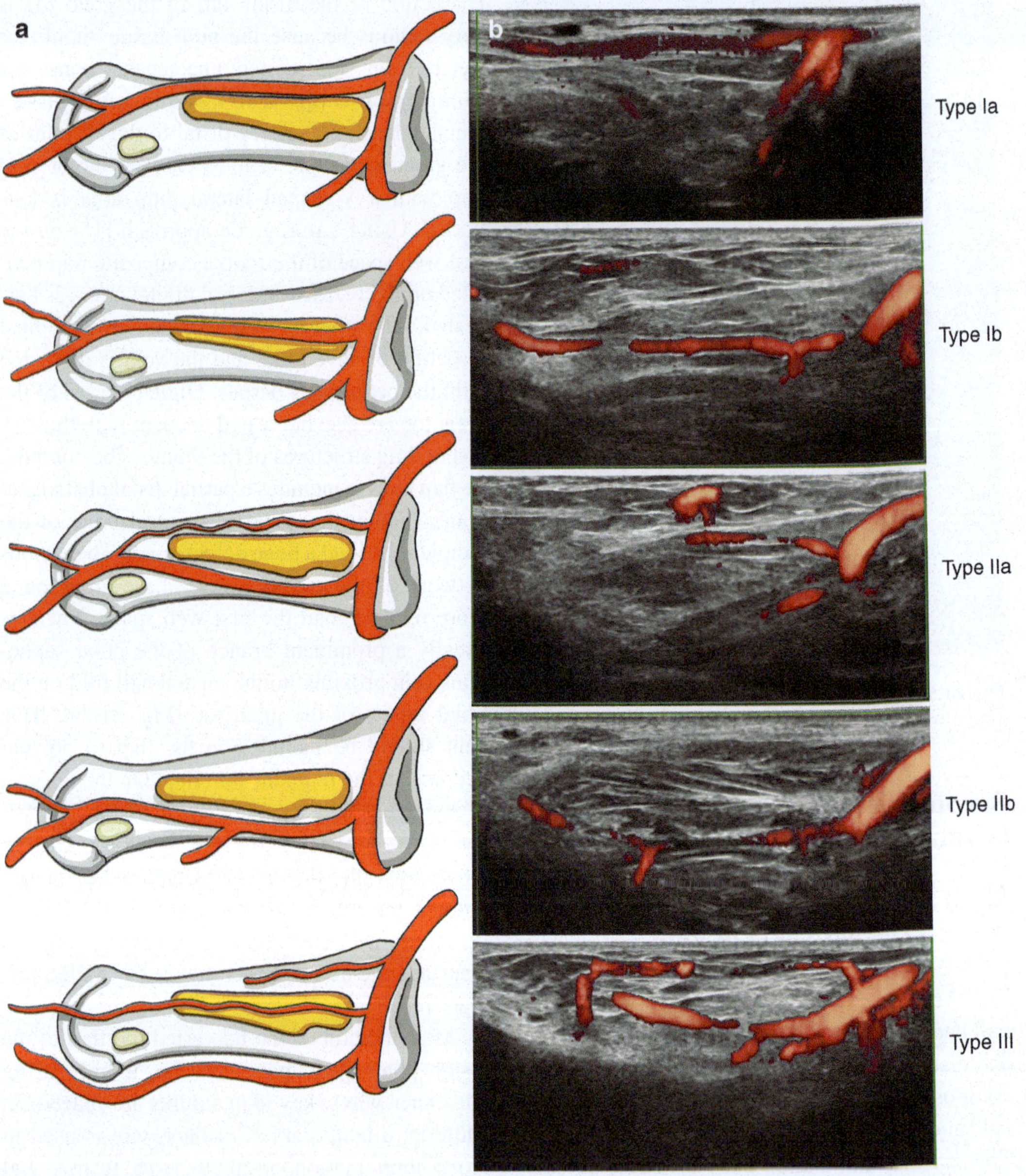


**Fig. 21.6** (**a**) Anatomical variation of the first dorsal metatarsal artery (red) in relation with the interosseous muscle (yellow) and intermetatarsal ligament (beige) on the metatarsal bone (gray) based on Gilbert's classification. (**b**) A power Doppler ultrasonography with longitudinal scan at foot dorsum checked by Medison RS80A (Samsung, Korea). (**c**) Intraoperative dissection shows dominant artery at the first web space through the retrograde approach. Dorsal approach is preferable in type I, which is superficial to the muscle. (**d**) In type II, dominant first plantar metatarsal artery needs plantar approach

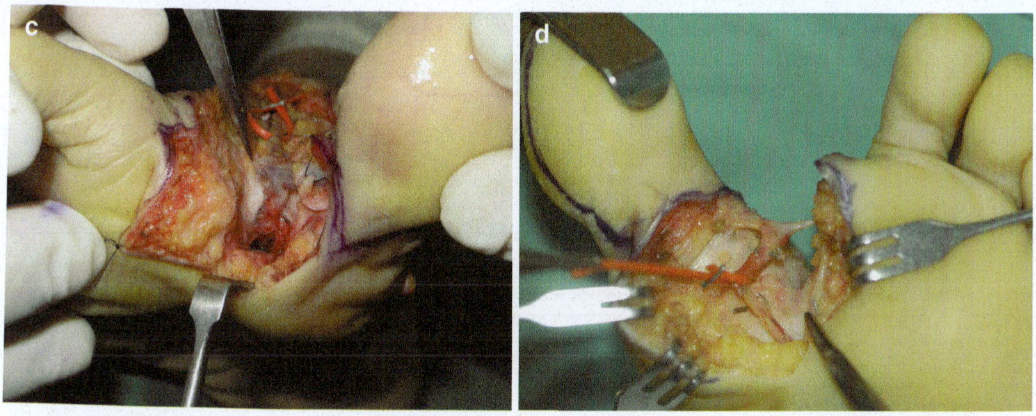


**Fig. 21.6** (continued)

splitting or ridge formation. Even if the nail defect is vertical or straight, it should be converted into an oblique one. Afterward, the nail bed repair is performed from the eponychium proximally through an extended incision upon it. Smooth, normal-appearing nail growth might be induced by the tight compression of the artificial nail on the repaired nail bed.

Arterial anastomosis is performed with the ulnar digital artery at the proximal phalanx, princeps pollicis artery, dorsalis pollicis artery at the first web space, or superficial radial artery at the anatomical snuffbox, depending on the strength of the pulsation of the recipient artery of the hand. When the arterial anastomosis is performed at the anatomical snuffbox, a subcutaneous tunnel is made by intraoperative expansion with a Nelaton catheter or silastic drain between two incisions for passage of the vascular pedicle (Fig. 21.7b). This helps avoid the scarring caused by a long incision and the necessity to perform a skin graft on the reconstructed thumb. Venous anastomosis is performed with a superficial vein at the dorsal aspect of the thumb.

The purpose of very distal thumb reconstruction with toe transfer is more focused on cosmesis than on functional restoration. To reduce the postoperative scar on the new reconstructed thumb, short or relatively long dissection is better than long dissection of neurovascular pedicles. It avoids the long surgical time required for dissection of a lengthy vascular pedicle. However, anastomosis of vessels less than 0.8 mm in diameter is not reliable to guarantee sufficient arterial supply. In cases of dissection of the long vascular pedicle, if the vessels are not passed through the subcutaneous tunnel, a long linear scar or a skin graft on the reconstructed hand is inevitable. Therefore, a moderately long vascular pedicle is good for anastomosis of the vessels at the first web space of the thumb (Fig. 21.7c).

## Postoperative Management and Secondary Procedures

Intensive postoperative monitoring of the perfusion of the transferred toe and anticoagulation therapy with heparin, aspirin, and prostaglandin E1 is performed for 5–7 days. After removal of the temporary Kirschner wire used to block joint motion on the 14th day after operation, passive motion of the finger is begun. From the third week after the operation, rehabilitation therapy is started for restoration of sensation, and Coban (3M, St. Paul, Minn.) taping is applied to decrease edema of the transferred toe. At seventh to eighth week after the operation, the remaining Kirschner wires are removed. Secondary procedures such as pulp plasty, nail fold plasty, or scar revision can be carried out 3–6 months after surgery.

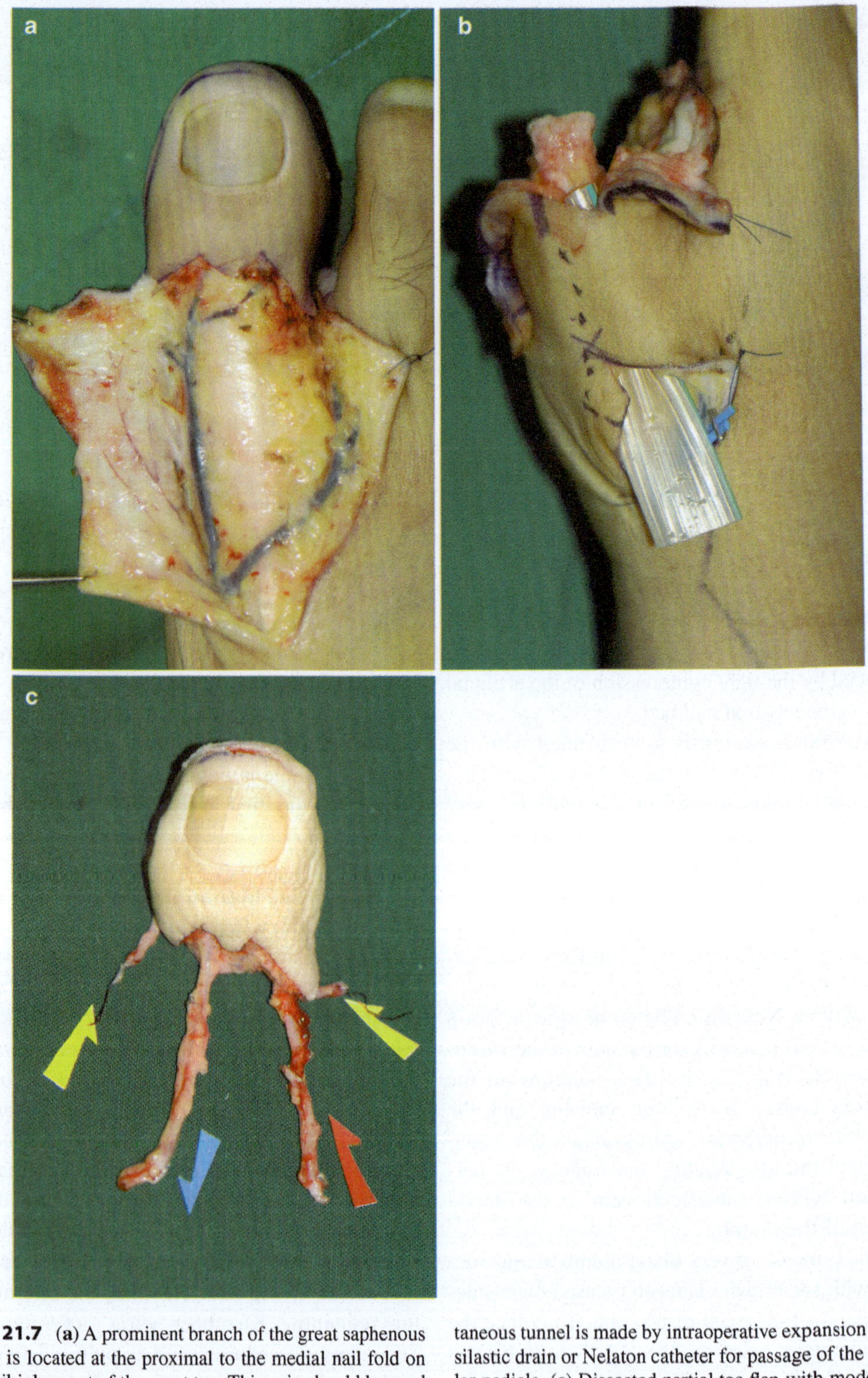


**Fig. 21.7** (**a**) A prominent branch of the great saphenous vein is located at the proximal to the medial nail fold on the tibial aspect of the great toe. This vein should be used for vein anastomosis. On the dorsum of the great toe, the subdermal venous plexus should be preserved in the dissected skin flap. (**b**) To avoid a long incision scar, a subcutaneous tunnel is made by intraoperative expansion with a silastic drain or Nelaton catheter for passage of the vascular pedicle. (**c**) Dissected partial toe flap with moderately long vascular pedicles. Yellow arrows show both digital nerves, the blue arrow points to superficial vein, and the red arrow points to first dorsal metatarsal artery

## Reconstruction Options of the Very Distal Amputation of the Thumb

Amputation of level Ia has defect of the pulp, partial nail bed, and dorsal skin involving less than 60% of the nail width, irrespective of a distal phalangeal bone fracture or defect. It is reconstructed with an osteo-onychocutaneous flap with a partial toenail from the great toe. The distal phalangeal bone under the nail bed is always included in the flap (Fig. 21.8).

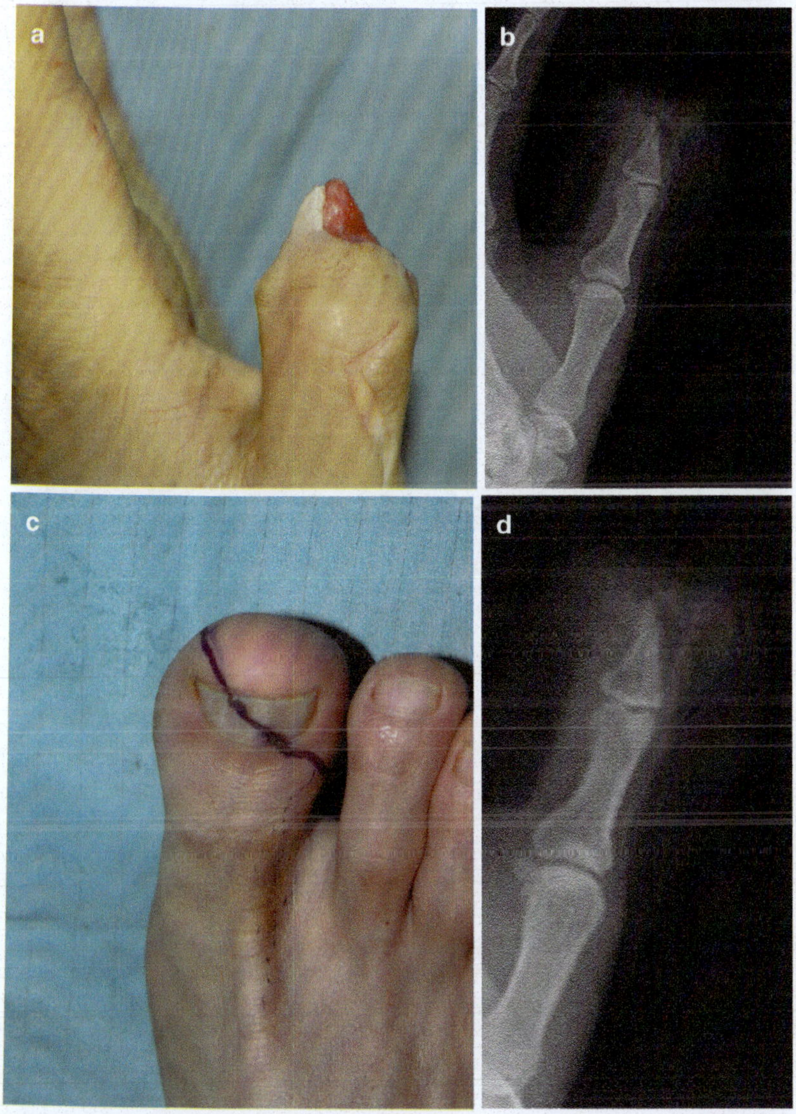


**Fig. 21.8** (**a, b**) Thumb defect at the level Ia has proximal part of the distal phalangeal bone and less than 60% defect of the nail bed. Remnant nail bed of the thumb is obliquely debrided. (**c, d**) Osteo-onychocutaneous flap is harvested from the great toe. (**e, f**) Immediate postoperation. After meticulous nail bed repair, nail plate is reinserted. Two K-wire is used to fix the distal phalangeal bone. (**g, h**) Postoperative view of the new thumb. I. Postoperative radiograph of the new thumb. J. Donor site of the left foot

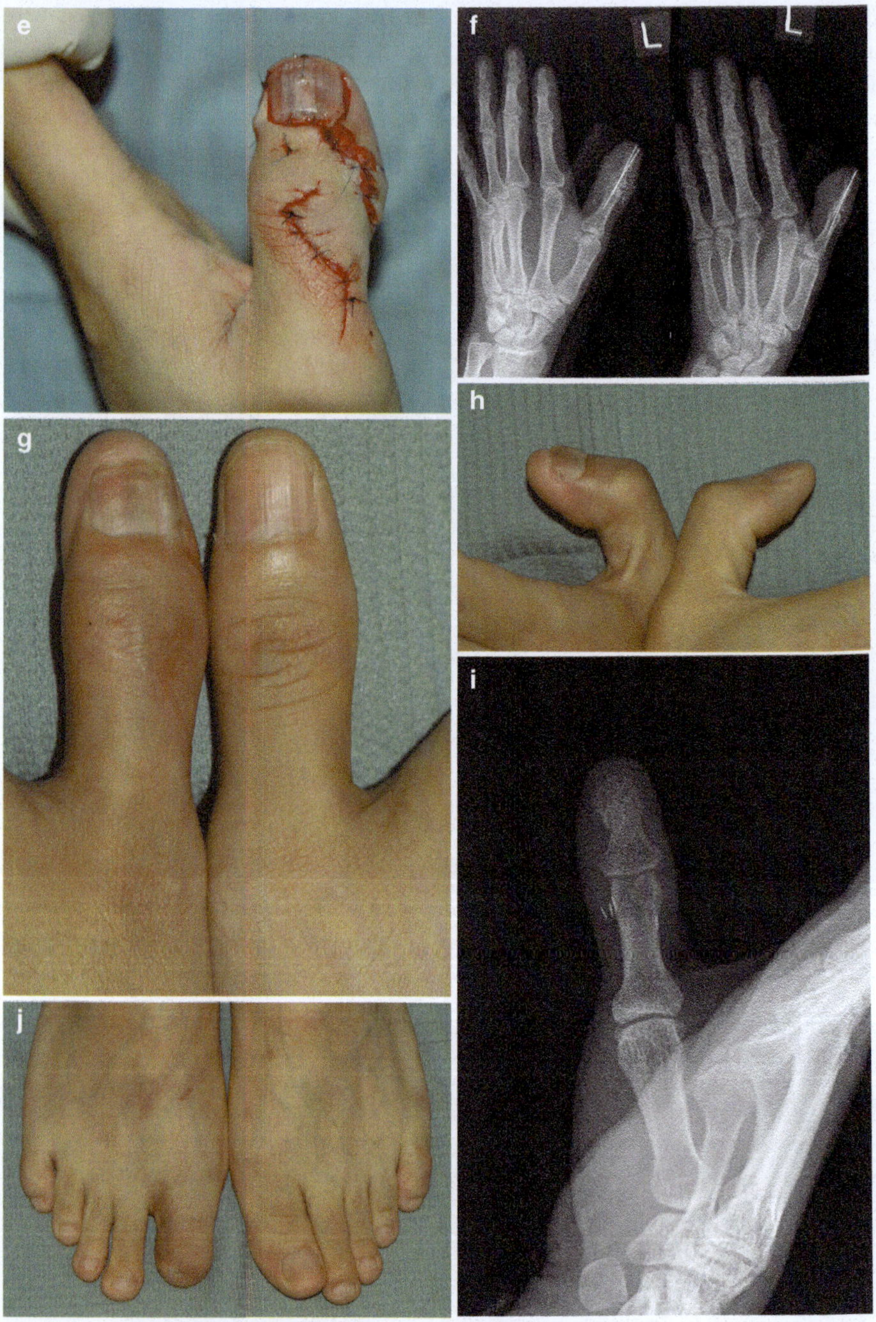


**Fig. 21.8** (continued)

In level Ib, an osteo-onychocutaneous flap with a whole toenail from the great toe is used to reconstruct nail bed defects involving more than 60% of the width. The IP joint of the thumb is preserved, and distal phalangeal bone of the toe should be fixed to the remnant of distal phalangeal bone of the thumb. After bone union of the distal phalangeal bone between toe and thumb, motion of the IP joint is almost possible (Fig. 21.9). A partial great toe transfer with an arthrodesis of the IP joint can be performed to reconstruct defects caused by amputation at the level of the IP joint in level III. In

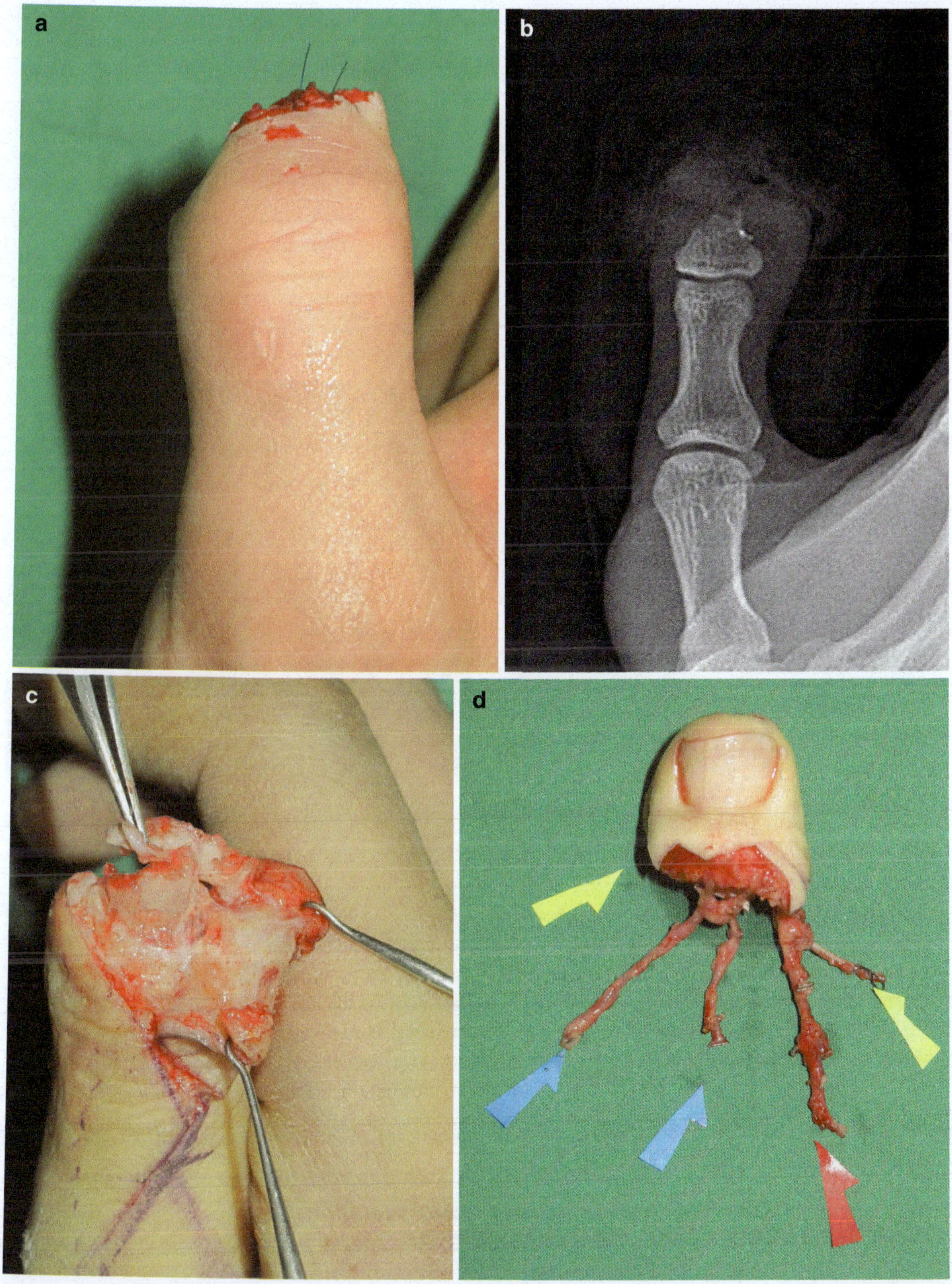

**Fig. 21.9** (**a**, **b**) Thumb defect at the level Ib has proximal part of the distal phalangeal bone and more than 60% defect of the nail bed. (**c**) Remnant nail bed is thoroughly removed to prevent nail growth from the thumb. (**d**) Partial great toe with whole nail is harvest at the distal phalangeal bone. (**e**, **f**) Postoperative view of the new thumb and range of motion of the interphalangeal joint. G. Postoperative radiograph of the thumb

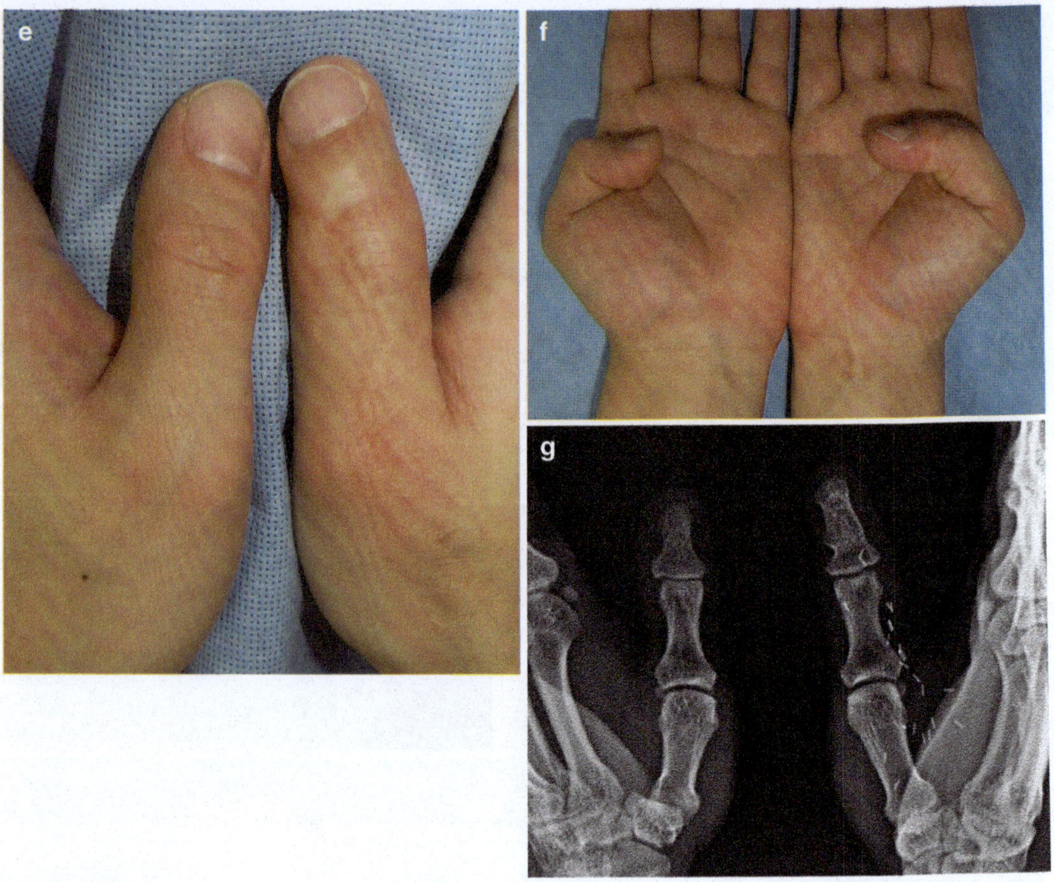


**Fig. 21.9** (continued)

cases where the difference of nail width between the thumb and the great toe is more than 3 mm, the great toe partial-nail-preserving transfer technique is useful [16].

In level Ic, there are various methods of great toe-to-hand transfer to restore the IP joint that play a critical role in key pinch and vice grip for larger objects [17]. The mini wraparound flap can be harvested from the great toe with arthrodesis of the IP joint [18]. Using a similar technique, key pinch and power grip can be achieved approximately 60–66% and 57% of the contralateral side, respectively [16]. With activities of daily life, the patients' complaint is not serious. Therefore, for the reconstruction of distal thumb defects at the IP joint with the intact MCP joint and carpometacarpal joint of the thumb, a simple procedure of arthrodesis at the IP joint is recommended over a complex design or difficult dissection involving both the great toe and the second toe (Fig. 21.10). Primary closure of the great toe with a medial skin flap from the remnant great toe is more acceptable after disarticulation at the IP joint to minimize the morbidity of the donor site.

## Level II. Reconstruction at Distal Subtotal Defect

In distal subtotal losses of the thumb where MCP joint function is still functioning, variable great toe transfer taken distal to the MTP joint is recommended. According to the Buncke's description [17], great toes make great thumbs. In cases of amputation at the proximal phalanx with an intact MTP joint, whole great toe transfer is one of the most acceptable indications. Compared with second toe transfer, it can provide a broad contact area of pulp with a strong grip and pinch power as well as optimal mobility. Donor site morbidity in function and appearance is the main pitfall.

The whole great toe can be transferred when the difference in nail width between the thumb and the great toe is less than 2–3 mm, in patients whose great toe is similar in size to the thumb (Fig. 21.11).

The modified wraparound flap [19] includes the skin, nail and nail bed, pulp, and part of the distal phalangeal bone from the great toe as well as a tri-cortical bone graft from the iliac crest. Neurovascular pedicle is based on the first dorsal metatarsal artery or dorsalis pedis artery, dorsal venous system, plantar digital nerves, and deep or superficial peroneal nerves. This technique is

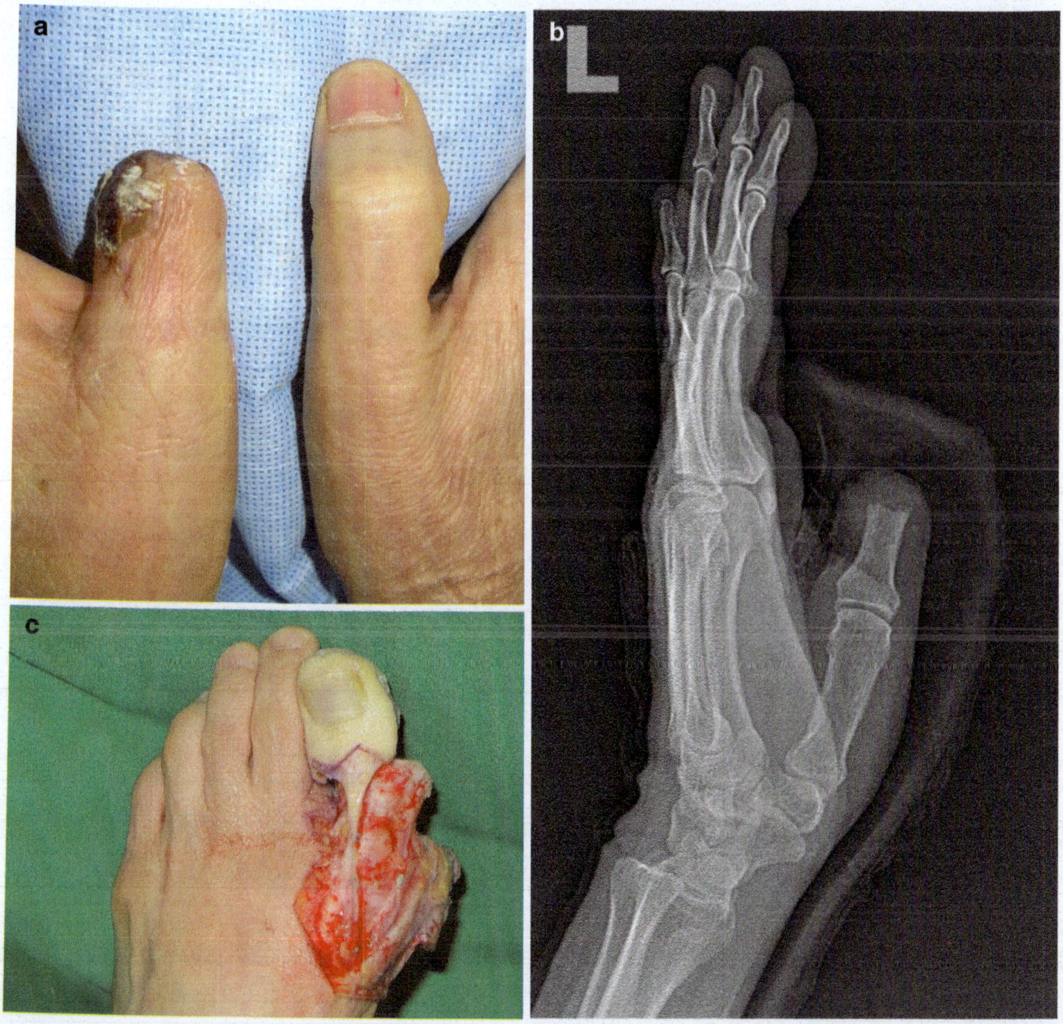


**Fig. 21.10** (**a**, **b**) Preoperative view of partial necrosis of the left thumb after crushing amputation. (**c**) Before division of the vascular pedicle, arterial perfusion of the dissected toe was not enough. (**d**) One day later, the color of the great toe was changed to pink very slowly. (**e**) Immediate after operation of partial great toe transfer with interphalangeal joint arthrodesis with 3 K-wire fixation. (**f**, **g**) Ten years postoperation. (**h**) Postoperative radiograph of the thumb

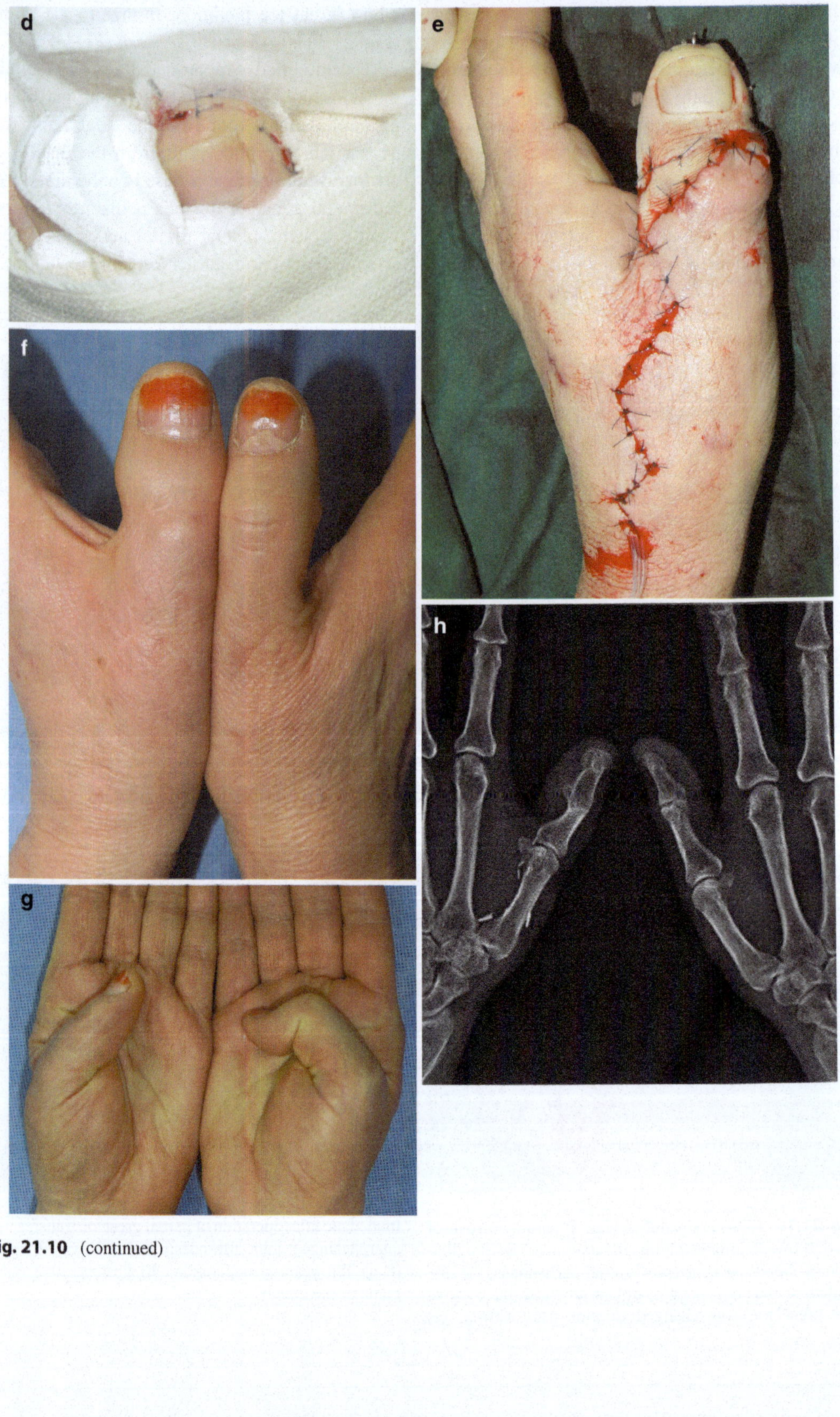


**Fig. 21.10** (continued)

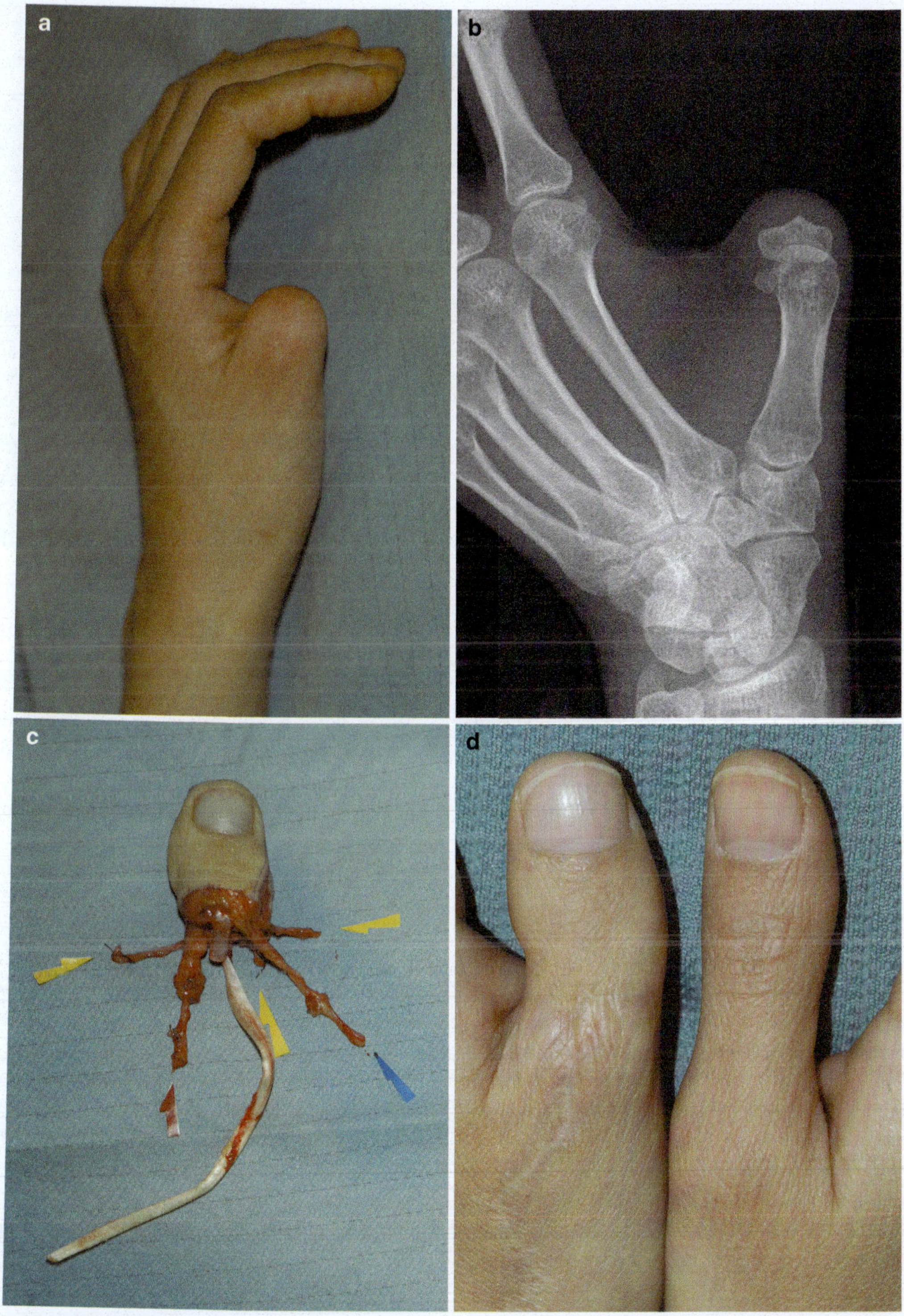

**Fig. 21.11** Whole great toe-to-thumb transfer. (**a**, **b**) Previous amputation of the thumb at the base of the proximal phalanx. (**c**) The whole great toe is harvested with a long flexor hallucis longus tendon from the mid-plantar area. Flexor pollicis longus tendon is repaired with flexor tendon of the great toe at wrist. (**d–f**) Clinical and radiographic results

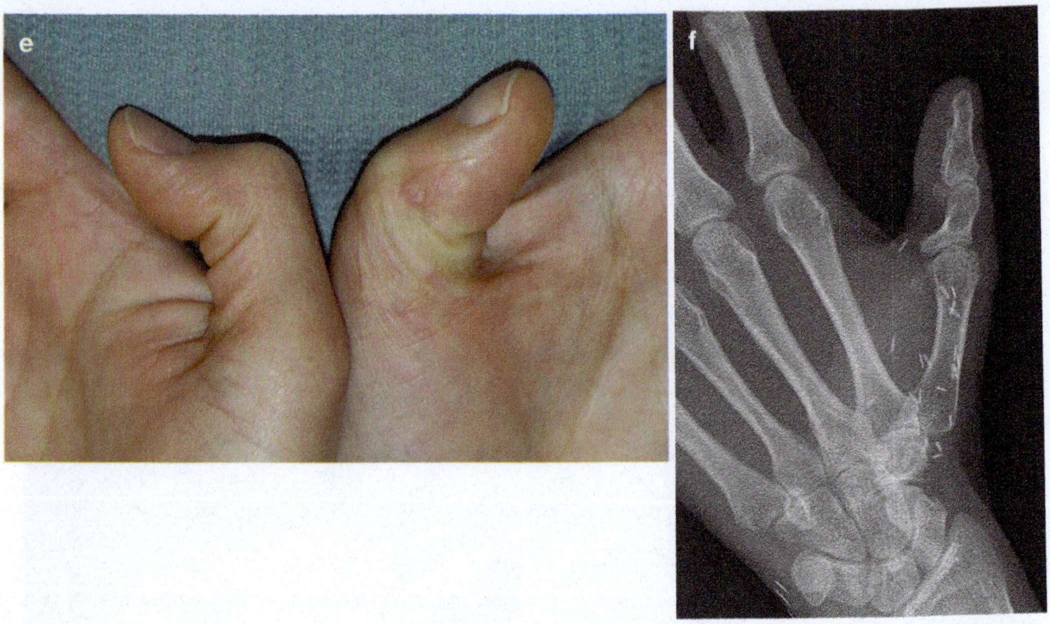


**Fig. 21.11** (continued)

most suitable for resurfacing the thumb with complete skin avulsion injuries but intact bone and tendons (Fig. 21.12). The main advantage of this flap is its well-matched size in relation to the contralateral normal thumb and a reduced morbidity at the donor site. A reconstructed thumb may have a limited range of motion, and a resorption of the bone graft may occur. The donor site needs to cover the defect with a cross-toe flap, arterialized venous flap, or dorsalis pedis free flap. A new modification technique of the wrap-around flap that preserves a plantar triangular flap of the great toe shows an excellent contour and functional outcome of the new thumb and reduced donor site morbidity [20, 21]. However, wrap-around flap is not useful for thumb reconstruction in children because of the lack of potential for growth.

When there is big difference in volume and nail width between the thumb and the great toe, trimmed great toe transfer is another modification. This technique includes a reduction of both the bony and soft tissues on the medial aspect of the great toe to create a more natural-looking thumb [22, 23]. To reduce the bony structure, a longitudinal osteotomy needs to be performed on the medial aspect of the distal and proximal phalangeal bone. The periosteum and medial collateral ligament of the IP joint of the great toe are harvested as is the proximally based flap. The stability of the new IP joint can be achieved by a simple repair of the periosteum, medial collateral ligament, and joint capsule. In exchange for a better cosmetic appearance, there is some loss of IP joint motion. The proximal remaining strip of the medial skin flap can be used to help close the

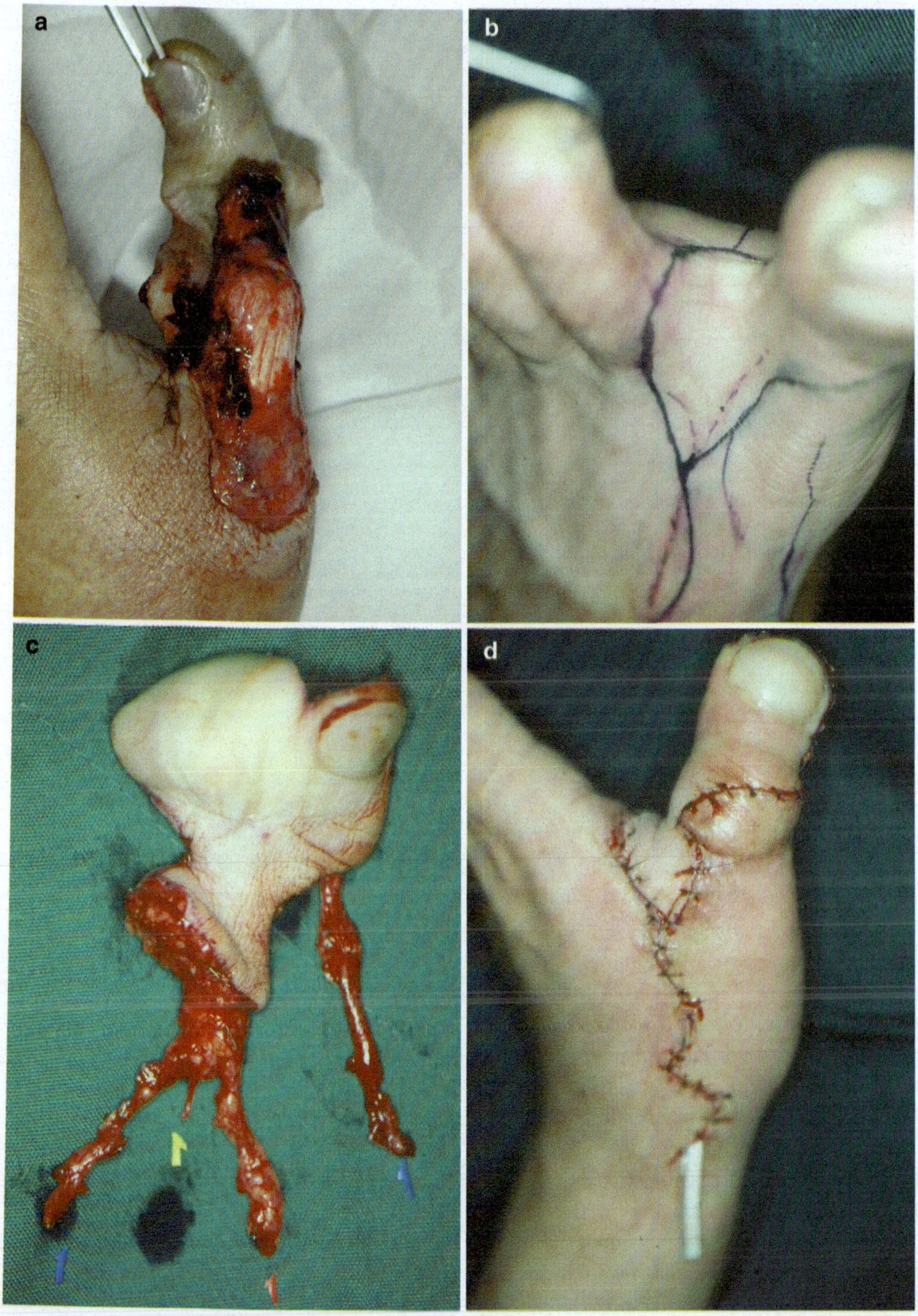


**Fig. 21.12** Wraparound flap transfer. (**a**) Avulsion amputation of the left thumb. (**b**, **c**) Design and harvested the wraparound flap combined with first web space flap. (**d**) Immediately after operation. (**e**) Postoperative view shows functional and cosmetic result compared with the contralateral thumb. (**f**) Donor site is covered with dorsalis pedis flap from the right foot

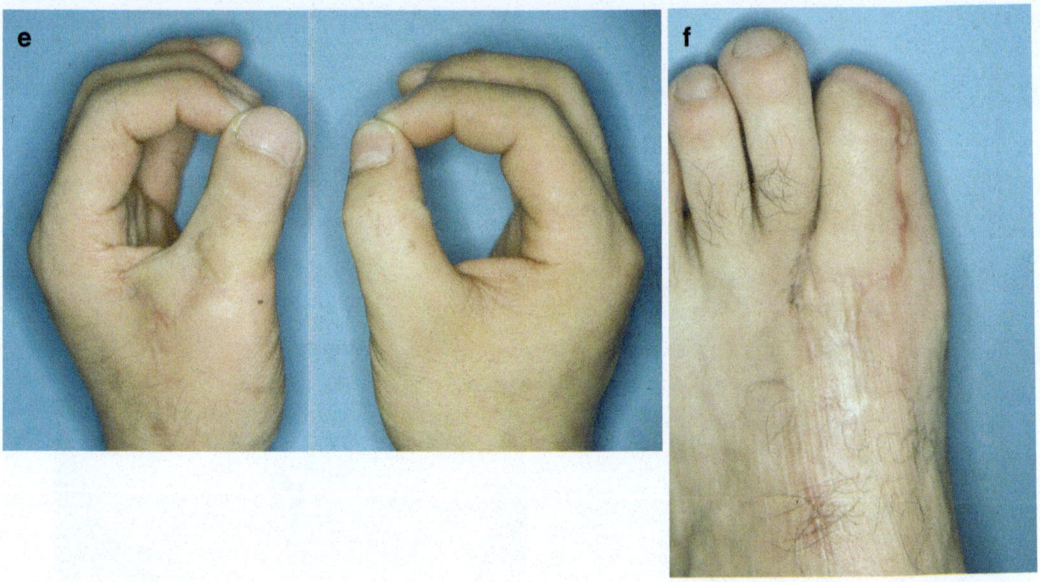


**Fig. 21.12** (continued)

donor defect, which is often quite tight. These modified procedures offer the aesthetic advantages of wraparound flaps while avoiding bone graft resorption and pulp mobility. To minimize the complications, at least 1–1.5 cm of the proximal phalanx in the great toe should be preserved. These modified procedures provide the aesthetic advantages of the wraparound flap while avoiding problems of bone graft resorption, pulp mobility, and a very difficult dissection.

Modified twisted-toe flap techniques [3, 24, 25] are also available for reconstruction. These techniques combine the wraparound flap technique with the vascularized joint transfer or neurovascular cutaneous flap and osteotendinous flap based on the single vascular pedicle. These procedures restore a more normal looking thumb, while preserving the epiphyses for future growth with reduced donor site morbidity. The modified twisted-toe technique by Kempny et al. [26] and Zhang et al. [27] reconstructs a very natural-appearing thumb with good stability and strength, together with a "new great toe" for the donor foot. Despite the many advantages, however, these techniques are not popular among surgeons, because their procedures are more complicated and time consuming than single-toe harvesting procedures.

## Level III. Reconstruction at Proximal Subtotal Defect at MP Joint

A thumb amputation through the metacarpal neck can be reconstructed with a trans-metatarsal transfer of the great toe or second toe. The range of motion in the MTP joint of the great toe and second toe is mainly extension. This should be corrected by an angled osteotomy of the metatarsal head, followed by a shortening of the plantar plate, with conversion of hyperextension of the MTP joint to flexion of the joint (Fig. 21.13). In cases of combined injury or previous amputation of the digits including the thumb, or for a laborer who needs a strong key pinch or grip, trans-metatarsal transfer of the great toe is recommended to overcome short remnant digits (Fig. 21.14). Trans-metatarsal great toe transfer should be applied with very limited indication because the sacrifice of the MTP joint of the great toe causes major donor site morbidity [28]. Preservation of the entire length of the first metatarsal as well as 1 cm of proximal phalangeal bone is just as important as the reconstruction of the thumb.

Compared with great toe transfer, trans-metatarsal second toe transfer is indicated at this level with the advantage of less donor site morbidity. Postoperative appearance and strength of the thumb are not as good as is the case with great toe transfer (Fig. 21.15). One's personal or cultural preference may be for the great toe to be preserved. A V-shaped incision is made on the both dorsal and plantar aspect of the foot. This provides adequate skin coverage for both donor and recipient sites. The procedure for foot dissection differs little from that of a great toe transfer. If there is not enough soft tissue coverage, the metatarsal bone should be harvested together with the interosseous muscle. A skin graft is always needed to cover the metatarsal bone. Regarding donor site closure, the intermetatarsal ligaments should be repaired between the great toe and third toe. Temporary K-wire fixation between metatarsals is needed to ensure a narrow interdigital web space and preserve the appearance of the donor site. In the second toe-to-thumb transfer, a modified technique reduces donor site

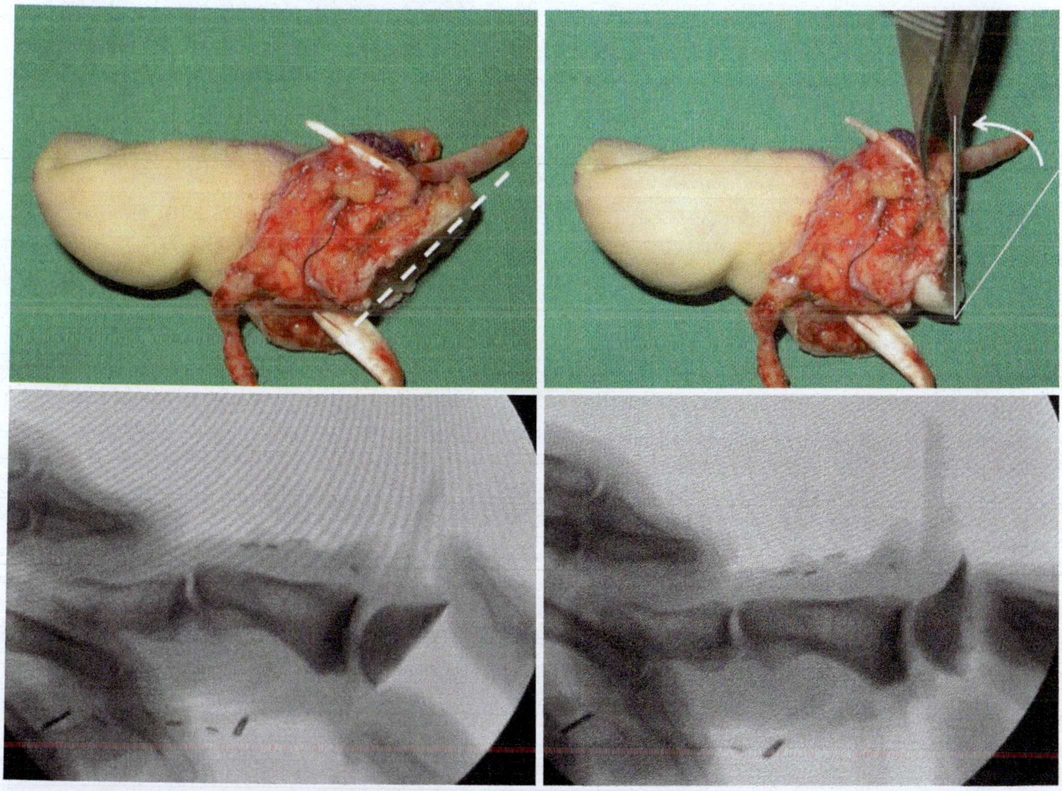

**Fig. 21.13** An oblique osteotomy (broken white line) at metatarsal head of the great toe converts hyperextension of the MTP joint into flexion of this joint. The white arrow shows changed angle

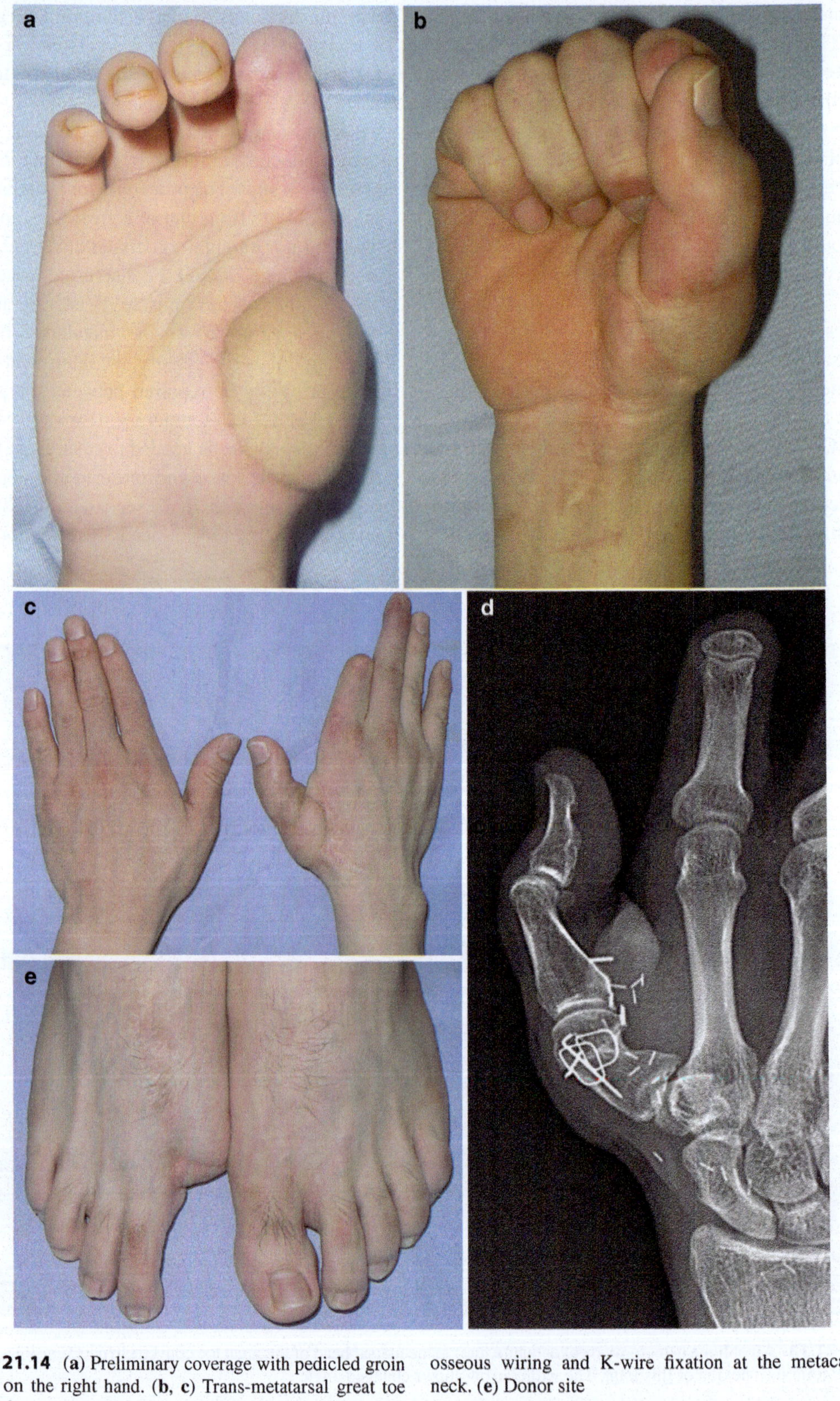


**Fig. 21.14** (**a**) Preliminary coverage with pedicled groin flap on the right hand. (**b**, **c**) Trans-metatarsal great toe transfer, postoperative view. (**d**) Bone fixation with interosseous wiring and K-wire fixation at the metacarpal neck. (**e**) Donor site

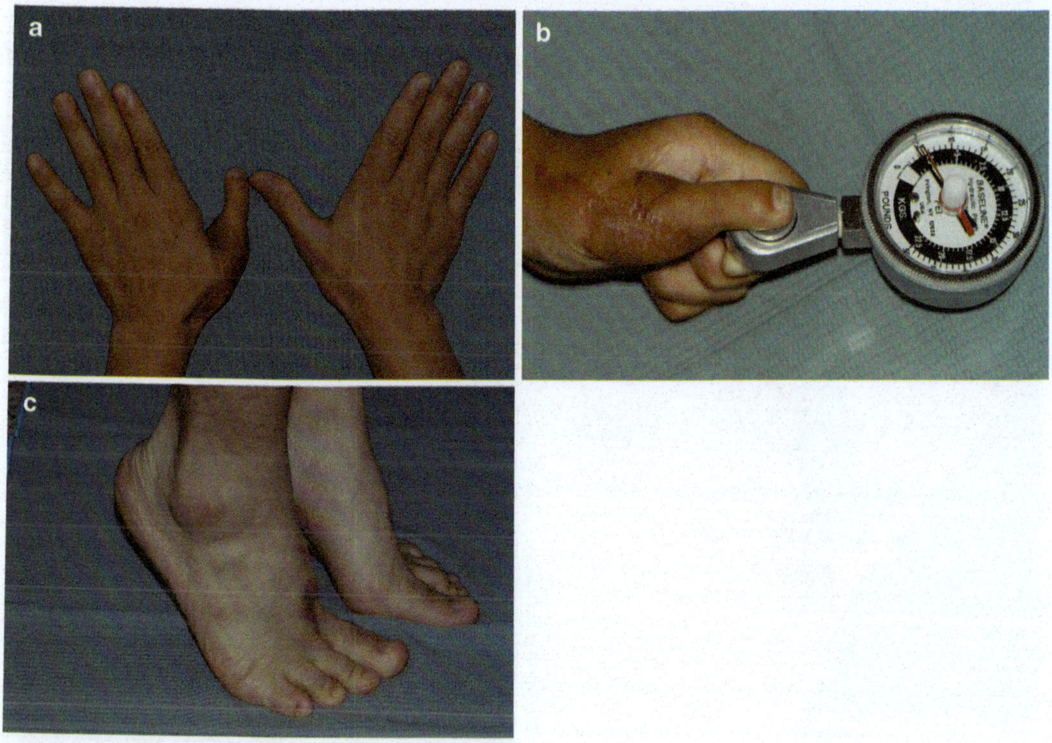

**Fig. 21.15** (**a**) Postoperative view of left thumb reconstruction with trans-metatarsal transfer of the second toe on the previous groin flap. The new thumb exhibits unattractive features, a narrow neck, a bulbous tip, and a short nail. (**b**) Key-pinch is 5 lbs, which is 35% of contralateral thumb. (**c**) Donor site of the right foot is aesthetically and functionally good

morbidity while providing an improved appearance of the new thumb [29]. This technique includes the harvesting of a flap from the lateral side of the great toe and inserting it into the volar aspect of the second toe to give more bulk. Skin excisions are then performed on each side of the tip to reduce the bulbous appearance. An eponychial flap increases the apparent lengthening of the nail [30].

## Level IV. Reconstruction for Total Defect of the Thumb

Amputation through the shaft of the metacarpal should be reconstructed in a two-stage procedure. At the first stage, a tri-cortical iliac bone graft is necessary to lengthen the metacarpal bone along with soft tissue coverage. Pedicled groin flap and a posterior interosseous reversed island flap are useful without damage of main vascular pedicle around the wrist. Three to 6 months later, a trans-metatarsal great toe or second toe transfer provides some motion for the new thumb's MCP joint. When the patient desires to preserve the MTP joint of the great toe, the great toe transfer can be harvested at the level of the proximal phalanx. In this case, the new thumb presents only two joints without an MCP joint (Fig. 21.16). Postoperatively, the functional results of the reconstructed thumb are not as good as reconstruction of the distal part of the thumb. When opting for the most suitable surgical procedure, the patient's aesthetic and functional expectations for the new thumb, as well as morbidity and appearance of the donor sites, should be carefully considered.

Amputation of the thumb through the proximal portion of the metacarpal or through the CMC joint is very disabling. Pollicization is the

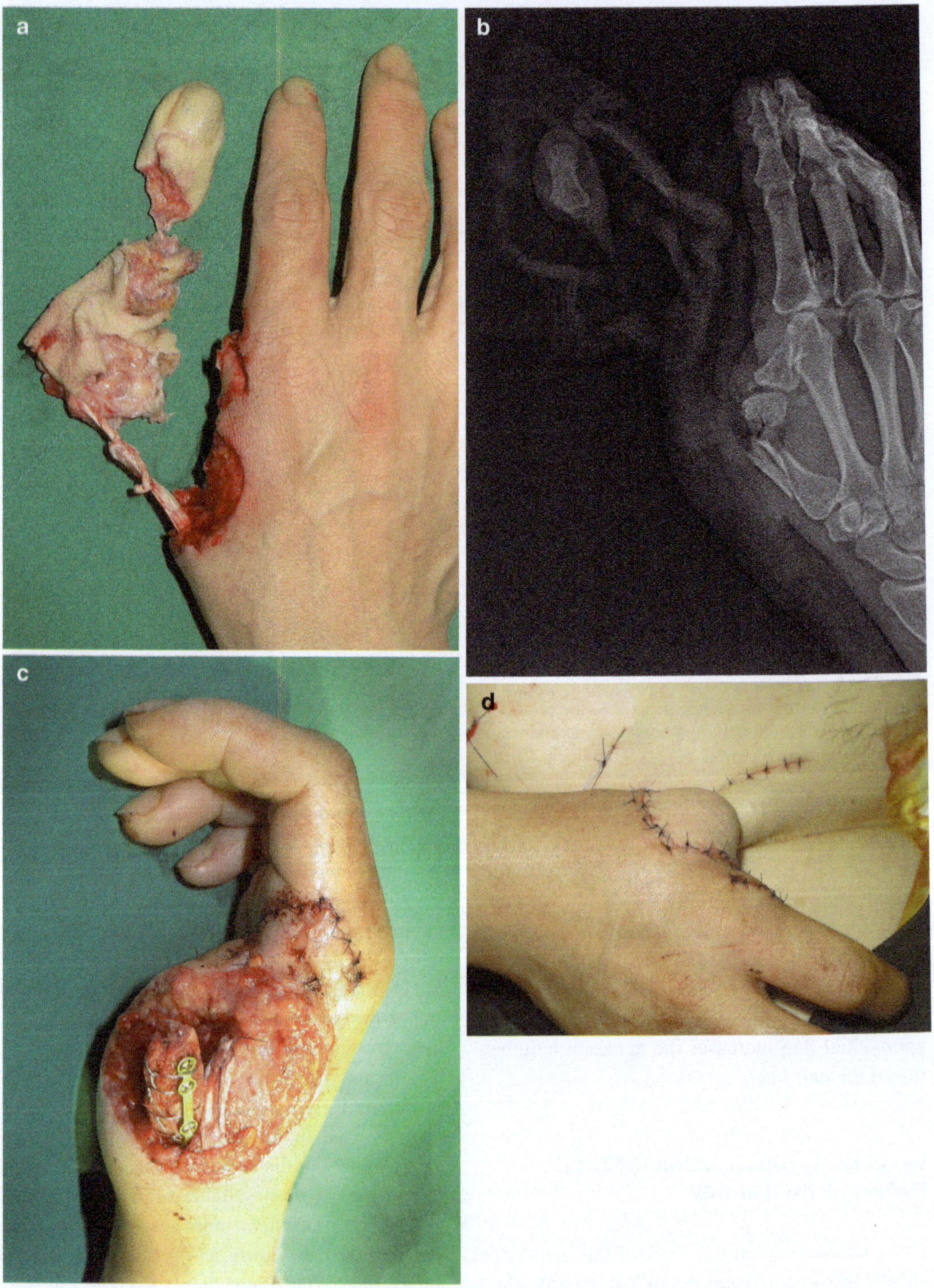


**Fig. 21.16** (**a**, **b**) Segmental crushing amputation of the right thumb at the mid-metacarpal shaft and radiograph. (**c**) Intraoperative view of interosseous wiring of the fractured metacarpal bone and 3-cortical autogenous iliac bone graft on it. (**d**, **e**) Pedicled groin flap to cover the bone graft and metacarpal bone and radiograph. (**f**, **g**) Six months later, whole great toe transfer on the lengthened metacarpal bone. (**h**, **i**) Nine years postoperation. Key-pinch is 6 lbs, which is 50% of contralateral side. (**j**, **k**) Postoperative radiograph of the right hand and foot

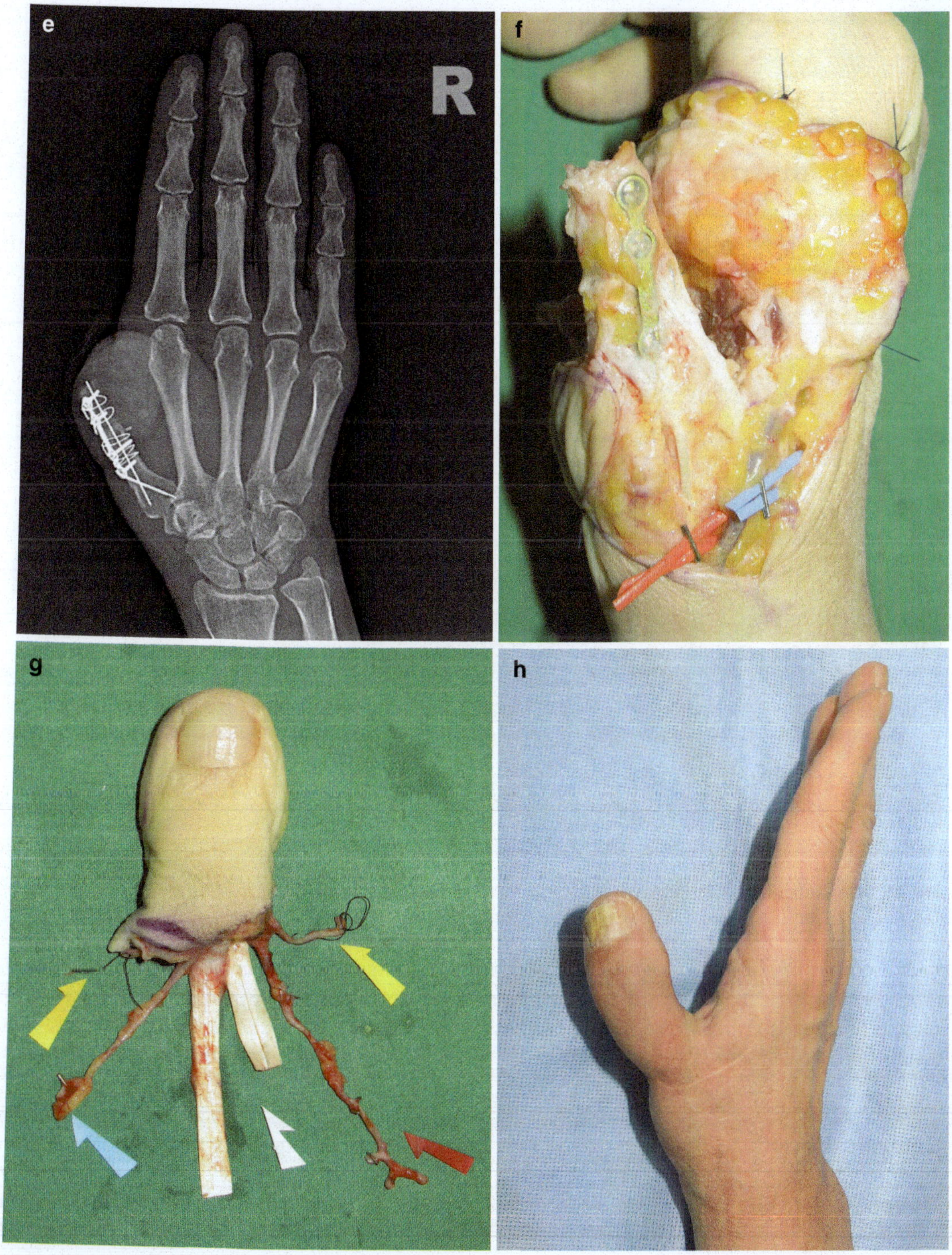


**Fig. 21.16** (continued)

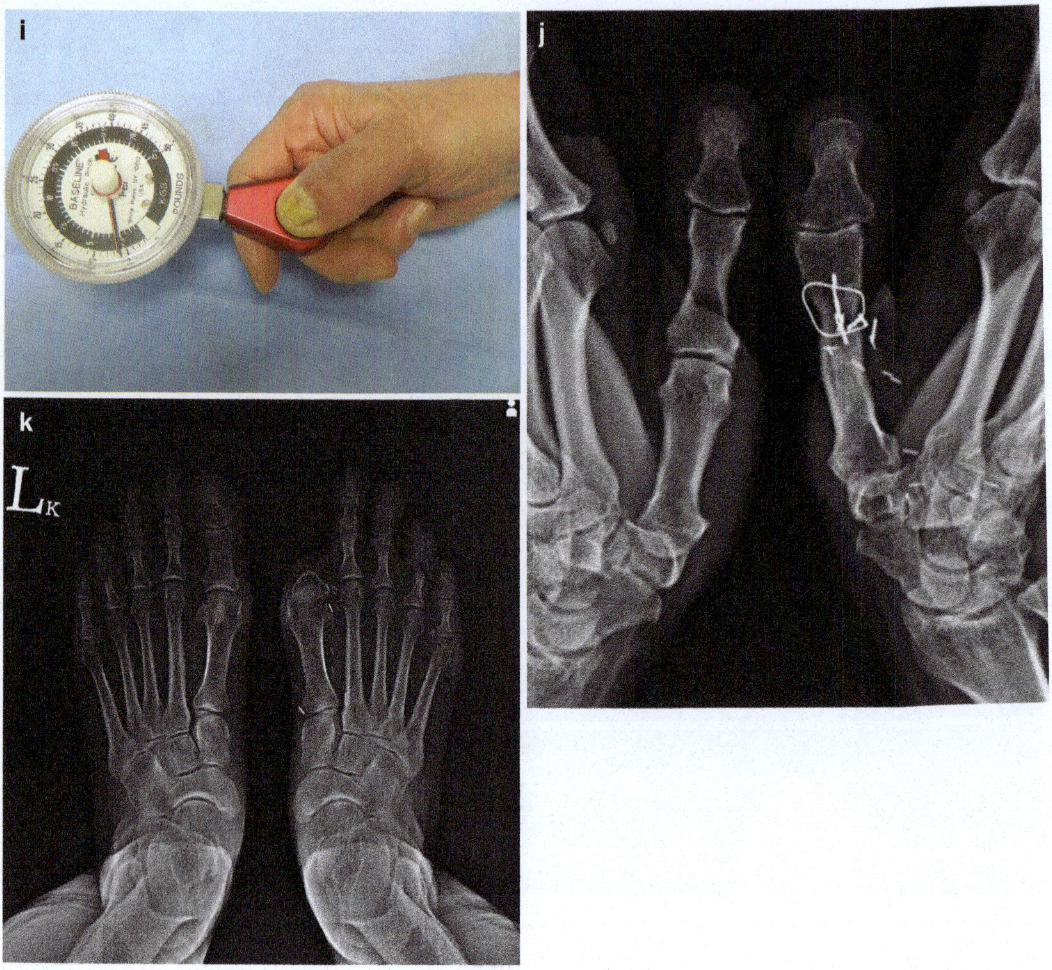


**Fig. 21.16** (continued)

most promising method of reconstruction (Fig. 21.17) [31, 32]. The presence of thenar muscle function is critical to obtain satisfactory results in pollicization [33].

## Complications

### Donor Site Problems

Even though a successful great toe transfer can provide satisfactory results both in function and appearance, donor site complications should be minimized. Donor site complications are categorized as wound dehiscence, infection, necrosis, pain or discomfort, and callosity (Fig. 21.18). The source of foot pain is localized to painful neuromas of the deep and superficial peroneal nerves and also to the saphenous nerve. Neuroma excision is identified through an incision in the non-weight-bearing portion of the foot. The proximal end of the nerve is implanted into the arch of the foot (Fig. 21.19).

The complications and donor site morbidity have historically been underestimated. Sosin et al. [34] showed that the overall rate of donor site complications was 22% in great toe transfers and 15% in second toe transfers. Some patients complain of occasional mild discomfort of the foot and intolerance to cold [35]. After a whole great toe transfer, the weight-bearing area shifts to the second and third metatarsal heads. There is

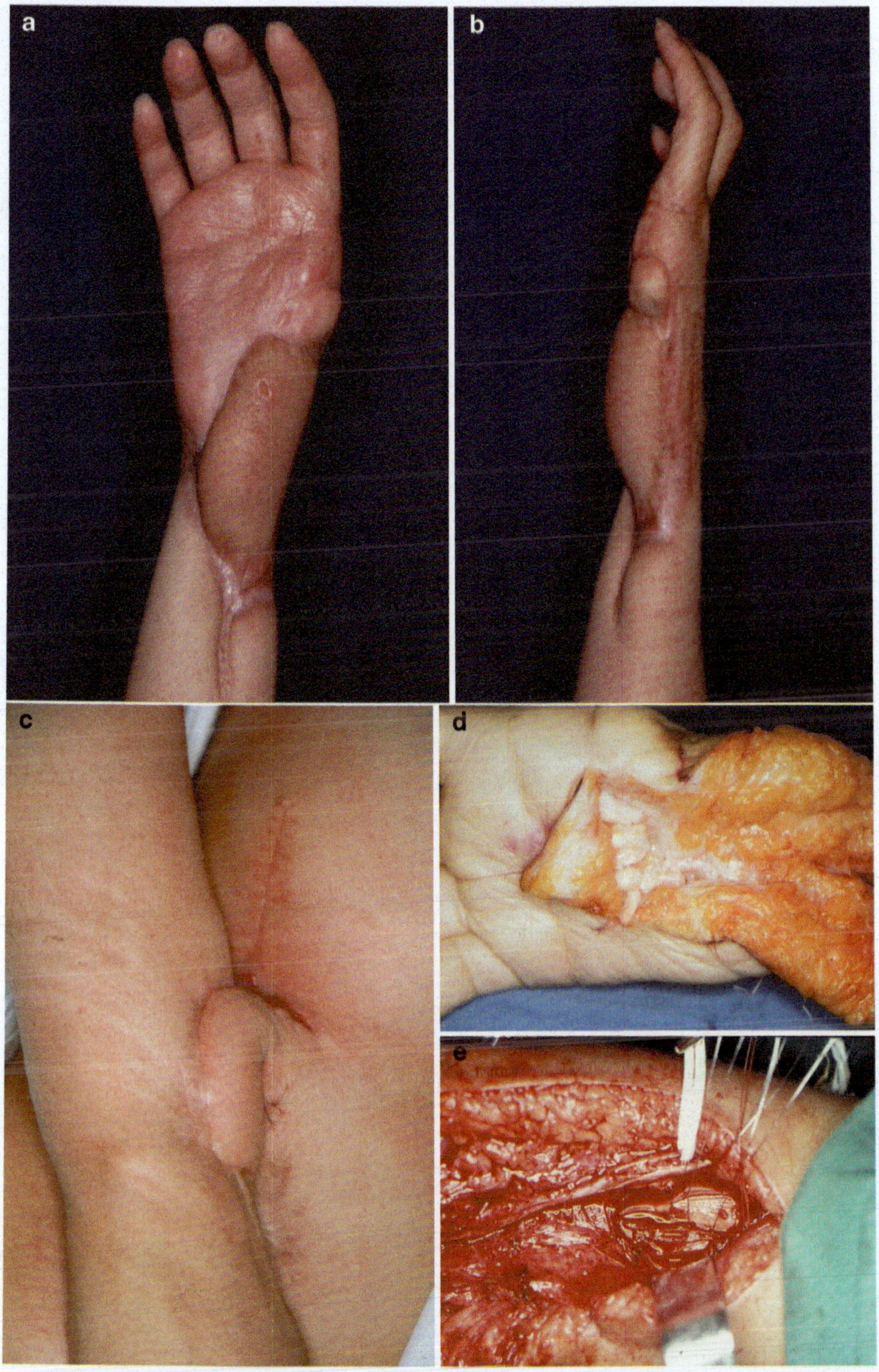

**Fig. 21.17** (**a**, **b**) Preoperative view shows amputation of the thumb and distant abdominal flap on the distal forearm. All four digits have no active motion. (**c**) Preliminary pedicled groin flap is made on the proximal border of the previous flap for passage of the new tendon. (**d**) Remnant flexor tendons are dissected at the palm for repair of the new tendon. (**e**) Medial epicondyle is prepared for fixation of the transferred muscle. (**f**) Dissected gracilis myocutaneous free flap with obturator nerve and vascular pedicle. (**g**) Postoperative view of free functioning muscle transfer. (**h**) Design for pollicization. (**i**, **j**) Postoperative view after 5 years shows powerful extension and flexion of the fingers with contraction of the transferred muscle. (**k**) Postoperative radiograph

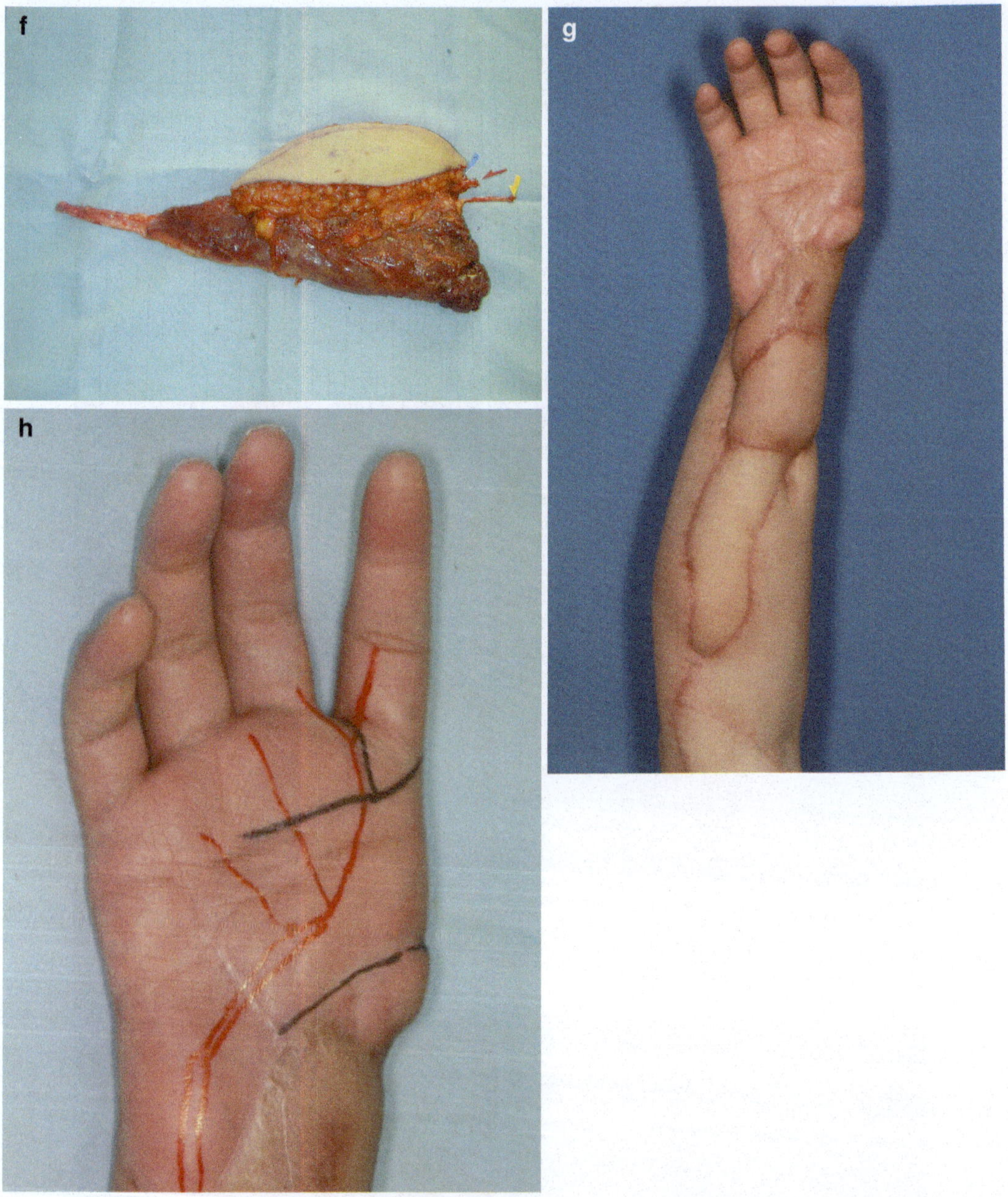


**Fig. 21.17** (continued)

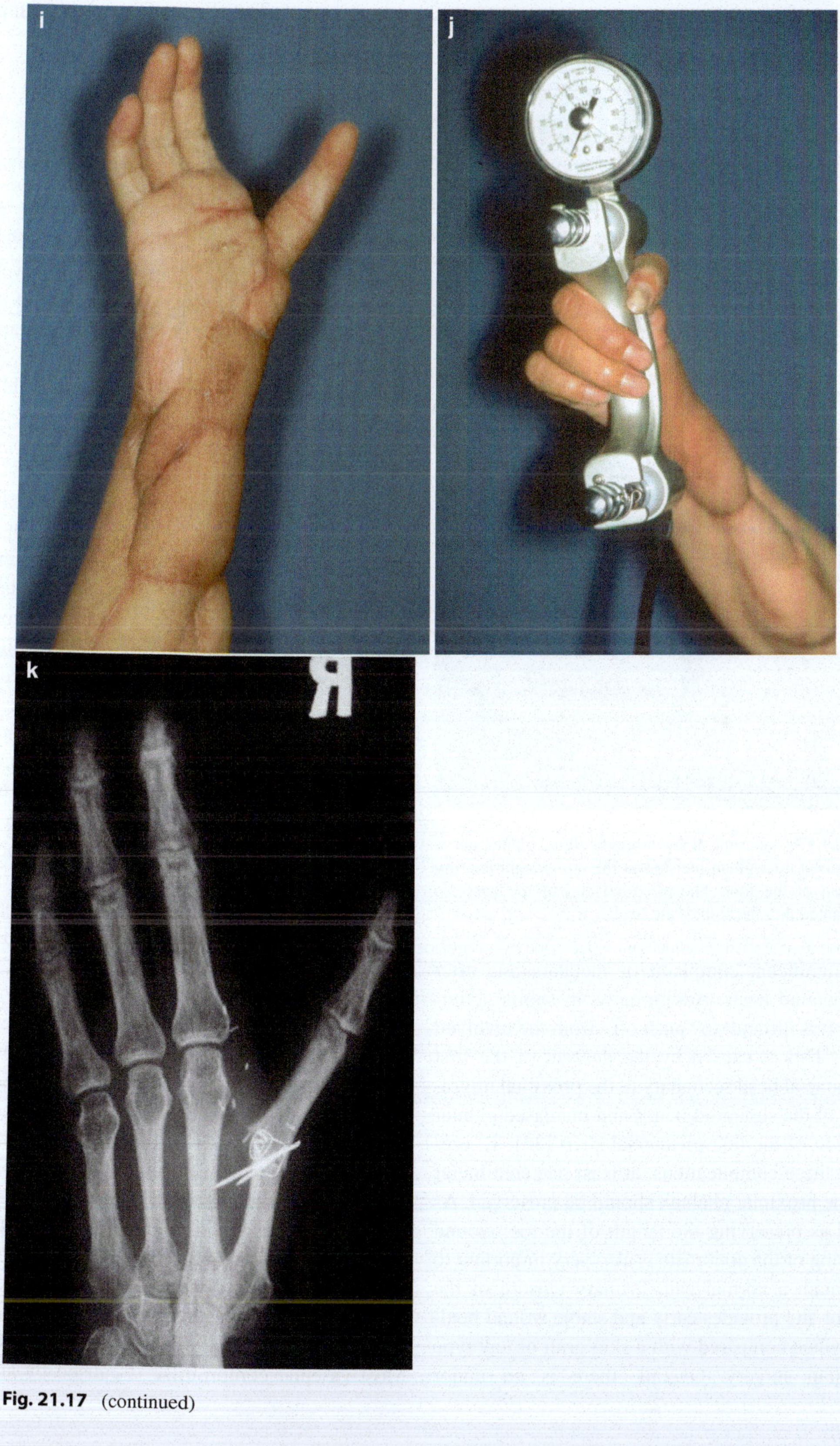


**Fig. 21.17** (continued)

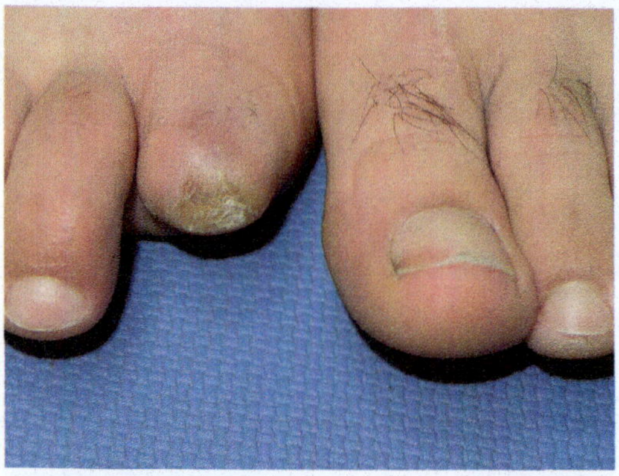

**Fig. 21.18** Callosity of the right great toe after toe transfer

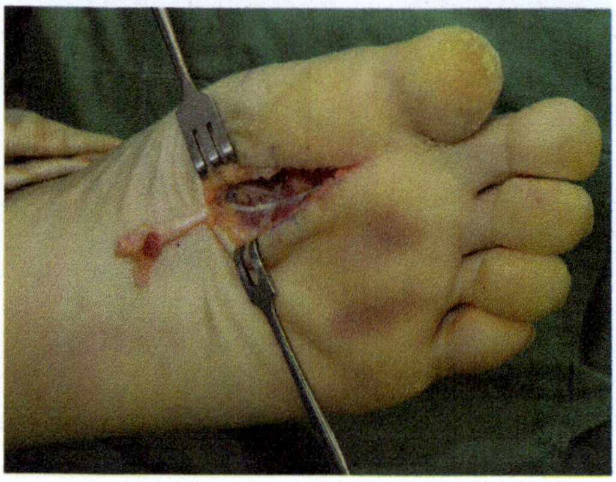

**Fig. 21.19** Neuroma of the common digital plantar nerve is excised through an incision in the non-weight-bearing portion of the foot. The proximal end of the nerve is implanted into the arch of the foot

no significant complaint of metatarsalgia after the wound heals. Additionally, in sports activities, it is difficult to "push off" from the involved foot. This is caused by the descent of the first metatarsal head secondary to the proximal migration of the sesamoid bones and increased plantar flexion of the first metatarsal shaft [36]. To prevent these complications, at least one centimeter of the proximal phalanx should be preserved. As well as preserving the length of the toe, wound healing of the donor site is also very important to maintain a normal gait. Primary closure of the donor site provides early and stable wound healing when compared with a skin graft or any type of flap surgery. Overall, there is no major objective disturbance in gait from elective amputation of the great toe.

## Flap Failure

The most disastrous complication of a toe-to-thumb transfer is flap failure (Fig. 21.20). The incidence of flap failure was reported in 0–7% of overall cases [37–39]. Up to the fifth or seventh day postoperatively, intensive monitoring of perfusion status is mandatory. To further guarantee complete survival of the transferred toe, the threshold determining re-exploration should be very low. Any circulatory problem or vessel condition should be checked under the microscope in an operating room immediately.

Recently, Lin et al. [40] demonstrated that the overall success rate of toe-to-hand transfer in 363 cases was 98%. Consequently, the diameter or anatomical location of the first dorsal metatarsal artery is no longer the main causative factor of the circulatory crisis resulting in flap failure. Even release of the tourniquet after toe dissection rarely results in a lack of reperfusion in the toe, even after 30 min. In this case, the dissection status of the main artery should be rechecked under a microscope. If any small branch of the main artery remains open, it should be ligated to prevent segmental spasm [41]. If there is no problem involving the vessels, warm saline irrigation is the best way to obtain reperfusion. Iatrogenic trauma of the vessel during dissection or drilling may cause vessel spasm or late thrombosis.

In the difficult case of a lack of perfusion even after perfect arterial anastomosis, first recheck the dissection status of the recipient artery proximally under a microscope. If a problem cannot be identified, a sympathetic block on the brachial plexus is needed to achieve vasodilatation. Awakening the patient from general anesthesia is another way to stimulate perfusion.

Operative failure is mainly due to failure to recognize and appropriately treat vascular compromise. Re-exploration should be carried out whenever vascular insufficiency is suspected or does not improve after bedside management. Most vascular compromise is caused by arterial

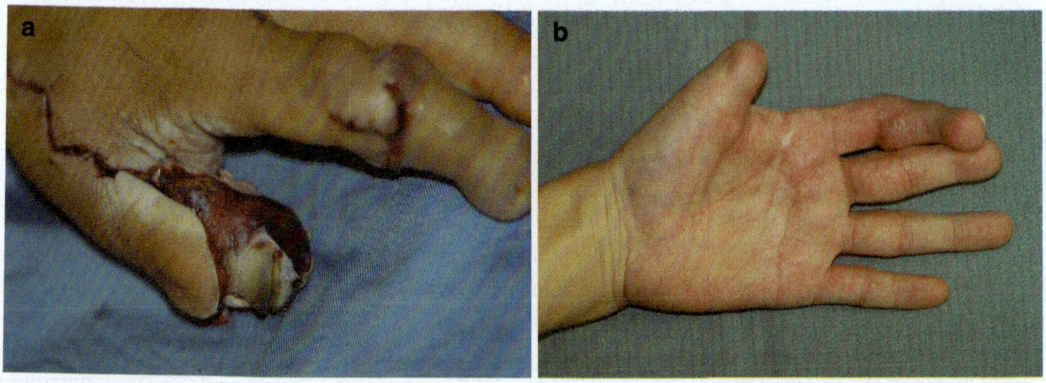

Fig. 21.20 (a) Transferred great toe had recal finger, transferred great toe had recalcitrant arterial spasm, even though arterial reanastomosis, vein graft, and artery transfer from common digital artery could not restore the arterial perfusion. (b) Postoperative view of revision amputation of transferred great toe

insufficiency within 72 h following surgery. During re-exploration, transfer of vascular structures from the adjacent finger may be an alternative means of creating a fresh recipient for arterial and venous structures rather than insisting on the revision of the previous recipient vessels [42]. To prevent vascular complications of the toe-to-hand transfer, meticulous dissection and ligation of the branch vessels, complete anastomosis of the vessels, and postoperative intensive monitoring of the transferred toe are mandatory.

Wound infection induces an inflammatory response and the release of inflammatory mediators. Previous injury and surgical procedures cause tissue fibrosis and adhesions. Postoperative wound infection is associated with an increased risk of re-exploration [40].

Unfortunately, even after all possible revision procedures to achieve normal circulation, circulatory problems may persist. In this case, a tubed groin flap can be the last resort to salvage the transplanted bone [42].

## Emergency Reconstruction of the Thumb

The concept of emergency toe-to-thumb transfer is based on both emergency free flap surgery for resurfacing in acute upper extremity injury and toe-to-hand transfer for thumb reconstruction. It is defined for the reconstruction of acute thumb injuries. It is indicated when replantation of the thumb is impossible or has failed [43–45]. First of all, the patient should have a strong desire for reconstruction of the thumb immediately following loss. The patient must also understand and accept the risks of operative failure, donor site morbidity, and functional limitations of the transferred toe. To endure prolonged anesthesia, the patient must be in good physical condition and have an overwhelming desire for hand reconstruction. Financial support or insurance coverage should be discussed before the operation.

Compared with elective toe transfer, radical debridement of the recipient site is necessary to prevent infection in acute amputation. In the case of necrosis of the replantation, serial debridement after amputation of the stump is necessary prior to toe transfer. The recipient vessel for anastomosis should be located outside the zone of injury.

Emergency toe transfer in acute injury of the thumb allows easy dissection of the intact neurovascular pedicles through the open wound, without fibrosis or scar adhesion, which results in a high operation success rate and a low incidence of emergency re-exploration [46, 47]. It also eliminates the need to shorten the exposed phalangeal bone and prevents the formation of tendon adhesions or atrophy, thus preserving the length of the finger and providing smooth gliding of the tendons to achieve greater total active range of motion. Immediate toe transfer is very efficient, from a socioeconomic point of view. It reduces the convalescent period by using single-stage reconstruction. In the series above, the duration of insurance coverage for patients who underwent emergency reconstruction was significantly shorter and their return to work earlier when compared with patients who underwent elective reconstruction. More patients who underwent immediate toe transfer maintained their original jobs following the operation, compared with electively treated patients, although the difference was not statistically significant.

A significant disadvantage of emergency toe transfer reconstruction is the lack of time to establish a good patient-surgeon rapport. If the patients do not understand the entire process of the operation and the probable postoperative functional results, disparate expectations might lead to legal action. In addition, the patients' subjective satisfaction with the postoperative function and appearance might be diminished as emergency reconstruction does not allow patients the necessary time to mourn the loss of their digits before toe transfer commences. Another disadvantage is the possibility of postoperative infections and flap failure that can happen if the contaminated wound or traumatized tissue is not debrided completely and thoroughly. To ensure successful immediate toe transfer, debridement should be aggressive. Because there are no statistically significant differences in the success rates, frequencies of complications, or ultimate functional results, emergency toe-to-thumb transfer is a safe and reliable procedure that is indicated for specific cases of thumb amputation.

## Rehabilitation and Functional Outcomes

The goals of rehabilitation are to increase the range of motion of the IP and MP joints, decrease postoperative edema, facilitate sensory restoration, and improve the coordination and dexterity of the reconstructed hand. Hand therapy essentially follows the same protocols as replantation. An aggressive rehabilitation program is likely to decrease the incidence and number of secondary procedures for tendon adhesions or joint stiffness. However, any exercise program should avoid deterioration of wound condition, bone fixation, or tendon suture.

Passive motion of the IP and MP joints usually starts at bed side 5–7 days after operation depending on the circulation and wound condition. Protected gentle active motion can start on the seventh day and no later than 14 days postoperatively. The motion starts at the wrist and thumb CMC joint with gradual and gentle passive and active motion of the MP and IP joints within 4 weeks postoperatively. During this period, passive and active exercise with a custom-made dynamic brace is initiated (Fig. 21.21). Exercise should always be carried out in a painless manner, avoiding excessive tension on repaired tendons, blood vessels, and nerves. After 6 weeks, neuromuscular electrical stimulation, blocking, and selective joint exercises are employed. After 2 months, light resistance and dynamic orthotic management are introduced and progressed according to bone consolidation and pain tolerance.

Functional outcome evaluations of toe transfers have traditionally been based on physical variables, including grip strength, pinch strength, and sensory recovery evaluations with two-point discrimination. Long-term functional results of toe-to-thumb reconstruction demonstrates 75% of pinch strength compared with the contralateral hand [48]. Grip strength can be restored to approximately 70% of the contralateral hand when performing an immediate second toe transfer, and up to 90% with osteo-onychocutaneous techniques [49]. Static 2-point discrimination can be achieved to 10 mm, and later sensory reorganization allows for ongoing improvements in perception of touch and interpretation of signals from the transferred digit. However, a recent systematic review of the literature failed to identify any differences in outcomes by technique, largely owing to the heterogeneity of current data, which are largely limited to smaller, single-center studies and case series(Table 21.1) [50]. Although microsurgical reconstruction of the thumb with toe transfer is lengthy, technically demanding,

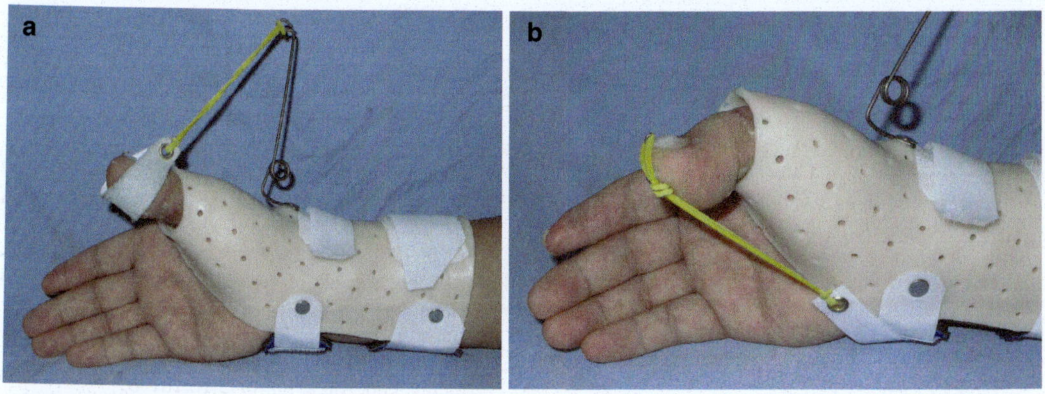


**Fig. 21.21** Functional rehabilitation of the reconstructed thumb with the early use of the dynamic crane outrigger splint. (**a**) Under passive extension with rubber band on the interphalangeal joint of the transferred great toe, patient starts gentle active flexion of the new thumb. (**b**) Under passive flexion with rubber band on the interphalangeal joint of the transferred great toe, patient starts gentle active extension of the new thumb

**Table 21.1** Comparison of available toe-to-thumb transfer techniques

| | Whole great toe | Trimmed great toe | Wrap-around | Second toe | Partial great toe |
|---|---|---|---|---|---|
| Function | | | | | |
| Mobility | ++++ | +++ | + | ++ | + |
| Sensation | ++++ | ++++ | ++++ | ++ | ++++ |
| Appearance | +++ | ++++ | ++++ | + | ++++ |
| Strength | ++++ | +++ | +++ | ++ | +++ |
| Donor site | | | | | |
| Function | + | ++ | +++ | ++++ | ++++ |
| Appearance | + | ++ | +++ | ++++ | +++ |
| Technical difficulty | Easy | Difficult | More difficult | Easy | Most difficult |
| Complication | None | None | Bone resorption no growth | Claw-finger | None |

+ poor, ++ fair, +++ good, ++++ excellent

and results in unavoidable donor site morbidity, postoperative results on both functional and aesthetic aspects are the most pleasing compared with other non-microsurgical techniques.

## References

1. Buncke HJ Jr, Buncke CM, Schulz WP. Immediate Nicoladoni procedure in the Rhesus monkey, or hallux-to-hand transplantation, utilising micro-miniature vascular anastomoses. Br J Plast Surg. 1966;19:332–7.
2. Cobbett JR. Free digital transfer. Report of a case of transfer of a great toe to replace an amputated thumb. J Bone Joint Surg Br. 1969;51:677–9.
3. Foucher G, Merle M, Maneaud M, et al. Microsurgical free partial toe transfer in hand reconstruction: a report of 12 cases. Plast Reconstr Surg. 1980;65:616–26.
4. Hirase Y, Kojima T, Matsui M. Aesthetic fingertip reconstruction with a free vascularized nail graft: a review of 60 flaps involving partial toe transfers. Plast Reconstr Surg. 1997;99:774–84.
5. Wei FC, Chen HC, Chuang DCC, et al. Aesthetic refinements in toe-to-hand transfer surgery. Plast Reconstr Surg. 1996;98:485–90.
6. Michon J, Merle M, Bouchon Y, et al. Functional comparison between pollicization and toe-to hand trans-

fer for thumb reconstruction. J Reconstr Microsurg. 1984;1:103–12.
7. Jones NF, Hansen SL, Bates SJ. Toe-to-hand transfers for congenital anomalies of the hand. Hand Clin. 2007;23:129–36.
8. Nguyen JT, Bakri K, Nguyen EC, et al. Surgical management of subungual melanoma: Mayo Clinic experience of 124 cases. Ann Plast Surg. 2013;71:346–54.
9. Kovachevich R, Giuffre JL, Shin AY, Bishop AT. Immediate great toe transfer for thumb reconstruction after tumor resection: report of 3 cases. Ann Plast Surg. 2016;76:280–4.
10. Morrison W, O'Brien BM, MacLeod AM. Experience with thumb reconstruction. J Hand Surg Br. 1984;9:223–33.
11. Gilbert A. Thumb reconstruction using microvascular techniques. In: Tubiana, editor. The hand, vol. III. Philadelphia: WB Saunders; 1988. p. P1142–51.
12. Zhu J, Hu B. Sonography of the first dorsal metatarsal artery of the foot. J Clin Ultrasound. 2006;34:1–4.
13. Xu L, Yang K, Wei P, et al. Computed tomography angiography allows the classification of the first dorsal metatarsal arteries. J Reconstr Microsurg. 2016;32:675–82.
14. Hou Z, Zou J, Wang Z, Zhong S. Anatomical classification of the first dorsal metatarsal artery and its clinical application. Plast Reconstr Surg. 2013;132:1028e–39e.
15. Wei FC, Silverman RT, Hsu WM. Retrograde dissection of the vascular pedicle in toe harvest. Plast Reconstr Surg. 1995;96:1211–4.
16. Woo SH, Seul JH. Distal thumb reconstruction with a great toe partial-nail preserving transfer technique. Plast Reconstr Surg. 1998;101:114–9.
17. Buncke HJ, Valauri FA. Reconstruction of the thumb with a trimmed-toe transfer technique (Discussion). Plast Reconstr Surg. 1988;82:514–5.
18. Adani R, Cardon LJ, Castagnetti C, Pinelli M. Distal thumb reconstruction using a mini wrap-around flap from the great toe. J Hand Surg Br. 1999;24:437–42.
19. Morrison WA, O'Brien BM, MacLeod AM. Thumb reconstruction with a free neurovascular wrap-around flap from the big toe. J Hand Surg [Am]. 1980;5:575–83.
20. Pan YW, Zhang L, Tian W, et al. Donor foot morbidity following modified wraparound flap for thumb reconstruction: a follow-up of 69 cases. J Hand Surg [Am]. 2011;36:493–501.
21. Shen XF, Mi JY, Xue MY, et al. Modified great toe wraparound flap with preservation of plantar triangular flap for reconstruction of degloving injuries of the thumb and fingers: long-term follow-up. Plast Reconstr Surg. 2016;138:155–63.
22. Wei FC, Chen HC, Chuang CC, et al. Reconstruction of the thumb with a trimmed-toe transfer technique. Plast Reconstr Surg. 1988;82:506–15.
23. Upton J, Mutimer K. A modification of the great-toe transfer for thumb reconstruction. Plast Reconstr Surg. 1988;82:535–8.
24. Tsai TM, Aziz W. Toe-to-thumb transfer: a new technique. Plast Reconstr Surg. 1991;88:149–53.
25. Iglesias M, Butron P, Serrano A. Thumb reconstruction with extended twisted toe flap. J Hand Surg [Am]. 1995;20:731–6.
26. Kempny T, Paroulek J, Marik V, et al. Further developments in the twisted-toe technique for isolated thumb reconstruction: our method of choice. Plast Reconstr Surg. 2013;131:871e–9e.
27. Zhang G, Ju J, Li L, et al. Combined foot flaps with iliac bone graft for reconstruction of the thumb. J Hand Surg Eur. 2016;41:745–52.
28. Barca F, Santi A, Tartoni PL, et al. Gait analysis of the donor foot in microsurgical reconstruction of the thumb. Foot Ankle Int. 1995;16:201–6.
29. Zhao J, Tien HY, Abdullah S, et al. Aesthetic refinements in second toe-to-thumb transfer surgery. Plast Reconstr Surg. 2010;126:2052–9.
30. del Piñal F, García-Bernal FJ, Regalado J, et al. A technique to improve foot appearance after trimmed toe or hallux harvesting. J Hand Surg [Am]. 2007;32:409–13.
31. Al-Qattan MM. Pollicization of the index finger requiring secondary fusion of the new metacarpophalangeal joint. J Hand Surg Eur. 2016;41:295–300.
32. Woo SH, Seul JH. Various functioning free muscle transfer for restoration of hand function. J Korean Soc Surg Hand. 2002;7:130–8.
33. Ishida O, Taniguchi Y, Sunagawa T, et al. Pollicization of the index finger for traumatic thumb amputation. Plast Reconstr Surg. 2006;117:909–14.
34. Sosin M, Lin CH, Steinberg J, et al. Functional donor site morbidity after vascularized toe transfer procedures: a review of the literature and biomechanical consideration for surgical site selection. Ann Plast Surg. 2016;76:735–42.
35. Lipton HA, May JW Jr, Simon SR. Preoperative and postoperative gait analyses of patients undergoing great toe-to-thumb transfer. J Hand Surg [Am]. 1987;12:66–9.
36. Poppen NK, Mann RA, O'Konski M, et al. Amputation of the great toe. Foot Ankle. 1981;1:333–7.
37. Buncke HJ, Buncke GM, Lineaweaver WC, et al. Bad results after large toe to thumb transplantation. Ann Chir Main Memb Super. 1991;10:513–6.
38. Graham DJ, Venkatramani H, Sabapathy SR. Current reconstruction options for traumatic thumb loss. J Hand Surg [Am]. 2016;41:1159–69.
39. Gu YD, Zhang GM, Chen DS, et al. Toe-to-hand transfer: an analysis of 14 failed cases. J Hand Surg [Am]. 1993;18:823–7.
40. Lin YT, Su ST, Lo S, et al. Risk factors for reexploration in toe-to-hand transfer: a multivariate analysis of 363 cases. Plast Reconstr Surg. 2015;135:501–6.
41. Lister GD, Kalisman M, Tsai TM. Reconstruction of the hand with free microneurovascular toe-to-hand transfer: experience with 54 toe transfers. Plast Reconstr Surg. 1983;71:371–86.
42. Ozkan O, Chen HC, Mardini S, et al. Principles for the management of toe-to-hand transfer in reexploration:

toe salvage with a tubed groin flap in the last step. Microsurgery. 2006;26:100–5.
43. Wei FC, Epstein MD, Chen HC, et al. Microsurgical reconstruction of distal digits following mutilating hand injuries: results in 121 patients. Br J Plast Surg. 1993;46:181–6.
44. Rose EH, Hendel P. Primary toe-to-thumb transfer in the acutely avulsed thumb. Plast Reconstr Surg. 1981;67:214–8.
45. Demirkan F, Wei FC, Jeng SF, et al. Toe transplantation for isolated index finger amputations distal to the proximal interphalangeal joint. Plast Reconstr Surg. 1999;103:499–507.
46. Woo SH, Kim JS, Seul JH. Immediate toe-to-hand transfer in acute hand injuries: overall results, compared with results for elective cases. Plast Reconstr Surg. 2004;113:882–92.
47. Woo SH, Lee GJ, Kim KC, et al. Immediate partial great toe transfer for the reconstruction of composite defects of the distal thumb. Plast Reconstr Surg. 2006;117:1906–15.
48. Kotkansalo T, Vilkki S, Elo P, et al. Long-term functional results of microvascular toe-to-thumb reconstruction. J Hand Surg Eur. 2011;36:194–204.
49. Huang D, Wang HG, Wu WZ, et al. Functional and aesthetic results of immediate reconstruction of traumatic thumb defects by toe-to-thumb transplantation. Int Orthop. 2011;35:543–7.
50. Waljee JF, Chung KC. Toe-to-hand transfer: evolving indications and relevant outcomes. J Hand Surg [Am]. 2013;38:1431–4.

# 22 Miscellaneous

Joo-Hak Kim and Jikang Park

## Infection of the Thumb

Hand and upper extremity infections have a wide range of clinical manifestations. They vary from simple superficial infections treatable by oral antibiotics to limb or life-threatening infection requiring a combination of surgical debridement and intravenous antibiotics. The thumb like other fingers, being constantly exposed to the environment, provides a wide variety of pathogens. An understanding of infectious pathogens, the clinical conditions they produce, and the appropriate treatment helps limit these potential debilitating conditions [1].

## General Principles

Several factors may predispose the thumb or hand to an infection. These include local wound conditions (crush injuries, contaminated puncture wounds, chronic edema), altered immune states, or host conditions. A careful medical history and physical examination should identify any additional infection risk factors, which may determine the need for more aggressive treatment. The successful treatment of thumb and hand infection requires an early recognition of the infection, the initiation of empiric and subsequent culture-directed antibiotic coverage, surgical debridement and irrigation for contaminated, devitalized tissue, and adequate follow-up care [2].

## Pathophysiology

Pathogens can be classified into five main groups: bacteria, fungi, viruses, protozoa, and metazoa. Resistance to infection occurs through several mechanisms, including nonspecific, or innate, immunity and specific immunity. Nonspecific immunity includes normal mechanical and physiologic properties of the host. Specific immunity includes a variety of defensive responses by the host to microorganisms [3].

## Clinical Evaluation

Bacterial infections unusually produce the normal signs of infection, including erythema, edema, and tenderness. Nonbacterial infections may present with innocuous swelling without significant erythema or pain. Included in the differential diagnosis of hand infection are gout,

J.-H. Kim (✉)
Department of Orthopaedic Surgery, Myongji Hospital, Hanyang University, College of Medicine, Goyang-si, Gyeonggi-do, South Korea

J. Park
Department of Orthopaedic Surgery, Chungbuk National University College of Medicine, Chungbuk National University Hospital, Cheongju-si, Chungcheongbuk-do, South Korea


S. H. Woo (ed.), *The Thumb*, https://doi.org/10.1007/978-981-10-4400-7_22

inflammatory conditions, collagen vascular disease, foreign body reaction, soft tissue calcifications, and neoplasm [4].

## Imaging Studies

Diagnostic studies should include radiographs to rule out a fracture, periosteal reaction, or osteomyelitis. Computed tomography (CT) can help determine the presence of septic arthritis and adjacent osteomyelitis. Magnetic resonance imaging (MRI) is helpful in the evaluation of musculoskeletal infections, providing excellent soft tissue contrast and bone marrow and joint involvement. Ultrasound can be used to evaluate area of edema, fluid accumulation, abscess formation, and osteomyelitis. Nuclear imaging is used to detect abscess, septic arthritis, and osteomyelitis [5].

## Laboratory Studies

### Complete Blood Cell Count with Differential White Blood Cell

Leukocytosis (white blood cell count of more than 12,000) and a left shift showing more immature polymorphonuclear leukocytes are signs of infectious process [5].

### Acute-Phase Protein

C-reactive protein (CRP), a commonly monitored acute-phase reactant, is produced in the liver. Its levels are rapidly elevated during the acute inflammatory phase in many bacterial and viral infections. Serum levels increase from 1 μg per milliliter by 100 to 1000 times within hours due to an induction in hepatic synthesis [5]. It is a disc-shaped pentameric molecule that readily binds a number of substances, including the C fraction of pneumococcal lysates, hence its name. In its bound form, it activates the complement cascade.

### Erythrocyte Sedimentation Rate

The viscosity of plasma is altered during inflammation secondary to protein change. The erythrocyte sedimentation rate (ESR) is the rate that red blood cells settle in anticoagulated blood left standing. The normal ESR is less than 20 mm per hour, rise to 30–50 per hour in acute infection, and can rise to 70–100 mm per hour in certain conditions (abscess, immunologic disease, atypical pneumonia). It can also be elevated with recent surgery of fracture; malignancy myocardial infraction; and gastrointestinal, thyroid, renal, and collagen vascular disease [6]. Both the ESR and CRP levels are nonspecific indicators of inflammatory change, with the ESR rising more slowly than the CRP levels.

## Nonoperative Management of Hand Infections

The initial medical treatment of open contaminated wounds should include the use of relatively broad-spectrum antibiotics covering the more commonly found aerobic and anaerobic pathogens [4].

## Surgical Management of Hand Infections

A biopsy is indicated in case of persistent signs of infections failing to respond to nonoperative management. Thc initial biopsy should include a deep wound sample of the infectious area. Sufficient tissue samples should be obtained for multiple cultures, including aerobic, anaerobic, mycobacterial, atypical mycobacterial, and fungal culture.

## Infections

### Paronychia

The perionychium is defined as the paronychium (border tissue around the nail) and the nail bed (germinal and sterile matrix). A paronychia is an infection of the lateral nail fold. When the infection extends to the eponychium (defined as the thin membrane distal to the nail wall at the base of the nail), it is properly termed an eponychia. When infection involves both lateral nail folds and eponychium, it is called a run-around infection [7]. In adults, *Staphylococcus aureus* is the most common pathogen. In children, there is often a mix of aerobic and anaerobic organism believed to be related to the finger-sucking and nail-biting habits of this young population.

Infections in the early stage can be treated with oral antibiotics, warm soaks, rest, and observation. Otherwise, surgical decompression is the treatment of choice for acute, established paronychia. Decompression is performed by carefully entering the abscess cavity between the nail plate and nail fold with a scalpel blade or hemostat. Aggressive decompression is needed with more established or resistant infections. Depending on the extent of the infection, a partial or complete nail plate removal with or without lateral nail fold relief incision is performed. The incision should be made perpendicular to the edge of the nail fold (Fig. 22.1). The wound is packed with a wick and subsequently changes, and intermittent warm saline soaks are started.

Subungual abscesses are treated with removal of a portion of or the entire nail. The abscess is carefully debrided while protecting the sterile and germinal matrices. Cultures should be obtained at the time of decompression, with initiation of empiric oral antibiotic therapy. The majority of these infections resolve without permanent sequelae, including nail dystrophy.

Chronic paronychia occurs more commonly in individuals constantly exposed to moist environments. *Candida albicans* is a frequent offending organism. Marsupialization of the nail may be needed with chronic paronychias [8]. After digital block anesthesia, a small, crescent-shaped portion of the eponychial fold is removed and made proximal to the distal edge of the eponychial fold without injuring the germinal matrix. A 5 mm wedge of skin, extending to lateral margins of the nail fold, is removed (Fig. 22.2). Wound epithelialization gradually occurs over 2–3 weeks. Topical antifungal ointments are generally used 4–6 weeks.

## Felon

A felon is a deep space infection or abscess of the distal pulp of the finger or thumb. It differs from the superficial apical infection involving the distal portion of the pulp skin, which often responds to a small, deroofing incision [7].

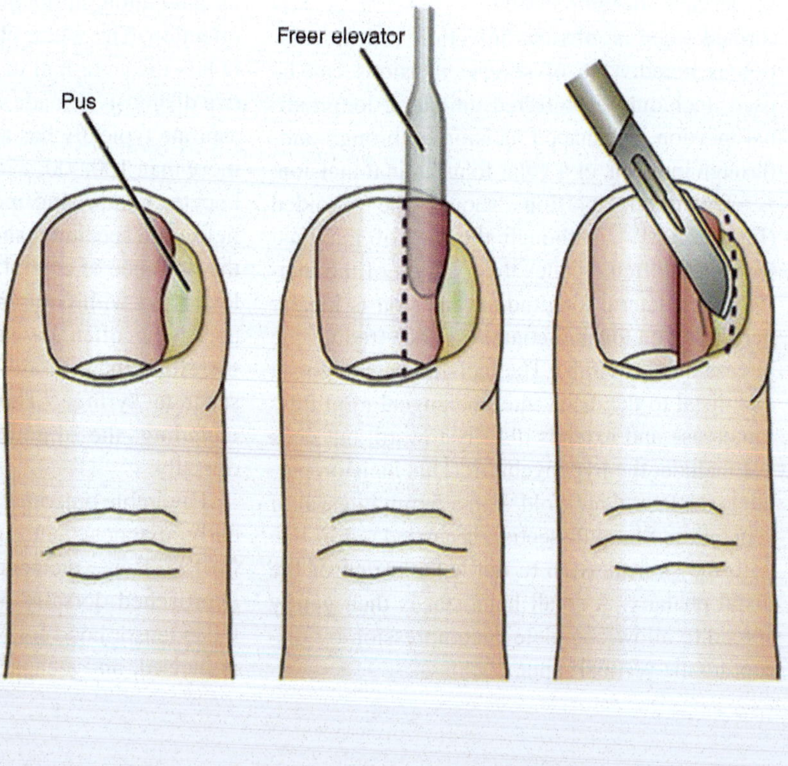


**Fig. 22.1** An infected lateral and proximal nail fold can be elevated by an elevator or scalpel. For extensive infections, a relief incision is made perpendicular to the edge of the nail fold to allow for removal of a portion or all of the nail plate

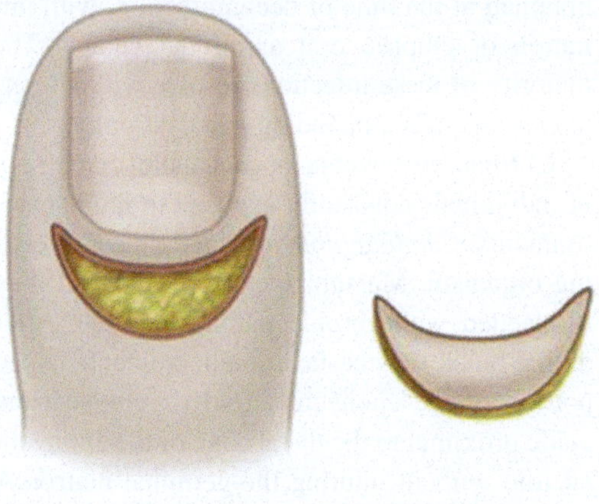

**Fig. 22.2** Eponychial marsupialization is performed by removing a small, crescent-shaped portion of the eponychial fold proximal to the distal edge of the eponychial fold. Care is taken not to injure the underlying germinal matrix

The pulp is composed of multiple vertical septa extending from the skin to the palmar distal phalanx, creating multiple small enclosed compartments in the pulp. Penetrating trauma serves as the event introducing a bacterial load. With further progression, the infection can produce a septic arthritis of the distal interphalangeal joint or pyogenic tenosynovitis. The organism most frequently cultured from a pulp space is *S. aureus*.

Surgical decompression of a felon is performed when an obvious infection with fluctuation is noted. One of several incisions can be used, including a preferred unilateral longitudinal incision, a J-shaped incision, a through-and-through incision, or a volar longitudinal incision. A fishmouth incision should be avoided (Fig. 22.3) [9]. Although the site of maximal induration often dictates the location of the incision, a unilateral longitudinal incision is ideally performed on the non-contact surface (radial side in case of the thumb). The incision begins dorsal and distal to the distal interphalangeal joint flexion crease and extends distally toward, but does not include, the hyponychium. This incision parallels the lateral nail fold with a 5 mm interval of separation. Sharp dissection is carried out in line with the skin incision to the volar cortex of the distal phalanx. A small hemostat is then gently spread to allow complete decompression by disrupting the vertical septa.

A longitudinal central midline incision [9] is advocated in an attempt to avoid skin slough, digital nerve injury, or creation of an unstable fat pad. This incision is preferred in the presence of a sinus track, allowing incorporaton of the sinus track with incision. The J-shaped, fishmouth, and transverse palmar incisions are to be avoided due to their potential iatrogenic morbidity. With any of these incisions, care is taken not to injure the neurovascular structures or introduce an infection into the flexor tendon sheath. A common problem is using too small an incision to adequately decompress the infection. As with paronychias, cultures should be obtained at the time of decompression, and empiric oral antibiotics should be started.

## Septic Arthritis

Septic arthritis is an infection of a joint space that, if left untreated, progresses to joint destruction and osteomyelitis. The most common infecting organism is *S. aureus*, whereas *Streptococcus* species are the second most prevalent bacterial isolates in the hand [10].

Patients present with a painfully swollen joint with guarded limited motion. The ESR and CRP levels are sensitive laboratory indicators of inflammation, although they are not specific for infection. The white blood cell count is elevated in less than one-half of these patients. The definitive diagnosis is made with a joint aspiration. The aspirate typically has a white blood cell count of more than 100,000, with polymorphonuclear leukocytes comprising more than 75% of the total field. The specimen should also be evaluated for the presence of crystal, for glucose and uric acid level, and with Gram's stain and cultures. Local anesthetic often has an antiseptic preservative; therefore, the aspirate should be obtained with a separate syringe. The joints of a small joint including the thumb are typically aspirated dorsally.

Favorable outcomes are directly dependent on early diagnosis and prompt surgical drainage [10]. The metacarpophalangeal joint is approached dorsally often requiring splitting of the extensor hood for exposure. The sagittal band is incised, and a capsulotomy is performed. The

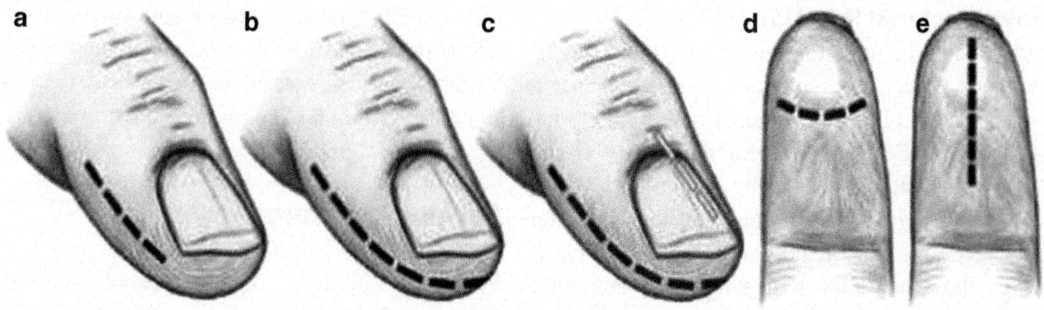


**Fig. 22.3** Incisions used for decompression of a felon. (**a**) Midlateral incision is preferred. (**b**) A J-shaped or hockey-stick incision. (**c**) A through-and-through incision. (**d** and **e**) A volar transverse or longitudinal incision

interphalangeal joints are best approached through midaxial incisions and release of the accessory collateral ligament, thereby avoiding dorsal disruption of the central slip. Intraoperative cultures are obtained, and the wound is frequently left open to heal by secondary intension. Conversely, loose closure over suction drain can be performed if adequate joint debridement can be obtained. Supervised early motion improves ultimate composite digit flexion.

## Osteomyelitis

Osteomyelitis infections occur secondary to an infection from an adjacent wound abscess, penetrating trauma, septic arthritis, pyogenic tenosynovitis, hematogenous seeding, or open fracture or after open treatment of closed fractures [11]. The hematogenous spread of an infection is uncommon. The most common pathogens are *S. aureus* and *Streptococcus* species.

Clinically, signs of infection including pain, erythema, swelling, and warmth are usually present. White blood cell count, ESR, CRP level are variably present. Radiographs may reveal lucencies, periosteal reaction or bone formation, osteolysis, or sequestrum formation. CT and MRI can help determine the extent of the infection. Nuclear imaging is helpful in detecting the infection earlier than in plain radiographs.

Treatment includes performing a biopsy to identify the pathogens, using antibiotics empirically until culture sensitivities have been obtained, and surgically draining the infection [11]. A midaxial incision is used for phalangeal infections, and a dorsal incision is used for metacarpal and carpal infection. Surgery should include removal of all of the infected bone and sequestra. Repeated surgical debridement and antibiotic-impregnated cement spacer may be needed. Severe infection may require an amputation. Late reconstruction may require flap coverage of skin grafting.

## Onychomycosis

Onychomycosis, or tiena unguium, is caused by a fungal infection of the nail plate resulting in destruction of the nail. The most common pathogens include dermatophytes, especially *Trichophyton rubrum*. The infection can also be caused by *C. albicans*. The infection can start in the hyponychium, in the eponychium, or on the nail plate surface [12]. The infection can begin with localized white or yellowish discoloration of the nail, progressing to involve the entire nail and gradual nail thickening. The infection can be treated with topical agents or oral agents. These systemic medications should be used with caution due to potential liver, renal, and bone marrow toxicity.

Extensively involved nails are removed using digital block anesthesia. Care is taken to protect the germinal and sterile matrix, which are gently scraped with a curette or scalpel. Topical antifungal agents are applied to the nail bed once or twice per day until a new nail grows (approximately 120–160 days).

## Mycobacterial Infection

Mycobacterial infection involves the skin, subcutaneous tissue, tenosynovium, joints, bone, or a combination of these structures. These infections have a predilection for synovium and produce caseating and noncaseating granuloma [13]. Although mycobacterial infection can simulate the appearance of rheumatoid arthritis tenosynovitis, the other clinical findings of rheumatoid arthritis are absent. The infections produced by typical and atypical mycobacterial infections are clinically similar. The diagnosis is confirmed by biopsy for histopathologic examination and cultures. Cutaneous infections are generally caused by inoculations and produce nodular or pustular lesions and abscess draining clear liquid. Lymphangitis is commonly present, but erythema, swelling, and cellulitis are less common. Tuberculous tenosynovitis involving the hand is common, and similar appearance of chronic tenosynovitis is seen with rheumatoid tenosynovitis. The flexor tendons are more commonly involved than the extensor tendons. Coexisting pulmonary or extrapulmonary tuberculosis is uncommon. Rice bodies or melon seeds are noted within synovial mass. Tuberculous osteomyelitis most commonly involves the phalanges and metacarpal. Concurrent pulmonary tuberculosis is uncommon. Painless digit or hand swelling without local inflammatory sign is noted. Adjacent tissue infection can occur.

## Complication

Complication arising from the treatment of infections includes surgical complications and complication related to antibiotic use [4]. Surgical complications include inadequate drainage of the infection resulting in continued infection or spread of the infection, complications related to the poor selection of incisions, and unnecessary surgery producing a secondary infection. Complications related to the use of antibiotics include inadequate antibiotic coverage resulting in residual infection and toxicity secondary to use of the antibiotics. Joint stiffness, loss of motion, and deformity occur with long-standing bone, joint, or soft tissue infections; prolonged immobilization or inadequate therapy can also contribute to the loss of hand function.

## Seymour Fracture

Pediatric Fractures of the Distal Phalanx (Seymour Fracture). A hyperflexion injury to the fingertip in a child is frequently mistaken for a mallet finger. In reality, the extensor tendon is still attached to the proximal dorsal metaphysis of the distal phalanx. The deformity is caused by an “open book” flexion fracture of the physis at the proximal end of the distal phalanx. In preadolescents, the fracture is either a Salter-Harris type 1 or 2; in adolescents, it is generally a type 3 pattern (Fig. 22.4). The diagnosis can be tricky in very small children, younger than 3 years, whose epiphysis may not be calcified. Because the FDP inserts on the distal phalanx distal to the fracture, it acts as a deforming force flexing the distal fragment.

If left untreated, growth arrest at the distal phalanx is virtually inevitable, and in young children, it will result in a shortened distal phalanx with stiffness in the DIP joint. These injuries, if closed, can be treated with simple reduction with or without K-wire fixation. However, most of these injuries are open with the physis herniated through the nail bed. As in adults, if the fracture is simply reduced without exposing the fracture and the sterile matrix, loss of reduction owing to the interposition of the proximal nail bed and infection can occur. Rogers and Labow described a 6-year-old child who was 3 years after a crush injury to the fingertip that was treated conservatively [14]. At 3 years, there was gross nail plate deformity overlying a nonunion at the distal phalanx. In order to minimize growth and nail bed deformity, treatment must include removal of the nail plate, careful debridement of the physis, removal of the interposed soft tissue, irrigation, fracture reduction, repair of the nail bed, and replacement of the cleaned nail plate under the eponychial fold to act as a stent to help hold the reduction.

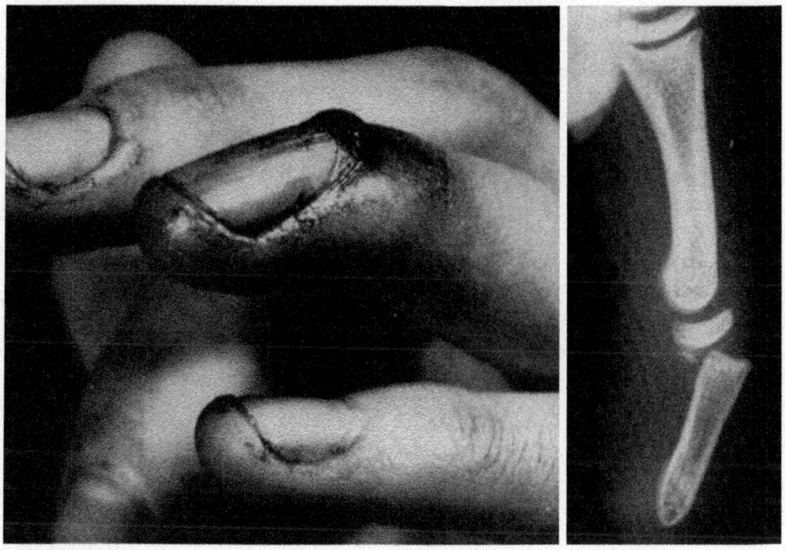

**Fig. 22.4** Seymour fracture (Salter type 2) of the distal phalanx. These are frequently open. Failed closed reduction of a Seymour fracture owing to soft tissue interposition, usually a fold of germinal matrix (Seymour N. Juxta-epiphyseal fracture of the terminal phalanx of the finger. J Bone Joint Surg 1966;48B:347–349 [15])

A longitudinal K-wire is placed across the fracture, if needed. Good results can be obtained with delayed presentation up to 1 month [15].

## Burned Thumb

Burn injuries to the hand and finger are a common occurrence [16, 17]. The first web space is critical for adequate circumduction and function of the thumb. The web space allows maximal abduction of the thumb to grasp large objects and also provides 80% of pinch strength [18]. Contracture of the first web space is a common consequence of hand burns that may reduce the hand's ability to grasp and diminish the ability of the thumb to function properly [19].

Surgical release of the first web is vital to restore hand function. Planning an adequate operation on an individual patient basis is important. There are some treatment algorithms for full-thickness burns of the first web space [20, 21]. Some studies recommended the use of Z-plasty for first-degree contractures, skin grafting and pedicled or free flaps for second-degree contractures, and distant or free flaps for third-degree contractures [22, 23].

Most recently, Yuste et al. have proposed a treatment algorithm. They conducted a review of the existing literature on the treatment of full-thickness burns of the first web space to develop a treatment algorithm that integrates the various currently available procedures [24]. In this paper, they divided the injuries into acute, chronic, and complex (those that presented bone lesions or associated digits). In the case of acute full-thickness injuries, treatment was based on the use of fasciocutaneous flaps and pedicled flaps in cases where there was enough tissue available. In the case of chronic contractures, those of patients who retained 50% or more of the original range of movement (ROM) were classified as mild, and severe contractures were those of patients who retained less than 50% of the ROM. In the case of the complex injuries, they included those procedures associated with a simultaneous thumb reconstruction, i.e., pollicization of the index finger or the transfer of a toe to the hand.

Various techniques have been described to manage web space contractures. Skin grafting and local flaps including Z-plasty, Y-V plasty, distant flap [25–28], island flap [29–36], or a free flap [37–40] are employed.

In mild cases, the adequate release of the first web space combined with skin grafting or local flap gives excellent results [41] (Fig. 22.5). However, in severe cases where a larger flap is needed, skin grafting or local flaps are insufficient

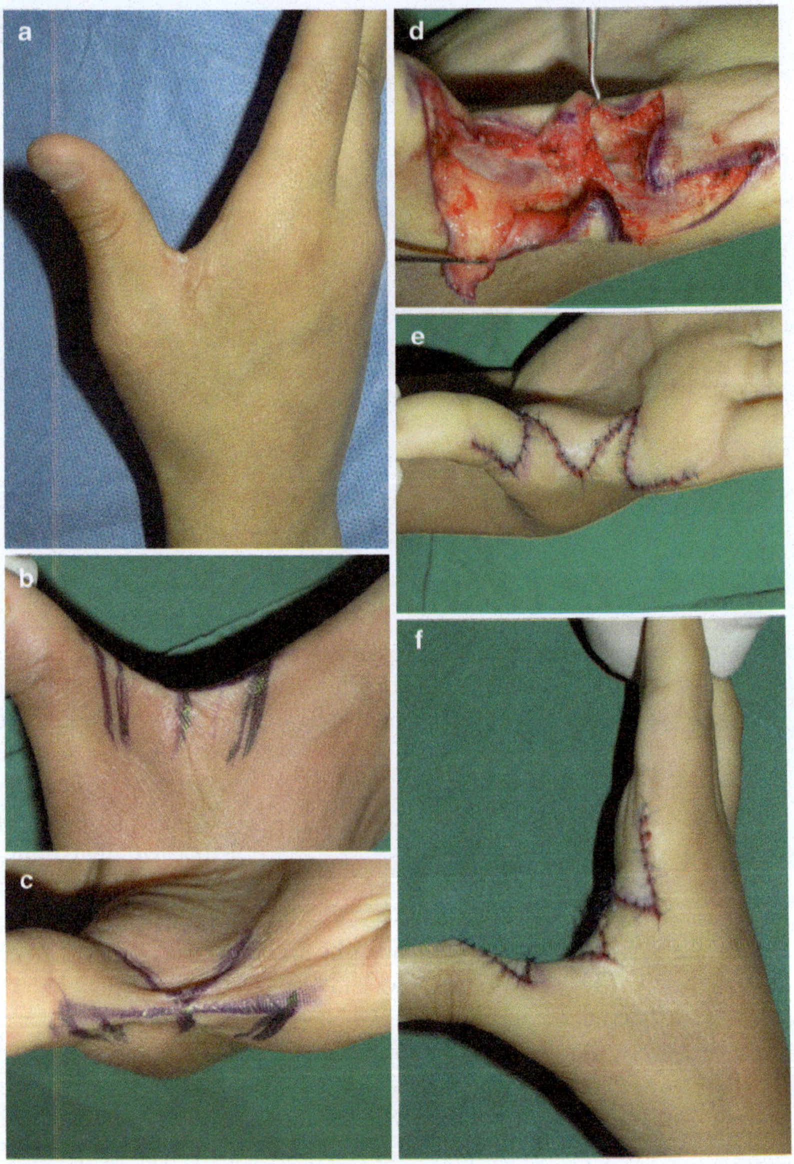

**Fig. 22.5** Five-flap Z-plasty with a Y-V advancement flap for the first web space contracture (Images courtesy of Dr. Woo SH, with original copyright holder's permission)

to achieve satisfactory reconstruction. In that cases, many studies have recommended the use of the reverse posterior interosseous flap in web space reconstruction [42–45]. Kai et al. report their experience in managing severe first web space contracture caused by various types of burns using the reverse posterior interosseous flap in patients with major burns [46]. In this paper, they describe the advantage of the reverse posterior interosseous flap that provides a thin, pliable tissue with adequate volume, a good color, and texture match. Moreover, it does not sacrifice a major artery of the hand.

The free flaps can be another option for reconstruction of large-sized defects (Fig. 22.6). Oh et al. recommend sensate neurovascular instep free flaps for resurfacing the skin after the release of severe contracture of the first web space [47].

These flaps were pliable, tough, and glabrous skin that were suitable for grasping and pinching movements. Recently, the development of perforator flaps has enabled the use of thinner flaps. The thinned anterolateral thigh flap provides a pliable tissue for first web space reconstruction [48].

To maintain thumb abduction and prevent contracture following reconstruction of the first web space, K-wires and external fixators have been positioned as useful tools [49, 50].

Harper et al. recommend a multiplanar external fixation technique. This technique allows for (1) prevention of thumb web space contractures without the need for labor-intensive splinting, (2) more control to position the thumb in space with the ability to easily manipulate or modify the construct in the postoperative course, and (3) can be used regardless of the soft tissue envelope [51].

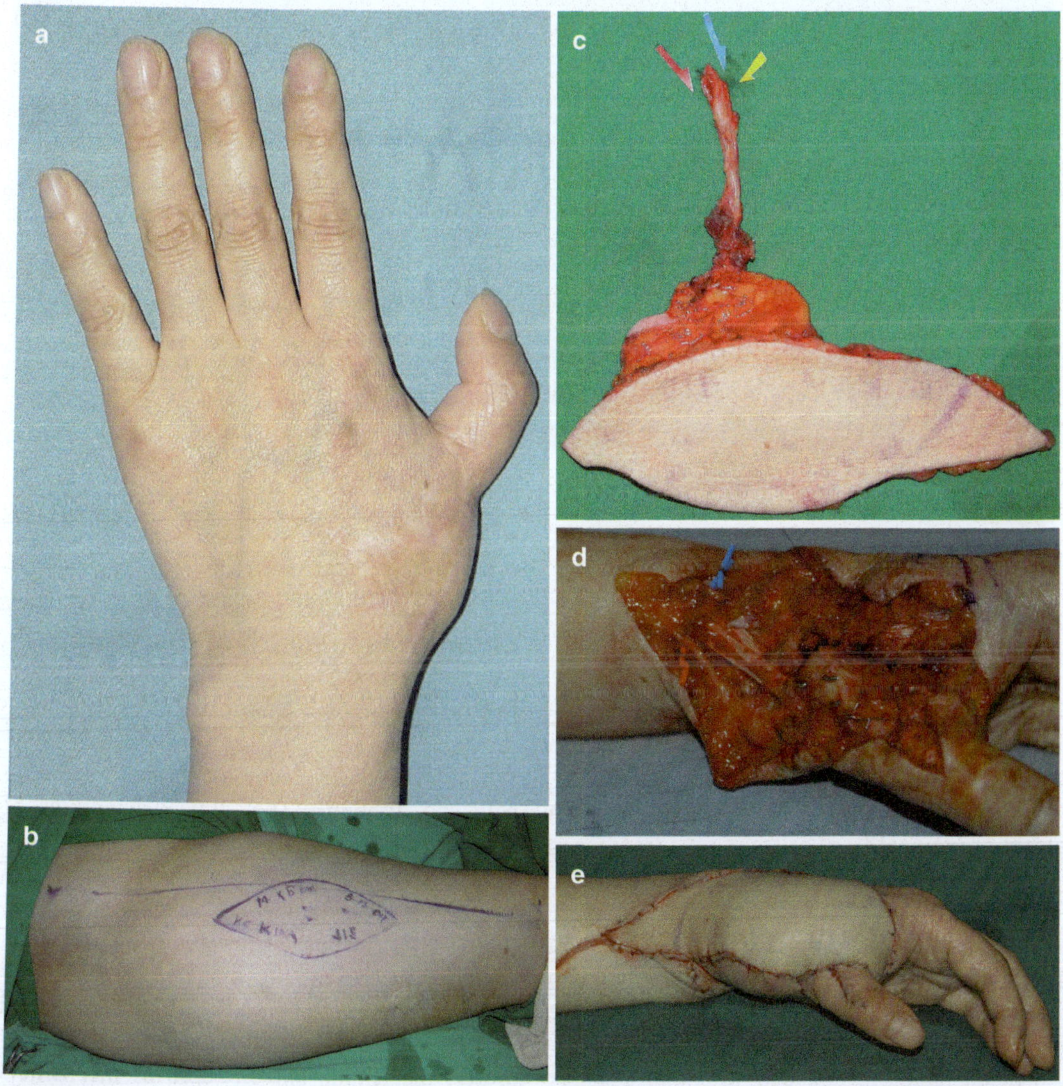


**Fig. 22.6** First web space reconstruction by the anterolateral thigh flap. (**a**) Preoperative view of a patient with adduction contracture caused by a burn. (**b–e**) The ALT flap in place. (**f–h**) Final outcome of the hand function (Images courtesy of Dr. Woo SH, with original copyright holder's permission)

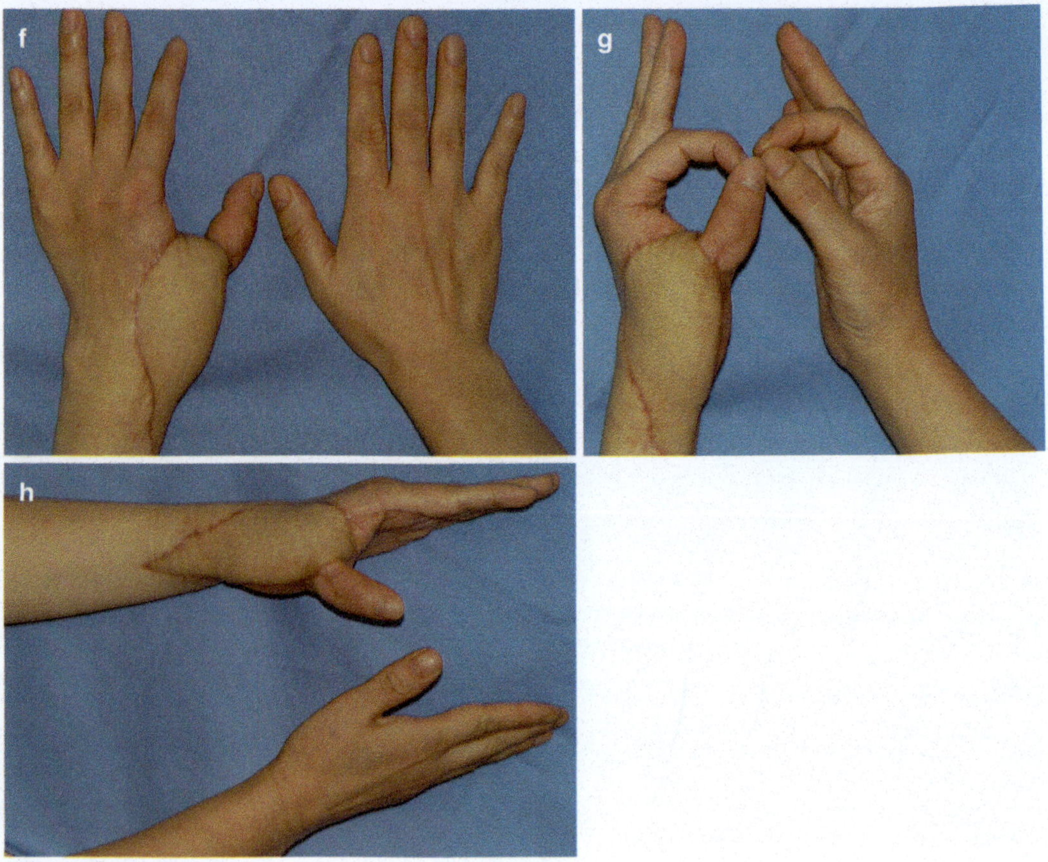


**Fig. 22.6** (continued)

## Thumb Amputation

In contrast to other fingers, revision amputation of the thumb at a more proximal level to obtain a primary closure is rarely indicated. The amputation wound should be closed with local or regional flaps or free tissue transfer to minimize loss of the length if possible (Fig. 22.7).

To cover the volar surface of the thumb, a groin or abdominal flap is contraindicated due to lack of fibrous septa which cause unstable touchpad.

If the thumb amputated proximal phalanx which remains a useful segment, deepening the first web space by Z-plasty may be a useful option.

## Chronic Sesamoiditis of the Thumb

### Introduction and Anatomy

Sesamoiditis is an uncommon cause of thumb pain and disability. The clinical symptoms of sesamoiditis are very similar to those of trigger thumb; several studies have reported on the trigger thumb related to the pathology of sesamoiditis [52–54]. Thus, differential diagnosis is essential to prevent the inadvertent A1 pulley releasing. Sesamoid bones are usually embedded in a tendon which is gliding over the joint. They protect the tendon and increase its mechanical effect by holding the tendon further away from the center of the joint thus increasing its lever arm. Furthermore, they modify the pressure,

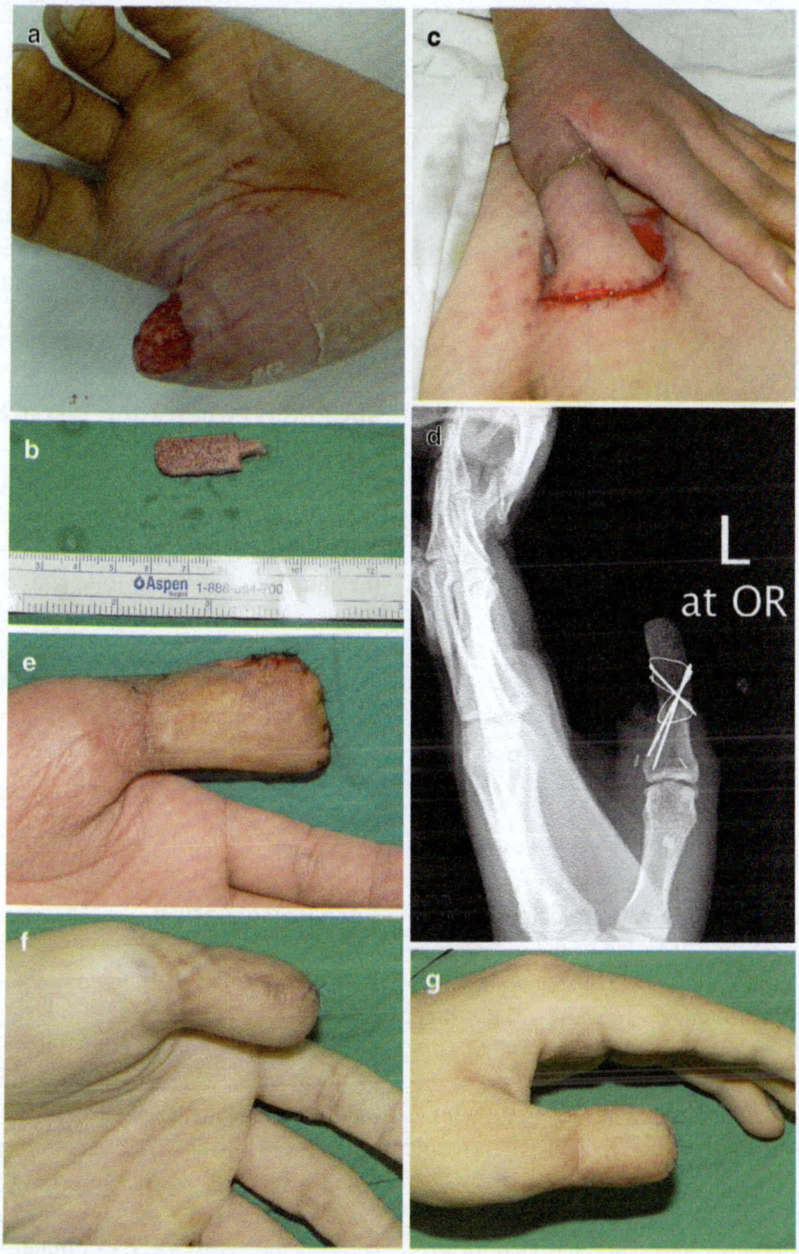


**Fig. 22.7** Composite osteocutaneous groin flap for thumb reconstruction

diminish the friction, and occasionally alter the direction of muscle pull [55, 56].

Most people have three sesamoid bones in the thumb, two at the metacarpophalangeal (MCP) joint and one at the interphalangeal (IP) joint [57]. Both sesamoid bones are embedded in the volar plate of the MCP joint and articulate with the volar condyles of the metacarpal head. The convex ulnar sesamoid articulates with a concavity in the ulnar condyle, while the concave radial sesamoid articulates with a convexity in the radial condyle (Fig. 22.8). The deep head of the flexor pollicis brevis tendon inserts on the radial sesamoid, and the transverse head of the adductor

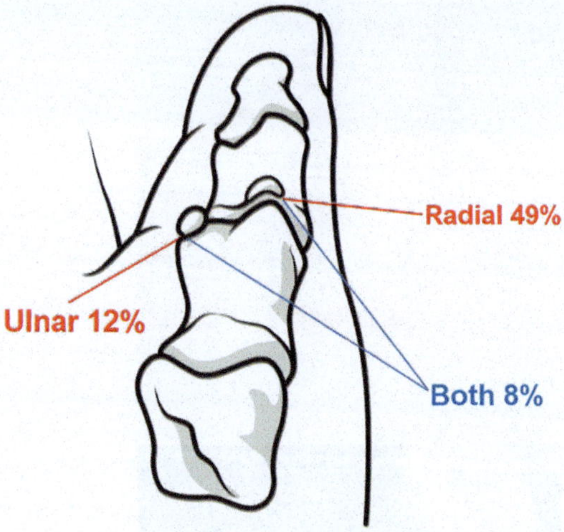


**Fig. 22.8** Thumb metacarpophalangeal (MCP) sesamoid anatomy and rate of subsesamoid arthritis

pollicis tendon inserts on the ulnar sesamoid [56, 58, 59].

## Diagnosis

The diagnosis may be difficult due to the small size of the sesamoid bones and subsesamoid joint. On physical examination, there was pain and swelling on the volar side of the metacarpophalangeal joint, limitation of motion, and decreased pinch strength. Because of the high incidence of arthritis involving the radial subsesamoid joint [56], tenderness on the volar radial side of the metacarpal head may be helpful to differentiate sesamoiditis from a trigger thumb (Fig. 22.8).

Trauma or degenerative change can cause chronic sesamoiditis [60]. Park and Hamlin [61] reported their experience in 25 patients with chronic sesamoiditis. All their patients had a history of blunt trauma and presented with pain which limited thumb function.

On the contrary, Chin et al. [62] reviewed their experience with 20 thumbs. In contrast to the previous series, the two-thirds of patients did not have a history of trauma.

And they suggest that the diagnosis of chronic sesamoiditis was made clinically based on the history, site of tenderness, and result of the sesamoid provocation test (SPT). In their study, all patients presented with chronic pain over the volar aspect of the thumb MCP joint that affected thumb function. On examination, all 20 thumbs had local tenderness over the radial and/or ulnar sesamoid(s) and a positive SPT [62].

## Sesamoid Provocation Test [62]

The test consists of two maneuvers. In the first maneuver, hold the patient's affected thumb maintaining the MCP joint in flexion, and ask the patient to flex the IP joint against resistance. In the second maneuver, maintain the thumb MCP joint in hyperextension, and ask the patient to flex the IP joint against resistance. The SPT is positive when the patient experiences little or no pain with the first maneuver and considerably more pain with the second maneuver.

## Case Presentation

A 45-year-old woman complained of persistent pain of her right thumb. She underwent A1 pulley release surgery 3 months ago. On physical examination, tenderness on the volar radial side of the metacarpophalangeal joint was detected. Plain radiographs of the affected thumb showed joint space narrowing of the subsesamoid joint and sclerotic change of the radial metacarpal head (Fig. 22.9a). With a CT examination, bony protrusion was present at the radial metacarpal head, causing compression of the radial sesamoid (Fig. 22.9b). She was diagnosed with a sesamoid arthritis, and surgical excision was performed. Intraoperatively, excised radial sesamoid showed cartilage denudation (Fig. 22.9c, d). At last follow-up, the patient had no pain and showed good function.

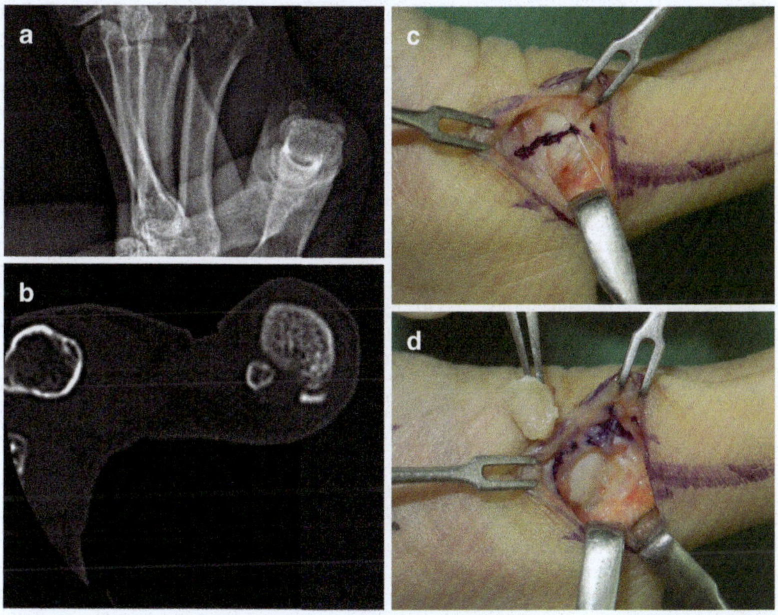


**Fig. 22.9** (**a**) Plain radiographs showed joint space narrowing of the subsesamoid joint and sclerotic changes of the metacarpal head. (**b**) Bony spur of radial metacarpal head was visible on CT scan. (**c**, **d**) The radial sesamoid bone was excised from the volar plate that showed cartilage denudation (Images courtesy of Dr. Woo SH, with original copyright holder's permission)

## Treatment

Trumble and Watson [60] performed sesamoidectomy in 36 patients with chronic sesamoiditis.

Fourteen patients had a good functional outcome (no residual symptoms), five patients had a fair result (residual symptoms not affecting return to work), and two patients required secondary surgery for persistent symptoms. Parks and Hamlin [61] also performed excision of both sesamoids in 20 patients and excision of 1 sesamoid in the remaining 5 patients. Twenty patients achieved good to excellent results (pain-free, no functional loss, and return to preinjury vocation), whereas the remaining five patients had residual pain and stiffness. Meanwhile, Chin et al. [62] suggested that a trial of nonoperative treatment is mandatory in all chronic sesamoiditis cases. They reported that steroid injection was an acceptable treatment modality with long-lasting effect. In their study, 13 out of 20 thumbs improved with steroid injection(s) and did not need any further treatment. Three out of the seven thumbs that failed conservative treatment were in patients with a nonsedentary occupation and with a history of prior trauma. The patients were successfully treated with sesamoidectomy.

## References


1. Bishop A. Infections. In: Manske P, editor. Hand surgery update. American Society for surgery of the hand. Rosemont, IL: American Academy of Orthopedic Surgeons; 1996. p. 395–404.
2. Abrams RA, Botte MJ. Hand infections: treatment recommendations for specific types. J Am Acad Orthop Surg. 1996;4:230.
3. Bannister BA, Begg NT, Gillespie SH. Infectious disease. 2nd ed. Oxford: Blackwell Science; 2000.
4. Szabo R, Palumbo C. Infections of the hand. In: Chapman M, editor. Chapman's orthopedic surgery. 3rd ed. Philadelphia: Lippincott Williams & Wilkins; 2001. p. 1989–2008.
5. Lahiji A, Esterhai JL Jr. Principles of treatment of infection an antimicrobial therapy. In: Chapman M, editor. Chapman's orthopedic surgery. 3rd ed. Philadelphia: Lippincott Williams & Wilkins; 2001. p. 3505–32.
6. Covey DC, Albright JA. Clinical significance of the erythrocyte sedimentation rate in orthopedic surgery. J Bone Joint Surg Am. 1987;69:148.
7. Jebson PJL. Infections of the fingertips. Paronychia and felons. Hand Clin. 1998;14:547–55.

8. Bednar MS, Lane LB. Eponychial marsupialization and nail removal for surgical treatment of chronic paronychia. J Hand Surg Am. 1991;16:314–7.
9. Kilgore ES Jr, Brown LG, Newmeyer WL, et al. Treatment of felons. Am J Surg. 1975;130:194–7.
10. Murray PM. Septic arthritis of the hand and wrist. Hand Clin. 1998;14:579–52.
11. Barbieri RA, Freeland AE. Osteomyelitis of the hand. Hand Clin. 1998;14:589–603.
12. Zaias N. Onychomycosis. Dermatol Clin. 1985;3:445–60.
13. Patel M. Chronic infections. In: Green D, Hotchkiss R, Pederson W, editors. Green's operative hand surgery. 4th ed. New York: Churchill Livingstone; 1999. p. 1048–93.
14. Rogers GF, Labow BI. Diaphyseal non-union in the distal phalanx of a child. J Hand Surg. 2007;32E:85–7.
15. Seymour N. Juxta-epiphyseal fracture of the terminal phalanx of the finger. J Bone Joint Surg. 1966;48B:347–9.
16. Dobbs ER, Curreri PW. Burns: analysis of results of physical therapy in 681 patients. J Trauma. 1972;12:242–8.
17. Schneider JC, Holavanahalli R, Helm P, O'Neil C, Goldstein R, Kowalske K. Contractures in burn injury part II: investigating joints of the hand. J Burn Care Res. 2008;29:606–13.
18. Hastings H II, Davidson S. Tendon transfer for ulnar nerve palsy: evaluation of results and practical treatment considerations. Hand Clin. 1988;4:167–78.
19. Jensen CB, Rayan GM, Davidson R. First web space contracture and hand function. J Hand Surg Am. 1993;18:516–20.
20. Hudson D, Renshaw A. An algorithm for the release of burn contractures of the extremities. Burns. 2006;32(6):663–8.
21. Oguz M, Seven E. The non-algorithmic nature of the hand burn contractures. Burns. 2007;33(8):1046–50.
22. Jain V, Wei FCH. Proposed classification of first web space contracture and management with ipsilateral lateral arm flap. J Reconstr Microsurg. 2002;18:455.
23. Choi TH, Son DG, Han K. Classification and reconstructive strategies of first web space contracture. J Korean Soc Plast Reconstr Surg. 2001;28:522–30.
24. Yuste V, Delgado J, Agullo A, Sampietro JM. Development of an integrative algorithm for the treatment of various stages of full-thickness burns of the first commissure of the hand. Burns. 2017 Jun;43(4):812–8.
25. Miura T. Use of paired abdominal flaps for release of adduction contractures of the thumb. Plast Reconstr Surg. 1979;63:242–4.
26. McGregor IA, Jackson IT. The groin flap. Br J Plast Surg. 1972;25:3–16.
27. Mutz SB. Thumb web contracture. Hand. 1972;4:236–46.
28. Bonola A, Fiocchi R. Cross-arm double flap in the repair of severe adduction contracture of the thumb. Hand. 1975;7:287–90.
29. Foucher G, Van Genechten F, Merle M, Michon J. A compound radial artery forearm flap in hand surgery: an original modification of the Chinese forearm flap. Br J Plast Surg. 1984;37:139–48.
30. Braun FM, Hoang P, Merle M, Van Genechten F, Foucher G. Technique and indications of the forearm flap in hand surgery: report of thirty-three cases. Ann Chir Main. 1985;4:85–97.
31. Akyurek M, Safak T, Kecik A. Coverage of thumb wound and correction of first web space contracture using a longitudinally split reverse radial forearm flap. Ann Plast Surg. 2001;47:453–7.
32. Prakash V, Mishra A. Management of adduction contracture of the thumb with a prefabricated radial fascial flap. Plast Reconstr Surg. 2004;114:1681–2.
33. Zancolli EA, Angrigiani C. Posterior interosseous island forearm flap. J Hand Surg. 1988;13B:130–5.
34. Costa H, Soutar DS. The distally based island posterior interosseous flap. Br J Plast Surg. 1988;41:221–7.
35. Buchler U, Frey HP. Retrograde posterior interosseous flap. J Hand Surg. 1991;16A:283–92.
36. Lu LJ, Gong X, Liu ZG, Zhang ZX. Antebrachial reverse island flap with pedicle of posterior interosseous artery: a report of 90 cases. Br J Plast Surg. 2004;57:645–52.
37. Scheker LR, Lister GD, Wolff TW. The lateral arm free flap in releasing severe contracture of the first web space. J Hand Surg. 1988;13B:146–50.
38. Schoofs M, Leps P, Millot F. The value of the free external brachial flap in surgery of the hand. Ann Chir Main. 1989;8:217–22.
39. Tonkin MA, Stern H. The posterior interosseous artery free flap. J Hand Surg. 1989;14B:215–7.
40. Woo SH, Choi BC, Oh SJ, Seul JH. Classification of the first web space free flap of the foot and its applications in reconstruction of the hand. Plast Reconstr Surg. 1999;103:508–17.
41. Bhattacharya S, Bhatnagar SK, Pandey SD, Chandra R. Management of burn contractures of the first web space of the hand. Burns. 1992;18:54–7.
42. Magdy A, Shaker A, Hassan MK. Reconstruction of the severely contracted first web space using the posterior interosseous artery flap. Egypt J Plast Reconstr Surg. 2003;27:53–60.
43. Gong X, Lu LJ. Reconstruction of severe contracture of the first web space using the reverse posterior interosseous artery flap. J Trauma. 2011;71:1745–9.
44. Zhu L, Dai C, Dong J. Reconstruction of the first web space in severely burned hand by the reverse posterior interosseous flap. Eur J Plast Surg. 2008;31:293–7.
45. Cheema TA, Lakshman S, Cheema MA, Durrani SF. Reverse-flow posterior interosseous flap—a review of 68 cases. Hand. 2007;2:112–6.
46. Kai S, Zhao J, Jin Z, Wu W, Yang M, Wang Y, Xie C, Yu J. Release of severe post-burn contracture of the first web space using the reverse posterior interosseous flap: our experience with 12 cases. Burns. 2013 Sep;39(6):1285–9.

47. Oh SJ, Koh SH, Chung CH. Wide thumb and the first web reconstruction using a neurovascularised instep free flap. J Plast Reconstr Aesthet Surg. 2010;63(9):1565–8.
48. Adani R, Tarallo L, Marcoccio I, Fregni U. First web-space reconstruction by the anterolateral thigh flap. J Hand Surg Am. 2006;31(4):640–6.
49. Araico J, Valdes JL, Ortiz JM. An internal wire splint for adduction contracture of the thumb. Plast Reconstr Surg. 1971;48:339–42.
50. Kamath BJ, Bhardwaj P. Adjustable distractor for management of thumb web contracture. Burns. 2009;35:274–9.
51. Harper CM, Iorio ML. Prevention of thumb web space contracture with multiplanar external fixation. Tech Hand Up Extrem Surg. 2016;20(3):91–5.
52. Seybold EA, Warhold LG. Impingement of the flexor pollicis longus tendon by an enlarged radial sesamoid causing trigger thumb: a case report. J Hand Surg Am. 1996;21(4):619–20.
53. Brown M, Manktelow RT. A new cause of trigger thumb. J Hand Surg Am. 1992;17(4):688–90.
54. Kim JY, Sung JH, Seo JG. Sesamoid arthritis mimicking trigger thumb. Orthopedics. 2011;34(3):228.
55. Sarin VK, Erickson GM, Giori NJ, Bergman AG, Carter DR. Coincident development of sesamoid bones and clues to their evolution. Anat Rec. 1999;257(5):174–80.
56. Goldberg I, Nathan H. Anatomy and pathology of the sesamoid bones. The hand compared to the foot. Int Orthop. 1987;11:141–7.
57. Wood VE. The sesamoid bones of the hand and their pathology. J Hand Surg Br. 1984;9:261–4.
58. Mohler LR, Trumble TE. Disorders of the thumb sesamoids. Hand Clin. 2001;17(2):291–301.
59. Gibeault JD, Saba P, Hoenecke H, Graham A. The sesamoids of the metacarpo-phalangeal joint of the thumb: an anatomical and clinical study. J Hand Surg Br. 1989;14(2):244–7.
60. Trumble TE, Watson HK. Post-traumatic sesamoid arthritis of the metacarpophalangeal joint of the thumb. J Hand Surg Am. 1985;10(1):94–100.
61. Parks BJ, Hamlin C. Chronic sesamoiditis of the thumb: pathomechanics and treatment. J Hand Surg Am. 1986;11(2):237–40.
62. Chin AY, Sebastin SJ, Wong M, Teoh LC. Long-term results using a treatment algorithm for chronic sesamoiditis of the thumb metacarpophalangeal joint. J Hand Surg Am. 2013;38(2):316–21.

# Index




S. H. Woo (ed.), *The Thumb*, https://doi.org/10.1007/978-981-10-4400-7

The manufacturer's authorised representative in the EU is Springer Nature Customer Service Centre GmbH, Europaplatz 3, 69115 Heidelberg, Germany. If you have any concerns regarding our products, please contact ProductSafety@springernature.com

Printed and bound by CPI Group (UK) Ltd, Croydon, CR0 4YY
30/09/2026
02225445-0019